Clinical Immunotoxicology

Clinical Immunotoxicology

Editor-in-Chief

David S. Newcombe, M.D.

Professor
Department of Environmental Health Sciences
Department of Medicine
Johns Hopkins Medical Institution
Baltimore, Maryland

Editors

Noel R. Rose, M.D., Ph.D.

Professor and Chairman
Department of Immunology and
Infectious Diseases
School of Hygiene and Public Health
Johns Hopkins University
Baltimore, Maryland

John C. Bloom, V.M.D., Ph.D.

Head, Clinical Laboratory Medicine
Lilly Research Laboratories
Indianapolis, Indiana

Raven Press   New York

Raven Press, Ltd., 1185 Avenue of the Americas, New York, New York 10036

Made in the United States of America

Library of Congress Cataloging-in-Publication Data
Clinical immunotoxicology / editor-in-chief, David S. Newcombe ;
  editors, Noel R. Rose, John C. Bloom.
     p. cm.
   Includes bibliographical references and index.
   ISBN 0–88167–830–9 (hardcover)
   1. Immunotoxicology. I. Newcombe, David S., 1929–   II. Rose,
Noel R. III. Bloom, John C.
   [DNLM: 1. Drugs—toxicity. 2. Immunity—drug effects.
3. Immunologic Diseases—chemically induced. 4. Xenobiotics—
metabolism. QV 600 C6384]
RC582.17.C55 1992
616.97′071—dc20
DNLM/DLC
for Library of Congress   91-31269
                                        CIP

Contents

Contributors

Ira Berkower
*Department of Biochemistry and
    Biophysics*
*Office of Biologics, Food and Drug
    Administration*
National Institutes of Health
Building 29, Room 523
8800 Rockville Pike
Bethesda, Maryland   20892

I. Leonard Bernstein
Division of Immunology
Department of Medicine
University of Cincinnati Medical Center
231 Bethesda Avenue, ML 563
Cincinnati, Ohio   45267

Roger B. Cohen
Division of Cytokine Biology
*Center for Biologics Evaluation and
    Research*
Food and Drug Administration
Building 29A, Room 3B24
Bethesda, Maryland   20892

Wafik S. El-Deiry
Department of Medicine
The Johns Hopkins Hospital
Oncology Center
600 N. Wolfe Street, Room 128
Baltimore, Maryland   21205

Ahmed H. Esa
Bone Marrow Transplantation Unit
Oncology Center
Johns Hopkins University
School of Medicine
600 N. Wolfe Street
Baltimore, Maryland   21205

Stephen J. Galli
Department of Pathology
Beth Israel Hospital
330 Brookline Avenue
Boston, Massachusetts   02215

Allan D. Hess
Bone Marrow Transplantation Unit
Oncology Center
Johns Hopkins University
School of Medicine
600 N. Wolfe Street
Baltimore, Maryland   21205

Richard E. Hoffman
Colorado Department of Health
4210 E. 11th Avenue
Denver, Colorado   80220

Kent Holland
Oncology Center
Johns Hopkins University
School of Medicine
600 N. Wolfe Street
Baltimore, Maryland   21205

Michael Kowolenko
Division of Investigative Toxicology
Bristol-Myers Squibb
Pharmaceutical Research Institute
P.O. Box 4755
Syracuse, New York   13221

Christian Grønhøj Larsen
Department of Dermatology
University of Aarhus
Marselisborg Hospital
DK-8000 Aarhus C., Denmark

David A. Lawrence
Department of Microbiology and
* Immunology*
The Neil Hellman Medical Research
* Building, A-68*
The Albany Medical College
47 New Scotland Avenue
Albany, New York   12208

Joseph B. Margolick
Department of Environmental Health
* Sciences*
Johns Hopkins University
School of Hygiene and Public Health
615 N. Wolfe Street, Room 7032
Baltimore, Maryland   21205

Jackie L. Martin
Department of Anesthesiology and Critical
* Care Medicine*
The Johns Hopkins Hospital
711 Tower
600 N. Wolfe Street
Baltimore, Maryland   21205

Michael J. McCabe, Jr.
Karolinska Institute
Department of Toxicology
P.O. Box 60400
S-10401 Stockholm, Sweden

David S. Newcombe
Department of Environmental Health
* Sciences*
Johns Hopkins University
School of Hygiene and Public Health
615 N. Wolfe Street, Room 2712
Baltimore, Maryland   21205

Dov H. Pluznik
Division of Cytokine Biology
Center for Biologics Evaluation and
* Research*
Food and Drug Administration
Building 29A, Room 3B24
Bethesda, Maryland   29082

Raj K. Puri
Division of Cytokine Biology
Center for Biologics Evaluation and
* Research*
Food and Drug Administration
Building 29A, Room 3B24
Bethesda, Maryland   29082

Jørgen Rønnevig
Department of Dermatology
University of Oslo
Rikshospitalet
Oslo-1, Norway

Noel R. Rose
Department of Immunology and Infectious
* Diseases*
Johns Hopkins University
School of Hygiene and Public Health
615 N. Wolfe Street, Room 4013
Baltimore, Maryland   21205

Ali M. Saboori
Department of Environmental Health
* Sciences*
Johns Hopkins University
School of Hygiene and Public Health
615 N. Wolfe Street, Room 2712
Baltimore, Maryland   21205

Jay P. Siegel
Division of Cytokine Biology
Center for Biologics Evaluation and
* Research*
Food and Drug Administration
Building 29A, Room 3B24
Bethesda, Maryland   20892

Jerry L. Spivak
Division of Hematology
Department of Medicine
Johns Hopkins University
School of Medicine
Blalock 1033
600 N. Wolfe Street
Baltimore, Maryland   21205

Peter B. Terry
Asthma and Allergy Center
Francis Scott Key Medical Center
301 Bayview Boulevard, 4B-72
Baltimore, Maryland   21224

Kristian Thestrup-Pedersen
Department of Dermatology
University of Aarhus
Marselisborg Hospital
DK-8000 Aarhus C., Denmark

Peter A. Ward
Department of Pathology
University of Michigan Medical School
1301 Catherine Street
5240 Medical Science Building 1
Ann Arbor, Michigan   48109-0602

Barry K. Wershil
Department of Pathology
Beth Israel Hospital
330 Brookline Avenue
Boston, Massachusetts   02215

Preface

Immunopharmacologic agents have been used for decades by physicians as a means of altering the pathologic immune responses of some diseases. As a consequence, toxic responses of the immune system to such agents have been well documented. Recently, occupational and environmental exposures to chemical, biological, and physical elements have been recognized as possible mediators of immune dysfunction. The potential for these elements to alter host defense functions has extended the spectrum of immunoactive agents and focused increased attention and concern on the health effects of such substances from environmental or industrial sources. Recognizing the immune system as a significant target organ subject to toxic insult has fostered the growth of a new discipline, immunotoxicology.

Clinical immunotoxicology emphasizes the detection and expression of alterations in the human immune system caused by toxic substances. Understanding such immune dysfunctions requires a knowledge of the organization, cellular expression, and regulation of the human immune system. Further, the immune system has a unique role in the assessment of toxicity since xenobiotic metabolism can occur via pathways of its cellular components and products of immune cell activity may alter the structure and effects of xenobiotics presented to these cells. The initial chapters of this book provide the reader with an overview of the principles of immunotoxicology and xenobiotic metabolism so that the mechanisms of toxicity and their clinical expression can be appreciated.

Xenobiotic-induced interruptions or inappropriate modifications of the essential cell-to-cell communications circuitry of the immune system by foreign substances may result in immunotoxic responses. A variety of vectors (antibodies, viruses, cytokines) provoke immunopathologic responses and provide excellent models for the characterization and elucidation of the mechanisms by which immunotoxic agents result in immune dysfunction. These models also emphasize the potential role of xenobiotics in the dissection of interactions within the immune system. Several models are detailed in the second section of this book.

The remainder of the text focuses on certain well characterized immunological dysfunctions associated with exposure to pharmacologic agents and environmental pollutants. The immunotoxic conditions related to common xenobiotic target organs such as the lung and skin as well as the immunotoxicity of pharmacologic agents which have special relevance to specific medical specialties (hematology, anesthesiology, oncology, and transplantation surgery) are described in some detail. Where relevant data exist, the mechanisms of toxic action of cell- and organ-specific agents are discussed, and in the case of the lung, immunopathogenesis and bronchoalveolar lavage findings are delineated for a variety of xenobiotic-mediated conditions.

The ever widening role of scientists, industrialists, government agencies, and the general population in the recognition and documentation of the effects of toxic substances should make this book a useful resource for studying the mechanisms of immunotoxic substances and the diversity of clinical expressions xenobiotics have in humans. Special attention is given to the inaccurate predictions that may be associated with extrapolation from animal to man and the possible role of low dose exposures, chronic immunosuppression, and cancer. We hope that the contents of this book will enrich the knowledge base of students of medicine, toxicology, immunology, cell and molecular biology, and especially those individuals faced with the awesome task of assessing the health effects and safety of both new and old chemicals and biologicals. The rapidly expanding number of these substances in today's technology-driven world places enormous responsibility on physicians who monitor the health of individuals exposed to a variety of patent and prescribed medicines as well as xenobiotics in their workplace and home environments. Early recognition of host defense dysfunctions, which can only come through a full understanding of their pathogenesis, is the key to the intercession and control of these disorders.

David S. Newcombe, M.D.

Clinical Immunotoxicology, edited by
D. S. Newcombe, N. R. Rose, and J. C. Bloom.
Raven Press, Ltd., New York © 1992.

1

Immunotoxicology: A New Challenge

David S. Newcombe

*Department of Environmental Health Sciences, Johns Hopkins University, School of
Hygiene and Public Health, 615 N. Wolfe Street, Room 2712, Baltimore, MD 21205*

In the past two decades there has been an extraordinary focus on diseases caused by chemical substances; this focus has been fostered, in part, by extensive press coverage of accidental chemical spills and misuse. The worldwide nature of this problem is evident from the publicity received after the human consumption of beef and milk contaminated with polybrominated biphenyls in Michigan, the human toxicity to polyhalogenated biphenyls reported in Japan and Taiwan, the purported contamination of troops with 2,4-dichlorophenoxyacetic acid and 2,4,5-trichlorophenoxyacetic acid (Agent Orange) during the Vietnam War, the methyl isocyanate leak in Bhopal, India, the 2,3,7,8-tetrachlorodibenzo-*p*-dioxin spill in Seveso, Italy, and the occurrence of asbestosis in shipworkers and construction workers and others exposed to asbestos throughout the industrialized world (1–13). Even though physicians and pharmacologists have long been aware of the capacity of drugs to cause disease, environmental contaminants and their health effects have been a primary force propelling the science of toxicology toward more innovative approaches to its practice and research in the 20th century. Unfortunately, such innovation is often constrained by classic toxicological concepts and regulatory impediments. Nonetheless, toxicology, the science dealing with chemicals that cause disease, has recently experienced significant growth as a scientific discipline and the inevitable subspecialization that accompanies growth in science. Technological advances have been made in animal breeding to produce pure breeds for use in toxicological testing, and automated procedures have been developed for rapid toxicological analyses. In comparison with these advances, relatively little progress has taken place in the assessment of human toxins. The content of this book deals with two toxicological subdisciplines, immunotoxicology and *in vitro* toxicology, disciplines likely to make significant contributions to human toxicology based on the rapidly expanding clinical and basic knowledge related to these fields.

In preparing a book to introduce these relatively new subdisciplines to scientists, our objectives are to characterize the spectrum of immunologically mediated disorders that could affect the individual after chemical exposures, to address the new problems associated with the toxicity testing of biological products such as lymphokines and antibodies, and to characterize to some degree the similarities and differences between toxicological studies for drug development and industrial chemical use. In a broader sense, our goal is to encourage a renaissance in toxicology supported by the many opportunities for creative clinical and basic research in the young subdiscipline immunotoxicology as well as in other areas of toxicology.

Certainly, in developing drugs careful consideration of the potential for therapeutic agents to induce damage to human organ systems, including the immune system, must be considered in any panel of toxicological tests. The identification of such detrimental properties should be made early in the development of a drug, so that the expenses of further development can either be curtailed or be shifted to a different compound. Similar arguments can be made for industrial chemicals that have the potential to impair host defense functions. Thus, toxicological investigations must be performed early in the development of new chemicals and drugs. Such studies should not be considered and initiated in depth only after human injury has occurred. The early detection of toxic properties represents not only sound practices of experimental toxicology but also curtails significant costs that may be incurred in the construction of a manufacturing facility for the production or use of a substance with significant human toxicity.

Unfortunately, industrial exposures offer no opportunity for the use of risk:benefit ratios to determine whether it is appropriate or justifiable to expose an individual to an industrial chemical, as is done with therapeutic drugs and at times used as a rationale for medical treatment. The clinical trial of a drug almost always follows extensive preclinical studies including human studies using volunteers, whereas exposure in the industrial environment during the manufacturing process is comparable to a clinical drug trial but it occurs late in the process of new chemical assessment and is most often not preceded by extensive preclinical human studies. Thus, environmental exposures should be preceded by extensive studies to characterize the chemical and physical properties of an agent, to determine its portals of entry, and to describe, through animal studies, including trans-species evaluations, the pharmacokinetic properties and metabolic pathways used by the agent. In the last case, whenever possible these fundamental studies should include evaluations of the parameters in the monkey, whose metabolism most often resembles that of humans. Simple extrapolation of nonprimate animal experimental data to the human often leads to inappropriate conclusions and to the unexpected occurrence of toxic responses when humans are eventually exposed.

Even with extensive toxicological evaluations, interindividual variations in the metabolism of a chemical that may identify hosts or ethnic groups with increased susceptibility to the toxic effects of specific chemicals cannot be excluded. Similarly, individuals with impaired renal function are probably best excluded from industrial exposures when metabolism and excretion of a chemical are either poorly characterized or are known to occur through the kidney. Individuals with renal impairment may retain significant quantities of toxic metabolites that would normally be excreted by those with adequate renal function. Similar concerns exist for chemicals excreted primarily by the lung and the exposure to them of individuals with decreased lung function.

Another significant variable not often considered in toxicological evaluations is the potential for toxicity resulting from chemical-chemical or chemical-drug interactions. Such chemical interactions are well characterized for pharmacological agents, but little attention has been given to their occurrence in industry. Thus, some attention should be given to the possibility that a nontoxic industrial chemical exposure could result in toxicity when combined with another chemical or drug. For example, an industrial chemical with immunotoxic properties at very high concentrations but little effect at the ambient concentrations observed in the workplace could cause immunotoxicity and serious health effects in workers who are being treated with immunosuppressive doses of corticosteroids or other such immunoactive drugs if additive or synergistic effects between such chemicals occur. Interactions of this type could be the cause of human disease in workers who are exposed outside the work environment to drugs or chemicals that have the capacity to alter the properties of chemicals in the workplace. For these and other reasons, there is an increasing need to develop new and alternative approaches to the toxicological evaluation of industrial chemicals in conjunction with the development of sensitive and specific means for measuring both environmental and human exposures and the products of metabolism. It would appear that industrial exposures should be evaluated in a manner similar to that established for the testing of new therapeutic agents, and there is a real need to establish guidelines and principles for industrial (occupational) toxicology such as have been carefully established for clinical pharmacology. If a system could be developed that would encourage the professional responsibility of reporting adverse chemical responses not only to the government but also to the scientific community at large without impinging on the privileged nature of many industrial chemical processes, the possibilities for characterizing the mechanisms of such toxic responses and designing alternative chemicals would be significantly increased.

The epidemic of tumors observed in association with acquired immunodeficiency syndrome (AIDS) has emphasized the role of immunosuppression as a cause of cancer and focused on another important reason for evaluating the effects of chemicals on the immune system (14–17). There is also other evidence, although less dramatic than the AIDS problem, that links the immune system with cancer. The rare congenital immunodeficiency syndromes (severe combined immunodeficiency, DiGeorge's syndrome, ataxia telangiectasia, Bruton's sex-linked hypogammaglobulinemia, Wiskott-Aldrich syndrome, common variable immunodeficiency, X-linked lymphoproliferative syndrome) also have an increased frequency of cancer associated with their clinical expression (18), especially non–Hodgkin's lymphoma and acute lymphoblastic leukemia. The increased risk of developing gastric carcinoma in immunologically mediated chronic atrophic gastritis and the increased frequency of intestinial lymphoma in celiac sprue add further credence to the concept that immune-mediated damage can result in cancer (19–21). Renal transplant patients probably represent the best characterized and quantified group of patients in whom immunosuppression is linked with an excess risk of cancer (22–29). In these patients with drug-induced immunodeficiency, the risk of non–Hodgkin's lymphoma is 25 to 50 times higher than expected (22,24). Squamous cell cancer of the skin is also found in excess in renal transplant patients (21,28). Similar data have been acquired from the clinical analyses of rheumatic disease patients who have been treated with immunosuppressive drugs (30). Thus, clinical evidence clearly links cancer and immune dysfunction.

The mechanisms by which such immune dysfunction result in cancer are not completely understood, but in renal transplant patients the risk of cancer is related both to the degree of immunosuppression and to the level of antigen stimulation (24). Further, the high prevalence of infections with hepatitis B virus and perhaps other viruses infecting the immunocompromised host may contribute to the development of specific cancers. Clearly, such hosts lose the capacity to resist, by immune mechanisms, the development of neoplasia. Thus, chemical carcinogenesis may be expressed as alterations in the immune system that lead to cancer as opposed to the other mechanisms postulated for chemical carcinogenesis (31). Once chemicals with immunoactivity are identified, careful monitoring of exposed populations for those malignancies observed and documented in association with clinical immune disorders appears to be warranted.

One approach that holds some promise for toxicological testing of chemicals is the use of human peripheral blood cells for the detection of adverse effects associated with environmental exposures. Such use is especially relevant to immune cells because they circulate throughout the body, make contact with all the body's major organ systems, control many host defense functions, and can metabolize xenobiotics. A number of chemicals and drugs (benzene, halogenated aromatic hydrocarbons, polycyclic aromatic hydrocarbons, urethrane, phorbol diesters, insecticides, ozone, lead, organotin, cadmium, mercury, and a variety of therapeutic agents) have been shown to elicit toxic responses of the immune system (32,33), but the total impact of industrial chemicals on the human immune system in terms of health effects remains to be completely determined. Since immune cells also contain phase I and phase II xenobiotic metabolizing enzymes, it is not unreasonable to suggest that some chemicals are metabolized by monocytes and lymphocytes and others are detoxified primarily by other organs, with immune cell enzymes representing secondary routes of xenobiotic metabolism. Further, since no systematic evaluations have been performed to compare hepatic and immune cell xenobiotic metabolism, it is impossible at this stage to predict how representative the complement of phase I and II enzymes in monocytes and lymphocytes is when used to predict xenobiotic metabolism in major biotransforming organs such as the liver. Monocytes or macrophages have often been referred to as "wandering hepatocytes," and in some instances these cells may be found to handle foreign compounds in a manner similar if not identical to that of the liver.

In addition to their capacity to metabolize xenobiotics, cells of the immune system also offer a unique opportunity to assess host defense functions whose impairment by chemicals could lead to significant health effects. Hypersensitivity reactions, autoimmune responses, and immunosuppression induced by chemical agents can all be assessed *in vitro* using human immune cells either cultured in the presense of industrial chemicals or examined directly after *in vivo* exposure has occurred.

Further, immunotoxicology represents the only discipline where *in vivo* immunology can be studied without extensive ethical justification with regard to human experimentation.

Investigations of the human immune system circumvent the high costs of animal testing and avoid the often inappropriate extrapolations of animal data to humans. Evaluations of the human immune system can easily be performed with mononuclear cells recovered from healthy human blood donors and treated *in vitro* with putative toxic chemicals. Such experiments can be complemented by the examination of immune cells from exposed populations to confirm or refute *in vitro* data. To supplement such human data, animals can be used to develop models of human exposures and to determine whether host resistance has been impaired, especially with respect to infectious agents.

In addition to evaluating immune responses in the presence of putative chemical toxicants, xenobiotic metabolism by immune cells can be examined using viable *in vitro* cell systems. Even though immune cell xenobiotic metabolism may differ in some ways from hepatic cell metabolism data, relatively few pathways of xenobiotic conversion have been compared in immune and hepatic cells. Immune cells, especially activated immune cells, may be found to be an important tool for the measurement of xenobiotic metabolism and the identification of chemical metabolites derived from phase I and II reactions. Mononuclear cells may also provide a means for selecting appropriate animals for the validation of toxicological testing panels. Since human hepatocytes are short-lived in culture and difficult to obtain on a routine basis, readily available peripheral blood immune cells offer a reasonable alternative source for human toxicological testing.

Despite careful toxicological analysis, individual variation in the metabolism and response to chemicals cannot be avoided. Such variation has been clearly documented for therapeutic drugs by pharmacogenetic studies, but less well-characterized interindividual variations have been recognized as causes of the toxic responses to industrial chemicals and environmental contaminants. Nonetheless, the genetic polymorphisms observed for paraoxonase, *N*-acetyltransferase, aryl hydrocarbon hydroxylase, and other enzymes involved in chemical metabolism have clearly established the discipline ecogenetics, which studies the role of genetically determined variation in the susceptibility of exposed hosts to environmental agents (34). Such interindividual variation has also been extended to ethnically distinct populations expressing susceptibility to drugs and chemicals (35). Identification of individual and ethnic variation may be a significant factor in the selection of construction sites for new manufacturing plants and in the introduction of chemical processes to the Third World. Since the number of polymorphic (variant) genes in the human is estimated to be between 20,000 and 25,000, it has been calculated that fewer than 1 percent of such genes have been identified to date (36). Based on the fact that individual variation in chemical metabolism exists and is likely to be expressed as toxic responses in some individuals, the use of human mononuclear cells to investigate detoxification pathways represents an easily accessible way for the identification of such "aberrant" metabolic pathways when immune cells are major routes of xenobiotic biotransformation. It also seems realistic to expect that in time there will be sufficient population data to warrant the screening of labor forces for genetic and ethnic variations in chemical metabolism as a means of preventing undesirable health effects following environmental or chemical exposures. Certainly, such screening would make for better job training and placement.

In summary, all these concepts provide a sound rationale for further evaluation of the immune system both as a target for toxic chemicals and as a tool for the study of metabolism of such chemicals. In the quest for ways to improve sensitivity and specificity in the detection of toxic responses, evaluation of the interactions between chemicals and the human immune system deserves increased attention.

The subdiscipline of immunotoxicology includes not only the development of protocols for the evaluation of the effects of chemicals on the immune system but also the use of the immunological laboratory for the detection and quantitation of chemicals in the tissues and blood of the exposed host. The generation of either polyclonal or monoclonal antibodies against specific chemical epitopes permits the use of such antibodies for the sensitive and specific detection of xenobiotics in the serum of exposed individuals as well as in their fixed tissues by immunoperoxidase techniques. Haptens in the form of chemicals or environmental contaminants of low molecular weight (200 to 300 daltons) can easily be coupled with carrier proteins, which results in hapten-protein complexes, molecules that may be intensely immunogenic. The use of two different carrier proteins (one for immunization and the other for immunoassay) avoids the detection of antibodies reacting with the carrier protein when immunoassays for a specific epitope are preformed. It is not beyond the realm of possibility that chemicals will provoke the production of autoantibodies against host tissues. Since drug-induced causes of disease such as lupus erythematosus and hemolytic anemia have clearly been identified, we can fully expect additional chemical-induced autoimmune diseases to be characterized in the future. In fact, we believe that a whole new industry will grow from the use of immunoassays for the detection of chemicals and chemical-induced antibodies in humans. Together with this technology, another laboratory-based industry will develop using antibodies as environmental sensors for chemicals. Further, there is a burgeoning use of antibodies for the detection of adducts formed between chemicals and nucleic acids. Such technology not only permits the documentation of adduct formation but also addresses the mechanisms by which such adducts may alter genetic information and its translation into functional proteins. It also provides a way of monitoring chemical exposure and nucleic acid damage. The next century may see the immunization of humans to protect exposed populations against chemical-induced injury.

Finally, a significant benefit to be accrued from the subdiscipline of immunotoxicology is likely to be the identification of chemicals with specificity for biochemical pathways used for the synthesis of immunoregulatory substances. The characterization of such chemicals offers a unique opportunity to dissect the mechanisms by which immune responses are mediated and controlled. Indeed, identification of chemicals with specificity for immunological pathways also provides an opportunity for the development of new therapeutic agents for immunologically mediated diseases.

Some of the major public health problems of the next few decades, such as substance abuse (tobacco, alcohol, and drugs), AIDS, chronic disease prevention (e.g., cancer, respiratory disease), unbalanced dietary intake and nutrition, and diseases created by the industrialization of the Third World, relate in one way or another to studies of the immune system and the development of the new discipline, immunotoxicology. One seminal problem pertinent to the development of this new discipline is the design of the educational programs essential for the training in immunotoxicology of scientists who will assume positions of responsibility in industry, government, and academia in the future. Progress in this new field depends on attracting young investigators with sound training and fresh ideas. The first step is a sound understanding of the cellular and molecular basis of immunological specificity. Next must come insight into the highly integrated nature of the immune response depending on the interactions of a variety of cells and their soluble products. Finally, students must appreciate the far-reaching effects of shifts in immunological homeostasis that can result from exposure to chemicals and drugs. In undertaking the preparation of this book, we wish to bring the challenging problems of immunotoxicology to the attention of students.

REFERENCES

1. Kay, K. (1977): Polybrominated biphenyls (PBB) environmental contamination in Michigan, 1973–1976. *Environ. Res.*, 13:74.
2. Bekesi, J. G., Holland, J. F., Anderson, H. A., et al. (1978): Lymphocyte function of Michigan dairy farmers exposed to polybrominated biphenyls. *Science*, 199:1207.
3. Chang, K., Hsieh, K., Lee, T., et al. (1981): Immunologic evaluation of patients with polychlorinated biphenyl poisoning: Determination of lymphocyte subpopulations. *Toxicol. Appl. Pharmacol.*, 61:58.
4. Chang, K., Hsieh, K., Lee, T., et al. (1982): Immunologic evaluation of patients with polychlorinated biphenyl poisoning: Determination of phagocytic Fc and complement receptors. *Environ. Res.*, 28:329.
5. Kashimoto, T., Miyata, H., Kunita, S., et al. (1981): Role of polychlorinated dibenzafuran in Yusho (PCB) poisoning. *Arch. Environ. Health*, 36:321.
6. Donovan, J. W., MacLennan, R., and Adena, M. (1984): Vietnam service and the risk of congenital abnormalities: A case control study. *Med. J. Aust.* 140:394.
7. Erickson, J. D., Mulinare, J., McClain, P. W., et al. (1984): Vietnam veterans risks for fathering babies with birth defects. *J.A.M.A.*, 252:903.
8. Patterson, D. G. Jr., Hampton, L., Lapeza, C. R. Jr., et al. (1987): High resolution gas chromatography/high-resolution mass spectrometric analysis of human serum on a whole-weight and lipid basis for 2,3,7,8-tetrachlorodibenzo-p-dioxin. *Anal. Chem.*, 59:2000.
9. Reggiani, G. (1983): Anatomy of a TCDD spill: The Seveso accident. *Hazard Ass. Chem. Curr. Dev.*, 2:269.
10. Reggiani, G. (1980): Acute human exposure to TCDD in Seveso, Italy. *J. Toxicol. Environ. Health*, 6:27.
11. Kilburn, K. H., Warshaw, R., and Thornton, J. C. (1986): Asbestos diseases and pulmonary symptoms and signs in shipyard workers and their families in Los Angeles. *Arch. Intern. Med.*, 146:2213.
12. Frumkin, I. T., Egilman, D., Kelly, M., et al. (1984): Asbestos-related diseases *J.A.M.A.*, 254:1307.
13. Muller, K., and Brown, R. C. (1985): The immune system and asbestos-associated disease. In Immunotoxicology and Immunopharmacology, edited by J. H. Dean, M. I. Luster, A. E. Munson, and H. Amos, pp. 429–440. Raven Press, New York.

14. Friedman-Kien, A. E., Laubenstein, L. J., Rubinstein, P., et al. (1982): Disseminated Kaposi's sarcoma in homosexual men. *Ann. Intern. Med.*, 96:693.
15. Ziegler, J. L., Drew, W. L., Mimer, R. C., et al. (1982): Outbreak of Burkitt's-like lymphoma in homosexual men. *Lancet*, 2:631.
16. Fauci, A. S., Macher, A. M., Longo, D. L., et al. (1984): Acquired immunodeficiency syndrome: Epidemiologic, clinical, immunologic, and therapeutic complications. *Ann. Intern. Med.*, 100:92.
17. Levine, A. M., Meyer, R. P., Begandy, M. K., et al. (1984): Development of B-cell lymphoma in homosexual men. Clinical and immunologic findings. *Ann. Intern. Med.*, 100:7.
18. Spector, B. D., Perry, G. S., and Kersey, J. H. (1978): Genetically determined immunodeficiency disease (GDID) and malignancy: Report from the Immunodeficiency-Cancer Registry. *Clin. Immunol. Immunopathol.*, 11:12.
19. Borch, K. (1986): Epidemiologic, clinicopathologic, and economic aspects of gastroscopic screening of patients with pernicious anemia. *Scand. J. Gastroenterol.*, 21:21.
20. Sipponen, P., Kikki, M., Haapakoski, J., et al. (1985): Gastric cancer risk in chronic atrophic gastritis: Statistical calculations of cross-sectional data. *Int. J. Cancer*, 35:173.
21. Morgan, D. R., Holgate, C. S., Dixon, M. F., and Bird, C. C. (1985): Primary small intestinal lymphoma: A study of 39 cases. *J. Pathol.*, 147:211.
22. Hoover, R., and Fraumeni, J. F. (1973): Risk of cancer in renal transplant recipients. *Lancet*, 2:55.
23. Penn, I., and Starzl, T. E. (1972): Malignant tumors arising de novo in immunosuppressed organ transplant recipients. *Transplantation*, 14:407.
24. Kinlen, L. J. (1982): Immunosuppressive therapy and cancer. *Cancer Surv.*, 1:565.
25. Porreco, R., Penn, I., Droeqemvellar, W., et al. (1975): Gynecologic malignancies in immunosuppressed homograft recipients. *Obstet. Gynecol.*, 45:359.
26. Penn, I. (1979): Kaposi's sarcoma in organ transplant recipients: Report of 20 cases. *Transplantation*, 27:8.
27. Penn, I. (1978): Tumors arising in organ transplant recipients. *Adv. Cancer Res.*, 28:31.
28. Koranda, F. C., Dehmel, E. M., Kahn, G., and Penn. I. (1974): Cutaneous complications in immunosuppressed renal homograft recipients. *J.A.M.A.*, 229:419.
29. Kinlen, L. J., Scheil, A. G. R., Peto, J., et al. (1979): Collaborative United Kingdom-Australasian study of cancer in patients treated with immunosuppressive drugs. *Br. Med. J.*, 2:1461.
30. Fraumeni, J. F. and Hoover, R. N. (1977): Immunosurveillance and cancer: Epidemiologic observations. *Natl. Cancer Inst. Monogr.*, 47:121.
31. Pitot, H. C. (1986): Fundamentals of Oncology, pp. 34–138. Third Edition. Marcel Dekker, Inc., New York.
32. Dean, J. H., Murray, M. J., and Ward, E. C. (1986): Toxic responses of the immune system. In Casarett and Doull's Toxicology. The Basic Science of Poisons, edited by C. D. Klaassen, M. O. Amdur, and J. Doull, pp. 245–285. Macmillan Publishing Company, New York.
33. Dean, J. H., Luster, M. I., Munson, A. E., and Amos, H. (1985): Immunotoxicology and Immunopharmacology. Raven Press, New York.
34. Omenn, G. S., and Gelboin, H. V. (1984): Banbury Report 16. Genetic Variability in Responses to Chemicals. Cold Spring Harbor Laboratory, Cold Spring Harbor, New York.
35. Kalow, W., Goedde, H. W., and Agarwal, D. P. (1986): Ethnic Differences in Reactions to Drugs and Xenobiotics. Alan R. Liss, Inc., New York.
36. Omenn, G. S. (1984): Risk assessment, pharmacogenetics, and ecogenetics. In Banbury Report 16. Genetic Variability in Responses to Chemical Exposure, edited by G. S. Omenn and H. V. Gelboin, Cold Spring Harbor Laboratory, Cold Spring Harbor, New York, p. 11.

Clinical Immunotoxicology, edited by
D. S. Newcombe, N. R. Rose, and J. C. Bloom.
Raven Press, Ltd., New York © 1992.

2

The Immunological Assessment of Immunotoxic Effects in Man

Noel R. Rose* and Joseph B. Margolick†

*Department of Immunology and Infectious Diseases, The Johns Hopkins University,
School of Hygiene and Public Health, Baltimore, Maryland 21205;
†Department of Environmental Health Sciences, The Johns Hopkins University,
School of Hygiene and Public Health, Baltimore, Maryland 21205*

This chapter approaches immunotoxicology from the vantage point of the patient. In an industrial or regulatory setting, immunotoxicologic investigations frequently begin with a specific chemical, such as a drug or environmental pollutant, and attempt to define the toxicity of that chemical on the immune system. For clinical assessment of individual patients, however, a different situation arises in which either (a) we start with evidence of an immunological deficit or dysfunction in the patient and then seek to attribute this effect to a particular drug or toxic agent, or, more commonly (b) we start with a known or suspected exposure to a potentially toxic agent and ask whether the immune system has been adversely affected or compromised. The process of answering the second question is known as immune assessment.

Much of the literature on immune assessment concerns severe immune deficiency, the first clinical evidence of which may be frequent or prolonged infections. Such deficiencies can be acquired or congenital, and excellent reviews of the assessment of each type are available (1,2). In these situations, it is likely that a specific area of immune deficiency can be found. Similarly, in cases of hypersensitivity reactions to specific compounds, it is frequently possible to identify the offending agent. However, much of the current interest in the area of immunotoxicology concerns the possibility of subtle defects that may exert their adverse effects only over a very long period of time, such as is required for the development of cancer or of *clinically important* autoimmunity. This situation is infinitely more controversial and difficult to understand, especially in an individual patient; rather, studies of an entire community may be needed when a number of individuals show characteristic immunological alterations in their immune response and some environmental pollutant is suspected.

This chapter illustrates a systematic approach to the assessment of immune competence in humans and to the understanding of where defects in the immune system may have occurred. Preferably, this approach begins with the simplest studies, which are relatively inexpensive and readily available, and proceeds to the use of more elaborate and expensive tests, as needed, to identify more precisely the location of the defect. As will be seen, the more severe the defect, the easier it is to delineate; conversely, the milder the defect, the more difficult it is either to confirm or to exclude.

COMPOSITION OF THE IMMUNE SYSTEM

Figure 1 presents an overview of the immune system. It includes organized lymphoid tissues, such as the spleen and lymph nodes; it also includes lymphoid cells that are widely distributed throughout the body and that permit immunological surveillance. The functions of the normal immune system depend on many specialized cell types and soluble factors that mediate interactions among these cells. The assessment of these various populations of cells and of their regulatory factors is the task of the clinical immunology laboratory.

A pluripotential stem cell is the source of almost all of the cells that are involved in immunological responses. The same stem cell gives rise to the cells of the hematopoietic system, including erythrocytes and platelets, as well as the families of immunologically active cells. The polymorphonuclear neutrophils represent the major population of circulating phagocytes, whereas basophils and eosinophils are involved in hypersensitivity reactions and resistance to parasitic infections. The circulating monocyte and the tissue macrophage are important both as phagocytic cells and as antigen-processing and antigen-presenting cells. The progenitor of the lymphocyte family, the lymphoid precursor, gives rise to two main populations, T cells and B cells. The effector or cytotoxic T cells and their soluble products, the lymphokines, are responsible for cell-mediated immunity. The helper-inducer T cell is necessary for the proper initiation and regulation of both humoral and cellular immunity. Finally, the memory T cell is responsible for the anamnestic response that is characteristic of adaptive immunity.

The helper-inducer T cell is capable of recognizing fragments of antigen presented in the context of class II histocompatibility (Ia) antigens of antigen-processing cells. Ia antigens are surface glycoproteins encoded by class II histocompatibility genes. Interleukin-1, a product of the antigen-presenting cell, triggers proliferation of T cells and stimulates production of interleukin-2, a T-cell growth factor. The B cell, usually following interaction with a T cell, is responsible for producing the antibodies found in the bloodstream and bodily secretions. T cell-B cell interaction is restricted by the class II products of the major histocompatibility complex and is promoted by interleukins produced by the T cells. These interactions direct the differentiation of the B cell into the plasma cell, which is essentially a cellular factory for producing and secreting antibodies. The B cell can also act as an antigen-presenting cell.

A third family of immunologically active cells, natural killer or NK cells, is

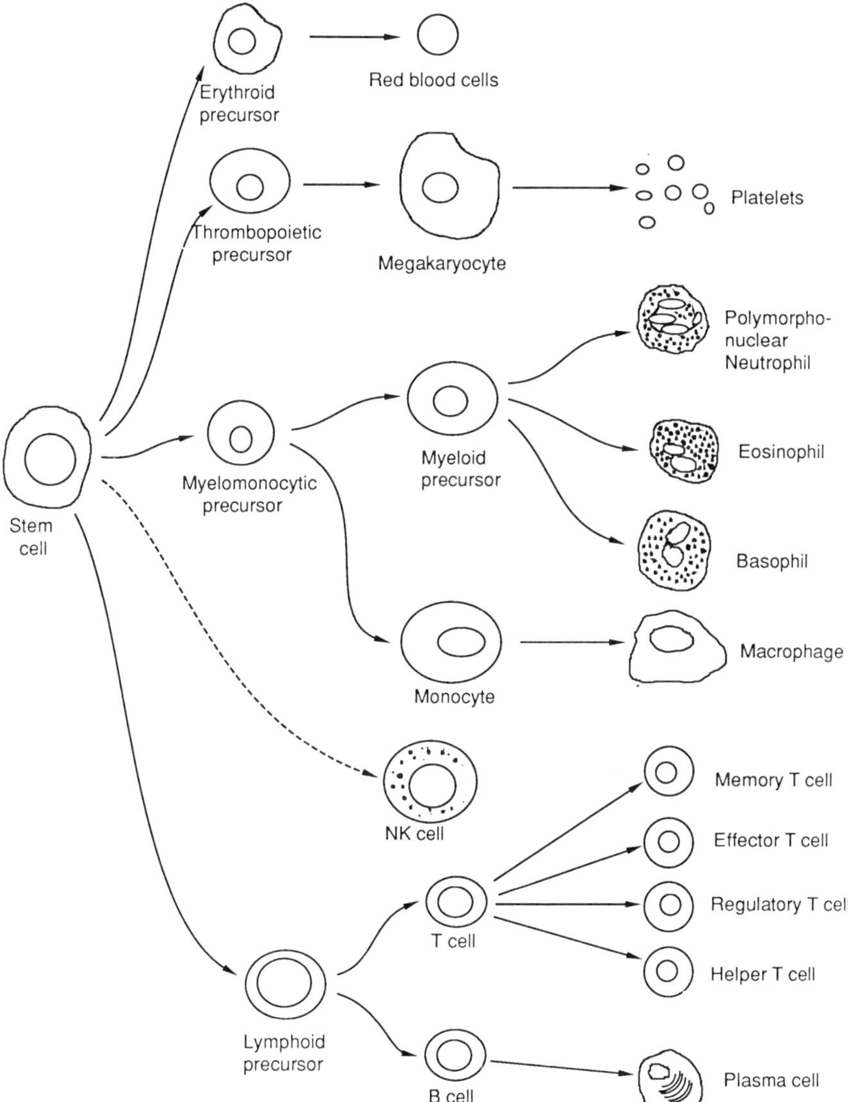

FIG. 1. Cellular components of the immune system.

found among the large granular lymphocytes, Their ontogenetic origin is still unknown. They are stimulated by lymphokines produced by helper T cells, such as interleukin-2 and interferon-γ.

MANIFESTATIONS OF IMMUNOTOXIC EFFECTS

Classically, immunotoxic effects are divided into three categories: immune suppression, hypersensitivity, and autoimmunity (Table 1). Each of these effects depends on the dysfunction or inhibition of specific populations of the cells discussed above.

Immune Suppression

Depression of the immune response may result in decreased host resistance to infection and malignancy. If the deficiency occurs in the T-cell lineage and therefore in the cell-mediated arm of the immune response, it characteristically presents clinically as repeated infections by intracellular pathogens, including some protozoan parasites (e.g., *Pneumocystis* and *Toxoplasma*), pathogenic fungi (e.g., *Candida*), viruses (e.g., varicella zoster, herpes simplex, cytomegalovirus), and certain bacteria (e.g., *Mycobacteria, Listeria*). Because the T cell also seems to play a role in resistance to certain malignancies, either directly through the action of cytotoxic T cells or indirectly through the production of lymphokines, an increased incidence of malignancy may also be a manifestation of cellular immune deficiency. However, it should be noted that no environmental exposure has yet been shown to have caused a cellular immune deficiency severe enough to manifest itself as opportunistic infection or neoplasm. In addition, the neoplasms that occur with increased frequency in immunocompromised humans tend to be derived from cells of the immune system, making it difficult to determine if the immune defect is responsible for the neoplasms or whether some other factor is causing both the neoplasms and the immune deficiency.

TABLE 1. *Possible immunotoxic effects*

Decreased host resistance
T-cell deficiency
B-cell deficiency
Complement deficiency
Phagocytosis defects
Hypersensitivity
Antibody-mediated (immediate)
Cell-mediated (delayed)
Autoimmunity
Altered self-antigen
Immune dysregulation

B-cell deficiency produces a distinct clinical syndrome characterized by increased susceptibility to acute infections with pyogenic bacteria, such as recurrent pneumonia, meningitis, or abscesses, against which antibody is the main protective mechanism. It can be seen that individuals with B-cell deficiency have quite a different clinical presentation from those with a T-cell defect; thus, the clinical picture itself is a major clue to the nature of the immunodeficiency.

Complement deficiencies show many similarities with B-cell deficiencies, but there are also some interesting differences. Complement deficiencies involving C6 and C8 characteristically predispose to infections with gram-negative cocci, such as meningitis or arthritis due to meningococcal infection. Here, it is the recurrent pattern of an unusual infection that provides the clue that there is an underlying immune deficiency. It is noteworthy that this deficiency would be missed by all the routine screening tests generally employed for immune deficiency and would be identified only when specifically tested for.

The manifestations of defects in phagocytes overlap with those of B-cell deficiency because of the important role of opsonins in facilitating Fcγ-dependent phagocytosis, but there are several significant differences between the two defects. For example, neutrophils from persons with chronic granulomatous disease phagocytize normally but are incapable of producing an oxidative burst in metabolism following phagocytosis. These individuals are prone to chronic infections (such as osteomyelitis attributable to *Klebsiella* or *Serratia* organisms) because the phagocytes can ingest these common organisms but cannot digest and kill them.

Although the importance of NK cells for human health is not as well established as that of B cells and T cells, they are believed to be important in host defense against viruses and tumors (3). This belief is supported by a recent case report describing a patient with recurrent herpesvirus infections who was shown to have a selective absence of NK cells (4).

Immunosuppressive agents may compromise one or both branches of the immune response. Some patients have symptoms mimicking genetic deficiencies of either T cells or B cells. In one study, for example, 30% of cardiac transplant patients receiving the drug cyclosporine developed pulmonary infections caused by *Pneumocystis carinii*, *Aspergillus*, or cytomegalovirus (5). Concurrent hematological deficiencies involving erythrocytes, platelets, or leukocytes implicate toxic effects on the stem cell. Chronic benzene exposure may induce pancytopenia by a direct effect on bone marrow (6).

Hypersensitivity Reactions

Hypersensitivity reactions are subdivided into those that are antibody-mediated (particularly IgE antibody-mediated reactions) or those that are T-cell–mediated and are associated with delayed hypersensitivity responses. The antibody–mediated hypersensitivity reactions include allergic rhinitis, asthma, atopic dermatitis, and some forms of gastrointestinal food intolerance. Among the T-cell–mediated reactions are contact dermatitis and hypersensitivity granulomas.

Autoimmunity

Autoimmunity may be another consequence of chemical exposure. Classic examples are the drug-induced hemolytic anemias. Lupus-like disease may also be induced by drugs. Investigations into this problem may represent a major growth area in immunotoxicology research. At least two basically different biological mechanisms can be proposed by which autoimmunity may result from chemical exposure. One mechanism is the alteration of self-constituents by the action of a chemical or a drug that converts a self-antigen to a foreign antigen. Alpha-methyldopa binding to erythrocytes, for example, induces the formation of antierythrocyte antibodies that recognize determinants derived from both normal proteins and the drug (7). A second mechanism is that some drugs interfere with immune regulation, thus giving rise to an inappropriate immune response. As an example, thyroiditis and hypothyroidism have been reported in patients receiving interleukin-2 therapy for malignancies (8,9).

Diagnosis of Immunotoxic Events

This very brief overview of the immune system illustrates three essential points that must be remembered in the context of immunotoxicological assessment. First, the immune system contains many different kinds of cells that perform many disparate but related functions. Therefore, abnormalities may be quite specific and localized, and the fact that some functions are normal does not mean that others are not impaired. Second, the immune system contains many redundancies and backups, so that any given abnormality may be compensated for by other functional pathways. Thus, it is possible that an abnormality may be present but not clinically manifest unless a pathway of compensation becomes compromised or a severe challenge occurs. Third, the division of immunotoxic effects into immune suppression, hypersensitivity, and autoimmunity is a clinically convenient classification that may not reflect underlying mechanisms. For example, hypersensitivity or autoimmunity may actually reflect suppression of normal inhibitory mechanisms.

A final question regarding immune deficiency is how much a given function must be compromised before a toxic effect is considered to have occurred. This question cannot necessarily be answered by study of congenital immune deficiencies. It depends on the health of the individual, the status of related immune pathways, and the status of the pathway in question to begin with. Similarly, how exaggerated hypersensitivity or autoimmune responses must be to cause clinical manifestations depends on other aspects of host immune regulation. All of these factors make immunotoxicology a very difficult field for which to define specific criteria for clinical immune assessment.

As mentioned previously, often the first indication of an immunotoxic effect is from the clinical history. This may be a history of immunodeficiency, hypersensitivity, or autoimmunity.

For immunodeficiency, the history is that of increased susceptibility to infection, either by an increased incidence of infections or by decreased ability to overcome or clear an infection. Whether an increased incidence of neoplasms can be a manifestation of immunodeficiency is not as clear. The role of the immune system in immunological surveillance of tumors is still a controversial subject, but some individuals deprived of their immune response develop an increased incidence of malignant disease. Persons with acquired immunodeficiency syndrome, for example, have an increased incidence of non-Hodgkin's lymphoma as well as Kaposi's sarcoma (10); in addition, transplantation patients undergoing chronic immunosuppression therapy develop malignancies, especially those of the lymphoid system, at higher than normal rates (11). These instances indicate that the immune system may play a role in resistance to tumors.

Dermatitis, as evidence of contact hypersensitivity, and respiratory distress, as evidence of immediate hypersensitivity in the bronchial tree, are discussed in other chapters of this book.

The clinical manifestations of autoimmunity are highly variable. Systemic diseases such as lupus erythematosus may appear as a characteristic skin rash, kidney failure, or cardiovascular disease. Patients with hemolytic anemia are typically pale and jaundiced. Other autoimmune diseases produce effects on particular organs, such as the hyperglycemia of diabetes or the hyperthyroidism of Graves' disease.

LABORATORY ASSESSMENT OF IMMUNOTOXIC EFFECTS

Once an immunotoxic effect is suspected, generally on the basis of the history of the patient or group of patients, many tests may assist in this diagnosis. The principal types of tests that are available to analyze general and specific immunological functions are summarized in Table 2. These tests are performed either *in vitro* using specimens obtained from the patients, e.g., peripheral blood, or *in vivo*, on the patients themselves.

Sequence of Immunopathologic Tests

Since investigation of immunological defects should begin with the simple procedures and then proceed to the more complex and expensive ones, and since the peripheral blood is the tissue most accessible to the immunologist, a good starting point is laboratory measurement of circulating immune cells in the peripheral blood, such as the complete blood counts and differential (Table 3). This inexpensive test

TABLE 2. *Types of immunotoxicity tests*

Immunopathology
Humoral immunity
Cell-mediated immunity
Nonspecific immunity
Hypersensitivity
Host challenge
Autoimmunity

provides essential information in determining whether there is a significant decrease in the cells that produce the immune response. A differential blood count assesses the quantity of the major categories of white blood cells (i.e., granulocytes, monocytes, and lymphocytes); differential counts are generally most accurately performed by automated methods counting at least 10,000 cells. In some circumstances it may be important to quantify eosinophils and basophils, which are not specifically distinguished from neutrophils by some automated methods. Although the total lymphocyte count (= white blood cells × % lymphocytes on differential count) is very important, it is also important to quantify the major categories of mononuclear cells, which can most accurately be done using fluorescent-labeled monoclonal antibodies and flow cytometry, as discussed in detail elsewhere in this volume. In brief,

TABLE 3. *Sequence of Immunopathologic Tests*

Clinical signs
   Infections
   Tumors
   Dermatitis
   Respiratory difficulties
Hematology
   Complete blood count
   Differential blood count
   Monoclonal antibody staining (immunophenotyping)
      T cells and subsets
      B cells and precursors
      Monocytes/macrophages
      Natural killer cells
      Other populations
Organ size
   Thymus
   Spleen
   Peripheral lymph nodes
Organ histology (biopsy)
   Lymph node
   Bone marrow
   Intestine
   Thymus
   Spleen

the number of circulating T cells in blood, formerly determined by the sheep cell rosette method, is best quantified by using anti-CD3 monoclonal antibodies. Further classification of the T cells is performed using CD4 antibodies, which usually identify helper-inducer T cells and CD8 antibodies, which react with cytotoxic T cells.

Direct measurement of the status of the main lymphoid organs can provide useful information when available, but in humans, unlike experimental animals, this is rarely the case in practice. We can determine splenomegaly and enlargement of peripheral lymph nodes by palpation, the dimensions of the thymus can be estimated by x-ray studies in infants, and at postmortem examination we can actually measure these organs. Invasive procedures are normally permitted only when there is persuasive clinical evidence of immunotoxicity, as described above, and noninvasive methods fail to establish a diagnosis. Histological examination of the lymphoid organs, when possible, can provide information about the nature of an immunological deficit, since the T cells populate the paracortical regions, whereas the B cells inhabit the follicles and germinal centers. Similarly, bone marrow samples permit assessment of the status of progenitor cells, providing an indication of the ability of the immunological system to recover from an insult. Finally, rectal biopsies are useful for the evaluation of plasma cells, and intestinal biopsies reveal Peyer's patches. Such biopsies are relatively easily performed and should not be overlooked as ways of gaining valuable immunological information. In most immunotoxicological investigations, the procedures listed here are considered too invasive to be useful.

Assays of Humoral Immunity

Measurements of total levels of immunoglobulins (Table 4) are now widely available in clinical laboratories using radial diffusion radioimmunoassay or laser nephelometry. There are five classes (isotypes) of immunoglobulins—IgM, IgG, IgA, IgD, and IgE; in addition, there are four subclasses of IgG and two subclasses of IgA. Levels of each class or subclass can be measured separately in serum, using antisera specific for the particular immunoglobulin heavy chain. Patients may manifest a deficiency in all classes of immunoglobulins or in only a single class. Measurement of IgA in body fluids such as saliva, if properly done, is used to assess secretory immunity. Some observers have associated low levels of secretory IgA with frequent respiratory tract infections. It has been reported that some patients with a deficiency of secretory IgA have increased secretion of IgM, possibly providing a compensatory mechanism (19).

Since normal immunoglobulin levels depend upon age as well as health, control values must be appropriately selected. Of concern is not only the level of immunoglobulins at one point in time but also the kinetics of the immunoglobulin disappearance, because a distinction needs to be made between defects in the synthesis of immunoglobulins, on the one hand, and inordinate loss of immunoglobulins, on the

TABLE 4. *Humoral immunity*

Immunoglobulin in serum, saliva, or other body fluids
Levels
Half-life
Clonality
Monoclonal gammopathy
Immunoglobulin gene rearrangements—restriction fragments
Antibody formation *in vitro*
Immunoglobulin synthesis
Plaque-forming cells
B-cell quantitation
B-cell response to mitogens
Antibody production *in vitro*
Natural
Induced
Complement
Classic pathway
Alternative pathway
Immune complexes
Circulating
Localized (*in situ*)

other hand. Plasma proteins may be lost through the intestine in patients with protein-losing enteropathy or even through the kidney in cases of nephrotic syndrome. The latter condition sometimes results from the action of toxic agents on the kidney, whereas the former may be associated with hypersensitive or idiosyncratic reactions to foods. An important feature of abnormal immunoglobulins is monoclonality, which is detected by the presence of a "spike" or "M-component" in the zonal electrophoresis test. Determination of the ratio of kappa to lambda light chains can be used to recognize monoclonal hypergammaglobulinemia. When appropriate, immunoglobulin gene rearrangements can be evaluated for evidence of clonal proliferation of B cells.

B lymphocytes in blood can be enumerated using immunofluorescence with antisera to surface immunoglobulin or with monoclonal antibodies to characteristic B-cell antigens such as CD19 and CD20. Pre–B cells in bone marrow can be identified by antibodies to cytoplasmic IgM heavy chains without surface immunoglobulin. The presence of pre-B cells in the bone marrrow in the face of low numbers of mature B cells in the peripheral blood suggests maturation arrest, that is, a toxic agent may interrupt the normal differentiation of the B cell series.

A more searching analysis of B-cell maturation involves studies of the biosynthesis of total immunoglobulin in the test tube by stimulating the cells with a polyclonal activator such as pokeweed mitogen. Evidence of immunoglobulin secretion *in vitro* may be found by the reverse hemolytic plaque technique or by measurement of secreted immunoglobulins in the culture supernatant.

To measure the so-called natural antibodies, such as blood group and heterophil antibodies, simple agglutination tests with appropriate human and sheep red blood cells are performed. Absence of these antibodies may indicate profound defects in immunoglobulin production. Immunologically normal individuals also have antibodies to common bacteria, such as streptococci or *Escherichia coli*. The ability of the subject to produce antibodies following immunization with an inert approved antigen (such as tetanus toxoid or diphtheria toxoid) can be ascertained. To measure antibody responses to carbohydrate antigens, pneumococcal or meningococcal capsular polysaccharides are used. These tests have the important advantages of testing immune function *in vivo* and covering a wide spectrum of functions, including antigen presentation and processing, T-cell recognition and help, and B-cell differentiation and antibody synthesis. In this regard, measurement of a primary immune response (e.g., to a new antigen) is a more sensitive indicator of insult than is measurement of a secondary response.

The total levels of complement and some of the components of the complement system are assayed by immunochemical or functional assays. Total hemolytic complement is measured by the ability of the serum sample to lyse a standard suspension of sensitized sheep red blood cells. Titrations of individual components are performed with sheep cell preparations with all components except the one to be measured. Antibodies specific for each of the complement proteins are available, permitting their measurement by radial diffusion or nephelometric immunoassays. Defects may occur either in the classic system of complement activation or the alternative (properdin) pathway.

Finally, the presence of immune complexes can be ascertained. Circulating complexes are determined by their ability to bind complement by Clq binding, by the Raji cell test, or by binding to rheumatoid factor. Localized immune complexes are frequently demonstrable by immunofluorescence or immunoperoxidase methods in tissues, such as kidney, lung, or skin.

Tests of Cell-Mediated Immunity

Assessment of cell-mediated immunity (Table 5) often starts with the delayed (24 to 72 hours) skin tests because they are simple, inexpensive, and one of the few procedures that test immune function *in vivo*. Most normal individuals develop delayed hypersensitivity reactions to common fungi, such as to *Candida albicans* or the tricophyton group, and to common bacteria, such as streptococci. A positive reaction to intradermal application of an antigen is denoted by induration after approximately 48 hours and indicates that the person tested is capable of recognizing the antigen and generating a cellular infiltrate at the site of the injection. Although the probability of an individual's reacting to a given antigen is highly variable, a reaction to any antigen proves the point; this fact has been used in the development of panels of six or eight common antigens, and most healthy persons will react to at least one (12). If no reaction is observed, delayed sensitivity can still be tested by deliberately attempting to induce a reaction with percutaneous application of simple chemicals, such as dinitrochlorobenzene, followed by rechallenge 2 weeks later.

TABLE 5. *Cell-mediated immunity*

Delayed hypersensitivity skin test
Preexisting
Induced
T-cell quantitation
T-cell response to mitogens
T-cell response to antigens
Foreign antigens
Alloantigens—mixed lymphocyte response
Lymphokine production
Macrophage inhibiting factor, leukocyte inhibitory
factor
Interleukin-1
Interleukin-2, interleukin-2R
Interleukin-3
Interleukin-4
Interleukin-5
Interleukin-6
Interferon-gamma
Suppressor cell assays
Cytotoxic T-cell cytolysis
Allogeneic target
Virus-infected target
Malignant cell target
Antibody-dependent cell-mediated cytolysis

Contact dermatitis elicited locally by this chemical is indicative of delayed hypersensitivity.

Delayed hypersensitivity skin tests are highly informative when carefully done and controlled; unfortunately, it is not a trivial matter to standardize all aspects of these tests, such as their application and reading, especially when large numbers of subjects are being studied. For example, in the investigation of potential dioxin-exposed trailer park residents in Missouri, approximately one half of the skin test results was considered unreliable (13). Moreover, almost all of the subjects who had decreased skin test responses at the time of the study had normal responses when retested 12 to 18 months later; recovery of previously impaired responses was not considered a likely explanation for this finding (14). Because of problems such as these, delayed hypersensitivity skin tests were recently classified as "not recommended" for immune biomarker studies by a task force reviewing this issue (15).

For the *in vitro* functional responses of T cells, T-cell mitogens such as concanavalin A and phytohemagglutinin are used to induce transformation of lymphocytes into proliferating lymphoblasts. Lymphocyte proliferation assays can also be performed with specific antigens, such as tetanus toxoid, as stimuli rather than mitogens. The proliferation response in either case is measured by ^{3}H-labeled thymidine incorporation or by the release of mediators such as interleukin-2. These tests have been used for many years and have documented decreased lymphocyte responsiveness in humans with known toxic exposures compared with controls, [e.g., (16)]. T-cell blast formation can also be assessed directly by activation markers, such as the interleukin-2 receptor, transferrin receptor, or class II major histocompatibility complex molecules.

Proliferation of lymphocytes in the above lymphoproliferation tests requires the normal function of monocytes. Therefore, in principle these tests could be used to evaluate monocyte function. However, in healthy individuals there is a great excess of monocytes, so that this approach is rather insensitive. Despite this, experiments adjusting the number of monocytes in the cultures have been used to study certain types of immunodeficiency (17).

Another test of T-cell function, the response to major histocompatibility alloantigens as measured by mixed lymphocyte reactions, may be a more discerning test of T-cell response because it combines some of the more desirable features of mitogen- and antigen-induced lymphocyte proliferative responses. It is more specific and physiological than mitogen-induced proliferation, but because most lymphocytes have alloreactivity, it is normally much more vigorous than the response to a given foreign antigen. A deficiency in mixed lymphocyte reactions, therefore, is considered a sensitive test of T-cell competence.

Other tests that have been used to measure other functions of T cells in humans are listed in Table 5. The reverse hemolytic plaque technique with stimulated B cells can be used to estimate helper-inducer functions of T cells. Soluble factors (lymphokines) serve as hormone-like messengers within the immune system, and several can readily be measured in the clinical immunology laboratory (see Table 5). The receptor for interleukin-2 is another valuable indicator of the activation of the T cell and can be measured by immunofluorescence using a monoclonal antibody. Nonspecific suppressor T cells can be generated with agents such as concanavalin A and measured for their ability to interfere with pokeweed-mitogen–induced B–cell lymphocyte proliferation or immunoglobulin synthesis. Among other tests of cell-mediated immunity, specific T-cell cytotoxic effects on allogeneic target lymphoblasts can be detected (i.e., by using an assay jointly with the mixed lymphocyte reaction), or the ability of antigen-specific T cells to destroy virus-infected or malignant target cells can be measured. Antibody-dependent cell-mediated cytolysis, which involves the combined action of antibody with Fc receptor–bearing large lymphocytes or macrophages on specific target cells, is another measurable function. *However, the application of these tests to the field of immunotoxicology and human immune assessment is still in the future.*

Nonspecific Immunity

Natural killer cells, which contribute to resistance to viral infections and to malignancies, can be measured by their cytotoxic effects on standard target cells (Table 6). The standard NK cell assays depend upon lysis of K562 human erythroleukemia cells. The proportion of NK cells can be measured with appropriate monoclonal antibodies, such as CD56 with or without coexpression of CD16; cells that coexpress CD3 and CD56, however, are T cells and not NK cells. NK activity can

TABLE 6. *Nonspecific immunity*

Natural killer cell activity
Phagocytosis
    Count and morphology
    Metabolism (nitroblue tetrazolium, chemiluminescence)
    Ingestion
    Bactericidal activity
    Chemotaxis
    Special leukocyte enzymes—myeloperoxidase

be augmented *in vitro* by incubating the effector lymphocytes with interferon-gamma or interleukin-2.

Neutrophil and Macrophage Function

Appropriate tests of macrophage function assess phagocytosis and intracellular killing.

Neutrophils or macrophages can be tested for phagocytosis. The number and morphological appearance of the leukocytes and their metabolism with respect to the respiratory bursts are examined by the nitroblue tetrazolium test, or by chemi-luminescence, but more specific tests for the generation of oxygen-free radicals are now becoming available. It is possible to quantify the ability of phagocytes to ingest particles, to kill ingested microorganisms, and to respond to chemotactic stimuli *in vitro*. Characteristic leukocyte or myelocyte enzymes, such as myeloperoxidase or nonspecific esterase, may be deficient owing to the action of toxic chemicals. This topic is discussed in more detail in Chapter 17.

Immediate Hypersensitivity

A first step in the diagnosis of immediate hypersensitivity (Table 7) is the demon-stration of cell-binding (homocytotropic) antibody which, in humans, is of the IgE

TABLE 7. *Immediate hypersensitivity*

Serum IgE and IgG subclass levels
    Total
    Antigen-specific (RAST)
Basophil degranulation
Histamine release
Arachidonic acid metabolism
Passive transfer
    Prausnitz-Küstner
    Passive cutaneous anaphylaxis
Passive sensitization of human leukocytes

or occasionally the IgG$_4$ class. The total IgE level may or may not be elevated, but the diagnosis of immediate hypersensitivity requires demonstration of antigen-specific IgE. The simple immediate skin test remains the gold standard for this purpose. If this cannot be done, several *in vitro* tests are available. RAST (radioallergosorbent tests) can demonstrate binding of IgE to an antigen-coated paper. Allergic responses, such as basophil degranulation and histamine release, may be demonstrated *in vitro*; for example, biochemical assays of the products of arachidonic acid metabolism, including the leukotrienes, are now becoming widely employed. Finally, hypersensitivity may be demonstrated by transfer experiments. The Prausnitz-Küstner passive transfer reaction to the human skin, which is now not done for safety reasons, was the definitive test of human homocytotropic antibody. Passive cutaneous anaphylaxis in primates, such as the rhesus or cynomolgus monkey, can be performed under special laboratory conditions to look for human homocytotropic antibody. An *in vitro* analogue is offered by passive sensitization of human leukocytes.

Challenge Tests

We rarely have the opportunity to test a human being directly for his or her immune status, as is frequently done in animal studies.

Although in humans not much can be done by means of infectious challenge tests, bronchial inhalation tests are used in immediate hypersensitivity reactions of the respiratory system. The elimination diet, a very difficult approach, is sometimes an aid in the diagnosis of intolerance or allergy to constituents of food products (18).

Chemically Induced Autoimmunity

A new chapter in immunotoxicology is the study of autoimmunity (Table 8). The first step in diagnosing autoimmune disease is to document the presence of an immune response to a self-antigen. The demonstration of specific antibody to a relevant tissue usually is the first step, because it is technically easier than demonstrating T lymphocytes reactive to self-antigens. The second step is to identify the responsible antigen. Usually this step requires fractionating an extract of the tissue and testing the individual fractions with antiserum or lymphocytes from affected patients. Often we are unable to determine if autoantibodies play any role in causing disease. After identification of the antigen, it is possible to isolate the equivalent antigen in experimental animals and to see whether it is capable of inducing an autoimmune disease. In the case of chemically induced autoimmune disease, the suspected antigen may be injected into the animal either in its native form or after combination with the incriminated drug or chemical agent in an effort to induce an autoimmune response accompanied by reproduction of the characteristic lesions in the form of tissue damage or functional impairment.

TABLE 8. *Steps for establishing the autoimmune basis of human disease*

Demonstration of autoantibodies or T cells
Identification of antigen
Experimental immunization with equivalent antigen
Reproduction of disease

SUMMARY

In summary, a great number of laboratory procedures are now available to assess the immune response in individuals suspected to be suffering from toxic effects of chemical agents. If in the course of clinical and epidemiological investigations there is reason to suspect that an individual has a depressed or an overactive immune response caused by environmental exposure, the clinical immunology laboratory is called upon to investigate, in a systematic manner, where the lesion resides and whether or not, in fact, an authentic immunotoxic effect is the culprit. In the absence of clinical evidence of disease or laboratory abnormalities whose meaning is well understood, results of immunological tests must be interpreted with great caution.

ACKNOWLEDGMENT

The authors' work was supported in part by NIEHS Center grant ES03819.

GENERAL REFERENCE

Further information on specific laboratory tests can be found in Rose, N. R., Friedman, H., and Fahey, J. L. (eds) (1986). Manual of Clinical Laboratory Immunology, Third Edition, 427 pp. American Society for Microbiology, Washington, D.C.

REFERENCES

1. Stiehm, E. R. (1989): Immunologic Disorders in Infants and Children. W. B. Saunders Company, Philadelphia,.
2. Samter, M. (1988): Immunological Diseases. Little, Brown, Boston.
3. Whiteside, T. L., and Herberman, R. B. (1989). The role of natural killer cells in human disease. *Clin. Immunol. Immunopathol.*, 53:1–23.
4. Biron, C. A., Byron, K. S., and Sullivan, J. L. (1990): Severe herpesvirus infections in an adolescent without natural killer cells. *N. Engl. J. Med.*, 320:1731–1735.
5. Austin, J. H., Schulman, L. L., and Mastrobattista, J. D. (1989): Pulmonary infection after cardiac transplantation: Clinical and radiological correlations. *Radiology*, 172:259–265.
6. Snyder, R. (1984). The benzene problem in historical perspective. *Appl. Toxicol.*, 4:692–699.
7. LoBuglio, A. F., and Jandl, J. H. (1967): The nature of alpha-methyldopa red cell antibody. *N. Engl. J. Med.*, 276:658.

8. Atkins, M. B., Mier, J. W., Parkinson, D. R., Gould, J. A., Berkman, E. M., and Kaplan, M. M. (1988): Hypothyroidism after treatment with interleukin-2 and lymphokine-activated killer cells. *N. Engl. J. Med.*, 318:1557–1563.

9. Mattijssen, V. J. M., DeMulder, P. H. M., Van Liessum, P. A., Corstens, F. H. M., Franks, C. R., and Wagener, D. J. T. (1990). Hypothyroidism and goiter in a patient during treatment with interleukin-2. *Cancer*, 65:2686–2688.

10. Ziegler, J. L. (1989): Lymphomas and other neoplasms associated with AIDS. In AIDS Pathogenesis and Treatment, edited by J. A. Levy, p. 359. Marcel Dekker, Inc., New York.

11. Penn, I. (1981): Depressed immunity and the development of cancer. *Clin. Exp. Immunol.*, 46:459–474.

12. Frazer, I. H., Collins, E. J., Fox, J. S., Jones, B., Oliphant, R. C., and Mackay, I. R. (1985): Assessment of delayed-type hypersensitivity in man: A comparison of the "Multitest" and conventional intradermal injection of six antigens. *Clin. Immunol. Immunopathol.*, 35:182–190.

13. Hoffman, R. E., Stehr-Green, P. A., Webb, K. B., Evans, R. G., Knutse, A. P., Schramm, W. F., Staake, J. L., Gibson, B. B., and Steinberg, K. K. (1986): Health effects of long-term exposure to 2,3,7,8-tetrachlorodibenzo-p-dioxin. *J.A.M.A.*, 255:2031–2038.

14. Evans, R. G., Webb, K. B., Knutsen, A. P., Rodman, S. T., Roberts, D. W., Bagby, J. R., Garrett, W. A., and Andrews, J. S. (1988): A medical follow-up of the health effects of long-term exposure to 2,3,7,8-tetrachlorodibenzo-p-dioxin. *Arch. Environ. Health*, 43:273–278.

15. Agency for Toxic Substances and Disease Registry. (1990): Biomarkers of organ damage or dysfunction for the renal, hepatobiliary and immune systems, Centers for Disease Control.

16. Bekesi, J. G., Holland, J. F., Anderson, H. A., Fischbein, A. S., Rom, W., Wolff, M. S., and Selikoff, I. J. (1978): Lymphocyte function of Michigan dairy farmers exposed to polybrominated biphenyls. *Science*, 199:1207–1209.

17. Prince, H. E., Moody, D. J., Shubin, B. I., and Fahey, J. L. (1985): Defective monocyte function in acquired immune deficiency syndrome (AIDS): Evidence from a monocyte-dependent T cell proliferation system. *J. Clin. Immunol.*, 5:21–25.

18. Jewett, D. L., Phil, D., Fein, G., and Greenberg, M. H. (1990): A double-blind study of symptom provocation to determine food sensitivity. *N. Engl. J. Med.*, 323:429–433.

19. Webster, A. D. B. (1976): "Immunodeficiency." In Immunology in Medicine, edited by E. J. Holboren and W. G. Reeves. Grune and Stratton, New York.

Clinical Immunotoxicology, edited by
D. S. Newcombe, N. R. Rose, and J. C. Bloom.
Raven Press, Ltd., New York © 1992.

3

The Immune System: An Appropriate and Specific Target for Toxic Chemicals

David S. Newcombe

*Department of Environmental Health Sciences, Johns Hopkins University,
School of Hygiene and Public Health, 615 N. Wolfe Street, Room 2712,
Baltimore, MD 21205*

Organs and cells of the immune system modulate interactions between the host and its environment and are strategically located both to monitor xenobiotic portals of entry and to participate in the absorption, distribution, and biotransformation of toxic substances. Cells of the myeloid and lymphoid lineage are also the first line of defense against infectious agents and conduct immunosurveillance against neoplastic transformation; therefore damage to these cells may cause disease. After interacting with immunocompetent cells, chemicals and drugs have clearly been shown to alter immune responses (1–5). Thus there is little question that xenobiotics may cause immunotoxic responses; immunosuppression, autoimmunity, or hypersensitivity reactions in humans and animals may result from xenobiotic exposures (1–5). For these reasons, immunotoxicological manifestations have been increasingly sought in both humans and animals. This review emphasizes the following factors of relevance to immunotoxic reactions: the anatomical location of the organs and cells of the immune system, the special functional capacities of immunocompetent cells, and the biotransformation pathways present in such cells.

In humans, the primary lymphoid tissue responsible for lymphopoiesis and monocytopoiesis is the bone marrow from which pluripotent stem cells originate. Such pluripotent cells are precursors of either mature cellular elements of the immune system or immature cells; which then migrate to another primary lymphopoietic organ, the thymus gland. The thymus gland contains immature lymphocytes (thymocytes) in its outer cortex; these proliferate and eventually reside as mature T lymphocytes in the inner medulla. Interdigitating cells expressing self-antigens are also derived from the bone marrow and are dispersed throughout the thymic epithelium, where they play a major role in the recognition and elimination of T cells that react with self-antigens. Fetal liver and bone marrow and mature bone marrow are also sources of B lymphocytes. The bone marrow, the liver, and the thymus gland do not reside in an anatomical location where chemical or drug exposure can affect them directly. On the other hand, secondary lymphoid organs such as tonsils, adenoids, and mucosa-associated lymphoid tissues provide protection to the mucosal and submucosal areas of the gastrointestinal and respiratory tracts and are in direct apposition to major portals of entry for toxicants. In contrast, the skin, another portal of entry for toxic substances, has a multicellular epidermal layer that forms a continuous barrier to the entry of foreign substances except for either highly lipid-soluble or small water-soluble compounds. Absorption through the skin is enhanced by epidermal abrasions, which occur frequently in many occupations. Such abrasions disrupt the stratum corneum and permit direct exposure to the vascularized dermis. In this setting, skin can become a significant site for toxicant absorption. Dendritic cells (Langerhans' cells) account for roughly 2 to 10% of the epidermal cellular content, and like other mesenchymally derived cells (e.g., monocytes or macrophages), they have the capacity to process antigens (6,7). Combined with epidermal or dermal lymphocytes, dendritic cells may account for skin-dependent immune responses. The vascularized dermis also provides a route of absorption for toxicants leading directly into the vascular spaces. It is important to recognize that regional variation in skin absorptive capacity for chemicals and drugs exists, the scrotal skin being most permeable and thickened and keratinized soles being the least penetrable (6).

The respiratory system and the gastrointestinal tract also represent major routes of entry for toxic substances, either by inhalation or ingestion. Absorption of toxicants by the respiratory tract usually includes three separate regions: nasopharyngeal, tracheobronchial, and pulmonary. Each of these sites can influence toxicant absorption in a different manner on the basis of its structural and functional capacities. The nasopharynx consists of highly vascularized, ciliated columnar epithelium, including interspersed mucus glands. The tracheobronchial tree is also lined with ciliated epithelium and contains goblet and other mucus-secreting cells. The pulmonary segment consists of respiratory bronchioles lined with either ciliated or nonciliated cuboidal epithelium leading to alveolar ducts and sacs that are covered with thin squamous epithelium and septal cells. Lying in direct contact with the alveolar epithelial cells (types I and II pneumocytes) are freely motile alveolar macrophages. The thickness of the alveolar wall is 9 μm, with only epithelium, a basement membrane, and loose connective tissue separating the alveolar sacs from the network of capillaries bathing the alveolus for gas exchange. The cells of greatest significance to the action of toxicants are ciliated epithelial cells, nonciliated bronchiolar cells (Clara cells), type II pneumocytes, and alveolar macrophages. Ciliated epithelium serves to move fluid and/or particles from the lung to the nasopharynx by a mucociliary escalator; this can represent a major route for toxicant removal. Clara cells are the major target of toxic substances that require metabolic activation by the P-450 system (8). Lung injury may result from activation of xenobiotics by these enzymes. Type II pneumocytes are cells designed to proliferate and differentiate after the occurrence of subtle lesions involving the alveolus (9–11). These cells differentiate into type I cells in the reconstitution of a damaged alveolus. Alveolar macrophages are phagocytic cells that serve both to ingest foreign substances and to scavenge dead cells. These cells are derived from blood monocytes and have the capacity, under certain conditions, to present antigen to lymphocytes. Further, monocytes and macrophages can biotransform certain toxicants using the enzymatic pathways present in these cells.

In general, the lung is highly permeable to volatile and lipid-soluble compounds that are rapidly absorbed by passive diffusion. Particulates with or without absorbed toxicants can be phagocytosed by alveolar and pulmonary macrophages, and these same cells can also ingest toxicants as cellular debris. Barriers to toxicant absorption include the mucociliary escalator, the mucus layers (5–10 μm thick) lining the various epithelial cells of the respiratory tract, and possibly the nasopharyngeal mucosa, which is a relatively weak barrier to water-soluble toxicants preventing their toxicity to the lower respiratory system by absorption in the nasopharynx. Further, on the basis of cellular and tissue damage diseased lungs may be more susceptible to toxicant absorption and its resultant injurious effects.

The gastrointestinal tract, the other major portal of entry for toxic substances, is exposed to toxicants through the direct ingestion of such substances, indirectly from contaminants present in food or from material swallowed after recovery from the tracheobronchial tree. Absorption in the gut is primarily dependent on the lipid solubility of the toxicant and its state of ionization. Substances that are ionized are usually unable to penetrate cell membranes, and the ionization state of compounds is highly dependent on the pH of the surrounding milieu. Thus, in the stomach where an acid pH exists, lipid-soluble, weak acids are readily absorbed since they are nonionized at a low pH, whereas in the blood plasma they become ionized at a neutral pH, maintaining a gradient between the transported form and the plasma component. In the small bowel where the pH is more alkaline, weak bases are more likely to be absorbed in a pH-dependent fashion where the nonionized form is maintained.

From the standpoint of environmental toxicants, the skin, gastrointestinal tract, and respiratory tract are primary sites of absorption. Of course, pharmacological agents can be administered by other routes (e.g., intravenous, subcutaneous, intramuscular), but such portals of entry are not those usually associated with environmental exposures. Drug abusers, especially narcotics addicts, are prone to exposure from a variety of toxic substances contaminating preparations thought to contain pure narcotics (e.g., heroin, cocaine), and under such conditions, serious toxic exposures may occur because the toxicant may be administered along with the drug directly into the bloodstream.

When considering toxicants with the potential to affect the immune system, the offending substance(s) must reach the bloodstream, the lymphatic system, or the portal circulation in order to be distributed to immune cells or lymphatic organs. For this reason, the plasma, portal, or lymphatic concentration of a toxicant is most significant, since it can be related to the toxicant dose delivered to its site of action. Blood circulates to almost every tissue in the body, whereas the portal circulation empties into the liver and provides nutrition for hepatocytes and Kupffer cells as well as other components of the hepatic acinus. The lymphatic circulation, together with the bloodstream, controls the circulation of cells of the immune system.

In most cases, an equilibrium is established between the circulatory system and tissues with respect to toxicants. The factors that influence absorption also play a major role in the regulation of toxicant distribution to tissues, especially the physiochemical properties of the toxic substance. In addition, certain specific properties relating directly to the transport of chemicals from the blood to extravascular compartments are important. These include capillary pore size, degree of plasma protein binding, the chemical and structural characteristics of the organ(s) perfused, the plasma pH, and the rate of toxicant excretion. Chemicals of low molecular weight, either in the ionized or nonionized state, can traverse most capillary pores and gain access to the extravascular space. Capillary pores vary in size depending on the particular capillary bed being evaluated, but in general small molecules (molecular weight 100 to 300 daltons) gain easy access to the extravascular spaces through pores 4 μm in diameter, whereas large molecules (molecular weight 10,000 daltons or greater) traverse such pores very slowly. The extremes in pore size are represented by brain capillaries, which are relatively impermeable, and the glomerulus, where the capillary pore size is 70 μm and permits large molecules (molecular weight 60,000 daltons) to pass to the extravascular space.

Many drugs and chemicals are bound extensively to plasma proteins, especially to albumin (12). Hydrogen and ionic bonds as well as Van der Waals forces contribute to such binding, providing the bound chemicals with important properties. Since such bonding is not covalent, molecules can be displaced readily by other chemicals that have greater affinity for a specific binding site. An equilibrium is established between the bound and the free compound, and only the free compound has access to the extravascular spaces, unless large capillary pores or damaged membranes permit the protein-bound chemical to traverse the capillary wall. Although passive diffusion may be regulated by plasma protein binding, active membrane transport systems appear not to be altered or restricted by protein binding. On the basis of these parameters, plasma protein binding affects tissue distribution and toxicity, since plasma protein binding will prolong the half-life of a chemical. Toxicity may be increased either by the release of free chemical over prolonged periods of time or by the massive displacement of a toxic substance by another chemical or drug with greater affinity for the binding site. Plasma protein binding provides a threshold dose for toxicity, since exceeding the capacity for binding by plasma proteins increases the concentration of free chemical, which may be the toxic species.

Uptake, metabolism, or storage of a chemical in a specific organ system, as noted previously, depends not only on its physiochemical characteristics but also on the properties of the organ system *per se*. As has been pointed out, nonionizable compounds are able to cross membranes more readily, and lipid solubility enhances the capacity of such compounds to gain access to the internal milieu of a cell. Thus, organs with a high fat content are likely to retain nonpolar compounds that are soluble in lipids (high octanol:water partition coefficient). Another factor that may result in the sequestration of specific chemicals by an organ is the affinity of a macromolecule for such chemicals. For example, diethylstilbestrol may exert its immunosuppressive actions via estrogen receptors present on lymphocytes and thymic epithelial cells; however, the evidence for this mechanism is controversial (13–

17). Thus, distribution is dependent, in part, on the chemical composition of the organ system and cell as well as the affinity of toxicants for specialized structures of the cell or organ. With respect to the immune system, particular attention should be given to the membrane receptors on monocytes, T lymphocytes, and B lymphocytes, since they are critical for the initiation and regulation of immune responses. Further, if toxic components become bound to cell structures directly, such toxicants may remain with the cell as it migrates to tissue sites of function or destruction.

The pH of plasma is also a significant factor controlling the distribution of toxic substances, since the ionization of chemicals is dependent on pH. Because plasma pH is tightly regulated in the healthy host, changes in pH are likely to affect alterations in toxicant distribution in disease states in which plasma pH may truly change the proportion of a toxic chemical in the nonionized state. Thus, clinical disorders associated with either acidosis or alkalosis may affect the potential toxicity of chemicals (Table 1).

Finally, the rate of excretion of a toxicant clearly influences plasma concentrations of a substance and its distribution. The more rapid the rate of excretion, the less likely it is that a toxicant will be distributed in high concentrations to tissues. Many toxic chemicals have to be transformed into water-soluble compounds prior to their excretion; therefore biotransformation pathways also play an important role in

TABLE 1. *Disorders associated with acidosis or alkalosis*

Respiratory Acidosis
    Reduced neurogenic transmission
    Regional alveolar hypoventilation
Respiratory Alkalosis
    Hypoxemia
    Fever
    Endotoxemia
    Hepatic failure
    Salicylate intoxication
    Brain stem lesions
Metabolic Acidosis
    Diabetic ketoacidosis
    Renal acidosis
    Lactic acidosis (e.g., convulsions, alcoholism, carbon monoxide)
    Acid generation (e.g., ammonium chloride, methyl alcohol, ethylene glycol)
    Acid ingestion
    Hypoaldosteronism
    Hyperparathyroidism
    Nonrenal bicarbonate loss
Metabolic Acidosis
    Loss of acid (e.g., vomiting, diarrhea)
    Renal tubular dysfunction (chloride deficiency, potassium deficiency,
      increased sodium delivery to the distal tubules)
    Excessive ingestion of base
    Contraction of blood volume
    Posthypercapneic metabolic acidosis
    Conversion of organic acids to bicarbonate

the rate of excretion of toxic substances. The kidney is a major route of excretion for many toxic substances. Here again, nonionizable, lipid-soluble compounds readily cross the glomerular membrane if they have a molecular weight of less than 60,000 to 70,000 daltons. Compounds with a high lipid-to-water partition coefficient are reabsorbed, whereas ionized, polar compounds are excreted rapidly by diffusion across the glomerular membrane. In urine with an acid pH, bases are excreted more rapidly than acids, and the reverse is true for alkaline urine. Active renal tubular secretory systems also exist for both organic acids and bases. In addition to urinary excretion, the lungs, bile, gastrointestinal tract, milk, sweat, and saliva all represent potential routes for the excretion of toxic substances. In general, large, polar compounds are excreted by the biliary route, whereas gases and volatile substances are excreted by the lungs. The gastrointestinal tract may be a major route of elimination for weak bases, insecticides (organochlorines), dioxin, and polychlorinated biphenyls. Toxic substances may also be metabolized and transformed by gut bacteria. Milk represents a potential source of toxic substances presented to the neonate, and sweat and saliva are relatively minor routes of elimination. Any of these routes of excretion may be significantly compromised by disease such that the rate of elimination is significantly decreased, perhaps increasing the potential for toxicity. Furthermore, toxic substances excreted by a particular route may cause a disease. For example, compounds excreted in the sweat may cause dermatitis (18).

The age of the exposed host also influences the rate of elimination of toxic substances. For example, the incompletely developed kidney in a newborn is often unable to handle the excretion of specific toxicants. Similarly, kidney function that is compromised by the aging process may clearly decrease the glomerular filtration rate and the rate of elimination of toxicants filtered by the glomerulus. Of course, toxic substances eliminated by a mother's milk may express their toxicity in the neonate.

The functional properties of immune cells have particular relevance to their role in the handling of xenobiotics. The most significant property is clearly the capacity of these cells to metabolize xenobiotics. Phase I and II enzymes have been documented in monocytes, lymphocytes, and other immune cells, and these enzyme pathways can metabolize a variety of xenobiotics. Since these enzyme systems play such an important role in xenobiotic handling, they are discussed in detail subsequently. Many other immune cell functions may be pertinent to discuss in relation to xenobiotic exposures, but only a few cellular properties that represent unique functions are emphasized here. These include cellular migration, phagocytosis, receptor-mediated ingestion, cell activation, and release of immunoregulatory substances.

Cells of the immune system can migrate to a variety of tissue and organ sites in the exposed host. Cell migration is dependent upon the integrity of cellular receptors that interact with specific chemoattractants, and occupancy of such receptors or damage to a receptor could significantly impair the response of the host to chemoattractant signals and subsequent cell migration. A variety of other receptors are present on immune cells, including those regulating phagocytosis, which could potentially be altered by xenobiotics. Lipoprotein receptors are especially important because chlorinated hydrocarbons, biphenyls, and other lipophilic substances are associated with lipoproteins (19–27). Thus, lipophilic xenobiotics not only become partitioned into serum lipoproteins (which may then be distributed throughout the lymphatic and circulatory systems) but also can be ingested by lymphocytes, monocytes, and fibroblasts using a lipoprotein receptor-mediated process (24,25). Such internalized xenobiotics can be further metabolized to either an activated or an inactivated state by phase I and phase II enzyme systems.

Phagocytosis is a unique and highly specialized function of certain immune cells such as neutrophils, basophils, monocytes, and macrophages. This function plays a key role in host defense, since phagocytosis is essential both for the presentation of antigen to lymphocytes and for the scavenging of effete cells and tissues and foreign substances. During the process of phagocytosis, xenobiotics may be ingested and metabolized, as these cells act as scavengers of dead and damaged tissues. Thus, xenobiotic-damaged tissues may serve as a source for the further disposition and metabolism of such compounds, since phagocytic cells can ingest the cellular debris associated with such xenobiotic-induced injury and transport it to various sites within the body.

The state of activation of monocytes, macrophages, neutrophils, and lymphocytes also influences the metabolism and disposition of xenobiotics. Toxic substances can induce drug-metabolizing enzymes and enhance the conversion of chemical toxicants to active or inactive chemical metabolites (26–29). Further, activation of cells by nontoxic agonists such as interferon-gamma or mitogens can also alter the activity of drug-metabolizing enzymes, resulting in differences in the metabolic conversion of toxicants when compared with resting cells (30–32). In many cases, activated cells express increased levels of drug-metabolizing enzymes enhancing the metabolism and disposition of xenobiotics, but decreases in these enzymes have also been observed, with immune cell activation leading to a decrease in xenobiotic metabolism (33).

The release of immunoregulatory substances from immune cells, especially arachidonic acid and its active metabolites, is of some significance to xenobiotic handling by cells. Prostaglandin synthesis can result in the cooxidation of xenobiotics catalyzed by the peroxidase component of the enzyme system, prostaglandin H synthase (34). This peroxidase has a broad substrate specificity and can cooxidize a large number of xenobiotics, including aromatic amines, phenols, furans, sulfides, polycyclic hydrocarbons, and others (34). Thus, certain xenobiotics, such as acrolein, which have the capacity to trigger arachidonic acid metabolism, may concurrently cooxidize other xenobiotics to electrophilic substances (35). An acrolein-induced cooxidation process may be especially important in the cigarette smoker, since cigarette smoke contains significant quantities of acrolein (36). Such electrophils can, of course, bind to cellular macromolecules, which may lead to a variety of toxic responses, including carcinogenesis and mutagenesis.

Undoubtedly, other immune cell functions may prove to be significant targets of xenobiotics, but such target molecules remain to be characterized in further detail.

Little is known about the role of xenobiotic metabolism and disposition by some immune cell types such as the basophil, natural killer cells, and the plasma cell. Further, almost nothing is known about the differences between monocyte or T-lymphocyte subsets in their capacity to metabolize xenobiotics. The emergence of data showing that "nonimmunologic" cells exposed to immunoregulatory substances can perform certain immune functions is another significant parameter extending the potential for immunotoxicity. For example, endothelial cells exposed to interferon-gamma can be induced to express class II major histocompatibility complex antigens and can then act as antigen-presenting cells (37). Here again, little is known about the relationships between such "pseudoimmune" cells and xenobiotics.

Probably the most significant parameter related to immunotoxicity is the capacity of immune cells to metabolize xenobiotics. Mononuclear cells have been shown to contain both phase I and phase II enzymes that convert lipophilic xenobiotics to more water-soluble compounds that can then be excreted. Phase I enzymes modify xenobiotics by oxidation, reduction, or hydrolysis, primarily by adding or exposing hydroxy, sulfhydryl, amine, or carboxyl groups, whereas phase II enzymes conjugate xenobiotics to make them more water-soluble or permit ionization of the xenobiotic or its metabolite. The enzymes responsible for phase I reactions are usually found in the endoplasmic reticulum and are termed microsomal enzymes, but some phase I enzymes are also found in the cell cytosol (e.g., alcohol dehydrogenase, monoamine oxidase, xanthine oxidase). Phase II enzymes are usually cytosolic, but there are prominent exceptions such as glucuronyl transferases and minor fractions of glutathione-*S*-transferases. The primary enzymes of detoxification acting on a variety of functional groups contained on xenobiotics are listed in Table 2.

Xenobiotic metabolism may occur via different routes or may occur as a result of sequential enzyme reactions. As is shown in Tables 3 and 4, most phase I and II enzymes documented in the liver have also been observed in mononuclear cells

TABLE 2. *Enzymes of detoxication*

Acetyltransacetylase	Esterases/amidases
Alcohol sulfotransferase	Flavin-containing monooxygenases
Alcohol dehydrogenase	Glutathione peroxidase
Aldehyde dehydrogenase	Glutathione transferase
Aldehyde oxidase	P-450–dependent monooxygenases
Amine *N*-methyltransferase	Phenol sulfotransferase
Amine *N*-sulfotransferase	Quinone reductase
D-Amino acid oxidase	Rhodanese
Carbonyl reductase	Thiol transferase
Catechol *O*-methyltransferase	Thiol *S*-methyltransferase
Cysteine conjugate *N*-acetyltransferase	Tyrosine-ester sulfotransferase
Dihydrodiol dehydrogenase	Uridine diphosphate-glucuronyl transferase
Epoxide hydrolase	Xanthine oxidase

Reproduced in modified form from W. B. Jacoby and D. M. Ziegler (1990): The enzymes of detoxication. *J. Biol. Chem.* 1990 Minireview Compendium, p. 20176. Reprinted with permission.

TABLE 3. *Selected phase I reactions*

---

*Cytochrome P-450 (aryl hydrocarbon hydroxylase)
*Nicotinamide-adenine dinucleotide-b5 reductase
*Nicotinamide-adenine dinucleotide phosphate-P-450 reductase
 Amine oxidase (flavin-containing monooxygenase)
*Epoxide hydrolase
*Esterases
 Amidohydrolases (amidases)
*Aldehyde/ketone reductase
 Alcohol oxidoreductase (alcohol dehydrogenase)
 Aldehyde oxidoreductase (aldehyde dehydrogenase)
*Epoxide hydrolase
*Monoamine oxidase (mitochondrial enzyme)
*Diamine oxidase (histaminase)
 Xanthine oxidase
 Aldehyde oxidoreductase (aldehyde oxidase)

Asterisks indicate that the enzyme activity has been measured in mononuclear cells.

(monocytes and/or lymphocytes). Even though such enzyme activities have been measured in mononuclear cells, the substrate specificity and basal activity may differ from what is observed in the liver, which is considered the primary site of xenobiotic metabolism and detoxification (31,38–40). As has been discussed previously, xenobiotic metabolism occurring in mononuclear cells may not always result in detoxification, since in some instances these biotransformation enzymes may convert "inactive" xenobiotics to active metabolites that are more toxic than the parent compound.

Obviously, this process is dependent upon the presence of activating enzymes and is, therefore, likely to be organ- or cell-specific. Further, active xenobiotic metabolites are often reactive toward intracellular macromolecules, and such reactions may disrupt normal cellular functions. On the other hand, cellular functions are preserved in most instances, since protective mechanisms exist in cells to prevent tissue damage by these active metabolites.

In addition to the conversion of an inactive and nontoxic xenobiotic to active and

TABLE 4. *Selected phase II conjugation reactions*

---

*Uridine diphosphate glucuronyl transferase
 Cytosolic sulfotransferases
*Catechol-*O*-methyltransferase
*Thiopurine methyltransferase
 Thiol methyltransferase
N-acetyltransferase
 Amino acid conjugases (glycine, glutamine, cysteine)
*Glutathione-*S*-transferase

Asterisks indicate that enzyme activity has been measured in mononuclear cells.

reactive metabolites, cellular enzyme systems may convert a xenobiotic by a one electron reduction to a free radical, which then may react with molecular oxygen (O_2) to regenerate the parent compound and form reactive intermediates such as superoxide (O_2^-). These reactive oxygen species may then be converted to hydrogen peroxide, hydroxy radicals (OH), and other oxidants, which can then act as mediators of tissue and cell damage. As is known from cell biology, phagocytic cells are rich in enzymes responsible for the generation and metabolism of oxidants, but such cells usually have sufficient intracellular mechanisms to protect them from oxygen-induced damage (41,42). Thus, compromised antioxidant defense mechanisms may be significant factors in the expression of free radical–induced tissue injury.

Many factors govern the degree of expression of these phase I and phase II enzymes and therefore the metabolism and toxicity of xenobiotics. These include dietary intake, age, sex, drug ingestion, environmental exposures, genetic constitution, and the presence of pathological conditions. The nutritional status of humans is likely to play a prominent role in their capacity to metabolize xenobiotics, and little knowledge exists concerning the role of nutrients on xenobiotic metabolism. Immune cells are easily accessible from the peripheral blood and could be useful in the study of dietary effects on xenobiotic metabolism and immunotoxicity. Since dietary deficiencies are associated with the suppression of immunity, exposure to environmental toxicants could aggravate such a state. Impaired drug metabolism has been clearly documented in severe malnutrition (kwashiorkor and marasmus); however few data are available concerning xenobiotic metabolism in moderate degrees of undernutrition (43). Protein deficiency in animals has clearly been shown to alter drug metabolism (43,44) and has been associated with increased xenobiotic toxicity, but specific dietary deficiencies have been incompletely investigated in the human. Zinc deficiency has clearly been shown to decrease drug biotransformations in adults (43), but additional studies relating toxicity to nutritional status are needed, and analyses of phase I and II enzymes from peripheral blood mononuclear cells may contribute a significant data base to such studies.

Interestingly, immune responses are modified both in the young and the aged; toxicity to pharmacological and environmental agents also has a higher incidence in these same groups. Certain phase I and II enzymes are reduced in newborns, such as cytochrome P-450, glutathione-*S*-transferase, and uridine diphosphate-glucuronyl transferase (33,44). Similarly, the aged population may have reduced levels of these enzymes. This decrease in phase I and phase II enzymes may lead to either increased or decreased toxicity, depending on whether the chemical must be activated by these drug-metabolizing enzymes to express toxicity or whether these enzymes are primarily responsible for detoxifying the parent chemical. Here again, immune cells and their drug-metabolizing enzymes could provide significant advances in our understanding of the possible relationships between chronological age and immunotoxicity. Similarly, xenobiotic metabolism may be influenced by sex, as has been shown definitively in animals. Unfortunately, little evidence exists to demonstrate that changes in xenobiotic metabolism are influenced by sex or male or female hormones in the human.

Phase I and phase II enzymes are also induced by a variety of drugs and environmental factors. Cytochrome P-450 monooxygenases, glucuronyl transferases, glutathione-*S*-transferases, and esterases are the best characterized enzymes observed to be induced by drugs and/or chemicals (33,44–48). In humans, several common environmental agents such as cigarette smoke, dietary polycyclic hydrocarbons (grilled steak), and ethanol can induce biotransformation enzymes (33,44–49). These agents induce not only hepatic but also extrahepatic biotransforming enzymes. The induction of these microsomal enzymes may markedly increase the toxicity of a variety of chemicals. Although this theory is controversial at this time, there is a significant body of evidence that lung cancer patients belong to genetic groups with high to moderate inducibility of aryl hydrocarbon hydroxylase (50–57). Clearly, evidence exists to support the induction of aryl hydrocarbon hydroxylase in cigarette smokers' pulmonary alveolar macrophages when compared with the enzyme activity in nonsmokers' macrophages (49). Investigations of aryl hydrocarbon hydroxylase activity in peripheral blood monocytes and lymphocytes as well as pulmonary alveolar macrophages provide a unique source of information regarding xenobiotic metabolism and may be able to characterize populations susceptible to chemically induced mutagenesis and carcinogenesis. It is also important to recognize that mitogens induce drug-metabolizing enzymes in lymphocytes, and it is entirely possible that other immunoregulatory molecules may also induce these same enzymes and thus alter xenobiotic metabolism and toxicity.

Enzyme inhibition is also an important mechanism that influences xenobiotic metabolism and toxicity. Two examples demonstrate the significance of inhibition of phase I reactions. Allopurinol, a hypoxanthine analogue with potent xanthine oxidase inhibitory properties, blocks a major pathway of 6-mercaptopurine metabolism (58). In the normal setting, 6-mercaptopurine would be oxidized by xanthine oxidase to 6-thiouric acid, an inactive metabolite (59–61). In the absence of xanthine oxidase activity (allopurinol-mediated), 6-mercaptopurine levels remain elevated, and significant increments in toxicity, including immunosuppression, are observed unless the dose of the drug is reduced. In the cases in which exposure to organophosphates has occurred, increased toxicity may be observed when a dual exposure occurs and one of the chemicals cannot be detoxified by cellular esterases (62–68). Thus, esterase inhibition significantly prolongs the half-life of a second xenobiotic that is dependent on esterase for its detoxification. On the other hand, esterase inhibition may protect the host from the toxic effects of a chemical that requires esterase-mediated metabolism to produce toxic metabolites.

Inherited variations and deficiencies in phase I and phase II enzymes have also been observed in a number of instances. Paraoxonase is an aryl esterase that hydrolyzes a number of substrates, including organophosphates such as diisopropyl fluorophosphate, isopropylmethylphosphonofluoridate, ethyl-*N*-dimethylphosphoroamidocyanidate, phenylacetate, 4-nitrophenylacetate, and diethyl-*p*-nitrophenyl phosphate (Paraoxon) (69–71). This enzyme is polymorphic, expressing two allelic genes on the same autosome. One of these isoenzymes hydrolyzes substrates rapidly, whereas the other metabolizes substrates at a much slower rate. This inherited enzyme polymorphism suggests that the isoenzyme catalyzing the slow conversion of Paraoxon may be responsible for an increased susceptibility to the toxic effects of organophosphates such as Parathion, whose intermediate toxic metabolite is not detoxified rapidly by paraoxonase (72). Similarly, a single gene difference accounts for variations in the capacity of individuals to acetylate a variety of substrates metabolized by *N*-acetyltransferase (73). This enzyme is responsible for the inactivation of arylamines such as 2-napthylamine, benzidine, 4-aminobiphenyl, and 4-nitrophenyl (73,74). All these chemicals are potent carcinogens, and evidence is accumulating to suggest that arylamine-induced bladder cancer may be highly associated with slow acetylation rates. Benzidine is immunosuppressive in mice and a potent carcinogen (75). These dual properties relate chemical carcinogens to the immune system (75). Other chemical agents, including chemotherapeutic drugs with immunosuppressive properties, further emphasize relationships between immunity and carcinogenesis, since tumors may occur in higher frequency in patients treated with such drugs. Paraoxonase and *N*-acetyltransferase polymorphisms represent only two genetic abnormalities that may affect the toxicity of chemicals and be related to immune functions. Others have been described, and more will undoubtedly be characterized in the future, since only a small fraction of the predicted protein polymorphisms have been discovered (76).

Clearly, a deficiency in phase I and phase II enzymes may also affect chemical toxicity. For example, glucuronyl transferase deficiencies exist in animals and humans that can be detected by measurements of the enzyme activity using immune cells (77–79). Thus, individuals with Gilbert's syndrome or the Crigler-Najjar syndrome who are deficient in glucuronyl transferase are likely to express serious chemical toxicity when exposed to agents that are detoxified by this pathway (79). Such genetic factors regulating susceptibility and resistance clearly suggest that genetic screening of workers may protect the labor force from expensive and preventable disease.

Underlying pathological conditions may also alter chemical metabolism by the human host. Such organ dysfunctions may be caused by the use of drugs that result in organ or tissue dysfunction or by other disease-producing factors. The most significant changes that affect biotransformation are those involving the liver, the primary site of chemical metabolism, and the kidney, a major route of toxicant excretion. Liver disease may shift chemical biotransformation to secondary organs that represent minor detoxification pathways in the healthy host. The consequences of such a shift are obvious. In severe hepatitis and/or cirrhosis, cytochrome P-450 activity is reduced by half the normal level (44). In renal failure from any cause, there is usually a significant decrease in the excretion of toxic substances, which prolongs the half-life of the chemical or drug and may increase its toxicity. Further, renal diseases associated with a significant loss of protein may reduce the binding capacity for toxic chemicals, resulting in an increase in the level of circulating unbound chemical. If the free chemical is toxic, such individuals are at increased risk for toxicity secondary to a decrease in plasma protein concentrations.

In addition to renal and liver disease, disorders that affect the immune system directly may have the potential to increase the risk of toxicity to chemicals whose target organ is the immune system. Such risk could occur either as a direct effect on an immune system with decreased functional capacity or by a synergistic effect between an immunological disease, an immunotoxic chemical, and an immuno-active drug (e.g., glucocorticoids).

Finally, the immune system also represents an important tool for the detection of toxicants. The use of immunoassays for detection and quantitation of specific drug and chemical toxicants is a significant advance (80–85). Even chemicals with relatively small epitopes have been used to raise specific antibodies for use in immunoassays designed to detect the toxic chemical in tissues or blood (83,84). Thus, the animal immune system can be used to raise specific antibodies against xenobiotics, and such antibodies can be used in sensitive and specific immunoassays both for the detection of chemical toxicants and for monitoring exposed populations. Whether such antibodies will be useful in protecting the host who is exposed or overexposed to toxic substances remains to be determined.

REFERENCES

1. Mullen, P. W. (1984): Immunotoxicology: A Current Perspective of Principles and Practice. North Atlantic Treaty Organization, Scientific Affairs Division, Springer-Verlag, New York.
2. Descotes, J. (1986): Immunotoxicology of Drugs and Chemicals. Elsevier Science Publishing Co., New York.
3. Gibson, G. G., Hubbard, R., and Parke, D. V. (1983): Immunotoxicology: Proceedings of the First International Symposium on Immunotoxicology. Academic Press, New York.
4. Exon, J. H. (1985): The immunotoxicology of selected environmental chemicals, pesticides and heavy metals. *Prog. Clin. Biol. Res.*, 161:355–368.
5. Dean, J. H., Luster, M. I., Munson, A. E., and Amos, H. (1985): Immunotoxicology and Immunopharmacology. Raven Press, New York.
6. Emmett, E. A. (1986): Toxic responses of the skin. In Casarett and Doull's Toxicology. The Basic Science of Poisons, edited by C. D. Klassen, M. O. Ander, and J. Doull, pp. 412–431. Macmillan Publishing Company, New York.
7. Braathen, L. R., and Thorsby, E. (1980): Studies of human Langerhans cells. I. Allo-activating and antigen-presenting capacity. *Scand. J. Immunol.*, 11:401–408.
8. Boyd, M. R., Statham, C. M., and Longo, N. S.: The pulmonary Clara cells as a target for toxic chemicals requiring metabolic activation: Studies with carbon tetrachloride. *J. Pharmacol. Exp. Ther.*, 212:109–114.
9. Bowden, D. H., and Adamson, I. Y. R. (1971): Reparative changes following pulmonary cell injury. Ultrastructural, cytodynamic, and surfactant studies in mice after oxygen exposure. *Arch. Pathol.*, 92:279–283.
10. Carrington, C. B., and Green, T. J. (1970): Granular pneumocytes in early repair of diffuse alveolar injury. *Arch. Intern. Med.*, 126:464–465.
11. Kapanci, Y., Weibel, E. R., Kaplan, H. P., and Robinson, F. R. (1969): Pathogenesis and reversibility of the pulmonary lesion of oxygen toxicity in monkeys. II. Ultrastructural and morphometric studies. *Lab. Invest.*, 20:101–108.
12. Goldstein, A., Arnow, L., and Kalman, S. M. (1968): Principles of Drug Action. Harper & Row, New York.
13. Danel, L., Souweine, G., Monier, J. C., and Saez, S. (1983): Specific estrogen binding sites in human lymphoid cells and thymic cells. *J. Steroid. Biochem.*, 18:559–563.
14. Grossman, C. J., Sholiton, L. J., and Nathen, B. (1979): Rat thymic estrogen receptor. I. Preparation, location and physiochemical properties. *J. Steroid Biochem.*, 11:1233–1240.

15. Raneletti, F. P., Carmignani, M., Marchetti, P., et al. (1979): Estrogen binding by neoplastic human thymus cytosol. *Eur. J. Cancer*, 16:951–955.
16. Neifeld, J. P., Kappman, M. E., and Tormey, D. C. (1977): Steroid hormone receptor in normal lymphocytes: Induction of glucocorticoid receptors by phytohaemagglutinin stimulation. *J. Biol. Chem.*, 252:2972–2977.
17. Kalland, T. (1985): Immunotoxicity of diethylstilbestrol in man. In Immunotoxicology and Immunopharmacology, edited by J. H. Dean, M. I. Luster, A. E. Munson, and H. Amos, pp. 407–414. Raven Press, New York.
18. Flynn, T. C., Harrist, T. J., Murphy, G. F., et al. (1984): Neutrophilic eccrine hidradenitis: A distinctive rash associated with cytarabine therapy and acute leukemia. J. Am. Acad. Dermatol., 11:584–590.
19. Malival, B. P., and Guthrie, F. E. (1981): Interactions of insecticides with human plasma lipoproteins. *Chem. Biol. Interactions*, 35:177–188.
20. Skalsky, H. L., and Guthrie, F. E. (1978): Binding of insecticides to human serum proteins. *Toxicol. Appl. Pharmacol.*, 43:229–235.
21. Moss, J. A., and Hathway, D. E. (1964): Transport of organic compounds in the mammal. Partition of dieldrin and telodrin between the cellular components and soluble proteins of blood. *Biochem. J.*, 91:384–393.
22. Mick, D. L., Long, K. R., Dretchen, J. S., and Bonderman, D. P. (1971): Aldrin and dieldrin in human blood components. *Arch. Environ. Health*, 23:177–180.
23. Matthews, H. B., Surles, J. R., Carver, J. G., and Anderson, M. W. (1977): Poly-chlorinated biphenyl transport by blood components. *Toxicol. Appl. Pharmacol.*, 41:201.
24. Maliwal, B. P., and Guthrie, F. E. (1982): In vitro uptake and transfer of chlorinated hydrocarbons among human lipoproteins. *J. Lipid Res.*, 23:474–479.
25. Karminski, N. E., Wells, D. S., Dauterman, W. C., et al. (1986): Macrophage uptake of a lipoprotein-sequestered toxicant: A potential route of immunotoxicity. *Toxicol. Appl. Pharmacol.*, 82:474–480.
26. Alvares, A. P., Pontuck, E. J., Kappas, A., and Conney, A. H. (1979): Regulation of drug metabolism in man by environmental factors. *Drug Metab. Rev.* 9:185–220.
27. Conney, A. H. (1967): Pharmacological implications of microsomal enzyme induction. *Pharmacol. Rev.*, 19:317–366.
28. Snyder, R., and Remmer, H. (1979): Classes of hepatic microsomal mixed function oxidase inducers. *Pharmacol. Ther.*, 7:203–244.
29. Von Bahr, C., Birgersson, C., Blanck, A., et al. (1984): Metabolism by human liver in relation to polymorphic drug oxidation. In Banbury Report 16. Genetic Variability in Responses to Chemical Exposure, edited by G. S. Omenn and H. V. Gelboin, pp. 107–115. Cold Spring Harbor Laboratory, Cold Spring Harbor, New York.
30. Glatt, H., Kaltenbach, E., and Oesch, F. (1980): Epoxide hydrolase activity in native and mitogen-stimulated lymphocytes of various donors. *Cancer Res.*, 40:2552–2556.
31. Lewis, J. G., and Adams, D. O. (1985): The mononuclear phagocyte system and its interactions with xenobiotics. In Immunotoxicology and Immunopharmacology, edited by J. H. Dean, M. I. Luster, A. E. Munson, and H. Amos, pp. 23–44. Raven Press, New York.
32. Newcombe, D. S., and Cassard, S. (1989): Unpublished data.
33. Sipes, I. G., and Gandolfi, A. J. (1986): Biotransformation of toxicants. In Casarett and Doull's Toxicology. The Basic Science of Poisons, edited by C. D. Klaassen, M. O. Ander, and J. Doull pp. 64–98. Macmillan Publishing Company, New York.
34. Marnet, L. J., and Eling, T. J. (1983): Cooxidation during prostaglandin biosynthesis: A pathway for the metabolic activation of xenobiotics. *Rev. Biochem. Toxicol.*, 5:135–172.
35. Grundfest, C. C., Chang, J., and Newcombe, D. S. (1982): Acrolein: A potent modulator of lung macrophage arachidonic acid metabolism. *Biochim. Biophys. Acta*, 713:149–159.
36. Beauchamp, R. O. Jr., Jelkovich, D. A., Kligerman, A. D., Morgan, K. T., and Heck, H. d'A. (1985): A critical review of the literature on acrolein toxicity. *CRC Crit. Rev. Toxicol.*, 14:309–380.
37. Pober, J. S., Gimbrone, M. A. Jr., Cotran, R. S., et al. (1983): Ia expression by vascular endothelium is inducible by activated T cell and human gamma interferon. *J. Exp. Med.*, 157:1339–1353.
38. Devereux, T. R., Hook, G. E. R., and Fouts, J. R. (1979): Foreign compound metabolism by isolated cells from rabbit lung. *Drug Metab. Dispos.*, 7:70–75.

39. Steinberg, P., Lafranconi, W. M., Wolf, C. R., et al. (1987): Xenobiotic metabolizing enzymes are not restricted to parenchymal cells in rat liver. *Mol. Pharmacol.*, 32:463–470.

40. Selkirk, J. K., Croy, R. G., Whitlock, J. P. Jr., and Gelboin, H. V. (1975): *In vitro* metabolism of benzo (a) pyrene by human liver microsomes and lymphocytes. *Cancer Res.*, 35:3651–3655.

41. Bors, W., Saran, M., and Tait, D. (1984): Oxygen Radicals in Chemistry and Biology. Proceedings Third International Conference, pp. 1–993. Walter de Gruyer, Berlin.

42. Rotilo, G. (1986): Superoxide and Superoxide Dismutase in Chemistry, Biology and Medicine, pp. 1–681. Elsevier Science Publishers, New York.

43. Krishnaswamy, K. (1983): Drug metabolism and pharmacokinetics in malnutrition. *Trends Pharmacol. Sci.*, 4:295–299.

44. Timbrell, J. A. (1982): Principles of Biochemical Toxicology, 109–113. Taylor and Francis, Ltd., London.

45. Conney, A. H., and Burns, J. J. (1962): Factors influencing drug metabolism. *Adv. Pharmacol.*, 1:31–58.

46. Korza, G., and Ozols, J. (1986): Complete covalent structure of 60-kDa esterase isolated from 2,3,7,8-tetrachlorodibenzo-p-dioxin-induced rabbit liver microsomes. *J. Biol. Chem.*, 263:3486–3495.

47. Satoh, T. (1987): Role of carboxylesterases in xenobiotic metabolism. *Rev. Biochem. Toxicol.*, 6:155–181.

48. Ketterman, A. J., Pond, S. M., and Becker, C. E. (1987): The effects of differential induction of cytochrome P-450, carboxylesterase and glutathione S-transferase activities on malathion toxicity in mice. *Toxicol. Appl. Pharmacol.*, 87:389–392.

49. Cantrell, E. T., Warr, G. A., Busbee, D. L., and Martin, R. R. (1973): Induction of aryl hydrocarbon hydroxylase in human pulmonary alveolar macrophages by cigarette smoking. *J. Clin. Invest.*, 52:1881–1884.

50. Emery, A. E. H., (1978): Aryl-hydrocarbon-hydroxylase in patients with cancer. *Lancet*, 1:470–471.

51. Kellerman, G., Luyten-Kellermann, M., and Shaw, C. R. (1973): Genetic variation of aryl hydrocarbon hydroxylase in human lymphocytes. *Am. J. Hum. Genet.*, 25:327–331.

52. Kellerman, G., Shaw, C. R., Luyten-Kellermann, M. (1973): Aryl hydrocarbon hydroxylase inducibility and bronchogenic carcinoma. *N. Engl. J. Med.*, 289:934–937.

53. Kouri, R. E., McKinney, C. E., Slomiany, D. J., et al. (1982): Positive correlation between high aryl hydrocarbon hydroxylase activity and primary lung cancer as analyzed in cryopreserved lymphocytes. *Cancer Res.*, 42:5030–5037.

54. Nebert, D. W. (1979): The Ah locus. A gene with possible importance in cancer predictability. *Arch. Toxicol. Suppl.*, 3:195–207.

55. Pelkonen, O., Karki, N. T., and Sotaniemi, E. A. (1980): Determination of carcinogen-activating enzymes in the monitoring of high risk groups. In Human Cancer: Its Characterization and Treatment, edited by W. Davis, K. R. Harrap, and G. Stathopoulas, pp. 48–57. Excerpta Medica, Amsterdam.

56. Trell, L., Janzon, L., Korsgaard, R., et al. (1984): Smoking, carboxyhaemoglobin, carbon monoxide in expired air and aryl hydrocarbon hydroxylase inducibility. A cross-sectional study and antismoking application in middle-aged men. *Anticancer Res.*, 4:347–350.

57. Karki, N. T., Pokela, R., Nuutinen, L., and Pelkonen, O. (1987): Aryl hydrocarbon hydroxylase in lymphocytes and lung tissue from lung cancer patients and controls. *Int. J. Cancer*, 39:565–570.

58. Elion, G. B. (1966): Enzymatic and metabolic studies with allopurinol. *Ann. Rheum. Dis.*, 25:608–614.

59. Elion, G. B., Cullahan, S., Nathan, H., et al. (1963): Potentiation by inhibition of drug degradation: 6-substituted purines and xanthine oxidase. *Biochem. Pharmacol.*, 12:85–93.

60. Levine, A. S., Sharp, H. L., Mitchell, J., et al. (1969): Combination therapy with 6-mercaptopurine (NSC-755) and allopurinol (NSC-1390) during induction and maintenance of remission of acute leukemia in children. *Cancer Chemother. Rep.*, 53:53–57.

61. Ragab, A. H., Gilkerson, E., and Myers, M. (1974): The effect of 6-mercaptopurine and allopurinol on granulopoiesis. *Cancer Res.*, 34:2246–2249.

62. DuBois, K. (1961): Potentiation of the toxicity of organophosphorus compounds. *Adv. Pest Control Res.*, 4:117–151.

63. Milik, J. K., and Summer, K. H. (1982): Toxicity and metabolism of malathion and its impurities in isolated rat hepatocytes: Role of glutathione. *Toxicol. Appl. Pharmacol.*, 66:69–76.

64. Murphy, S. D., Anderson, R. L., and DuBois, K. P. (1959): Potentiation of toxicity of malathion by triorthotolyl phosphate. *Proc. Soc. Exp. Med. Biol.*, 100:483–487.
65. Lauwerys, R. R., and Murphy, S. D. (1969): Interaction between paraoxon and tri-o-tolyl phosphate in rats. *Toxicol. Appl. Pharmacol.*, 14:348–357.
66. Cohen, S. D., and Murphy, S. D. (1974): A simplified bioassay for organophosphate detoxification and interactions. *Toxicol. Appl. Pharmacol.*, 27:537–550.
67. DuBois, K. P. (1969): Combined effects of pesticides. *Can. Med. Assoc. J.*, 100:173–179.
68. Murphy, S. D. (1969): Mechanisms of pesticide interactions in vertebrates. *Residue Rev.*, 25:201–221.
69. LaDu, B. N., and Adkins, S. (1986): Analysis of the serum paraoxonase/arylesterase polymorphism in some Sudanese families. In Ethnic Differences in Reactions to Drugs and Xenobiotics, edited by W. Kalow, H. W. Goedde, and D. P. Argarwal, pp. 87–98. Alan R. Liss, Inc., New York.
70. LaDu, B. N., and Eckerson, H. W. (1984): Could the human paraoxonase account for different responses to certain environmental chemicals? Banbury Report 16. Genetic Variability in Responses to Chemical Exposure, edited by G. S. Omenn and H. V. Gelboin, pp. 167–175. Cold Spring Harbor Laboratory, Cold Spring Harbor, New York.
71. Ortigoza-Ferado, J., Richter, R., Furlong, C., and Motulsky, A. G. (1984): Biochemical genetics of paraoxonase. Banbury Report 16. Genetic Variability in Responses to Chemical Exposures, edited by G. S. Omenn and H. V. Gelboin, pp. 177–188. Cold Spring Harbor Laboratory, New York.
72. Butler, E. G., Eckerson, H. W., and LaDu, B. N. (1982): Human serum paraoxonase polymorphism and organophosphate toxicity implications. *Am. J. Hum. Genet.*, 34:47A.
73. Weber, W. W., and Hein, D. W. (1985): N-acetylation pharmacogenetics. *Pharmacol. Rev.*, 37:25–70.
74. Price-Evans, D. A., (1986): Acetylation. In Ethnic Differences in Reactions to Drugs and Xenobiotics, edited by W. Kalow, H. W. Goedde, and D. P. Argarwal, pp. 209–242. Alan R. Liss, Inc., New York.
75. Luster, M. I., Tucker, A. N., Hayes, H. T., et al. (1985): Immunosuppressive effects of benzidine in mice: Evidence of alterations in arachidonic acid metabolism. *J. Immunol.*, 135:2754–2761.
76. Omenn, G. S. (1984): Risk assessment, pharmacogenetics, and ecogenetics. Banbury Report 16. Genetic Variability in Responses to Chemical Exposure, edited by G. S. Omenn and H. V. Gelboin, pp. 3–13. Cold Spring Harbor Laboratory, Cold Spring Harbor, New York.
77. Wolkoff, A. W., Chowdhury, J. R., and Arias, I. M.: Hereditary jaundice and disorders of bilirubin metabolism. In The Metabolic Basis of Inherited Disease, Fifth Edition, edited by J. B. Stanbury, J. B. Wyngaarden, D. S. Fredrickson, J. L. Goldstein, and M. S. Brown, pp. 1385–1420. McGraw-Hill Book Company, New York.
78. Schmid, R., Axelrod, J., Hammaker, L., and Swarm, R. L. (1958): Congential jaundice in rats due to a defective glucuronide formation. *J. Clin. Invest.*, 37:1123–1130.
79. Gessner, T., Dresner, J. H., Freedman, H. J., and Gurtoo, H. L. (1978): Presence of glucuronyltransferase activity in human lymphocytes. *Res. Commun. Chem. Pathol. Pharmacol.*, 22:187–197.
80. Henderson, G. L., Frincke, J., and Leung, C. Y. (1975): Antibodies to fentanyl. *J. Pharmacol. Exp. Ther.*, 192:489–496.
81. Lenz, D. E., Brimfield, A. A., Hunter, K. W. Jr., et al. (1984): Studies using a monoclonal antibody against soman. *Fund. Appl. Toxicol.*, 4:5156–5164.
82. Wing, K. D., and Hammock, B. D. (1980): Immunochemical methods to detect pesticide residues. *Calif. Agriculture*, 34:34–35.
83. Hunter, K. W. Jr., Lenz, D. A., Brimfield, A. A., and Naylor, J. A.: (1982): Quantification of the organophosphorus nerve agent soman by competitive inhibition enzyme immunoassay using monoclonal antibody. *FEBS Lett.*, 149:147–151.
84. Hunter, K. W. Jr., and Lenz, D. A. (1982): Detection and quantification of the organophosphate insecticide paraoxon by competitive inhibition enzyme immunoassay. *Life Sci.*, 30:355–361.
85. Brimfield, A. A., Hunter, K. W. Jr., Lenz, D. A., et al. (1985): Structural and stereochemical specificity of mouse monoclonal antibodies to the organophosphorus cholinesterase inhibitor soman. *Mol. Pharmacol.*, 28:32–39.

Clinical Immunotoxicology, edited by
D. S. Newcombe, N. R. Rose, and J. C. Bloom.
Raven Press, Ltd., New York © 1992.

4

Flow Cytometric Analysis of the Immune and Phagocytic Cells

Peter A. Ward

*Department of Pathology, University of Michigan Medical School,
Ann Arbor, Michigan*

The linkage between the cellular immune system and the phagocytic cell system is well known. For instance, cytokine products of activated T cells have substantial functional effects on both macrophages and neutrophils, as reflected in enhanced microbicidal activity and oxygen radical responses. It is well known that macrophages may present antigen to T cells for subsequent cellular and/or humoral immune responses. Macrophages may also release cytokines that can directly or indirectly affect immune as well as functional responses of phagocytic cells. For instance, tumor necrosis factor (TNF), interleukin-1, and interleukin-8 can directly stimulate neutrophil oxygen radical responses and can "prime" macrophages (in a manner that does not initiate a response) for subsequent enhanced oxygen radical responses. Another example of interplay between the immune and phagocytic cell systems is found in the cytokine released from activated T cells, interleukin-2, which can interact both with other T cells (to bring about enhanced immune responses) and with macrophages (to initiate release of TNF). Accordingly, the status of the immune cellular system can affect the phagocytic cell system, and vice versa. There is a substantial body of clinical and experimental evidence indicating that defects in the cellular immune system can place the phagocytic cell system at risk for diminished function. Because of the synergy between the immune and the phagocytic cell systems, the ability to quantitatively assess both lymphocyte and phagocytic cell functions becomes important. The technology of flow cytometry is ideally suited for this purpose, although, as will be described, the constraints against excessive interpretation of the data need to be kept in mind.

ANALYSIS OF LYMPHOCYTIC CELLS

Phenotypic analysis of T and B cells based on cell surface markers is a well-developed technique that is constantly undergoing expansion and modification because of the development of new monoclonal antibodies. The classic subtyping of T cells (e.g., T4 helper cells, T8 suppressor cells) has now given way to additional classifications within almost all of the original subcategories. Perhaps the most interesting surface antigens on T cells are the "markers of activation." Among the first markers of T-cell activation to be recognized were Dr antigen and the receptor for interleukin-2. As indicated above, there is currently a rapidly increasing array of newly defined activation antigens expressed, whose biological and clinical relevance has yet to be determined. The availability of markers of T-cell activation has already found some clinical utility. For instance, transplant patients infected with cytomegalovirus demonstrate the presence of T8 cells in the blood bearing Dr antigen, a coincidence that is distinctly abnormal. These T cells bear the marker of cell activation as a consequence of the presence of an "opportunistic" virus, a condition that is secondary to a state of suppressed immune responsiveness. This example underscores the difficulty in interpreting data obtained from human patients with complex clinical problems.

It has been hoped that the ability to discriminate subclasses of T cells would result in patterns predictive either of the state of immunosuppression (as in patients with homotransplanted organs) or of the state of immunoactivation (as in transplant patients undergoing an acute immune response that threatens survival of the homograft). Our own extensive clinical studies have yet to demonstrate that this hope will be realized. First of all, to date we have not been able to demonstrate a predictive quantitative relationship between changes in T-cell subsets and the state of immunosuppression, the latter being defined by survival of homografts in patients undergoing immunosuppressive therapy that has been documented to result in a functional state of diminished immune responsiveness. It is possible that we have failed to define a matrix of T-cell subset changes (e.g., by employing multiparameter analysis) that collectively define a state of immunosuppression. Alternatively, we may have to wait for the development of new monoclonal antibodies to T-cell activation antigens. Either way, it is obvious that if phenotypic changes in T-cell subsets are linked to predictive correlations with the immune status, this has yet to be demonstrated. This conclusion has substantial implications in the area of immunotoxicology. It is important to stress that it is not to be implied that phenotypic analysis of T cells will not be useful; it only means that much more work is required before T-cell phenotyping as a measure of immune competence can be reliably employed.

The biological complexity of humans undergoing immunosuppressive therapy should not be understated. Virtually all patients receive multidrug immunosuppressive therapy. Some transplant centers still employ antithymocyte globulin, which blocks or otherwise interferes with phenotypic analysis of T cells. The lymphopenia that occurs frequently with the use of immunosuppressive drugs also complicates the technical accomplishment of phenotypic analysis. Finally, as indicated above, immunosuppressed humans frequently develop secondary infections with the herpes group of viruses (Epstein-Barr, cytomegalovirus, or herpes simplex), the result of which can alter the phenotypic pattern of T cells (see above). Perhaps it can be concluded that humans undergoing immunosuppressive therapy are simply too biologically complex for phenotypic analysis and that less severe perturbations in the immune system, as might be the case after exposure to immunotoxins, may provide more clear-cut patterns of phenotypic change; however, at present this is only speculative.

A functional approach to the status of T and B cells may be more informative. Functional activation of lymphocytes can be measured by flow cytometry either directly by ultraviolet light wave absorption or by the use of dyes that bind to DNA and emit fluorescent signals in a manner that is quantitatively related to DNA content. Cell cycling can be initiated by contact of T cells either with biologically relevant antigens (e.g., *Candida* antigen) or with nonspecific, plant-derived mitogenic agents such as concanavalin A. With flow cytometry, changes in DNA content occurring during the cell cycle (G_0, G_1, S, G_2 and mitotic phases) can be measured with fluorescent dyes bound to DNA in a highly sensitive and reproducible manner. Cell cycling analysis may yield useful, functional information that will correlate with alterations in immune function, but this awaits confirmation. DNA analysis of stimulated lymphocytes has two serious constraints. First, measuring cell cycling is a rather laborious and slow process, requiring 72 hours before the end-points are achieved. From a clinical point of view, this extended period of time is often unacceptable. Second, the problem of the relevant mitogenic stimulus is a concern. Ideally, antigens to which T cells from most individuals respond (e.g., *Candida* antigen, streptokinase/streptodornase) should be used, but the availability of reference standard data to which test results can be compared is a problem that has not been resolved. Plant-derived mitogens induce substantial T-cell responses that often correlate poorly with the blastogenic responses of T cells to naturally occurring antigens. Accordingly, plant-derived mitogens are not very useful in clinical testing except for detection of the most extreme states of T-cell dysfunction.

ANALYSIS OF PHAGOCYTIC CELLS

Flow cytometric analysis of phagocytic cells has been carried out with both blood cells (neutrophils, monocytes, eosinophils) and macrophages. The great advantage of this approach is the high sensitivity and reproducibility of the analysis, the need for relatively few cells, the ability to perform the assays with small volumes (0.1 ml) of unfractionated blood, and the opportunity to obtain rapid and consecutive measurements using the same donor of cells.

Formyl chemotactic peptide receptors on neutrophils can be quantitated using fluorescein-labeled peptide. In addition, it is possible to measure biochemical events (e.g., changes in intracellular Ca^{2+} using quin-2, fura-2, and indo-1 probes), degranulation (measuring either changes in light scatter of cells or the appearance of an enzyme such as elastase that has been released into the extracellular medium), and products of neutrophils activation such as hydrogen peroxide (H_2O_2). Most of our experience relates to the generation of H_2O_2 by activated neutrophils. In this assay, neutrophils are "preloaded" with $2'$-$7'$-dichlorofluorescein diacetate (DCFH-DA). DCFH-DA readily enters the cell, where it undergoes deacetylation to $2'$-$7'$-dichlorofluorescein (DCFH), which is compartmentalized within the cytosol. Upon cell activation H_2O_2 is produced and reacts with DCFH, apparently in the presence of peroxidase, to generate the fluorescent derivative, dichlorofluorescein (DCF), which can be readily quantitated in the flow cytometer. It is important to emphasize that the production of DCF, which is stoiciometrically related to H_2O_2 generation, occurs intracellularly. Thus, this assay measures *intracellular*, not *extracellular*, H_2O_2. Typically, after stimulation with phorbol ester human neutrophils generate 200 to 400 attomols H_2O_2 per cell as measured to dichlorofluorescein. The more traditional assays for oxygen products of stimulated human neutrophils record only what is extracellular to the neutrophil. Typically, in 15 minutes 5×10^5 human neutrophils will generate 35 nmol superoxide ($O_2{}^-$) and approximately 20 nmol H_2O_2, using the "bulk" assay featuring superoxide dismutase inhibitable reduction of ferricytochrome c or oxidation of substrates such as potassium ferrocyanate, scopoletin, or homovanillic acid. *It can be calculated that there is nearly a 10,000-fold discrepancy between the results of these two assays.* It is apparent that intracellular generation of oxidants does *not* necessarily equate to what can be measured in the extracellular medium. Since the enzyme (nicotinamide-adenine dinucleotide phosphate oxidase) directly responsible for neutrophil-dependent formation of $O_2{}^-$ is physically present in the cell membrane, the origin of the intracellular products being measured is not apparent. Do these products derive from the external cell surface and gain entry to the neutrophil by diffusion (H_2O_2) or transport via anionic channels ($O_2{}^-$) or are they formed by a separate intracellular source of nicotinamide-adenine dinucleotide phosphate oxidase, for which there is some evidence? The issue of the relationship between intracellular oxygen and extracellular oxygen products needs to be resolved in order to determine if the intracellular assay is quantitatively related to the standard assays that measure extracellular oxygen products. This is not to say that the DCFH-DA assay is not useful. For example, neutrophils from patients with chronic granulomatous disease of childhood are profoundly defective in H_2O_2 production, which is measured by either extracellular or intracellular assays. Cells deprived of calcium (which is required for optimal oxygen radical responses) show depressed H_2O_2 production in both analytical systems.

As indicated above, the flow cytometric method for H_2O_2 production permits the calculation of rates of H_2O_2 generation as well as its aggregate production. The ability to measure slight changes in rates of generation provides a sensitive tool for the probing of either enhanced or depressed oxygen radical responses. In experimental studies comparing H_2O_2 production in rat blood neutrophils to glycogen-induced peritoneal neutrophils obtained from the same animal, it is obvious that peritoneal neutrophils have substantially elevated (threefold) "basal" rates of H_2O_2 production when compared with those measured in blood neutrophils obtained from the same animals. These differences are much less discernible by the "bulk" assays employing the assay for extracellular $O_2{}^-$ or H_2O_2. Thus, it would appear that the flow-based analysis of oxidant production in neutrophils provides a dimension of sensitivity that is not currently available by more conventional analytical methodologies. The DCFH-DA assay for H_2O_2 in animal and human phagocytic cells has yet to reveal its full potential. It must be determined whether or not this assay will correlate with the bulk assay. The flow-based assay will permit tests to be done in nearly unlimited numbers employing minute amounts of whole blood. It seems reasonable that this assay can be used to monitor serially the functional integrity of phagocytic cells in humans and animals whether after their contact with various drugs or after exposure to any number of environmental agents. As described, analysis of phagocytic cells for H_2O_2 responses may reveal defective function attributable either to the direct effects of inhibitory agents or to indirect effects, such as inadequate cytokine formation resulting in depressed phagocytic cell function. Obviously, it will be necessary to determine by extensive analysis for both animal and human phagocytic cells to what extent the flow-based assay for H_2O_2 production correlates with the bulk assay.

REFERENCES

Bass, D. A., Parce, J. W., DeChatelet, L. R., Szeda, P., Seeds, M. C., and Thomas, M. T. (1983). Flow cytometric studies of oxidative product formation by neutrophils. *J. Immunol.*, 130:190–195.

Braylan, R. C., Benson, N. A., Nourse, V. A. (1984). Cellular DNA of human neoplastic B cells measured by flow cytometry. *Cancer*, 44:5010–5016.

Dafoe, D. C., Stoolman, L. M., Campbell, D. A. Jr., Lorber, M. I., Waskerwits, J., and Turcotte, J. G. (1987). T-cell subset patterns in cyclosporine-treated renal transplant recipients with primary CMV disease. *Transplantation*, 43:452.

Darzynkiewicz, Z., Traganos, F., Xue, S. B., Staino-Coico, L., and Melamed, M. R. (1981). Rapid analysis of drug effects on the cell cycle. *Cytometry*, 1:279–286.

Duque, R. E., Stoolman, L. M., Hudson, J. L., and Ward, P. A. (1985). Multiparameter analysis of immunohematological disorders of flow cytometry. *Surv. Synth. Pathol. Res.*, 4:323–340.

Duque, R. E., Ward, P. A., (1987). Quantitative assessment of neutrophil function by flow cytometry. *Anal. Quant. Cytol. Histol.*, 9(1):42–48.

Fantone, J. C., and Ward, P. A. (1982). Role of oxygen derived free radicals and metabolites in leukocyte dependent inflammatory reactions. *Am. J. Pathol.*, 107:395–418.

Robinson, J. P., Bruner, L. H., Bassoe, C-F, Hudson, J. L., Ward, P. A., and Phan, S. H. (1988). Measurement of intracellular fluorescence of human monocytes relative to oxidative metabolism. *J. Leukocyte Biol.*, 43:304–410.

Robinson, J. P., Duque, R. E., Boxer, L. A., Ward, P. A., and Hudson, J. L. (1987). Measurement of antineutrophil antibodies by flow cytometry: Simultaneous detection of antibodies against monocytes and lymphocytes. *Diagn. Clin. Immunol.*, 5:163–170.

Sentzer, D., Sawyer, T. A., Clifford, S. S., Chaudhuri, K., Gohara, A. F., and Selmar, S. H. (1985). Post-transplant immune monitoring with monoclonal antibodies. *Transplant. Proc.*, 17:2555.

Sklar, L. A., Finney, D. A., Oader, Z. G., Jesaitis, A. J., Painter, R. G., and Cochrane, C. G. (1984). The dynamics of ligand-receptor interactions. Real time analysis of association, disassociation, and internalization of an N-formyl peptide and its receptors on the human neutrophil. *J. Biol. Chem.*, 259:5661–5669.

Van Es, A., Baldwin, W. M., Oljans, P. J., Tanke, H. J., and Ploem, J. S. (1984). Expression of HLA/DR on T-lymphocytes following renal transplantation and association with graft-rejection episodes and cytomegalovirus infection. *Transplantation*, 37:65–69.

Clinical Immunotoxicology, edited by
D. S. Newcombe, N. R. Rose, and J. C. Bloom.
Raven Press, Ltd., New York © 1992.

5

An Approach for Analyzing the Role of Mast Cells in Immunotoxicological Processes and Other Biological Responses

Barry K. Wershil and Stephen J. Galli

*Department of Pathology, Beth Israel Hospital,
Boston, Massachusetts*

Any consideration of the contributions of mast cells to immunotoxicological processes and other biological responses must begin by defining the type of evidence required to implicate mast cells in the pathogenesis of a particular reaction. At one end of the spectrum of certainty, proof might be required that expression of the reaction *in vivo* differs significantly in tissues that are identical except in whether or not they contain mast cells. As illustrated below, this approach would permit discussion of a very limited number of reactions. Alternatively, one might discuss any process in which mast cells have been observed to exhibit morphological evidence of proliferation and/or of activation and mediator release, or in which the administration of antihistamines or other agents that antagonize the actions of mast cell–associated mediators has been shown to alter the expression of the reaction.

Our own position is to acknowledge that mast cells *might* participate in diverse biological processes but to reserve final judgment about any particular role until such a function has been demonstrated convincingly *in vivo*. We would like to defend this position by considering why it has been popular to propose that mast cells play critical roles in a bewildering variety of biological processes, discussing why it has been so difficult to prove that mast cells contribute significantly to these processes, and then describing the development of a new animal model that permits precise and quantitative definition of the actual contributions of mast cells to biological reactions *in vivo*.

The evidence that mast cells might participate in the expression of diverse biological responses—five lines of evidence, summarized in Table 1—is consistent with the idea that mast cells contribute significantly to many biological reactions.

TABLE 1. *Findings suggesting roles for mast cells in diverse biological responses*

Wide anatomical distribution
Ability to synthesize (and in some cases store) many biologically active mediators
Ability to release mediators in response to many immunological and nonimmunological stimuli
Ability to concentrate exogenous substances within cytoplasmic granules
Evidence of proliferation and/or activation during many different biological responses

Reprinted with permission from Galli, ref. 30.

1. Mast cells are distributed throughout essentially all vascularized tissues and may be particularly abundant beneath epithelial surfaces, in the vicinity of blood and lymphatic vessels, within and near peripheral nerves, and in certain species within peritoneal and pleural cavities (31,36,90,114). Mast cells thus are situated where they might interact with other cells and with extracellular elements, including the cells and products of the immune system. Furthermore, the wide distribution of mast cells beneath epithelial surfaces, such as in the skin, gastrointestinal tract, and respiratory system, places them in a favorable position to interact with exogenous antigens and toxins.

2. Mast cells can elaborate and release a great variety of potent, biologically active compounds (36,41,50,90,99,113,114). Some of these (e.g., biogenic amines such as histamine, and in murine rodents serotonin, sulfated proteoglycans, proteases) are stored in the cytoplasmic granules; others (e.g., lipid mediators such as platelet-activating factor/AGEPC and the products of arachidonic acid oxidation) are generated upon stimulation of the cell.

The nature of these mediators and their multiple biological effects have recently been reviewed in detail (31,41,45,50,90,113,114a), and new mast cell–associated mediators continue to be discovered. For example, we have reported that murine mast cells constitutively store tumor necrosis factor-alpha (TNF-α) and secrete it upon appropriate stimulation (51,137). Nevertheless, macrophage-derived TNF-α has been reported to have myriad biological activities in addition to cytolytic function (3,96). Testing the mast cell–associated, TNF product for these and other activities will be of great interest. Such work is likely to expand further our concepts of how mast cells *might* influence the expression of biological responses *in vivo*.

3. Mast cells can be induced to release biologically active mediators by a wide variety of stimuli. These include specific antigens (if the mast cells have been previously sensitized, e.g., by IgE class antibodies [61] or, possibly, by certain T-cell–derived factors distinct from IgE [70]); products generated during complement activation; many other basic substances, including some derived from leukocytes or animal venoms; certain neuropeptides; and, directly and/or indirectly, by the effects of many physical agents (e.g., mechanical injury, heat, cold, ultraviolet light) (36, 41,49,90,104,113,114). Some of these agents can cause mediator release by injuring or killing mast cells, but many of the stimuli provoke mediator release in the absence of detectable cell damage. Mast cells that release mediators in response to the latter agents may synthesize a new complement of cytoplasmic granules and

then participate in additional cycles of mediator release (reviewed in 36 and 90). Moreover, the extent, kinetics, and nature of the mast cell mediators released may be influenced by the type and concentration of stimulus (perhaps in part because of the activation of different mechanisms of mediator release, reviewed in 31 and 36), and/or by the presence of other agents that modulate mast cell function (41,77,99).

4. Mast cells can concentrate certain exogenous substances (including certain toxins or enzymes) within their granules, providing a mechanism whereby the mast cells can regulate the activity of these agents (21,98). For example, mast cells can take up eosinophil peroxidase from the ambient medium and store this substance in their cytoplasmic granules (21). This may permit agents that influence mast cell, as opposed to eosinophil, function to regulate expression of the biological effects of eosinophil peroxidase.

5. Finally, morphological studies have documented changes in the number and/ or cellular activity of mast cells during a bewildering variety of inflammatory, immunological, metabolic, reparative, toxic, and neoplastic responses (31,36,90, 114). A *partial* list of these proposed mast cell functions, abstracted from Selye's book (114) and more recent reviews (4,36,90,103) is presented in Table 2. It cannot be emphasized strongly enough that this list is presented solely to illustrate the broad range of biological processes that individual authors have suggested *might* involve participation by mast cells. In some cases, list entries are based on indirect lines of evidence derived from single unconfirmed reports. Many of the putative roles listed might be considered to be within the domain of immunotoxicology.

TABLE 2. *Proposed roles of mast cells in biological responses (an incomplete list)*[a]

Immunological:

Essential for expression of certain IgE-dependent reactions (e.g., passive cutaneous anaphylaxis reactions)[b]

Contribute to the expression of many other manifestations of immediate hypersensitivity (e.g., certain forms of asthma, anaphylaxis, urticaria)

Participate in protective immunity to certain parasites (in many instances, in conjuction with IgE)[b]

Participate in certain T-cell–mediated responses. (*Note*: hypotheses that mast cells are *essential* for elicitation of contact sensitivity responses or that they augment suppressor T-cell activity have not been confirmed *in vivo* [see text])[b]

Contribute to expression of "natural cytotoxicity" against certain tumors

Amplification of inflammation associated with immune responses (e.g., as a result of mast cell mediator release induced by products of complement activation)[b]

Inflammatory:

Augmentation of acute and chronic inflammation[b]

Suppression of acute and chronic inflammation

Limitation of the local or systemic toxicity of exogenous compounds

Promotion of gastrointestinal mucosal damage/ulceration (e.g., in reactions to toxins, peptic ulcer disease, inflammatory bowel disease)

(continued)

TABLE 2. *Continued*

Promotion (or suppression) of angiogenesis

Promotion (or suppression) of fibrosis in many different responses

Amplification (or suppression) of tissue damage secondary to physical agents (e.g., heat, cold, trauma, ultraviolet light, ionizing radiation)

Regulation of wound healing (through effects on interstitial substances, epithelial cells, fibroblasts, myofibroblasts, blood vessels and/or nerves)

Promotion of fibrin deposition and/or degradation[b]

Neoplastic:

Role in promotion or initiation of tumor development

Regulation of tumor-associated angiogenesis[b]

Inhibition of tumor metastasis

Mediation of direct (or indirect) tumoricidal or tumoristatic effects

Physiological (mast cells have been proposed to influence the following):

Nutrition of connective tissue

Fibroblast function

Angiogenesis

Bone remodeling

Cellular proliferation

Microvascular tone and permeability

Central and/or peripheral nervous system function

Blood pressure

Temperature

pH

Osmolarity of interstitial fluid

Epithelial function (e.g., ion transport)

Hair growth and pigmentation

[a]The list represents *some* of the roles that have been proposed for mast cells. In some instances, these hypotheses are based on indirect evidence and/or single unconfirmed reports.
[b]These hypotheses have been tested using WBB6F$_1$-*W/W*^{v} mice locally reconstituted with cultured mast cells of WBB6F$_1$-+/+ origin (see text).

Why is it still unclear what mast cells actually do? We have pointed out that there is no shortage of hypotheses, some of them quite imaginative, concerning the roles of mast cells *in vivo.* Yet the precise contribution of mast cells to the great majority of the biological responses listed in Table 2 remains obscure. This state of confusion concerning the mast cell's functions can be understood, at least in part, by considering the following facts (Table 3).

1. Many mast cell–associated mediators (or molecules with biological activities similar to those of mast cell–associated mediators (79,109) are also produced by

TABLE 3. *Problems with defining the precise contribution of mast cells to biological responses*

1. Many mast cell–associated mediators or molecules with similar biological activities can also be produced by other cell types
2. Mast cell activation usually results in release of multiple different mediators, which can interact with each other and with other cells and mediators to orchestrate potentially complex biological effects
3. Drugs influencing mast cells or antagonizing the effects of mast cell–associated mediators may also have other significant biological effects
4. Mast cells of different phenotypes may have different functions

Modified after Galli, ref. 30; used with permission.

other cell types (reviewed in 31,34,36,50,68,90,113). Indeed, the possibility should be entertained that non–mast cell sources of mediators identical or very similar to those of mast cells may eventually be found for all mast cell–associated mediators, with the possible exception of certain proteases. As a result, even unequivocal evidence that a particular mast cell–associated *mediator* has a critical role in a given biological response may not necessarily prove that the *mast cell* participates in the response. A corollary of this point is that pharmacological approaches employing antagonists of particular mast cell–associated mediators may provide important information about the roles of these mediators (and/or the effects of these drugs) in the process under study without necessarily clarifying the role of the mast cell itself (e.g., see 1,34,39,88).

2. Mast cell activation results in the elaboration of multiple mediators, each of which can have diverse and sometimes opposing biological effects (1,34,36, 41,90,99,113). The *net* biological consequences of the combined activities of all of these mediators thus may be very difficult to predict.

3. Drugs such as disodium cromoglycate, which can inhibit mediator release from certain mast cells, are not effective on all mast cell subpopulations and may have important effects on biological processes that actually are independent of the agents' actions on mast cells (4,77).

4. As will be considered at greater length below, mast cell phenotype (morphology, mediator content, response to drugs and secretogogues) may vary according to the cells' stage of maturation and/or anatomical location (4,12,25,29,31,41, 54,100,121). Such mast cell heterogeneity has raised the interesting possibility that mast cells of different phenotypes might have distinctly different roles in health and disease.

DEVELOPMENT OF NEW APPROACHES FOR THE ANALYSIS OF MAST CELL HETEROGENEITY AND FUNCTION

Despite the problems summarized in Table 3, it is now possible to identify and quantitate the mast cell's contribution to the expression of particular biological responses *in vivo*. The development of an approach for performing such studies was based on the convergence of two important advances in the field of mast cell biology. One of these was the recognition that certain mutant mice virtually lack mast cells (46,64,65). The other was the development of techniques to grow mouse mast cells *in vitro*.

Genetically Mast Cell–Deficient Mice

The biology and special advantages of genetically mast cell–deficient mice have recently been described in detail (40,44,66,67,93) but may be summarized briefly here. A double dose of mutant alleles at either the W locus on chromosome 5 or the Sl locus on chromosome 10 produces pleiotropic effects, including macrocytic anemia, sterility, and lack of hair pigmentation (53,110). Kitamura and colleagues found that W/W^v and Sl/Sl^d mice also express a profound deficiency of mast cells (67,93). The number of morphologically identifiable mast cells in the normal skin of adult WBB6F$_1$-W/W^v or WCB6F$_1$-Sl/Sl^d mice is <1% (~0.3%) of the number present in the congenic normal ($+/+$) mice; no mast cells are present in the normal W/W^v or Sl/Sl^d bone marrow, spleen, thymus, brain, heart, lung, kidney, urinary bladder, liver, stomach, ileum, cecum, mesentery, peritoneal cavity, hind limb skeletal muscle, or uterus (40).

Despite the similarities of their phenotype, W/W^v and Sl/Sl^d mice differ significantly in the susceptibility of their mast cell deficiency to repair by transplantation of genetically compatible bone marrow cells derived from mice with normal numbers of mast cells. The hematological defects in W/W^v mice reflect an intrinsic defect in hematopoietic stem cells (CFU-S) (76,83), whereas transplantation studies demonstrate that Sl/Sl^d mice apparently have normal hematopoietic stem cells (83). As a result, bone marrow transplantation from congenic $+/+$ mice (or from semisyngeneic C57BL/6-bg/bg [beige] mice) cures both the anemia and the mast cell deficiency of W/W^v mice (65). By contrast, the WCB6F$_1$- Sl/Sl^d mouse fails to develop mature mast cells after either systemic or local injection of WCB6F$_1$-$+/+$ cell populations containing mast cell precursors (64). Because mast cells derived from beige mice can be recognized on the basis of their giant cytoplasmic granules (11), the mast cells that develop in WBB6F$_1$-W/W^v mice transplanted with B6-bg^J/bg^J bone marrow cells can be identified unambiguously as of donor origin. Indeed, this approach was used to establish that mouse mast cells develop from bone marrow–derived precursors (65) and that a common precursor cell can give rise to both mast cells and granulocytes (69).

Recently, the W locus was shown to encode the tyrosine kinase growth factor receptor, c-kit (46a). Because of the similarities of the phenotypic abnormalities of mice doubly mutant at either W or Sl, and because the defect in Sl/Sl^d mice was known to reside in the microenvironment required for mast cell development rather than in the mast cell lineage itself, it was suggested that Sl might encode the ligand for c-kit (46a). This hypothesis recently was confirmed. Zsebo and colleagues (141) showed that a newly recognized hematopoietic growth factor, stem cell factor, is encoded at Sl represents a ligand for c-kit, and when injected subcutaneously into

Sl/Sl^d mice daily for 3 weeks, repairs both the anemia and the local cutaneous mast cell deficiency of these animals. Recent data indicate that soluble recombinant stem cell factor can induce proliferation of both immature and mature mouse mast cells, can induce maturation of mouse mast cells, and at high concentrations, can induce mast cell mediator release (43,124a).

Growth of Mouse Mast Cells *in Vitro*

The seminal studies in this area were performed by Ginsburg and associates, who reported that mast cells developed in complex tissue culture systems incorporating embryonic fibroblasts and cells derived from lymphoid organs (47,48). In 1981, several groups independently discovered that apparently pure populations of cells with many of the features of mast cells could be generated in the absence of stromal monolayers by culturing normal mouse hematopoietic cells in media derived from mitogen-activated T cells, cloned $Ly1^+2^-$ inducer T cells, or WEHI-3B tumor cells (91,92,105,112,122). Although various names were proposed for these cells, we thought it most reasonable to identify them as mast cells: all of the cells' known characteristics were compatible with their membership in a lineage committed to expression of the mast cell phenotype, and they resembled mast cells, not basophils, by ultrastructure (22,29,37,35,91). These mast cell populations can be grown in large quantities and cloned, thus facilitating a variety of biochemical and functional studies.

In addition to their value for studies of mast cell biochemistry and function, cloned mouse mast cells have been used to clarify certain long-standing issues in mast cell biology. One of these was the question of whether the "T-cell–dependent" mast cell proliferation that occurred in the rat or mouse gastrointestinal mucosa during certain parasitic infections reflected the derivation of mast cells from T cells or the influence of a T-cell–derived factor(s) on mast cell proliferation (9). Because both the cells producing the factor(s) required for mast cell proliferation *in vitro* ($Ly1^+2^-$ "inducer" T cells) and the responding mast cells (which lacked surface structures and functions characteristic of mature T cells) could be cloned and characterized in detail (37,91), it was possible to explain T-cell–dependent mast cell proliferation without postulating that mast cells were derived from T cells. Further analysis of the products of cells capable of sustaining the growth of mast cell populations *in vitro* has helped in the characterization of the biological activities of two molecules that promote (IL-3) or augment (IL-4) mast cell proliferation and have a variety of other important effects (28,60,74,89,95,107,136).

Cultured Mast Cells and Mast Cell Heterogeneity

Growth factor–dependent cultured mast cells also may be used to analyze mast cell maturation and heterogeneity. As reviewed in detail elsewhere (29,31,41), it was apparent from the beginning that the phenotype of growth factor–dependent cultured mouse mast cells was not identical to that of mature peritoneal mast cells.

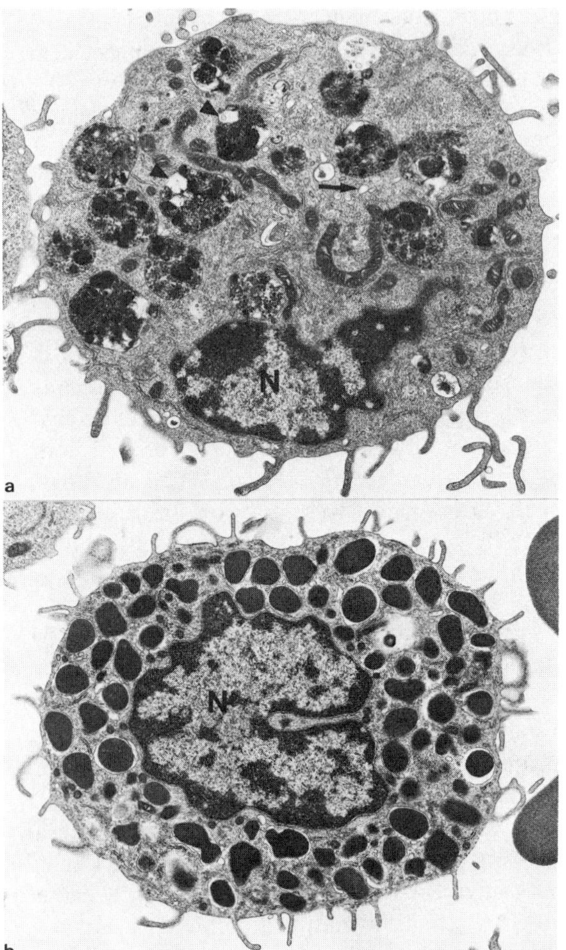

FIG. 1. (a) Typical immature mast cells from clone MC/9 derived from fetal liver. The cell exhibits numerous "immature" granules that appear as large, membrane-bound, focally electron-lucent (*solid arrowheads*) structures containing small vesicles and/or electron-dense material. Mitochondria and cytoplasmic vesicles (*solid arrow*) are also evident. The cell surface is covered with short, narrow, uniform processes. N, nucleus ($\times$11,700). **(b)** Mature peritoneal mast cell from adult C57BL/6J mouse. Short, narrow surface processes appear similar to those of cultured mast cells in **(a)**, but the cytoplasmic granules of this cell are more homogeneously electron-dense than those of the cultured mast cell. N, nucleus ($\times$10,000). (Reproduced with permission from Galli et al., ref. 35.)

In part because they are relatively easy to isolate and study, peritoneal mast cells represented the best-characterized mouse mast cell population for comparison with the growth factor–dependent cells grown *in vitro*. And these two populations expressed differences in ultrastructure (Fig. 1;37,91,122), content of histamine (37, 91,92,105,112,118) and serotonin (125), content of sulfated glycosaminoglycans (37,106,118), number of high affinity receptors for IgE (37), and responsiveness to secretogogues (118). On the other hand, several groups noted that growth factor–dependent mouse mast cells were similar in some respects to the mucosal mast cells that proliferate in the intestinal lamina propria of rats and mice during certain T-cell–dependent responses to intestinal parasites (29,37,118,121).

Unfortunately, mouse mucosal mast cells had not been purified, and little was known about their mediator content. As a result, there could be little direct comparison of the properties of cultured mouse mast cells with the mucosal mast cells of the same species. Techniques for purifying rat mucosal mast cells had been described (2), however, as had methods for growing rat mast cells *in vitro* either in the absence (62) or the presence (16) of T cells activated by specific antigen. Moreover, it was known that rat mucosal and connective tissue-type mast cells could be distinguished on the basis of their predominant cytoplasmic granule-associated chymotryptic protease (73,131–133,139). Haig and colleagues showed that rat mast cells generated *in vitro* in media conditioned by antigen-activated T cells expressed a number of properties shared by rat mucosal mast cells, including synthesis of similar or identical chymotryptic protease (56,57). These studies complemented and extended those performed with mouse cells in calling attention to certain remarkable parallels between the phenotype of murine growth factor–dependent mast cells and that of mucosal mast cells.

However, other findings indicated that it might be premature to conclude that growth factor–dependent cultured mast cells were irrevocably committed to expression of a mucosal mast cell phenotype. Thus, several earlier morphological and histochemical studies showed that populations of classic murine connective tissue-type mast cells, such as those in the skin and peritoneal cavity, were themselves heterogeneous with respect to morphology, proliferative ability, histochemistry, and density (12,100). Moreover, certain features of immature connective tissue or peritoneal mast cells resembled those of mucosal mast cells (reviewed in 29,37,41, 138).

Taken together, these considerations suggested that the phenotype of growth factor–dependent mouse mast cells might reflect their immaturity (29,35,37,91, 138). It should be stated that the word "immature" was used simply to indicate that the cultured mast cells exhibited ultrastructural features similar to those of certain other immature bone marrow–derived cells and to suggest that the cells might acquire, under appropriate circumstances, a phenotype more closely resembling that of mature connective tissue or peritoneal (serosal) mast cells. It is important to recognize, however, that even mature mast cells may exhibit considerably more phenotypic plasticity than certain other mature bone marrow–derived cells. For example, there is currently no evidence that fully mature circulating granulocytes can exhibit significant proliferative ability. By contrast, several lines of evidence indicate that differentiated mast cells retain proliferative ability (reviewed in 12,26,35,63,90, 114,116). Indeed, the mouse mast cell appears to have a very complex natural history, which may include expression of proliferative activity (and assumption of a less mature phenotype) at several points along its sequence of differentiation and maturation (29,31,67,93). In this respect, the mast cell lineage appears more similar to that of B cells than of granulocytes (29). Mast cells also differ from granulocytes (and resemble B cells, or cells in the monocyte/macrophage series [29,67,115]) in that full maturation generally occurs outside the bone marrow.

To evaluate whether cloned, growth factor–dependent cultured mast cells could be induced to mature *in vitro*, the cells were exposed to sodium butyrate (37,38), an agent known to increase development of cytoplasmic granules and storage of granule-associated mediators in mouse mastocytoma cells. Exposure to butyrate did induce partial maturation of cloned mast cells, as judged by ultrastructural criteria (Fig. 2) and increased storage of the granule-associated mediators histamine and ^{35}S-labeled chondroitin sulfates. These changes were accompanied by a marked diminution of the cells' proliferative ability (37). DuBuske and colleagues (18) confirmed the effect of butyrate on cultured mast cell histamine content and also showed that butyrate-treated mast cells stored increased quantities of cytoplasmic

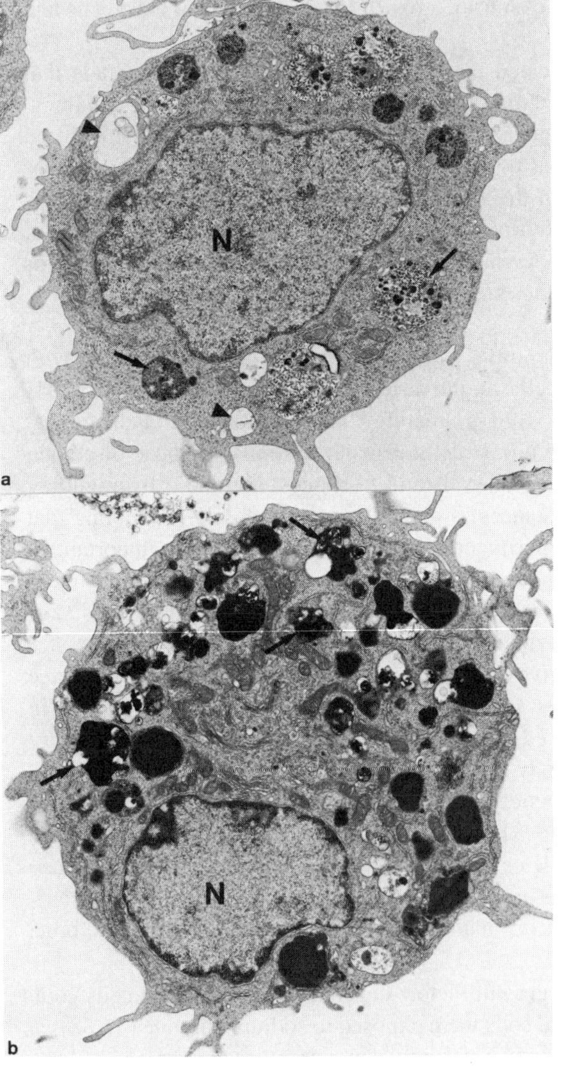

FIG. 2. Cloned mast cells (Cl.MC/9) derived from fetal liver and maintained in a medium supplemented with supernatant of cloned Ly1+2-inducer T cells. Cell in **(a)**, cultured without sodium butyrate, contains cytoplasmic vacuoles (*solid arrowheads*) and immature granules (*solid arrows*) with small vesicles and electron-dense particulate material. N, nucleus (×8,000). The cell in **(b)** was cultured for 5 days in the same medium as the cell in (a), except that the medium also contained 1 mM sodium butyrate. The cytoplasmic granules appear more "mature" than in (a), with abundant electron-dense granule content. N, nucleus (×8,700). However, several granules (*solid arrows*) have content that appears more heterogeneous than that of the granules of the mature peritoneal mast cell in Fig. 1b. (Reproduced with permission from Galli, Dvorak, and Dvorak, ref. 38.)

granule-associated serine neutral proteases. But butyrate treatment did not induce the cells to synthesize detectable quantities of ^{35}S-labeled heparin (37).

The apparent lack of heparin synthesis by growth factor–dependent mouse mast cells was regarded as a particularly important finding. Histochemical evidence suggested that rat mucosal mast cells contained little or no heparin (reviewed in 25), whereas heparin had been detected by biochemical analysis in both rat (7,72, 73,111,140) and mouse (7,37,106) peritoneal mast cells. The initial inability to detect heparin in growth factor–dependent mouse mast cells (37,106,118), and the recognition that the chondroitin sulfate proteoglycans produced by these cells included a species with 30 to 50% of its chondroitin sulfate disaccharides consisting of glucuronic acid $\rightarrow$ *N*-acetylgylucosamine-4,6-disulfate (chondroitin sulfate E) (106) therefore suggested that the detailed biochemical characterization of mast cell sulfated glycosaminoglycans might provide a basis for the classification of distinct mast cell subsets (121).

Use of Mast Cell–Deficient Mice to Study Mast Cell Heterogeneity

Even the demonstration of striking biochemical differences between two cell populations cannot exclude the possibility that these cells are in a single lineage. To return to the example of B cells, maturation of a single B cell clone is accompanied by a switch in immunoglobulin isotype as well as other remarkable alterations in phenotype such as the onset of Ig secretion and the development of a plasma cell morphology (13). In the case of mast cells, it was important to determine whether growth factor–dependent cultured mast cells were committed to expression of a phenotype resembling that of mucosal mast cells, or, alternatively, could give rise to mast cells with a phenotype resembling that of mature connective tissue or peritoneal mast cells. This issue was addressed by a combination of the *in vitro* and *in vivo* approaches to mast cell differentiation and maturation outlined above, *i.e.*, analysis of the phenotype of the mast cells that developed in genetically mast cell–deficient WBB6F$_1$- *W/W^v* mice after systemic or local injection of genetically compatible mast cell populations expanded *in vitro* (94).

This strategy was based on a straightforward assumption. Since the WBB6F$_1$-*W/W^v* mouse provides an environment suitable for the development of both connective tissue (65) and mucosal (14) mast cells from pluripotent bone marrow–derived precursors, it should also be able to reveal potential for phenotypic change in more differentiated cells in the mast cell lineage, such as populations of growth factor–dependent mast cells. In the initial studies, mast cell phenotype was assessed according to ultrastructure, histamine content, staining with Alcian blue and safranin O, and staining with the cationic fluorescent dye, berberine sulfate (94). Berberine sulfate binds to phosphate- and/or sulfate-containing polyanions, including DNA and heparin (24). The binding to DNA and heparin are distinguishable according to the characteristics of the fluorescence, the subcellular localization of the fluorescence, and, most critically, the sensitivity of the staining to treatment with heparinase (24,94).

Growth factor–dependent, bone marrow–derived mast cell populations whose phenotypes resembled those of mucosal mast cells gave rise to two phenotypically distinct populations of mast cells in $WBB6F_1$-W/W^v recipients (94). In anatomical sites that in $WBB6F_1$-$+/+$ mice ordinarily contain berberine sulfate–positive (heparin-rich) mast cells (dermis, peritoneal cavity, muscularis propria of the stomach), the adoptively transferred mast cells were berberine sulfate–positive and expressed other phenotypic characteristics of mature connective tissue-type mast cells. A representative experiment is shown in Table 4. But in anatomical sites populated in $WBB6F_1$-$+/+$ mice by berberine sulfate–negative mucosal mast cells (e.g., gastric mucosa), the adoptively transferred mast cells in $WBB6F_1$-W/W^v recipients were negative for berberine sulfate. These results were obtained with cultured mast cells derived either from $WBB6F_1$-$+/+$ or $C57BL/6$-$bg^J bg^J$ mice. Mast cells of the latter ("beige") genotype could be identified unambiguously because of their giant granules, proving that the berberine sulfate–positive mast cells that developed in $WBB6F_1$-W/W^v recipients were of donor origin. In a subsequent study, biochemical analysis confirmed that heparin represented the predominant ^{35}S-proteoglycan in the berberine sulfate–positive mast cells that developed in the peritoneal cavities of $WBB6F_1$-W/W^v mice injected 15 weeks earlier with cultured $WBB6F_1$-$+/+$ bone marrow–derived mast cells (97). The latter population, examined before injection into W/W^v mice, contained predominantly chondroitin sulfates rather than heparin (97).

Findings similar to those obtained with cultured mast cells were obtained when partially purified, berberine sulfate–positive, connective tissue-type mast cells derived from the peritoneal cavities of $WBB6F_1$-$+/+$ mice were injected into $WBB6F_1$-W/W^v mice (94). This result suggested that peritoneal mast cells themselves, a classic example of a heparin-rich mast cell, might give rise to mast cell populations phenotypically similar to either the connective tissue or mucosal type

TABLE 4. *Proportion of berberine sulfate–positive cells and histamine content of mast cells recovered from the peritoneal cavity of $WBB6F_1$-W/W^v mice after intraperitoneal injection of 10^6 cultured mast cells derived from $WBB6F_1$-$+/+$ mouse bone marrow cells*

Type of cells	Berberine sulfate–positive cells as a percentage of alcian blue–positive cells[a]	Histamine content of peritoneal cells[a] (ng/10^6 mast cells)
Cultured mast cells		
Before intraperitoneal injection	<0.1 (7)[b]	120 ± 9 (4)
1 week after	<0.1 (7)[b]	430 ± 100 (4)
3 weeks after	5 ± 1 (6)[c]	470 ± 130 (7)
5 weeks after	60 ± 11 (5)[c]	1,540 ± 310 (6)[c]
10 weeks after	93 ± 3 (10)[c]	2,730 ± 140 (8)[c]
Peritoneal mast cells of $WBB6F_1$-$+/+$ mice	98 ± 5 (5)	13,800 ± 2,100 (7)[c]

Reprinted with permission from Nakano et al., ref. 94.
[a]Mean ± SE; number of mice is shown in parenthesis.
[b]No berberine sulfate–positive cells seen in >1,000 Alcian blue–positive cells.
[c]$p<0.01$, when compared with the value listed above by Student's *t*-test.

mast cells. This possibility has now been confirmed using single peritoneal mast cells (63,117). Indeed, recent evidence suggests that clonal populations of mast cells derived from single peritoneal mast cells have the potential to exhibit bidirectional alterations of phenotype between the connective tissue and mucosal types (63).

Taken together, these observations supported the concept that mast cell phenotype (and, by implication, mast cell function) might be regulated, at least in part, by the tissue microenvironment. They also established that, in appropriate environments, growth factor–dependent cultured mast cell populations with phenotypic similarities to mucosal mast cells can give rise to mast cells with a phenotype similar to that of mature, connective tissue–type mast cells, and vice versa. Finally, because the alterations of mast cell phenotype were produced *in vivo,* this work established that microenvironmental regulation of mast cell differentiation/maturation represented a phenomenon of clear biological relevance.

However, the specific microenvironmental factors influencing mast cell phenotype and the mechanisms by which such effects are exerted remain to be fully defined. As developed in more detail elsewhere (29,31) and summarized in Table 5, mast cell phenotype theoretically can be influenced in at least four ways: (a) by factors that induce irrevocable commitment to different branches of mast cell differentiation and maturation (it is not clear whether such branching occurs within the mast cell lineage); (b) by factors affecting maturation within single (or multiple) vectors of mast cell development; (c) by factors affecting mast cell function (e.g., mast cells stimulated to degranulate can have histochemical characteristics different from those of control mast cells [108]); and (d) by products of other cells that are taken up by mast cells and stored in their granules, such as eosinophil peroxidase (23). The last mechanism provides a means by which mast cell phenotype can be altered indirectly, by factors influencing the functional activity or viability of other cells in the mast cells' environment. Clearly, any of these factors may operate systemically or in particular anatomical microenvironments or both and may act singly or in concert.

TABLE 5. *Mechanisms influencing the expression of mast cell phenotype*[a]

Factors promoting branching within the mast cell linkage (if this occurs)
Factors influencing differentiation and maturation (within single or multiple pathways)
Factors modulating mast cell function
Factors influencing the local concentrations of exogenous substances taken up and stored in mast cell granules

Reprinted with permission from Galli, ref. 30.

[a]Variation in mast cell phenotype may include differences in the amounts and/or the nature of surface structures, granule-associated mediators, products of cell activation, morphology, and sensitivity to stimuli of activation and/or drugs. The factors listed may include soluble products, or direct contact with certain cells or structures or other agents, and these may act singly or in concert.

Identifying how these multiple mechanisms might interact to regulate mast cell phenotype *in vivo* constitutes a significant challenge. A useful first step, as initially developed by Ginsburg and associates using heterogeneous stromal cell populations (6,15,47,48) and by Austen and associates using pure populations of fibroblasts (75,121) is to employ tissue culture systems to define cell-cell interactions that can regulate mast cell phenotype *in vitro*.

Clearly, performing such studies with cells derived from W/W^v and Sl/Sl^d mice and the congenic normal (+ / +) animals is of particular value in elucidating mechanisms of mast cell differentiation and maturation (66,44). Such studies, together with the identification of stem cell factor as a product of *Sl* and a ligand for c-kit (reviewed in 44), strongly indicate that interactions between c-kit and its ligand represent a major mechanism by which the microenvironment can regulate mast cell proliferation, phenotype, and perhaps function in the mouse. Indeed, it is possible that such interactions represent the major determinant of expression of the connective tissue phenotype by mouse mast cells *in vivo* (reviewed in 44). The extent to which interactions between c-kit and its ligand influence mast cell proliferation and maturation in humans remains to be determined.

USE OF MAST CELL–DEFICIENT MICE TO EVALUATE MAST CELL FUNCTION *IN VIVO*

Rationale

Even a complete understanding of the mechanisms regulating mast cell differentiation and phenotypic variation would not explain the mast cell's roles in health and disease. It is fortunate, therefore, that the combination of *in vitro* and *in vivo* approaches that already has provided important information concerning mast cell differentiation and maturation also appears to represent a useful new approach for analyzing mast cell function. A general scheme for evaluating mast cell function *in vivo*, which incorporates this approach, is outlined in Table 6.

TABLE 6. *General scheme for investigating mouse mast cell function* in vivo

1. Search for quantitative differences in the expression of biological responses in genetically mast cell–deficient WBB6F$_1$-W/W^v, and Sl/Sl^d mice and the congenic normal (+ / +) mice.[a]

2. Compare the responses in W/W^v mice and W/W^v mice that have received bone marrow transplants from congenic + / + mice.

3. Analyze the responses in W/W^v mice selectively reconstituted with mast cells.[b]

4. Define the mechanisms by which mast cells influence the responses.

Modified after Galli, ref. 30; used with permission.

[a] It is important to rule out the possibility that the biological response being studied induces the development of mast cells in the genetically mast cell–deficient mice (see Galli et al. 1987a; 52).

[b] A useful approach is to test the expression of the response in paired anatomical sites in the same mice, one site selectively reconstituted with mast cells and the other not.

The first step is to search for quantitative differences in the expression of a biological response in mast cell–deficient mice and their congenic normal litter mates. The two best studied mast cell–deficient mutants (WBB6F$_1$-*W/W^v* and WCB6F$_1$-*Sl/ Sl^d* mice) express a profound mast cell deficiency based on the effects of distinct mutations involving different chromosomes (40,44,66). Yet mast cell deficiency is not their only abnormality; both mutants lack cutaneous melanocytes, express a macrocytic anemia, and are sterile (40,66). As a result, the demonstration of differences in the biological responses of the mast cell–deficient mutants and their normal litter mates does not prove that these differences are mast cell–dependent.

Because the mast cell deficiency of the WBB6F$_1$-*W/W^v* animals can be cured by bone marrow transplantation from congenic +/+ mice (65), a reasonable second step is to evaluate the biological response in +/+ bone marrow–reconstituted *W/W^v* mice. But bone marrow reconstitution also cures the mutants' anemia and theoretically might influence the expression of biological responses through effects on other bone marrow–derived cells as well (40,66). These considerations can complicate the interpretation of experiments performed with bone marrow–reconstituted WBB6F$_1$-*W/W^v* mice, particularly in the case of biological responses not involving IgE (42,68). However, cultured mast cell populations exhibit much more stringent lineage commitment than do normal bone marrow cells (31,36,37,94). We therefore suggested that transplantation of these cells into various anatomical compartments of WBB6F$_1$-*W/W^v* mice represented an attractive strategy for selectively reconstituting mast cell populations in these animals and for analyzing the contribution of mast cells to biological responses *in vivo* (94). As illustrated below, this approach already is beginning to define the contribution of mast cells to a variety of cutaneous immune or inflammatory responses.

Mast Cell Function in IgE-Dependent Cutaneous Reactions

Many lines of evidence indicated that mast cells were critical for the local expression of IgE-mediated immediate hypersensitivity reactions (reviewed in 36,61, 113,128). However, it had not actually been demonstrated that restoring a population of phenotypically mature cutaneous mast cells to skin ordinarily devoid of this population would permit such skin to express IgE-dependent reactions.

We therefore investigated IgE-dependent passive cutaneous anaphylaxis (PCA) reactions in mast cell-deficient, mast cell-reconstituted, and normal mice, using an assay of ^{125}I-fibrin deposition to detect and quantitate alterations in local vascular permeability (23,85). For these studies, monoclonal mouse anti-DNP IgE antibodies (78) were injected intradermally, and the next day ^{125}I-guinea pig fibrinogen was administered intravenously 10 to 30 minutes before intravenous antigen (DNP$_{10}$ -HSA) challenge. In normal mice, 2-hour PCA reactions were associated with substantial leakage of ^{125}I-fibrinogen and deposition of ^{125}I-fibrin: ears injected with IgE contained up to 6 times the total ^{125}I-cpm and up to 30 times the cross-linked ^{125}I-fibrin-associated ^{125}I-cpm than did control ears.

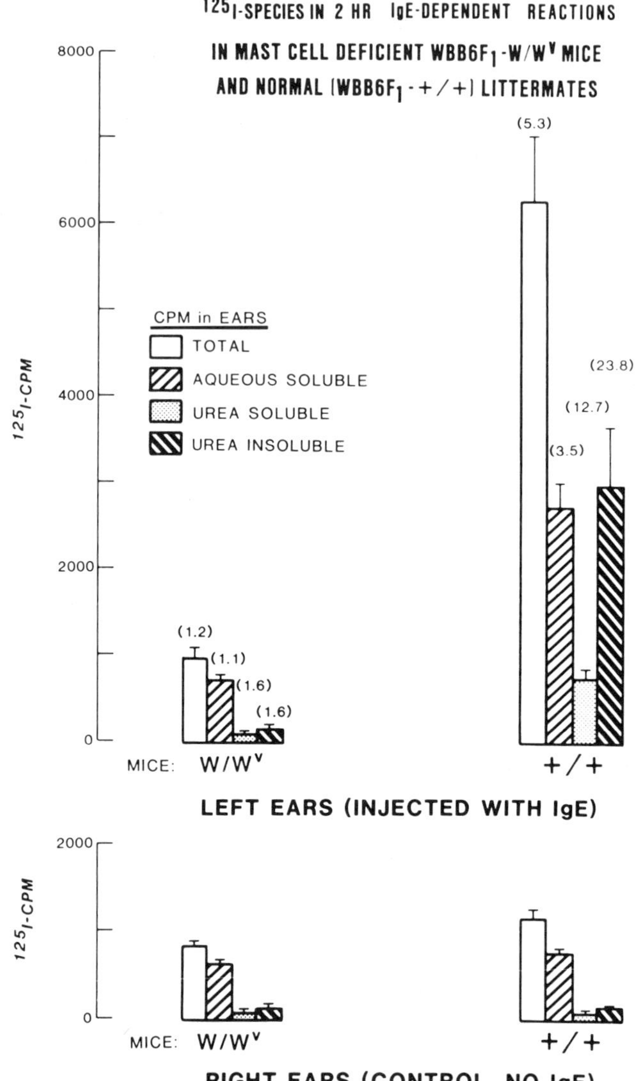

FIG. 3. ^{125}I-Species derived from ^{125}I-guinea pig fibrinogen in left ears injected with IgE anti-DNP and right (control) ears injected with vehicle alone in 6-month-old genetically mast cell–deficient WBB6F$_1$-*W/Wᵛ* mice and congenic normal (WBB6F$_1$-+/+) mice 2 hours after intravenous administration of DNP$_{10}$-HSA. The data are presented as mean ± SE cpm/ear (four to five mice per group). Each cpm value for the IgE-injected ears of +/+ mice is significantly greater than that for the IgE-injected ears of the *W/Wᵛ* mice ($p<0.001$, Student's *t*-test, two-tailed). *Numbers in parentheses above the bars* represent the ratio of cpm in that fraction for left (IgE-injected) as opposed to right (control) ears. The ear weight ratios (left/right) were 1.21 ± 0.05 for the WBB6F$_1$-+/+ mice and 1.02 ± 0.02 for the WBB6F$_1$-*W/Wᵛ* mice ($p<0.04$, Mann-Whitney U test, two-tailed). At the time of sacrifice, the ^{125}I-cpm in 50 µl of platelet-poor plasma was 32726 ± 3786 for the +/+ mice and 28473 ± 1009 for the *W/Wᵛ* mice. (Reproduced with permission from Wershil et al., ref. 128.)

TABLE 7. ^{125}I-species derived from ^{125}I-GPF two hours after intravenous antigen challenge in IgE-injected ears of WBB6F$_1$-W/W^v mice locally reconstituted with cultured mast cells 9–10 weeks earlier[a]

	IgE-dependent reactions			
	A. Left ears (mast cell–reconstituted)	B. Right ears (controls: mast cell–deficient)	left/right	p value a versus b
Experiment 1:				
Ear weight (mg)	60.2 ± 3.1	49.9 ± 1.0	1.21	$p<0.01$
Total cpm	3291 ± 593	286 ± 24	11.5	$p<0.001$
Aqueous-soluble cpm	795 ± 88	145 ± 55	5.5	$p<0.001$
Urea-soluble cpm	370 ± 87	30 ± 11	12.3	$p<0.001$
Urea-insoluble cpm	2905 ± 659	65 ± 11	44.7	$p<0.001$
Experiment 2:				
Ear weight (mg)	60.8 ± 2.4	51.8 ± 1.0	1.20	$p<0.01$
Total cpm	2831 ± 586	390 ± 28	7.3	$p<0.003$
Aqueous-soluble cpm	910 ± 143	294 ± 51	3.1	$p<0.003$
Urea-soluble cpm	248 ± 52	59 ± 47	4.2	$p<0.02$
Urea-insoluble cpm	1326 ± 555	62 ± 7	21.4	$p<0.03$
Experiment 3:				
Ear weight (mg)	66.2 ± 5.5	53.1 ± 1.6	1.29	$p<0.05$
Total cpm	2085 ± 727	400 ± 56	5.2	$p<0.03$
Aqueous-soluble cpm	781 ± 239	221 ± 21	3.5	$p<0.03$
Urea-soluble cpm	219 ± 91	27 ± 12	8.1	$p<0.03$
Urea-insoluble cpm	930 ± 384	60 ± 17	15.5	$p<0.03$

Reprinted with permission from Wershil et al., ref. 128.

[a] WBB6F$_1$-W/W^v mice (10 to 12 weeks old) received, to the left ear, 0.5×10^6 cultured mast cells derived from WBB6F$_1$-+/+ mice, and to the right ear medium alone (experiments 1 and 2) or (as a control cell population devoid of mast cells) 0.5×10^6 resident peritoneal cells from WBB6F$_1$-W/W^v mice (experiment 3). Nine to 10 weeks later, 20 µl of IgE anti-DNP (20 ng) was injected intradermally into each ear. The next day, the mice received an intravenous injection of ^{125}I-GPF, followed 20 minutes later by an intravenous injection of DNP$_{10}$-HSA (100 µg in 0.1 ml of 0.9% sodium chloride containing 1.0% Evans blue dye). Two hours later the mice were killed, and the reactions were evaluated. The ears were amputated and weighed. The sites of mast cell or medium injection (identified by the deposition of carbon particles that had been mixed with the injectate, and, in ears containing mast cells, by the extravasation of Evans blue dye) were then resected with a 6-mm skin punch biopsy for further processing (see 128). Data are presented as mean ± SE cpm/6-mm specimen. Results from measurements of mast cell–reconstituted (left) and control (right) ears were tested for statistical significance using Student's t-test (two-tailed). At the time of sacrifice, the ^{125}I-cpm in 50 µl of platelet-poor plasma was 63036 ± 2696 for experiment 1, 34714 ± 3004 for experiment 2, 38197 ± 3238 for experiment 3. The hematocrits of the mice were 37.9 ± 0.6% (n = 7) for experiment 1, 38.3 ± 0.5% (n = 4) for experiment 2, and 39.3 ± 0.8% (n = 4) for experiment 3, indicating that the adoptive transfer of a mast cell population into the left ears was not associated with correction of the recipients' hematocrit reading. Histological analysis confirmed that mast cell reconstitution was restricted to the left ears in all three experiments.

Several lines of evidence indicated that the ^{125}I-fibrin deposition associated with the PCA reactions was dependent on the activity of mast cells. (a) Mast cell degranulation occurred at sites of PCA reactions. (b) Antigen-induced influx of ^{125}I-fibrinogen and deposition of ^{125}I-fibrin were virtually abolished by heating the IgE (56°C, 1 hour) before intradermal injection (this maneuver abolishes the ability of the IgE to bind to high-affinity IgE receptors on the surface of mast cells (61). (c) Little or no IgE-dependent ^{125}I-fibrinogen influx of ^{125}I-fibrin deposition occurred in mast cell–deficient WBB6F$_1$-*W/W^v* (Fig. 3) or WCB6F$_1$-*Sl/Sl^d* mice. (d) The most convincing evidence that mast cells were critical to the expression of PCA was that adoptive transfer of cutaneous mast cell populations into WBB6F$_1$-*W/W^v* mice conferred on the recipients the ability to express the tissue swelling and the ^{125}I-fibrinogen influx and ^{125}I-fibrin deposition associated with PCA.

In the experiments shown in Table 7, cultured, phenotypically immature, WBB6F$_1$-+/+ bone marrow–derived mast cells were injected intradermally into the left ears of WBB6F$_1$-*W/W^v* mice, and medium or control cell preparations devoid of mast cells were injected into the right ears. When the experiments were performed 9 to 10 weeks later, the left ears but not the contralateral control ears had undergone reconstitution with populations of phenotypically mature, berberine sulfate–positive mast cells morphologically similar to the normal populations of mast cells present in the skin of WBB6F$_1$-+/+ mice. These adoptively transferred mast cells degranulated in response to IgE and specific antigen and conferred PCA reactivity to the mast cell–reconstituted ears (see Table 7). These data represented the first demonstration that ^{125}I-fibrinogen influx and ^{125}I-fibrin deposition occur in association with PCA reactions in the mouse; they also showed that the reaction is critically dependent on the function of cutaneous mast cells.

Mast Cell Function in Other Cutaneous Inflammatory Responses and in Ethanol-Induced Gastric Injury

WBB6F$_1$-*W/W^v* mice whose skin was locally reconstituted with phenotypically mature mast cells by the injection of mast cell populations generated *in vitro* have also been employed in the evaluation of mast cell function in four other biological responses: tick immunity, T-cell–mediated contact sensitivity, phorbol ester-induced acute inflammation, and inflammatory responses induced by intradermal injection of substance P.

Matsuda and coworkers (81) demonstrated that mast cells were required for the expression of immune resistance to the tick *Haemaphysalis longicornis* by *W/W^v* mice. The adoptively transferred mast cells at the tick feeding sites, like those at sites of passive cutaneous anaphylaxis (128), exhibited degranulation. As suggested by Matsuda and coworkers (81), this finding raised the possibility that mast cell function in resistance to *H. longicornis* is IgE-dependent. Recently, Matsuda and associates (82) demonstrated that this response indeed required IgE.

It should be noted, however, that the extent of mast cell involvement in the expression of tick resistance may vary according to the model system examined. DenHollander and Allen (17) reported that WBB6F₁-*W/Wᵛ* mice acquired strong resistance to the feeding of larval *Dermacentor variabilis* ticks, although the resistance expressed by *W/Wᵛ* mice during tertiary or quaternary infestations with this parasite was somewhat less than that expressed by the congenic +/+ mice ($p <$ 0.1). Recent morphological findings indicate that basophils may contribute significantly to the expression of immune resistance to *D. variabilis* by *W/Wᵛ* mice (120). Brown and colleagues (8) demonstrated in guinea pigs that ablation of basophils by intravenous injection of an antibasophil serum that had no effect on numbers of cutaneous mast cells abrogated acquired resistance to the feeding of larval *Amblyomma americanum* ticks. Taken together, these and other studies (reviewed in 8,17,33, and 120) indicate that the expression of immune resistance to tick feeding by mammalian hosts may involve multiple mechanisms, including IgE, mast cells, and basophils, with the particular factors contributing to reactions elicited by individual parasites varying according to species of host as well as species of tick. In contrast to the cutaneous mast cell's essential role in the expression of IgE-dependent PCA reactions (128) or acquired resistance to the feeding of larval *Haemaphysalis longicornis* ticks (81), experiments with WBB6F₁-*W/Wᵛ* mice locally reconstituted with cultured, bone marrow–derived WBB6F₁-+/+ mast cells indicate that mast cells have no detectable role in the expression of T-cell–dependent cutaneous contact sensitivity responses (84). These data support a large body of evidence indicating that genetically mast cell–deficient mice exhibit little or no detectable impairment in their ability to express T-cell–mediated responses (34,39,55,87, 123).

These negative findings are of some interest, since morphological evidence reviewed elsewhere indicates that mast cell degranulation can occur during certain T-cell–mediated reactions (34,84). Such degranulation might reflect the influence of any of a number of different factors, including IgE generated parallel with the T-cell response, complement products, T-cell–derived molecules, or products of leukocytes infiltrating the reaction (reviewed in 34,84). Thus, although mast cell activation is not required for the expression of experimental contact sensitivity responses, it is conceivable that in more complex reactions, particularly those incorporating both T-cell–dependent and IgE-dependent components (e.g., reactions to certain parasites), mast cells may be responsible for certain aspects of the reaction but not others. Indeed, WBB6F₁-*W/Wᵛ* mice locally reconstituted with cultured mast cells may be useful in the identification and detailed analysis of the mast cell–dependent or mast cell–independent components of such responses.

Our work with IgE-dependent and contact sensitivity responses may define two extremes of a spectrum of mast cell contributions to biological responses. The cells are essential for expression of PCA reactions but make no detectable contribution to the orchestration of the contact sensitivity response. It is likely, however, that in many biological responses the mast cell's contribution falls between these two extremes. We have demonstrated that both the acute gastric damage induced by oral ethanol (42) and the acute inflammation induced by epicutaneous application of

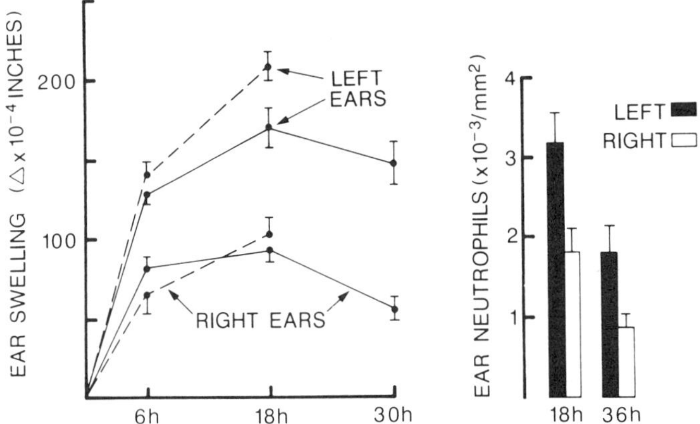

FIG. 4. Tissue swelling and neutrophil infiltration associated with phorbol 12-myristate 13-acetate–induced reactions in mast cell–reconstituted *left* ears and mast cell–deficient *right* ears of WBB6F$_1$-*W/W^v* mice. Results are of two experiments, one terminated at 18 hours (------) and the other at 36 hours (------). For both swelling and neutrophil infiltration, the values for left ears were significantly higher than those for right ears ($p<0.05$–0.001, paired Student's *t*-test, two-tailed) at all intervals examined. Total neutrophil counts in a full-thickness 50-μm length of the ears were, at 18 hours, L = 75.1 ± 12.8, R = 32.2 ± 5.1 ($p<0.001$), and at 36 hours, L = 33.4 ± 7.4, R = 12.8 ± 2.2 ($p<0.05$). Mast cell counts number per linear millimeter of skin) in the left and right ears were 15.9 ± 3.2 versus 0 (n = eight mice) at 18 hours, and 9.0 ± 0.9 versus 0.03 ± 0.03 (n = ten mice) at 36 hours ($p<0.001$ at either interval, Mann-Whitney U test, two-tailed). The hematocrits of these mice (38 ± 0.4%) were indistinguishable from those of age-matched, untreated *W/W^v* mice (39 ± 0.6%). (Reproduced with permission from Wershil et al., ref. 129.)

either croton oil (127) or phorbol 12-myristate 13-acetate (129) are significantly less severe in mast cell–deficient mice than in congenic normal ($+/+$) mice. In the cutaneous acute inflammatory responses, the contribution of mast cells to the augmentation of the responses has been confirmed by performing the experiments in WBB6F$_1$-*W/W^v* mice locally reconstituted with cultured $+/+$ mast cells (Fig. 4; 129).

Recently, the same approach was taken to show that virtually all of the augmentation of vascular permeability, infiltration of granulocytes, and augmentation of interstitial fibrin deposition associated with the intradermal injection of the neuropeptide substance P is mast cell–dependent (135). Matsuda and coworkers (80) showed that mast cells also greatly augment the granulocyte infiltration produced by injecting substance P into cutaneous air pouches in mice. However, other effects of substance P, such as the vascular changes induced by intravenous administration of the neuropeptide, may occur by mast cell–independent mechanisms (reviewed in 71,135).

Mast cell–reconstituted *W/W^v* mice have also been used to demonstrate that mast cells augment the neutrophil infiltration in thioglycolate– or immune complex–induced peritonitis in mice (101,102) and accelerate the development of blood vessels in association with the local growth of a melanoma cell line (119).

TABLE 8. *Hematocrit, gastric mast cell counts, and areas of ethanol-induced gastric injury in WBB6F$_1$-W/W^v mice 17 or 70 days after intravenous transplantation of WBB6F$_1$-+/+ bone marrow cells*[a]

	Interval after bone marrow transplantation (days)	Mice		
		A: +/+	B: W/W^v	C: +/+ → W/W^v
Mice used for mast cell counts				
Hematocrit (%) (number of mice)	17	48.0 ± 0.9 (6)	39.8 ± 1.1 (6) $p<0.02$ versus A,C	47.5 ± 0.8 (6) NS[b] versus A
	70	48.5 ± 0.6 (6)	40.0 ± 0.6 (6) $p<0.02$ versus A,C	48.6 ± 0.3 (6) NS versus A
Mast cells (number/mm^2)				
Glandular stomach, mucosa	17	40 ± 22	0	0.6 ± 0.7
	70	71 ± 33	0	67 ± 23 NS versus A
Glandular stomach, submucosa	17	64 ± 33	0	0
	70	47 ± 19	0	87 ± 29 $p<0.04$ versus A
Mice given oral ethanol				
Hematocrit (%)	17	48.8 ± 0.3 (10)	38.9 ± 0.8 (8) $p<0.02$ versus A,C	47.2 ± 0.5 (7) NS versus A
	70	ND[c]	37.6 ± 0.6 (6) $p<0.02$ versus A,C NS versus 17-day value	46.8 ± 0.9 (6) NS versus 17-day value
Area of mucosal lesions after 100% ethanol (% of glandular stomach)	17	9.2 ± 1.2	2.7 ± 0.8 $p<0.001$ versus A	2.7 ± 0.8 $p<0.001$ versus A, NS versus B
	70	ND	1.2 ± 0.8	11.7 ± 3.4 $p<0.01$ versus B $p<0.01$ versus 17-day value (C) NS versus 17-day value (A)

Reprinted with permission from Galli et al., ref. 42.

[a]Pooled litter mate WBB6F$_1$-+/+ mice were left untreated (group A) or were used as donors for bone marrow cells, which were administered intravenously (2.0 × 10^7 cells/mouse) to pooled litter mate WBB6F$_1$-W/W^v mice (group C). Other pooled litter mate W/W^v mice were left untreated (group B). Mice in groups A through C were sacrificed 17 or 70 days after transplantation in group C mice was carried out; some of the mice did not receive ethanol and were used for determination of hematocrit levels and quantitation of gastric mast cells; others were used for determination of hematocrit levels and quantitation of areas of ethanol-induced gastric mucosal injury (see ref. 42). The values are mean ± SE or, for mast cell counts, mean ± SD; tests for statistical significance of differences in values were by the Mann-Whitney U test (two-tailed).

[b]NS, not significant ($p>0.05$).

[c]ND, not done.

In the case of ethanol-induced gastric injury, the role of mast cells in the augmentation of the damage has not been demonstrated as directly. However, WBB6F$_1$-W/W^v mice transplanted with WBB6F$_1$-$+/+$ bone marrow cells responded to oral ethanol in the same manner as did W/W^v mice if the challenge was done 17 days after transplantation, when the recipients' hematocrit levels had been corrected but not their mast cell deficiencies. By contrast, when challenge was performed 70 days after transplantation, after correction of both the hematocrit and the mast cell deficiency of the recipients, the mice developed as much ethanol-induced damage as did the congenic normal animals (Table 8). In addition, mast cell disruption-degranulation occurred at sites of ethanol-induced injury in normal or mast cell–reconstituted mice (Fig. 5; 42), and the gastric damage induced by ethanol challenge was mark-

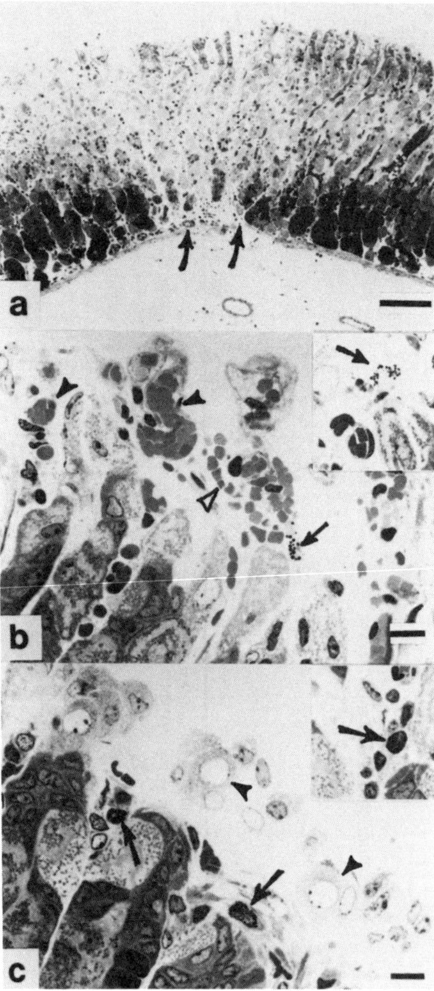

FIG. 5. Photomicrographs of the glandular stomach of a WCB6F$_1$-$+/+$ mouse that received 100% ethanol 1 hour before sacrifice. **(a)** A well-circumscribed region of mucosal injury that was evident upon gross examination of the fixed stomach. The area of damage, indicated by the loss of staining intensity of the affected epithelial cells, extends focally to the muscularis mucosa (*arrows*) (bar = 100 μ). **(b)** Higher magnification of the superficial mucosa at the periphery of an area of damage similar to that shown in (a). There is compaction of erythrocytes within superficial mucosal vessels (*solid arrowheads*), evidence of vascular stasis, and focal hemorrhage (*open arrowhead*). A mast cell (*arrow*) exhibits disruption, with release of cytoplasmic granules and loss of nuclear staining. *Inset*: Another disrupted mast cell (*arrow*) in a field adjacent to that in (b) (bar = 10μ). **(c)** Grossly normal-appearing area of superficial mucosa from the same stomach shown in (b). There are a few desquamated necrotic cells (*arrowheads*) but no other evidence of tissue injury. Two mast cells (*arrows*) near the mucosal surface appear intact. *Inset*: Another intact mast cell (*arrow*) in a field adjacent to that in (c). (a–c, 1-μ thick, Giemsa-stained, Epon-embedded sections) (bar = 10 μ) (Reproduced with permission from Galli et al., ref. 42.)

edly reduced by administration of antagonists of the H_1-dependent effects of histamine (126). Taken together, these findings strongly suggest that release of mast cell mediators induced by the direct or indirect effects of oral ethanol challenge contributed to the gastric damage elicited in this experimental model.

Can Mast Cells Suppress Reactions to Toxins?

Our studies in the skin and stomach provide evidence in support of the hypothesis that mast cells can augment the intensity of reactions elicited by exogenous toxins. Such a role has been established in the case of phorbol ester-induced acute cutaneous inflammation and is likely in the case of ethanol-induced gastric injury. But discussion of the contribution of mast cells to reactions induced by exogenous agents would not be complete without brief consideration of a very different function: the suppression of the response. Many authors have suggested that mast cells *might* down-regulate several different biological responses, including reactions to exogenous toxins (see Table 2). Although no such role has yet been proved by using W/W^v mice locally reconstituted with cultured mast cells, studies in mast cell–deficient mice have provided evidence that is *consistent* with a protective effect of mast cells in one toxic reaction.

It has been recognized for many years that the intravenous injection of commercial India ink can result in platelet aggregation (19,134), activation of the clotting system (27,58,59), and death (5,27,58,59). In collaboration with Kitamura and colleagues (68), we found that the intravenous injection of a 10% or 20% preparation of commercial India ink resulted in far greater mortality in mast cell–deficient $WBB6F_1$-W/W^v mice than in the congenic $+/+$ controls. In both W/W^v and $+/+$ mice, intravenous ink resulted in thrombocytopenia and markedly prolonged bleeding times as well as prolonged partial thromboplastin and prothrombin times and reduced fibrinogen concentrations. These effects were similar in W/W^v and $+/+$ mice, although the reduction in platelet counts was greater in W/W^v mice. In addition, the mortality associated with ink injection was significantly higher in W/W^v mice than in congenic $+/+$ mice. Most W/W^v mice that died first exhibited paralysis, and examination under the dissection microscope revealed that ink injection resulted in significantly more cerebral thromboembolism in W/W^v mice than in $+/+$ controls.

Bone marrow transplantation from $+/+$ mice corrected both the mast cell deficiency and the anemia of W/W^v mice and protected the W/W^v recipients from the adverse consequences of ink injection (Table 9). By contrast, $+/+$ mice rendered as anemic as W/W^v mice by bleeding did not exhibit increased morbidity and mortality after ink injection. Mast cell–deficient $WCB6F_1$-Sl/Sl^d mice also exhibited increased morbidity and mortality after intravenous ink injection (see Table 10). Finally, mixing the ink with commercial heparin prior to intravenous injection markedly reduced the incidence of cerebral thromboembolism and death in W/W^v mice.

Taken together, these findings suggested that the increased morbidity and mortal-

TABLE 9. *Effect of WBB6F$_1$-+/+ mouse bone marrow transplantation ("rescue") on number of cerebral thromboemboli and mortality of WBB6F$_1$-W/W^v mice injected with 10% India ink (0.04 ml/g body weight)*

Experiment number	Mice	Number of emboli at 4 hours (mean ± SE)[a]	Proportions of deaths within 24 hours
1	Untreated W/W^v	36 ± 5 (13)	NE[b]
	Rescued W/W^v	15 ± 4 (18)[c]	NE
	Untreated +/+	11 ± 3 (12)[c]	NE
2	Untreated W/W^v	NE	21/25 (84%)
	Rescued W/W^v	NE	2/15 (13%)[c]
	Untreated +/+	NE	1/17 (6%)[c]
3	Untreated W/W^v	NE	7/13 (54%)
	Rescued W/W^v	NE	2/22 (9%)[c]
	Untreated +/+	NE	1/11 (9%)[c]

Reprinted with permission from Kitamura et al., ref. 68.
[a]Number of mice is shown in parentheses.
[b]NE, not examined.
[c]$p<0.02$, when compared with the value of nontreated W/W^v mice by X^2 test.

ity exhibited by W/W^v and Sl/Sl^d mice injected with ink might be related to their mast cell deficiency rather than to their anemia. But measurement of the histamine content of the blood and various tissues of WBB6F$_1$-+/+ mice injected with ink and examination of their tissues in 1-μ sections showed that intravenous ink did not cause detectable mast cell degranulation. These findings indicate that the differences in ink-induced toxicity in W/W^v or Sl/Sl^d mice and their +/+ litter mates may be attributable to defects other than their lack of mast cells. Alternatively, we cannot exclude the possibility that mast cells protect +/+ mice from the adverse effects of intravenously injected ink by mechanisms other than degranulation and release of heparin.

Need for Caution in the Interpretation of Experiments Employing Mast Cell–Deficient Mice

Having presented examples of the usefulness of the approach shown in Table 6, it is only fair to strike a few cautionary notes. A positive result in the series of experi-

TABLE 10. *Mortality of WCB6F$_1$-Sl/Sl^d and -+/+ mice within 72 hours after injection of 20% India ink[a]*

Genotype	No. of mice injected	No. of mice that died at each interval after the injection[b]			
		0–8 hours	8–24 hours	24–72 hours	Total
Sl/Sl^d	11	5	6	0	11
+/+	9	0	0	0	0

Reprinted with permission from Kitamura et al., ref. 68.
[a]0.02 ml/g body weight, i.e., 0.32 mg carbon/g body weight.
[b]$p<0.01$, when distribution of death was compared in Sl/Sl^d versus +/+ mice by X^2 test.

ments outlined as steps 1 through 3 in the table can demonstrate that mast cells contribute to a particular biological response, but a negative result does not exclude such participation; it merely shows that the mast cells' contribution was not detected. This may reflect either the insensitivity of the assay system or the presence of redundancy in the cellular or mediator pathways influencing the response (34). For example, if a critical biological function in a given response can be provided either by mast cells or by another cell type, both populations might have to be ablated in order to detect a significant effect on the expression of that response. Other factors might contribute to a negative response as well. For example, the anatomical relationship of mast cells to other cells in the tissue microenvironment might not be precisely the same in $WBB6F_1$-W/W^v mice with adoptively transferred mast cell populations as in $WBB6F_1$-$+/+$ mice; the phenotype of native and adoptively transferred mast cell populations, although similar, may not be identical. These represent some of the theoretical considerations that might be invoked to explain an unexpected negative result. On the other hand, the demonstration that mast cell–deficient mice lacking adoptively transferred mast cells *can* express a particular biological response strongly suggests that mature mast cells are not essential for the response (34,39,44,84,86,88).

The last statement needs some qualification, however. We recently reported that phenotypically mature connective tissue-type mast cells appeared in the dermis of $WBB6F_1$-W/W^v mice at sites of inflammation associated with either spontaneously occurring chronic idiopathic dermatitis (32) or the chronic dermatitis induced by epicutaneous application of phorbol 12-myristate 13-acetate (52). Mast cell development appeared to represent a local effect of these two processes, since no mast cells appeared in uninvolved skin or in other tissues, nor was the anemia of the mice corrected. These represented the first and, to date, the only reported instances in which populations of connective tissue-type mast cells developed in W/W^v mice that had not received transplantation of hematopoietic or mast cells. Nevertheless, even the rare occurrence of this phenomenon indicates that when $WBB6F_1$-W/W^v mice are used for the evaluation of mast cell function, the investigator must rule out the possibility that the biological process under study actually induced the development of mast cells in the W/W^v animals.

In contrast to $WBB6F_1$-W/W^v mice, mast cell–deficient $WCB6F_1$-Sl/Sl^d mice did not develop detectable populations of dermal mast cells at sites of either idiopathic (32) or phorbol 12-myristate 13-acetate–induced (52) dermatitis. These findings suggest that for certain investigations of mast cell function, Sl/Sl^d mice may be more suitable than W/W^v mice.

CONCLUSIONS

We have illustrated how mast cell–deficient mice, and especially W/W^v mice locally reconstituted with mast cells by the injection of cultured mast cells derived from the congenic $+/+$ mice, can be used to define and quantitate the contribution of mast cells to biological responses expressed *in vivo*. Although such experiments represent an obligatory first step in characterizing the roles of mast cells in such responses, much additional work may be required to understand the mechanisms by which mast cells exert their influence. Mast cell–deficient, congenic normal, and mast cell–reconstituted mast cell–deficient mice can also be useful to efforts to elucidate the pathogenesis of reactions shown to require mast cells. For example, this approach recently was used to demonstrate that the neutrophil infiltration associated with IgE-dependent cutaneous responses is mast cell–dependent and that a substantial fraction of such leukocyte infiltration probably reflects the action of mast cell–derived tumor necrosis factor— (130).

It should be acknowledged that one of the more powerful forces driving research in mast cell biology is the belief that these cells play critical, if sometimes poorly understood, roles in human health and disease. Although it is axiomatic that results obtained in experimental animals cannot be extrapolated uncritically to humans, approaches employing genetically mast cell–deficient mice, like those based on mutant mice expressing other defects in immunological or hematopoietic cells, are convenient models for developing insights that may then be evaluated in other mammalian species, including humans.

Unfortunately, it is much more difficult to identify and quantitate the contribution of mast cells to biological responses in humans than in mice. To our knowledge, no genetic syndrome associated with profound mast cell deficiency has been reported in humans. In the absence of information from such an experiment of nature, how can one be certain that mast cells contribute significantly to a particular response in humans? Demonstrating that the response is dependent on IgE is useful but not sufficient. Basophils also elaborate a variety of potent mediators, many of them similar or identical to those of mast cells, upon stimulation with IgE and antigen (36,41,45,113). Platelets, monocytes, and eosinophils also may participate in at least some IgE-dependent reactions (reviewed in 10).

If detailed analysis of multiple cell types establishes that a particular mediator (perhaps a protease and/or cytokine) is absolutely specific for mast cells, does detection of increased levels of this mediator in tissues or fluids constitute proof that mast cells have an important role in the reaction? Not necessarily. Such evidence would show that the release of this mast cell–specific mediator had occurred in association with the reaction, but additional evidence would be required to prove that this mediator participated critically in the pathogenesis of the response in question. If the expression of the reaction were significantly influenced by the administration of an agent whose *sole* effect was to block the activity (or suppress the production) of the putative mast cell–specific mediator, most investigators probably would be satisfied that the mast cell's role in this reaction had been established. But how many agents (even monoclonal antibodies) have a single effect when administered *in vivo?*

On the other hand, the objective of therapy is to eliminate or at least ameliorate pathological processes and their sequelae. These goals often can be achieved even when the pathogenesis of these conditions is not fully understood. Agents that interfere with the production of and/or the end-organ effects of mast cell–associated mediators abound, and newer and possibly more effective compounds are being developed. Since absolute proof of an important role for the mast cell in any particular pathological process in humans may be virtually impossible to achieve, what sort of evidence can be used to justify trials of therapies directed at the mast cell and/or its products? Such evidence might include (a) proof, based on studies with mast cell–deficient mice, that the mast cell plays a critical role in the murine model of the human process; (b) morphological evidence that mast cells participate in the human condition (e.g., evidence of changes in mast cell numbers and/or evidence of anaphylactic or piecemeal [36] degranulation of mast cells); and (c) demonstration that mediators unique to or at least characteristic of the mast cell are released in association with the reaction in humans.

As noted above, many therapies directed against mast cells or their mediators may also be effective if basophils, rather than mast cells, play an important role in the disease process. Despite their many similarities, basophils may be distinguished from mast cells by morphological criteria in appropriately processed tissues and fluids (20,22,36). Human basophils and mast cells may also be distinguished by searching for mediators produced by one cell type but not the other (41). Thus, the morphological and biochemical studies recommended in points (b) and (c) above may, in some instances, implicate basophils in human reactions that have been shown to be mast cell–dependent in the mouse. Such a result would lend further support to the widely held view that basophils and mast cells may perform similar or complementary functions (reviewed in 36,41,90,113). If therapeutic approaches are developed that have more efficacy against the effects of one of these two cell types than the other, the accurate identification of whether a pathological process involves basophils, mast cells, or both populations will become of even greater interest.

ACKNOWLEDGMENTS

Supported in part by U.S.P.H.S. grants AI 22674, AI 23990, and P01 DK 33506, and Physician-Scientist Award (to B.K.W.) K11 DK01543. We thank Ann M. Dvorak, M.D., for the electron micrographs.

REFERENCES

1. Askenase, P. W. (1980): Immunopathology of parasitic disease: Involvement of basophils and mast cells. *Springer Semin. Immunopathol.*, 2:417–442.
2. Befus, A. D., Pearce, F. L., Gauldie, J., Horsewood, P., and Bienenstock, J. (1982): Mucosal mast cells. I. Isolation and functional characteristics of rat intestinal mast cells. *J. Immunol.*, 128:2475–2480.
3. Beutler, B., and Cerami, A. (1986): Cachectin and tumor necrosis factor as two sides of the same biological coin. *Nature*, 320:584–588.
4. Bienenstock, J., Befus, A. D., and Denburg, J. A. (1986): Mast cell heterogeneity: Basic questions and clinical implications. In Mast Cell Differentiation and Heterogeneity, edited by A. D. Befus, J. Bienenstock, and J. A. Denburg, pp. 391–402. Raven Press, New York.
5. Biozzi, G., Benacerraf, B., Mene, G., and Halpern, B. N. (1951): Etude quantitative de l'activite granulopexique du systeme reticulo-endothelial par l'injection intraveineuse d'encre de Chine chez les diverses especes animales. II. Relations entre les modifications de la coagulation du sang *in*

vitro sous l'effet de l'injection intraveineuse de doses croissantes d'encre de Chine et sa repartition dans l'organisme. *Ann. Inst. Pasteur*, 81:164–172.

6. Bland, E. C., Ginsburg, H., Silbert, E., and Metcalfe, D. D. (1982): Mouse heparin proteoglycan: Synthesis by mast cell fibroblast monolayers during lymphocyte-dependent mast cell proliferation. *J. Biol. Chem.*, 257:8661–8666.

7. Bloom G., and Ringertz, N. R. (1960): Acid polysaccharides of peritoneal mast cells of the rat and mouse. *Arkiv. Kemi.*, 16:51–56.

8. Brown, S. J., Galli, S. J., Gleich, G. J., and Askenase, P. W. (1982): Ablation of immunity to *Amblyomma americanum* by anti-basophil serum: Cooperation between basophils and eosinophils in expression of immunity to ectoparasites (ticks) in guinea pigs. *J. Immunol.*, 129:790–796.

9. Burnet, F. M. (1977): The probable relationship of some or all mast cells to the T-cell system. *Cell. Immunol.*, 30:358–360.

10. Capron, A., Dessaint, J. P., Capron, M., Joseph, M., Ameisen, J. C., and Tonnel, A. B. (1986): From parasites to allergy: The second receptor for IgE (Fc R2). *Immunol. Today*, 7:15–19.

11. Chi, E., and Lagunoff, D. (1975): Abnormal mast cell granules in the beige (Chédiak-Higashi syndrome) mouse. *J. Histochem. Cytochem.*, 23:117–122.

12. Combs, J. W., Lagunoff, D., and Benditt, E. P. (1965): Differentiation and proliferation of embryonic mast cells of the rat. *J. Cell Biol.*, 25:577–592.

13. Cooper, M. D., Kearney, J., and Scher, I. (1984): B lymphocytes. In Fundamental Immunology, edited by W. E. Paul, pp. 43–55. Raven Press, New York.

14. Crowle, P. K., and Reed, N. D. (1984): Bone marrow origin of mucosal mast cells. *Int. Arch. Allergy Appl. Immunol.*, 73:242–247.

15. Davidson, S., Kinarty, A., Coleman, R., Reshef, A., and Ginsburg, H. (1986): Fibroblasts are required for mast cell granule synthesis. In Mast Cell Differentiation and Heterogeneity, edited by A. D. Befus, J. Bienenstock, and J. A. Denburg, 115–124. Raven Press, New York.

16. Denburg, J. A., Befus, A. D., and Bienenstock, J. (1980): Growth and differentiation *in vitro* of mast cells from mesenteric lymph nodes of *Nippostrongylus brasiliensis*-infected rats. *Immunology*, 41:195–202.

17. den Hollander, N., and Allen, J. R. (1985): *Dermacentor variabilis:* Resistance to ticks acquired by mast cell-deficient and other strains of mice. *Exp. Parasitol.*, 59:169–179.

18. DuBuske, L., Austen, K. F., Czop, J., and Stevens, R. L. (1984): Granule-associated serine neutral proteases of the mouse bone marrow-derived mast cells that degrade fibronectin: Their increase after sodium butyrate treatment of the cells, *J. Immunol.*, 133:1535–1541.

19. Dudgeon, L. S., and Goadby, H. K. (1931). The examination of the tissues and some observations on the blood platelets of rabbits at intervals of five minutes, and later, after intravenous inoculations of *Staphylococcus aureus* and India ink. *J. Hyg.* (Cambridge), 31:247–256.

20. Dvorak, A. M., Dvorak, H. F., and Galli, S. J. (1983): Ultrastructural criteria for identification of mast cells and basophils in humans, guinea pigs, and mice. *Am. Rev. Respir. Dis.*, 128:S49–S52.

21. Dvorak, A. M., Klebanoff, S. J., Henderson, W. R., Monshan, R. A., Pyne, K., and Galli, S. J. (1985): Vesicular uptake of eosinophil peroxidase by guinea pig basophils and by cloned mouse mast cells and granule-containing lymphoid cells. *Am. J. Pathol.*, 118:425–438.

22. Dvorak, A. M., Nabel, G., Pyne, K., Cantor, H., Dvorak, H. F., and Galli, S. J. (1982): Ultrastructural identification of the mouse basophil. *Blood*, 59:1279–1285.

23. Dvorak, H. F., Senger, D. R., Dvorak, A. M., Harvey, V. S., and McDonagh, J. (1985). Regulation of extravascular coagulation by microvascular permeability. *Science*, 227:1059–1061.

24. Enerback, L. (1974): Berberine sulfate binding to mast cell polyanions: A cytofluorometric method for the quantitation of heparin. *Histochemistry*, 42:301–313.

25. Enerback, L. (1986): Mast cell heterogeneity: The evolution of the concept of a specific mucosal mast cell. In Mast Cell Differentiation and Heterogeneity, edited by A. D. Befus, J. Bienenstock, and J. A. Denburg, pp. 1–26. Raven Press, New York.

26. Enerback, L., and Rundquist, I. (1981): DNA distribution of mast cell populations in growing rats. *Histochemistry*, 71:521–531.

27. Foot, N. C. (1923): Studies of endothelial reactions. VII. Changes in the distribution of colloidal carbon noted in the lungs of rabbits following splenectomy. *J. Exp. Med.*, 37:139–152.

28. Fung, M. C., Hapel, A. J., Ymer, S., Cohen, D. R., Johnson, R. M., Campbell, H. D., and Yung, I. G. (1984): Molecular cloning of cDNA for murine interleukin-3. *Nature*, 307:233–237.

29. Galli, S. J. (1986): Mast cell heterogeneity: Can variation in mast cell phenotype be explained without postulating the existence of distinct mast cell lineages? In Mast Cell Differentiation and

Heterogeneity, edited by A. D. Befus, J. Bienenstock, and J. A. Denburg, pp. 167–182. Raven Press, New York.

30. Galli, S. J.: New approaches for the analysis of mast cell maturation, heterogeneity and function. *Fed. Proc.*, 46:1906–1914.
31. Galli, S. J. (1990): Biology of disease. New insights into "the riddle of the mast cells:" Microenvironmental regulation of mast cell development and phenotypic heterogeneity. *Lab. Invest.*, 62: 5–33.
32. Galli, S. J., Arizono, N., Murakami, T., Dvorak, A. M., and Fox, J. G. (1987a). Development of large numbers of mast cells at sites of idiopathic chronic dermatitis in genetically mast cell-deficient WBB6F$_1$-*W/W^v* mice. *Blood*, 69:16–26.
33. Galli, S. J., and Askenase, P. W. (1986): Cutaneous basophil hypersensitivity. In The Reticuloendothelial System: A Comprehensive Treatise. Volume IX: Hypersensitivity, edited by P. Abramoff, S. M. Phillips, and M. R. Escobar, pp. 321–369. Plenum Press, New York.
34. Galli, S. J., and Dvorak, A. M. (1984): What do mast cells have to do with delayed hypersensitivity? *Lab. Invest.*, 50:365–368.
35. Galli, S. J., Dvorak, A. M., and Dvorak, H. F. (1984): Mouse mast cells and other granulated leukocyte clones. Ultrastructure of cloned mouse leukocytes. *Monogr. Allergy*, 18:129–137.
36. Galli, S. J., Dvorak, A. M., and Dvorak, H. F. (1984): Basophils and mast cells: Morphologic insights into their biology, secretory patterns, and function. *Prog. Allergy*, 34:1–141.
37. Galli, S. J., Dvorak, A. M., Marcum, J. A., Ishizaka, T., Nabel, G., Der Simonian, H., Pyne, K., Goldin, J. M., Rosenberg, R. D., Cantor, H., and Dvorak, H. F. (1982). Mast cell clones: A model for the analysis of cellular maturation. *J. Cell Biol.*, 95:435–444.
38. Galli, S. J., Dvorak, A. M., Marcum, J. A., Nabel, G., Goldin, J. M., Rosenberg, R. D., Cantor, H., and Dvorak, H. F. (1983b). Mouse mast cell clones: Modulation of functional maturity *in vitro*. *Monogr. Allergy*, 18:166–170.
39. Galli, S. J., and Hammel, I. (1984): Unequivocal delayed hypersensitivity in mast cell-deficient and beige mice. *Science*, 226:710–713.
40. Galli, S. J., and Kitamura, Y. (1987): Animal model of human disease. Genetically mast cell-deficient *W/W^v* and *Sl/Sl^d* mice: Their value for the analysis of the roles of mast cells in biological responses *in vivo*. *Am. J. Pathol.*, 127:191–198.
41. Galli, S. J., and Lichtenstein, L. M. (1988): Biology of mast cells and basophils. In Allergy: Principles and Practice, Third Edition, edited by E. Middleton, Jr., L. E. Reed, E. F. Ellis, N. F. Adkinson, Jr., Y. W. Yunginger, pp. 106–134. Mosby, St. Louis.
42. Galli, S. J., Wershil, B. K., Bose, R. Walker, P. A., and Szabo, S. (1987b): Ethanol-induced acute gastric injury in mast cell-deficient and congenic normal mice: Evidence that mast cells can augment the area of damage. *Am. J. Pathol.*, 128:131–140.
43. Galli, S. J., Tsai, M., Langley, K. E., Zsebo, K. M., and Geisler, E. N. (1991): Stem cell factor (SCF), a ligand for *c-kit*, induces mediator release from some populations of mouse mast cells. *FASEB J.*, 5:A1092(abstract).
44. Galli, S. J., Geissler, E. N., Wershil, B. K., Gordon, J. R., Tsai, M., and Hammel, J.: Insights into mast cell development and function derived from analyses of mice carrying mutations at *beige*, *w/c-kit*, or *Sl/SCF* (*c-kit* ligand) loci. In The Role of the Mast Cell in Health and Disease, edited by M. A. Kaliner and D. D. Metcalfe. Marcel Dekker, New York, in press.
45. Galli, S. J., Wershil, B. K., Gordon, J. R., and Martin, T. R. (1989): Mast cells: Immunologically specific effectors and potential sources of multiple cytokines during IgE-dependent responses. In IgE, Mast Cells and the Allergic Response, Ciba Foundation Symposium No. 147, edited by D. Chadwick, D. Evered, and J. Whelan, pp. 53–73. John Wiley and Sons, Ltd., Chichester, UK.
46. Geissler, E. N., and Russell, E. S. (1983): Analysis of hematopoietic effects of new dominant spotting (*W*) mutants of the mouse. II. Effects on mast cell development. *Exp. Hematol.*, 11:461–466.
46a. Geissler, E. N., Ryan, M. A., and Housman, D. E. (1988): The dominant-white spotting (*W*) locus of the mouse encodes the *c-kit* proto-oncogene. *Cell*, 55:185–192.
47. Ginsburg, H. (1963): The *in vitro* differentiation and culture of normal mast cells from mouse thymus. *Ann. N.Y. Acad. Sci.*, 103:20–30.
48. Ginsburg, H., and Lagunoff, D. (1967): The *in vitro* differentiation of mast cells. Cultures of cells from immunized mouse lymph nodes and thoracic duct lymph on fibroblast monolayers. *J. Cell Biol.*, 35:685–697.

49. Goetzl, E. J., Charnov-Regan, T., Furuichi, K., Goetzl, L. M., Lee, J. Y., and Renold, F. (1986): Neuromodulation of mast cell and basophil formation. In Mast Cell Differentiation and Heterogeneity, edited by A. D. Befus, J. Bienenstock, and J. A. Denburg, pp. 223–229. Raven Press, New York.

50. Gordon, J. R., Burd, P. R., and Galli, S. J. (1990): Mast cells as a source of multifunctional cytokines. *Immunology Today*, 11:458–64.

51. Gordon, J. R., and Galli, S. J. (1990): Mast cells as a source of both preformed and immunologically inducible TNF-α/cachectin. *Nature*, 346:274–276.

52. Gordon, J. R., and Galli, S. J. (1990): Phorbol 12-myristate 13-acetate-induced development of functionally active mast cells in W/W^v but not Sl/Sl^d genetically mast cell-deficient mice. *Blood*, 75:1637–1645.

53. Green, M. C. (1966): Mutant genes and linkages. In Biology of the Laboratory Mouse, Second Edition, edited by E. L. Green, pp. 87–150. McGraw-Hill, New York.

54. Guy-Grand, D., Dy, M., Luffau, G., and Vassalli, P. (1984): Gut mucosal mast cells. *J. Exp. Med.*, 160:12–28.

55. Ha, T.-Y., Reed, N. D., and Crowle, P. K. (1986): Immunologic response potential of mast cell-deficient W/W^v mice. *Int. Arch. Allergy Appl. Immunol.*, 80:85–94.

56. Haig, D. M., McKee, T. A., Jarrett, E. E. E., Woodbury, R., and Miller, H. R. P. (1982): Generation of mucosal mast cells is stimulated *in vitro* by factors derived from T cells of helminth-infected rats. *Nature* (London), 300:188–190.

57. Haig, D. M., McMenamin, C., and Jarrett, E. E. E. (1986): Mast cell development in the rat. In Mast Cell Differentiation and Heterogeneity, edited by A. D. Befus, J. Bienenstock, and J. A. Denburg, pp. 55–62. Raven Press, New York.

58. Halpern, B.-N., Benacerraf, B., and Biozzi, G. (1953): Quantitative study of the granulopectic activity of the reticulo-endothelial system. I. The effect of the ingredients present in India ink and of substances affecting blood clotting *in vivo* on the fate of carbon particles administered intravenously in rats, mice and rabbits. *Br. J. Exp. Pathol.*, 34:426–440.

59. Halpern, B.-N., Biozzi, G., Mene, G., and Benacerraf, B. (1951): Etude quantitative de l'activite granulopexique du systeme reticulo-endothelial par l'injection intraveineuse d'encre de Chine chez les diverses especes animales. I. Methode d'etude quantitative de l'activite granulopexique du systeme reticulo-endothelial par l'injection intraveineuse de particules de carbone de dimension connues. *Ann. Inst. Pasteur*, 80:582–604.

60. Ihle, J. N., Keller, J., Oroszlan, S., Henderson, L. E., Copeland, T. D., Fitch, F., Prystowsky, M. B., Goldwasser, E., Schrader, J. W., Palaszynski, E., Dy, M., and Lebel, B. (1983): Biological properties of homogeneous interleukin-3. I. Demonstration of WEHI-3 growth-factor activity, mast cell growth-factor activity, P cell-stimulating factor activity, colony-stimulating factor activity, and histamine-producing cell-stimulating factor activity. *J. Immunol.*, 131:282–287.

61. Ishizaka, T., and Ishizaka, K. (1984): Activation of mast cells for mediator release through IgE receptors. *Prog. Allergy*, 34:188–235.

62. Ishizaka, T., Okudaira, H., Mauser, L. E., and Ishizaka, K. (1976): Development of rat mast cells *in vitro*. I. Differentiation of mast cells from thymus cells. *J. Immunol.*, 116:747–754.

63. Kanakura, Y., Thompson, H., Nakano, T., Yamamura, T., Asai, H., Kitamura, Y., Metcalfe, D. D., and Galli, S. J. (1988): Bidirectional alterations of phenotype and changes in proliferative potential during the passage of mouse peritoneal mast cells *in vitro* and *in vivo*. *Blood*, 72:877–885.

64. Kitamura, Y., and Go, S. (1979): Decreased production of mast cells in Sl/Sl^d anemic mice. *Blood*, 53:492–497.

65. Kitamura, Y., Go, S., and Hatanaka, S. (1978): Decrease of mast cells in W/W^v mice and their increase by bone marrow transplantation. *Blood*, 52:447–452.

66. Kitamura, Y., Nakayama, H., and Fujita, J. (1989): Mechanisms of mast cell deficiency in mutant mice of W/W^v and Sl/Sl^d genotype. In Mast Cell and Basophil Differentiation and Function in Health and Disease, edited by S. J. Galli and K. F. Austen, pp. 15–25. Raven Press, New York.

67. Kitamura, Y., Sonoda, T., and Yokoyama, M. (1983): Differentiation of tissue mast cells. In Hematopoietic Stem Cells, Alfred Benzon Symposium 18, edited by Sy-Aa Killmann, E. P. Cronkite, and C. N. Muller-Berat, pp. 350–361. Munkegaard, Copenhagen.

68. Kitamura, Y., Taguchi, T., Yokoyama, M., Yamatodani, A., Asano, H., Koyama, T., Kanamaru, A., Hatanaka, K., Wershil, B. K., and Galli, S. J. (1986): Higher susceptibility of mast cell-deficient W/W^v mutant mice to brain thromboembolism and death caused by intravenous injection of India ink. *Am. J. Pathol.*, 122:469–480.

69. Kitamura, Y., Yokoyama, M., Matsuda, H., Ohno, T., and Mori, K. J. (1981). Spleen colony-forming cell as common precursor for tissue mast cells and granulocytes. *Nature* (London), 291:159–160.
70. Kops, S. K., Ratzlaff, R. E., Meade, R., Iverson, G. M., and Askenase, P. W. (1986): Interaction of antigen-specific T cell factors with unique "receptors" on the surface of mast cells: Demonstration *in vitro* by an indirect rosetting technique. *J. Immunol.*, 136:4515–4524.
71. Kowalski, M. L., Sliwinska-Kowalska, M., and Kaliner, M. A. (1990): Neurogenic inflammation, vascular permeability, and mast cells. II. Additional evidence indicating that mast cells are not involved in neurogenic inflammation. *J. Immunol.*, 145:1214–1221.
72. Lagunoff, D. (1966): Structural aspects of histamine binding: The mast cell granule. In Mechanisms of Release of Biogenic Amines, pp. 79–94. Pergamon Press, Oxford.
73. Lagunoff, D., and Benditt, E. P. (1963): Proteolytic enzymes of mast cells. *Ann. N.Y. Acad. Sci.*, 103:185–197.
74. Lee, F., Yokota, T., Otsuka, T., Meyerson, P., Villaret, D., Coffman, R., Mosmann, T., Rennick, D., Roehm, N., Smith, C., Zlotnick, A., and Arai, K.-I. (1986): Isolation and characterization of a mouse interleukin cDNA clone that expresses B cell stimulatory factor 1 activities and T-cell- and mast cell-stimulating activities. *Proc. Natl. Acad. Sci. U.S.A.*, 83:2061–2065.
75. Levi-Schaffer, F., Austen, K. F., Gravallese, P. M., and Stevens, R. L. (1986): Coculture of interleukin 3-dependent mouse mast cells with fibroblasts results in a phenotypic change of the mast cells. *Proc. Natl. Acad. Sci. U.S.A.*, 83:6485–6488.
76. Lewis, J. P., O'Grady, L. F., Bernstein, S. E., Russell, E. S., and Trobaugh, F. E., Jr. (1967): Growth and differentiation of transplanted W/W^v marrow. *Blood*, 30:601–610.
77. Lichtenstein, L. M., Fox, C. C., Schleimer, R. P., Proud, D., Naclerio, R. M., and Kagey-Sobotka, A. (1986): Heterogeneity in human histamine-containing cells. In Mast Cell Differentiation and Heterogeneity, edited by A. D. Befus, Bienenstock, J., and Denburg, J. A., pp. 331–345. Raven Press, New York.
78. Liu, F.-T., Bohn, J. W., Ferry, E. L., Yamamoto, H., Molinaro, C. A., Sherman, L. A., Klinman, N. R., and Katz, D. H. (1980): Monoclonal dinitrophenol-specific murine IgE antibody: Preparation, isolation, and characterization. *J. Immunol.*, 124:2728–2737.
79. Marcum, J. A., McKenney, J. B., Galli, S. J., Jackman, R. W., and Rosenberg, R. D. (1986): Anticoagulantly active heparin-like molecules from mast cell-deficient mice. *Am. J. Physiol.*, 250:H879–H888.
80. Matsuda, H., Kawakita, K., Kiso, Y., Nakano, T., and Kitamura, Y. (1989): Substance P induces granulocyte infiltration through degranulation of mast cells. *J. Immunol.*, 142:927–931.
81. Matsuda, H., Nakano, T., Kiso, Y., and Kitamura, Y. (1987): Normalization of anti-tick response of mast cell-deficient W/W^v mice by intracutaneous injection of cultured mast cells. *J. Parasitol.*, 73:155–160.
82. Matsuda, H., Watanabe, N., Kiso, Y., Hirota, S., Ushio, H., Kannan, Y., Azuma, M., Koyama, H., and Kitamura, Y. (1990): Necessity of IgE antibodies and mast cells for manifestation of resistance against larval *Haemaphysalis longicornis* ticks in mice. *J. Immunol.*, 144:259–262.
83. McCulloch, E. A., Siminovitch, L., and Till, J. E. (1964): Spleen-colony formation in anemic mice of genotype *W/W*. *Science*, 144:844–846.
84. Mekori, Y. A., Chang, J. C. C., Wershil, B. K., and Galli, S. J. (1987): Studies of the role of mast cells in contact sensitivity responses: Passive transfer of the reaction into mast cell-deficient mice locally reconstituted with cultured mast cells; effect of reserpine on transfer of the reaction with DNP-specific cloned T cells. *Cell Immunol.*, 109:39–53.
85. Mekori, Y. A., Dvorak, H. F., and Galli, S. J. (1986): ^{125}I-fibrin deposition in contact sensitivity reactions in the mouse. Sensitivity of the assay for quantitating reactions after active or passive transfer. *J. Immunol.*, 136:2018–2025.
86. Mekori, Y. A., and Galli, S. J. (1985): Undiminished immunological tolerance to contact sensitivity in mast cell-deficient W/W^v and Sl/Sl^d mice. *J. Immunol.*, 135:879–885.
87. Mekori, Y. A., and Galli, S. J. (1990): [125I]Fibrin deposition occurs at both early and late intervals of IgE-dependent and contact sensitivity reactions elicited in mouse skin. Mast cell-dependent augmentation of fibrin deposition at early intervals in combined IgE-dependent and contact sensitivity reactions. *J. Immunol.*, in press.
88. Mekori, Y. A., Weitzman, G. L., and Galli, S. J. (1985): Reevaluation of reserpine-induced suppression of contact sensitivity. Evidence that reserpine interferes with T lymphocyte function independently of an effect on mast cells. *J. Exp. Med.*, 162:1935–1953.

89. Metcalf, D. (1986): The molecular biology and functions of the granulocyte-macrophage colony stimulating factors. *Blood*, 67:257–267.
90. Metcalfe, D. D., Kaliner, M., and Donlon, M. A. (1981): The mast cell. *CRC Crit. Rev. Immunol.*, 2:23–74.
91. Nabel, G., Galli, S. J., Dvorak, A. M., Dvorak, H. F., and Cantor, H. (1981): Inducer T lymphocytes synthesize a factor that stimulates proliferation of cloned mast cells. *Nature* (London), 291:332–334.
92. Nagao, K., Yokoro, K., and Aaronson, S. A. (1981): Continuous lines of basophil/mast cells derived from normal mouse bone marrow. *Science*, 212:333–335.
93. Nakano, T., Kanakura, Y., Nakahata, T., Matsuda, H., and Kitamura, Y. (1987): Genetically mast cell-deficient *W/W*ᵛ mice as a tool for investigations about differentiation and function of mast cells. *Fed. Proc.*, 46:1920–1923.
94. Nakano, T., Sonoda, T., Hayashi, C., Yamatodani, A., Kanayama, Y., Yamamura, T., Asai, H., Yonezawa, Y., Kitamura, Y., and Galli, S. J. (1985): Fate of bone marrow-derived cultured mast cells after intracutaneous, intraperitoneal and intravenous transfer into genetically mast cell-deficient *W/W*ᵛ mice. Evidence that cultured mast cells can give rise to both connective tissue-type and mucosal mast cells. *J. Exp. Med.*, 162:1025–1043.
95. Noma, Y., Sideras, P., Naito, T., Bergstedt-Lindquist, S., Azuma, C., Severinson, E., Tanabe, T., Kinashi, T., Matsuda, F., Yaoita, Y., and Honjo, T. (1986): Cloning of cDNA encoding the murine IgGl induction factor by a novel strategy using SP6 promoter. *Nature* (London), 319:640–646.
96. Old, L. J. (1985): Tumor necrosis factor (TNF). *Science*, 230:630–633.
97. Otsu, K., Nakano, I., Kanakura, Y., Asai, H., Katz, H. R., Austen, K. F., Stevens, R. L., Galli, S. J., and Kitamura, Y. (1987): Phenotypic changes of bone marrow-derived mast cells after intraperitoneal transfer into *W/W*ᵛ mice that are genetically deficient in mast cells. *J. Exp. Med.*, 165:615–627.
98. Padawer, J. (1979): The mast cell and immediate hypersensitivity. In Immediate Hypersensitivity, edited by M. K. Bach, pp. 301–367. Marcel Dekker, New York.
99. Parker, C. W. (1984): Mediators: Release and function. In Fundamental Immunology, edited by W. E. Paul, pp. 697–747. Raven Press, New York.
100. Pretlow, T. G., and Cassady, I. M. (1970): Separation of mast cells in successive stages of differentiation using programmed gradient sedimentation. *Am. J. Pathol.*, 61:323–338.
101. Qureshi, R., and Jakschik, B. A. (1988): The role of mast cells in thioglycollate-induced inflammation. *J. Immunol.*, 141:2090–2096.
102. Ramos, B. F., Qureshi, R., Olsen, K. M., and Jakschik, B. A. (1990): The importance of mast cells for the neutrophil influx in immune complex-induced peritonitis in mice. *J. Immunol.*, 145:1–6.
103. Ranadive, N. S., and Menon, I. A. (1986): Role of reactive oxygen species and free radicals from melanins in photoinduced cutaneous inflammations. *Pathol. Immunopathol. Res.*, 5:118–139.
104. Ranadive, N. S., Shirwadkar, S., Persad, S., and Menon, I. A. (1986): Effects of melanin-induced free radicals on the isolated rat peritoneal mast cells. *J. Invest. Dermatol.*, 86:503–507.
105. Razin, E., Cordon-Cardo, C., and Good, R. A. (1981): Growth of a pure population of mouse mast cells *in vitro* with conditioned medium derived from concanavalin A-stimulated splenocytes. *Proc. Natl. Acad. Sci. U.S.A.*, 28:2559–2561.
106. Razin, E., Stevens, R. L., Akiyama, F., Schmidt, K., and Austen, K. F. (1982): Culture from mouse bone marrow of a subclass of mast cells possessing a distinct chondroitin sulfate proteoglycan with glycosaminoglycans rich in N-acetylgalactosamine-4, 6-disulfate. *J. Biol. Chem.*, 257:7229–7236.
107. Rennick, D., Lee, F. D., Yokota, T., Arai, K.-I., Cantor, H., and Nabel, G. (1985): A cloned MCGF cDNA encodes a multilineage hematopoietic growth factor: Multiple activities of interleukin-3. *J. Immunol.*, 134:910–914.
108. Rohlich, P., and Csaba, G. (1972): Alcian blue-safranine staining and ultrastructure of rat mast cell granules during degranulation. *Acta Biol. Acad. Hung.*, 23:83–89.
109. Rosenberg, R. D., Marcum, J. A., and Reilly, C. F. (1986): The role of specific forms of heparin sulfate in regulating blood vessel wall function. *Prog. Hemost. Thromb.*, 9:185–215.
110. Russell, E. S. (1979): Hereditary anemias of the mouse: A review for geneticists. *Adv. Genet.*, 20:357–459.
111. Schiller, S., and Dorfman, A. (1959): The isolation of heparin from mast cells of the normal rat. *Biochim. Biophys. Acta*, 31:276–280.

112. Schrader, J. W. (1981): The *in vitro* production and cloning of the P cell, a bone marrow-derived null cell that expresses H-2 and Ia-antigens, has mast cell-like granules, and is regulated by a factor released by activated T cells. *J. Immunol.*, 126:452–458.
113. Schwartz, L. B., and Austen, K. F. (1984): Structure and function of the chemical mediators of mast cells. *Prog. Allergy*, 34:271–321.
114. Selye, H. (1965): The Mast Cells. Washington: Butterworths.
114a. Serafin, W. E., and Austen, K. F. (1987): Mediators of immediate hypersensitivity reactions. *N. Engl. J. Med.*, 317:30–34.
115. Shevach, E. M. (1984): Macrophages and other accessory cells. In Fundamental Immunology, edited by W. E. Paul, pp. 71–107. Raven Press, New York.
116. Sonoda, T., Kanayama, Y., Hara, H., Hayashi, C., Tadokoro, M., Yonezawa, T., and Kitamura, Y. (1984): Proliferation of peritoneal mast cells in the skin of W/W^v mice that genetically lack mast cells. *J. Exp. Med.*, 160:138–151.
117. Sonoda, S., Sonoda, T., Nakano, T., Kanayama, Y., Kanakura, Y., Asai, H., Yonezawa, T., and Kitamura, Y. (1986): Development of mucosal mast cells after injection of a single connective tissue-type mast cell in the stomach-mucosa of genetically mast cell-deficient W/W^v mice. *J. Immunol.*, 137:1319–1322.
118. Sredni, B., Friedman, M. M., Bland, C. E., and Metcalfe, D. D. (1983): Ultrastructural, biochemical and functional characteristics of histamine-containing cells cloned from mouse bone marrow: Tentative identification as mucosal mast cells. *J. Immunol.*, 131:915–922.
119. Starkey, J. R., Crowle, P. K., and Taubenberger, S. (1988): Mast cell-deficient W/W^v mice exhibit a decreased rate of tumor angiogenesis. *Int. J. Cancer*, 42:48–52.
120. Steeves, E. B. T., and Allen, J. R. (1990): Basophils in skin reactions of mast cell-deficient mice infested with *Dermacentor variabilis*. *Int. J. Pathol.*, 20:655–667.
121. Stevens, R. L., Katz, H. R., Seldin, D. S., and Austen, K. F. (1986): Biochemical characteristics distinguish subclasses of mammalian mast cells. In Mast Cell Differentiation and Heterogeneity, edited by A. D. Befus, J. Bienenstock, and J. A. Denburg, pp. 183–204. Raven Press, New York.
122. Tertian, G., Yung, Y.-P., Guy-Grand, D., and Moore, M. A. S. (1981): Long-term *in vitro* culture of murine mast cells. I. Description of a growth factor-dependent culture technique. *J. Immunol.*, 127:788–794.
123. Thomas, W. R., and Schrader, J. W. (1983): Delayed hypersensitivity in mast cell-deficient mice. *J. Immunol.*, 130:2565–2567.
124. Tsai, M, Takeishi, T., Thompson, H., Langley, K. E., Zsebo, K. M., Metcalfe, D. D., Geissler, E. N., and Galli, S. J. (1991): Induction of mast cell proliferation, maturation and heparin synthesis by the rat c-kit ligand, stem cell factor. *Proc. Natl. Acad. Sci. U.S.A.*, 88:6382–6386.
124a. Tsai, M., Shih, L.-S., Newlands, G. F. J., Takeishi, T., Langley, K. E., Zsebo, K. M., Miller, H. R. P., Geissler, E. N., and Galli, S. J. (1991): The rat c-kit ligand, stem cell factor, induces the development of connective tissue-type and mucosal mast cells in vivo. Analysis by anatomical distribution, histochemistry and protese phenotype. *J. Exp. Med.* 174:125–131.
125. Weitzman, G., Galli, S. J., Dvorak, A. M., and Hammel, I. (1985): Cloned mouse mast cells and normal mouse peritoneal mast cells. Determination of serotonin content and ability to synthesize serotonin *in vitro*. *Int. Arch. Allergy Appl. Immunol.*, 77:189–191.
126. Wershil, B. K., and Galli, S. J. (1986): Pathogenesis of acute gastric injury in mice: H1 but not H2 antihistamines diminish the augmented vascular permeability and hemorrhagic erosions produced by oral ethanol. *Gastroenterology*, 90:1688 (abstract).
127. Wershil, B. K., Mekori, Y. A., Murakami, T., and Galli, S. J. (1986): Diminished croton oil-induced acute inflammation in mast-cell-deficient (W/W^v and Sl/Sl^d) mice. *Fed. Proc.*, 45:1104 (abstract).
128. Wershil, B. K., Mekori, Y. A., Murakami, T., and Galli, S. J. (1987): ^{125}I-Fibrin deposition in IgE-dependent immediate hypersensitivity reactions in mouse skin. Demonstration of the role of mast cells using genetically mast cell-deficient mice locally reconstituted with cultured mast cells. *J. Immunol.*, 139:2605–2614.
129. Wershil, B. K., Murakami, T., and Galli, S. J. (1988): Mast cell-dependent amplification of an immunologically nonspecific inflammatory response. Mast cells are required for the full expression of cutaneous acute inflammation induced by phorbol 12-myristate 13-acetate. *J. Immunol.*, 140:2356–2360.
130. Wershil, B. K., Wang, Z-S, Gordon, J. R., and Galli, S. J. (1991): Recruitment of neutrophils during IgE-dependent cutaneous late phase responses in the mouse is mast cell dependent: Partial

inhibition of the reaction with antiserum against tumor necrosis factor-alpha. *J. Clin. Invest.*, 87:446–453.

131. Woodbury, R. G., Everitt, M., Katanuma, N., Lagunoff, D., and Neurath, H. (1978): A major serine protease in skeletal muscle. Evidence for its mast cell origin. *Proc. Natl. Acad. Sci. U.S.A.*, 75:5311–5313.

132. Woodbury, R. G., Gruzenski, G. M., and Lagunoff, D. (1978): Immunofluorescent localization of a serine protease in rat small intestine. *Proc. Natl. Acad. Sci. U.S.A.*, 75:2785–2789.

133. Woodbury, R. G., and Neurath, H. (1980): Structure, specificity and localization of the serine proteases of connective tissue. *FEBS Lett.*, 114:189–196.

134. Wright, H. D. (1927): Experimental pneumococcal septicemia and anti-pneumococcal immunity. *J. Pathol. Bacteriol.*, 30:185–252.

135. Yano, H., Wershil, B. K., Arizono, N., and Galli, S. J. (1989): Substance P-induced augmentation of cutaneous vascular permeability and granulocyte infiltration in mice is mast cell-dependent. *J. Clin. Invest.*, 84:1276–1286.

136. Yokota, T., Lee, F., Rennick, D., Hall, C., Arai, N., Mosman, T., Nabel, G., Cantor, H., and Arai, K. (1984): Isolation and characterization of a mouse cDNA clone that expresses mast-cell growth-factor activity in monkey cells. *Proc. Natl. Acad. Sci. U.S.A.*, 81:1070–1074.

137. Young, J. D.-E., Liu, C. C., Butler, G., Cohn, Z. A., and Galli, S. J. (1987): Identification, purification and characterization of a mast cell-associated cytolytic factor related to tumor necrosis factor. *Proc. Natl. Acad. Sci. U.S.A.*, 84:9175–9179.

138. Yung, Y.-P., and Moore, M. A. S. (1983): Mast cell growth factor. *Lymphokine Res.*, 2:127–131.

139. Yurt, R. W., and Austen, K. F. (1977): Preparative purification of rat mast cell chymase. Characterization and interaction with granule components. *J. Exp. Med.*, 146:1405–1419.

140. Yurt, R. W., Leid, R. W., Austen, K. F., and Silbert, J. E. (1977): Native heparin from rat peritoneal mast cells. *J. Biol. Chem.*, 252:518–521.

141. Zsebo, K. M., Williams, D. A., Geissler, E. N., Broudy, V., Martin, F. H., Atkins, H., Hsu, R.-Y., Birkett, N. C., Okino, K. H., Murdock, D., Jacobsen, F. W., Langley, K. E., Smith, K. A., Takeishi, T., Cattanach, B. M., Galli, S. J., and Suggs, S. V. (1990): Stem cell factor (SCF) is encoded at the *Sl* locus of the mouse and is the ligand for the *c-kit* tyrosine kinase receptor. *Cell*, 63:213–224.

Clinical Immunotoxicology, edited by
D. S. Newcombe, N. R. Rose, and J. C. Bloom.
Raven Press, Ltd., New York, 1992.

6

Toxicity of Monoclonal Antibodies and Conjugates

Ira Berkower

*Department of Biochemistry and Biophysics, Office of Biologics,
Food and Drug Administration, National Institutes of Health,
Bethesda, MD*

ADVANTAGES AND PROPOSED USES

Monoclonal antibodies have several potential advantages as specific reagents for a variety of diagnostic and therapeutic applications. First, the uniformity of the antibody ensures that it will behave essentially the same way each time it is used. If its safety and efficacy are proved in clinical trials, then substantially the same performance would be expected for subsequent clinical use. Second, hybridoma technology ensures a virtually limitless supply of the product. Third, it is possible to produce a monoclonal antibody that is specific for a cell surface antigen without purifying the antigen or absorbing a polyclonal serum. Finally, antibodies to a variety of cell surface markers can be generated without knowing in advance which antigens are selectively expressed by each cell type.

Monoclonal antibodies have been used alone or after chemical modification for diagnosis or treatment. In some cases, the unmodified monoclonal antibody can have a direct therapeutic effect such as depletion of a specific cell type simply by binding to the cell surface. In other cases, such as immunotherapy for cancer, destruction of cancer cells may require the additional activity of a toxin coupled to the antibody: antibody binding is followed by toxin-mediated killing of the target cells (1). Finally, diagnostic imaging has been attempted by labeling the monoclonal antibody with a radioisotope. Bound antibody emits a signal that reveals the size and location of the target tissue. Once specific labeling of a tumor can be demonstrated in this way, it is tempting to try to destroy the tumor cells by delivering a much higher local radiation dose via the monoclonal antibody or by using a toxin coupled to the same antibody.

LIMITATIONS

Despite these promising characteristics, there are several ways that toxicity or other undesirable effects can limit the clinical usefulness of monoclonals and their conjugates. First, monoclonality does not imply monospecificity. Thus, a monoclonal antibody specific for one cell type may also bind to a less differentiated stem cell in the same lineage, or it may even bind to an "unrelated" cell in another system. For example, there is significant cross-reactivity of antibodies to the murine T-cell marker Thy-1 on brain cells. The cross-reacting cells may express the same antigen at lower surface density, or they may express a slightly different antigen that is recognized by the same monoclonal antibody at lower affinity. In either case, cytotoxic therapy directed to one cell type could also affect the other cells.

Second, with regard to diagnostic imaging, the quality of the image depends on the physiology of the labeled monoclonal antibody, which is largely the same as for any foreign immunoglobulin (2). After injection, the monoclonal antibody distributes rapidly in the circulating blood volume. Early images simply reflect the blood flow to each organ. Over time, the labeled antibodies gradually leave the circulation to enter tissues and lymphatics. The redistribution to tissues is the rate-limiting step in the binding of antibodies to tumor cells for imaging. At the same time, unbound antibody is cleared steadily by the reticuloendothelial (RE) system, where it is degraded, and this releases the isotope in the liver and spleen. For a mouse monoclonal antibody given to a human, the half-life for intact IgG is about 5 to 7 days. Most images are taken during this time and reflect a mixture of the desired signal with the signal from unbound antibodies in the circulation, antibodies passing through normal tissues and lymphatics, and antibodies already degraded in the RE system of the liver and spleen. When imaging is performed at various time points, the signal from the tumor may be less than the background signal from these other sources. Detection of tumor metastases to the liver could be particularly difficult, because of the high background signal from immunoglobulins cleared by the RE system. One way to improve the signal is to use antibody fragments that leave the circulation and enter tissues more quickly and are cleared by different pathways. For example, antibodies can be cleaved to $F(ab')_2$ fragments that contain the variable regions and hence retain the antigen-binding sites but lack the Fc tails by which antibodies are removed from the circulation by the RE system. These fragments retain the high affinity of dimeric immunoglobulins but spend less time in the circulation (<1 day) and are cleared by the kidneys rather than the RE system. Thus, they could potentially be used for imaging the liver or highly perfused organs. Even smaller fragments such as Fab monomers (which are cleared from the circulation in hours) might work, but they suffer from a lower affinity than dimers of the same intrinsic affinity.

For diagnostic imaging, antibody physiology is also important in choosing an isotope that will give the greatest signal with the lowest tissue dose. The absorbed dose depends on the number of millicuries given and on the half-life of the conjugate: therefore a short half-life is desirable. The optimal conjugate is obtained when the physical half-life of the isotope matches the biological half-life of the labeled antibody (3). Thus, for intact immunoglobulins, the half-life of the isotope should be 1 week or less, and for $F(ab')_2$ fragments it should be 1 or 2 days. These considerations suggest that we switch away from using ^{125}I with a physical half-life of 60 days toward [131]I (half-life of 6 days), [111]In (half-life of 2.8 days), [123]I (half-life of 13 hours), or [99m]Tc (half-life of 6 hours).

The choice of isotope is particularly important when attempting to deliver therapeutic doses of radiation via labeled monoclonal antibodies. Besides matching the half-life of the carrier protein, the isotope becomes an internal source and should deliver the maximum radiation effect within the tumor and not to vital organs nearby. Thus, gamma radiation, which is good for imaging because the rays interact very little with tissues of water density, may not be optimal for therapy. However, radiation that interacts more strongly with tissues, i.e., has high linear energy transfer, is better for radiotherapy from an internal source of radiation. For example, alpha rays (which have both mass and charge, unlike gamma rays) readily transfer their energy to tissues, coursing extensive radiation damage over a short path length. Thus, alpha-emitting isotopes such as [212]Bi concentrate the radiation damage in a small volume around the target (4). When such isotopes are guided to a tumor by monoclonal antibodies, the therapeutic effect could be delivered precisely to the tumor cells plus a narrow layer of normal cells extending just a few cell diameters (50 to 80 μ, the width of a human hair) into the normal tissues surrounding the tumor. The total dose could be increased because less radiation reaches vital organs, and the entire dose would be received where it is needed. However, the short physical half-life of [212]Bi (60 minutes) suggests that it should be coupled to an antibody fragment so it can reach the tumor rapidly and deliver the full dose of radiation to the tumor cells.

The quality of a diagnostic image also depends on the nature of the chemical bond between the isotope and the immunoglobulin. Different bonds are degraded at different rates in different organs. The earliest labeling method for antibodies was iodination with [125]I. However, many tissues have a dehalogenase activity that uncouples the iodine label from the antibody. This reduces the specific labeling of the tumor and increases nonspecific labeling, particularly of the thyroid gland. Subsequently, labeling methods have been developed in which metal isotopes are bound by chelators that are covalently attached to the monoclonal antibody. For example, the chelator diethylenetriamine penta-acetic acid (DTPA) can be coupled to the monoclonal antibody, and it will take up ^{111}In with an affinity of 10^{-28}M. However, these conjugates are subject to loss of the metal ion due to transchelation, in which the metal ion is transferred to the carrier protein transferrin. Transferrin then efficiently transports the isotope to the liver and spleen, where it is taken up readily via the transferrin receptor. This results in significant nonspecific background labeling and makes it very difficult to scan the liver for metastases, which is often the point of the radiological study.

Similar considerations apply when the goal is to use antibody specificity as a guidance system to deliver toxins to tumor cells. Toxins such as ricin have been used to render tumor-specific monoclonal antibodies highly toxic (1, 5). Ricin is a very potent toxin, and one molecule is reportedly able to kill one cell. Native ricin normally consists of an A chain that turns off protein synthesis by inactivating the 60s ribosomal subunit and a B chain that has the binding affinity for the cell membrane and helps the A chain to translocate across membranes to gain access to the cytoplasm. By removing the B chain and coupling the A chain to a monoclonal antibody, the toxin gains the desired specificity. As with radionuclides, the coupling method is critical, since the bond must be strong enough to survive the trip through the serum but labile enough to allow ricin A chain to uncouple from the immunoglobulin chains inside the cell and to escape from endosomes into the cytoplasm, where it turns off protein synthesis. In addition, the coupling method must not damage the antibody (as this could interfere with antibody specificity and affinity) but must be complete enough that no free toxin remains in the product. At this time, the favored coupling method is via disulfide bonds between the ricin A chain and the monoclonal antibody, which appear to meet all the above requirements.

Even with a good toxin-antibody conjugate, there are still several hurdles to be overcome before an immunotoxin can be considered to have therapeutic potential. As mentioned above, the tumor antigen may be present on normal cells in the same or a different lineage. The enhanced toxicity of a ricin-antibody conjugate may prove too much for the normal tissue, particularly if the cross-reacting antigen is expressed on a small number of stem cells that are rapidly multiplying to replenish a larger pool of differentiated cells. Second, the normal metabolism of immunoglobulins by the RE system may release toxic levels of ricin A chain locally in the liver and spleen. This is compounded by the ability of free ricin A chain formed at other sites to bind to RE cells. Third, the ability of the antibody-toxin complex to reach the tumor may be limited by poor blood supply to the tumor or by the release of tumor antigens into the circulation; therefore the antibody is bound up in circulating complexes before it can reach the tumor. Fourth, the biology of the tumor itself may limit the effectiveness of immunotoxin therapy by varying the expression of the marker antigen among different clones of the tumor, modulating the antigen from the cell surface or metabolizing the toxin before it can kill the cells. Finally, the host immune response to the complex of two foreign proteins (antibody and toxin) may produce human antibodies to either component, which can block the cytotoxic effect of the complex.

CLINICAL TOXICITY

To date, monoclonal antibodies have been tested clinically in three different constructs, and each has its own toxic or untoward effects. Unmodified monoclonal antibodies specific for T cells have been found to cause marked depletion of T cells, resulting in profound suppression of cell-mediated immunity. This effect has been used to reverse the acute rejection of kidney allografts. Second, ricin A chains conjugated to antibodies specific for tumor antigens have been used to treat cancer. Third, radiolabeled monoclonals specific for tumor markers have been used to label tumors for diagnostic imaging. In each case, toxicity can result from an immediate direct effect of the monoclonal antibody, a delayed effect of the monoclonal antibody or its metabolites, or an effect of the host's immune response to the foreign protein.

OKT3 was the first monoclonal antibody licensed for human use. The antigen receptor complex of T cells is known to consist of at least six components (6), and OKT3 is specific for the 25 kilodaltons component known as the delta chain (7). Treatment of T cells *in vitro* with OKT3 results in modulation of the entire receptor complex, which causes immunological paralysis of the cells. *In vivo* treatment also results in marked and very rapid depletion of all circulating mature T cells. After the first 5-mg dose of OKT3, there are no detectable T cells within 5 minutes, and daily infusion of 5 mg results in no detectable T cells for up to 10 to 14 days (8). This is not simply owing to modulation of the T-cell receptor complex, since the number of cells bearing other T-cell markers such as CD4 and CD8 is also markedly reduced. Most renal transplantation is done with a kidney that is partially mismatched with the HLA histocompatibility antigens of the recipient. In the majority of cases, this results in acute rejection of the graft, which is mediated by host T cells responding to the foreign HLA antigens. Removal of all circulating T cells by OKT3 treatment reverses the acute rejection episode in about 90% of the cases (9).

The toxic effects of OKT3 therapy can be divided into acute and chronic (9). With the first or second dose, nearly all patients experience fever and chills. In some cases, these can be severe, and they may be accompanied by bronchospasm that may progress to pulmonary edema, particularly if the patient is well hydrated. Interestingly, this syndrome is not observed after subsequent doses of the monoclonal antibody, when the T cell numbers are already very low. It appears to be caused by the rapid destruction of circulating T cells, with the simultaneous release of numerous lymphokines and mediators of inflammation that are stored in these cells. Pulmonary edema can be prevented by ensuring that the patient is in good fluid balance (e.g., returned to his or her dry weight by dialysis if necessary) before the treatment is given. In addition, antihistamines and steroids are given prior to the first dose of OKT3 to minimize the effects of mediator release.

Not surprisingly for this extent of immunosuppression, opportunistic infections may occur, including the reactivation of latent viral infections. This may be manifested as acute nonbacterial meningitis (10), or the effects may occur long after the period of maximal immunosuppression of the host. Renal transplant patients treated with OKT3 have significant reactivation of Epstein-Barr virus as measured by rising titers of antibodies to the viral capsid antigen (11). Subsequently, they may develop a polyclonal B-cell lymphoproliferation syndrome with rapidly enlarging lymph nodes. In three cases that resulted from treatment with other monoclonals specific for T cells, the B cells contained Epstein-Barr virus DNA and expressed Epstein-Barr virus nuclear antigen (12). This syndrome strongly resembles the B-cell lymphoproliferation syndrome formerly observed when excessively high doses of cyclosporine A were used to treat graft rejection (13–15), although the latter proliferation could often be terminated by discontinuing the drug (16). It is unclear when the enlarging lymph nodes cease to be a reversible polyclonal proliferation and convert to an irreversible malignancy. Some physicians recommend acyclovir to prevent or treat the early phase of the lymphoproliferation syndrome, when its antiviral effect may block the Epstein-Barr virus–induced proliferation. These immunosuppressive effects of OKT3 and cyclosporine A can be mimicked *in vitro*, where either agent can greatly enhance the outgrowth of Epstein-Barr virus lines from peripheral blood lymphocytes (17). Fortunately, the lymphoproliferation syndrome is quite rare at the dose used in renal allograft rejection, and to some extent this may reflect the care and moderation of the physicians who are inducing the immunosuppressed state.

However, at the higher levels of immunosuppression used to treat cardiac allograft rejection, the tumorigenic potential of this treatment becomes more apparent (18). In these cases, the B-cell lymphoproliferative syndrome may occur in as many as 11% of patients, with rapid onset of disseminated disease within 1 to 2 months after the transplant followed by rapid progression to organ failure, sepsis, and death. The B-cell tumors may be either polyclonal or monoclonal, and the role of Epstein-Barr virus is suggested by finding Epstein-Barr viral DNA in all tumors tested. Both the incidence and rapidity of onset of tumors appear to be related to the dose and duration of OKT3. Thus, OKT3 shows significant potential for contributing to this syndrome, and the intensity and duration of immunosuppression should be adjusted to avoid this toxicity.

The antigen bound by OKT3 is expressed on all T cells, not just those that are causing the rejection episode. This may not be the theoretical optimal treatment for acute rejection, since it destroys all circulating T cells, most of which are not responding to the foreign HLA antigens of the allograft and are not participating in the acute rejection. Thus, other T cells that are needed to protect the host from infection are removed unnecessarily by OKT3. More selective therapy would be desirable, if it could target only those cells participating in the rejection episode. For example, T-cell activation antigens that are expressed only on activated T cells after exposure to antigen would be a better target for monoclonal antibody therapy. T cells express the receptor for interleukin-2 only after they are activated by antigen. A monoclonal antibody specific for the interleukin-2 receptor would target activated T cells exclusively, which would include most of the T cells participating in acute rejection. The potential effectiveness of this type of selective monoclonal therapy was illustrated in mice receiving cardiac allografts (19). A monoclonal antibody directed against the interleukin-2 receptor prevented graft rejection in four out of six mice without causing immune paralysis.

The main factor limiting the duration of immunotherapy with OKT3 is the appearance of human antibodies to OKT3 in about 80% of the patients by 10 to 14 days of treatment (20). These antibodies are most often directed against the variable regions of OKT3 and therefore can interfere with the binding site. This blocks OKT3 from binding to T cells and eliminates any further therapeutic effect. In contrast, true IgE–mediated reactions to mouse immunoglobulins are rare. Once a patient makes an immune response to one mouse monoclonal antibody, it is unclear whether he or she would be able to receive other mouse monoclonals with different specificities. It seems likely that the response to the first monoclonal would include helper T cells specific for the constant regions of mouse immunoglobulins, and these would accelerate and enhance the response to subsequent monoclonals. On the other hand, the immunosuppression induced by OKT3 itself may delay the onset of blocking antibodies by reducing the number of available T-helper cells.

A second clinical application for monoclonals is in the form of an immunotoxin conjugate: the binding site of the monoclonal antibody provides the specificity and is chemically coupled to a toxin that provides the cytotoxic effect. One of the first immunotoxin conjugates to be tested in humans is an antimelanoma antibody coupled to the ricin A chain for use in patients with disseminated melanoma (21). About one quarter of the patients treated with the conjugate showed some objective improvement in their disease. However, nearly all patients showed toxicity manifested by a significant decrease in serum albumin levels, falling below 3.0 g 8/100 mL for about a week after treatment, with concomitant edema and weight gain. The hypoalbuminemia may be caused by liver toxicity of the conjugate. The mechanism could be hepatic uptake of free ricin A chain via the oligosaccharide side chains of ricin binding to cells with mannose receptors (1) or uptake of conjugated immunotoxin via the RE system, with the release of free toxin to nearby hepatic parenchymal cells. Since ricin is a ribosomal inhibitor, one of the first signs of its effects would be the shutdown of albumin synthesis. Proteinuria was not observed, and there was no suggestion of protein-losing enteropathy, but capillary leak syndrome is another possible mechanism of this toxicity. In each case, the hypoalbuminemia reverted to normal within about a week after stopping therapy, and there were no other signs of significant liver injury. In addition, most of the patients made antibodies to both the monoclonal antibody and ricin A chain.

The observed toxic effect of this conjugate serves as a reminder that even when the chemical coupling is stable and the conjugate is not contaminated with free toxin, the toxin may still exert its own side effects. Modification of the mannose-rich oligosaccharide side chains may help by reducing hepatic uptake of free ricin A chain. In addition, the potency of ricin is known to be increased in the presence of endosomal protease inhibitors such as ammonium chloride, and these may help to increase the antitumor effect of a given dose of conjugate, especially if timed to coincide with the peak of tumor binding.

A third clinical application for monoclonal antibodies is in the form of a radiolabeled conjugate for diagnostic imaging or as a vehicle to deliver radiotherapy directly to tumors. In one example (22) an ^{111}In-labeled monoclonal antibody was used to detect a tumor implanted in a nude mouse, and the amount of labeled antibody bound per gram of tumor versus normal tissues was measured. On days 1 to 3, the radioactivity per gram of tumor was 25% to 27% of the total dose per gram of mouse, whereas for the liver and spleen it was 15%, declining to 11% on day 3. However, when multiplied by the weight of each tissue, the liver and spleen gave off more radiation than the tumor itself. By day 5, uptake of ^{111}In by the liver and spleen had increased further, to 20% of the total dose per gram, whereas that of the tumor had decreased to 10%. Thus, imaging studies with ^{111}In labeled antibodies can be thought of as a race between three processes: the labeled antibody must reach the tumor before the label is removed by transchelation and before labeled antibody is removed from the circulation and metabolized by the RE system. Otherwise, the nonspecific background will be stronger than the signal from the tumor itself. Converting from intact immunoglobulin to F(ab')$_2$ fragments would speed up tumor labeling and delay RE clearance. However, to overcome transchelation may require the use of other isotopes that are not carried by transferrin, or it may be reduced by saturating the metal binding sites of transferrin.

SUMMARY

Monoclonal antibodies are highly useful research tools because of their specificity and reproducibility. However, their clinical applications for purposes such as immunosuppression, immunotoxin therapy, diagnostic imaging, and radiotherapy need to be approached with considerable care. In the future, immunosuppression should be possible with reagents specific for markers on activated T cells without causing the destruction of all mature T cells (including resting memory T cells) that results from currently available monoclonals. Immunotoxins should be designed with consideration for the metabolic fate of the conjugate, with the goal of directing the toxin away from the RE system. Radionuclides with shorter physical half-lives will be coupled to antibody subunits such as $F(ab')_2$ fragments that have shorter biological half-lives. In this way, we will use antibody physiology to improve the quality and safety of diagnostic imaging. Different chemical bonds between antibody and isotope may be able to direct the isotope away from the RE system to reduce the nonspecific signal from the liver and the spleen. Immunoradiotherapy may not be feasible unless isotopes with short physical half-lives and high linear energy transfer are used so the dose to the tumor will be quick and lethal, without overdosing the vital organs over time.

REFERENCES

1. Vitetta, E. S., and Uhr, J. W. (1985): Immunotoxins. *Ann. Rev. Immunol.*, 3:197.
2. Waldmann, T. A., and Strober, W. (1969): Metabolism of immunoglobulins. *Prog. Allergy*, 13:1.
3. National Council on Radiation Protection and Measurements (1982): NCRP Report No. 70. Nuclear Medicine—factors influencing the choice and use of radionuclides in diagnosis and therapy. NCRP, Bethesda, MD.
4. Macklis, R. M., Kinsey, B. M., Kassis, A. I., Ferrara, J. L. M., Atcher, R. W., Hines, J. J., Coleman, C. N., Adelstein, S. J., and Burakoff, S. J. (1988): Radioimmunotherapy with alpha-particle-emitting immunoconjugates. *Science*, 240:1024.
5. Uhr, J. W. (1984): Immunotoxins: Harnessing nature's poisons. *J. Immunol.*, 133:i.
6. Samelson, L. E., Harford, J. B., and Klausner, R. D. (1985): Identification of the components of the murine T cell antigen receptor complex. *Cell*, 43:223.
7. van den Elsen, P., Shepley, B.-A., Cho, M., and Terhorst, C. (1985): Isolation and characterization of a cDNA clone encoding the murine homologue of the human 20K T3/T-cell receptor glycoprotein. *Nature*, 314:542.
8. Cosimi, A. B., Colvin, R. B., Burton, R. C., Rubin, R. H., Goldstein, G., Kung, P. C., Hansen, W. P., Delmonico, F. L., and Russell, P. S. (1981): Use of monoclonal antibodies to T-cell subsets for immunologic monitoring and treatment in recipients of renal allografts. *N. Engl. J. Med.*, 305:308.
9. Goldstein, G., and Ortho Multicenter Transplant Study Group (1985): A randomized clinical trial of OKT3 monoclonal antibody for acute rejection of cadaveric renal transplants. *N. Engl. J. Med.*, 313:337.
10. Massanari, R., Martin, M., Smith, J., Nghiem, D., Corry, K. J., Flanigan, M., Emmons, C., and Wintermayer, L. A. (1986). Aseptic meningitis among kidney transplant recipients receiving a

newly marketed murine monoclonal antibody preparation. *Morbidity and Mortality Weekly Report*, 35:551.

11. Schooley, R. T., Arbit, D. I., Henle, W., and Hirsch, M. S. (1984): T-lymphocyte subset interactions in the cell-mediated immune response to Epstein-Barr virus. *Cell. Immunol.*, 86:402.
12. Martin, P. J., Shulman, H. M, Schubach, W. H., Hansen, J. A., Fefer, A., Miller, G., and Thomas, E. D. (1984): Fatal Epstein-Barr-virus-associated proliferation of donor B cells after treatment of acute graft-versus-host disease with a murine anti-T-cell antibody. *Ann. Intern. Med.*, 101:310.
13. Miller, G. (1984): Latent herpesviruses of humans: Epstein-Barr virus, M. C. Jordan, moderator. *Ann. Intern. Med.*, 100:872.
14. Penn, I. (1983): Lymphomas complicating organ transplantation. *Transplantation Proc.*, 15:2790.
15. Thiru, S., Calne, R. Y., and Nagington, J. (1981): Lymphoma in renal allograft patients treated with cyclosporin-A as one of the immunosuppressive agents. *Transplantation Proc.*, 13:359.
16. Starzl, T. E., Nalesnik, M. A., and Porter, K. A. (1984): Reversibility of lymphomas and lymphoproliferative lesions developing under cyclosporin-steroid therapy. *Lancet*, 1:583.
17. Tosato, G., and Blaese, R. M. (1985): Epstein-Barr virus infection and immunoregulation in man. *Adv. Immunol.*, 37:99.
18. Swinnen, L. J., Costanzo-Nordin, M. R., Fisher, S. G., O'Sullivan, E. J., Johnson, M. R., Heroux, A. L., Dizikes, G. J., Pifarre, R., and Fisher, R. I. (1990): Increased incidence of lymphoproliferative disorder after immunosuppression with the monoclonal antibody OKT3 in cardiac-transplant recipients. *N. Engl. J. Med.*, 323:1723.
19. Kirkman, R. L., Barrett, L. V., Gaulton, G. N., Kelley, V. E., Ythier, A., and Strom, T. B., (1985): Administration of an anti-interleukin 2 receptor monoclonal antibody prolongs cardiac allograft survival in mice. *J. Exp. Med.*, 162:358.
20. Chatenoud, L., Baudrihaye, M. F., Chkoff, N., Kreis, H., Goldstein, G., and Bach, J.-F. (1986): Restriction of the human *in vivo* immune response against the mouse monoclonal antibody OKT3. *J. Immunol.*, 137:830.
21. Spitler, L. E., del Rio, M., Khentigan, A., Wedel, N. I., Brophy, N. A., Miller, L. L., Horkonen, W. S., Rosendorf, L. L., Lee, H. M., Mischak, R. P., Kawahata, R. T., Stoudemire, J. B., Fradkin, L. B., Bautista, E. E., and Scannon, P. J. (1987): Therapy of patients with malignant melanoma using a monoclonal antimelanoma antibody-ricin A chain immunotoxin. *Cancer Res.*, 47:1717.
22. Khaw, B. A., Cooney, J., Edgington, T., and Strauss, H. W. (1986): Differences in experimental tumor localization of dual-labeled monoclonal antibody. *J. Nucl. Med.*, 27:1293.

Clinical Immunotoxicology, edited by
D. S. Newcombe, N. R. Rose, and J. C. Bloom.
Raven Press, Ltd., New York, 1992.

7

The Immunotoxicology of Cytokines

Roger B. Cohen, Jay P. Siegel, Raj K. Puri, and Dov H. Pluznik

*Division of Cytokine Biology, Center for Biologics Evaluation and Research,
Food and Drug Administration, Bethesda, Maryland
The contents of this article are the views of the authors and do not necessarily reflect
the official views of the U.S. Food and Drug Administration.*

Over the past two decades a large number of soluble factors have been described that regulate cell growth, the immune response, and hematopoiesis. Many of these factors were first described as lymphokines and interleukins (ILs) and were believed to be involved mainly in the regulation of the immune response (76,77). At the same time, another set of glycoproteins was described that regulates hematopoiesis, namely, the colony stimulating factors (CSFs). It is now apparent that there is considerable overlap in the cellular origins and functions of the CSFs, ILs, and lymphokines. In fact, at least five of the ILs—IL-1 (hemopoietin-1), IL-3, IL-4, IL-5, and IL-6—are now known to act as hematopoietic growth factors either directly or indirectly (reviewed in 58,59,76,77). Consequently, many in the field now feel that the term cytokine best characterizes all of these factors and has the advantage of emphasizing their production by many cell types besides T lymphocytes, including fibroblasts, monocytes, and endothelial cells (17) as well as their functional diversity with effects on the immune response, hematopoiesis, cell growth, and coagulation. The term cytokine also includes growth factors such as epidermal growth factor, nerve growth factor, transforming growth factors-alpha and -beta, and platelet-derived growth factor (which regulate the growth and replication of nonhematopoietic cells) as well as erythropoietin, tumor necrosis factor, and the interferons.

At the present time, the following cytokines, involved in the immune response and/or hematopoiesis, have been isolated and characterized: ILs 1 through 8 (76, 77), interferons-alpha, -beta, and -gamma (83), tumor necrosis factor-alpha (80), the CSFs (55,58,59), and erythropoietin (27). Following their biochemical purification, many have now been molecularly cloned, thus permitting large-scale production (22,57) and clinical studies. At present, IL-1, IL-2, and IL-3, granulocyte-CSF (G-CSF), granulocyte-macrophage-CSF (GM-CSF), tumor necrosis factor-alpha, and the interferons are under intensive study for clinical use in humans. Interferon-alpha has received Food and Drug Administration approval for use in the treatment of hairy cell leukemia, condylomata acuminata, and Kaposi's sarcoma. Final approval is near for its use in treating chronic non-A-non-B hepatitis. Food and Drug Administration approval has been granted for the use of interferon-gamma for decreasing infections in patients with chronic granulomatous disease. In an attempt to elucidate some of the general principles that apply to the study of cytokine immunotoxicology, this chapter focuses mainly on the clinical use of the CSFs and IL-2 in humans and the immunologically mediated toxicities their use has revealed. This group of cytokines has been sufficiently tested in animals and humans to provide significant data, although many questions remain unanswered. We will consider the use of IL-2 and the CSFs against the background of more extensive data regarding the clinical use and toxicology of interferons, which have been reviewed extensively elsewhere (4,29).

BIOLOGICAL ACTIVITIES AND CLINICAL UTILIZATION OF CYTOKINES

The widest clinical experience to date with the ILs has been with IL-2. IL-2 is a broad-spectrum immunomodulator that is a growth and differentiation factor for activated T cells and cells with nonspecific cytotoxicity (76,77). Interleukin-2 can also stimulate B cells to differentiate and secrete antibody and can promote activation and differentiation of monocytes. Most studies have used IL-2 in patients with cancer. There is also growing interest in the use of IL-2 in the treatment or prevention of infectious diseases. At present IL-2 is being investigated as part of a novel form of immunotherapy for cancer, either by itself or in conjunction with activated lymphocytes. A wide variety of activated lymphocyte therapies are being evaluated in combination with IL-2. Most commonly these use lymphocytes from blood that have been activated with IL-2 for 3 to 6 days (lymphokine-activated killer cells) (91) or lymphocytes derived from tumor biopsies that have been expanded and activated with IL-2 *in vitro* for several weeks (tumor-infiltrating lymphocytes) (92).

The CSFs are being investigated for use in a diverse group of patients who have in common hematological cytopenias attributable to a variety of causes. There are four classic subclasses of CSF: G-CSF, GM-CSF, M-CSF, and IL-3 (or multi-CSF) (55,61). Their primary function is the regulation of hematopoiesis, a process in which bone marrow progenitor cells proliferate and differentiate and acquire the characteristics of mature blood cells. Interestingly, three of the four classic CSFs (GM-CSF, M-CSF, and IL-3) are linked on human chromosome 5, and their linkage may be responsible for coordinate patterns of gene expression in certain tissues (reviewed in 73). In addition, IL-5, the M-CSF receptor (*c-fms*; 115), IL-4, platelet-derived growth factor, the beta-adrenergic receptor, and endothelial cell growth factor are also located on this chromosomal arm (48). The biological activity of the CSFs is assessed according to their ability to stimulate progenitor cells to give rise to colonies of differentiated cells in soft agar cultures (12,86,87). All four of the classic, or myeloid, CSFs have been purified to homogeneity and molecularly cloned, so that large quantities of each are available for laboratory and clinical trials. Interestingly, whether the recombinant product is glycosylated or not does not seem to significantly affect the clinical response, toxicity, or immunogenicity

(11). Many of the CSFs (GM-CSF is a good example) are also highly species-specific (56).

The actions of G-CSF appear to be restricted primarily to granulocyte precursors, causing them to proliferate and differentiate into mature neutrophils. M-CSF causes proliferation and differentiation of monocyte and macrophage precursors. GM-CSF has a much broader function and stimulates the differentiation of granulocyte, macrophage, megakaryocytic, eosinophilic, and erythroid precursors. Interleukin-3, or multi-CSF, has the broadest spectrum and can stimulate all of the preceding classes of progenitor cells as well as mast cells, multipotential stem cells, and lymphocytes (31,57,60,73). In addition to their interactions with hematopoietic precursors, the CSFs also influence the function of mature immune effector cells. Effects on chemotaxis, expression of membrane surface antigens, phagocytosis, superoxide production, killing of microorganisms, and tumor cell killing are well described (reviewed in 22,73,102) as well as effects on endothelial cell growth and migration (16). It is likely that to some extent toxicity may be related to the type and number of cell lineages that are targets of a particular cytokine. Of the CSFs, recombinant G-CSF and GM-CSF have received the greatest attention in preclinical and clinical studies. Studies with natural M-CSF (45,66) and IL-3 (31,32) are still at an early stage. We anticipate that many aspects of the experience with G-CSF and GM-CSF will be repeated as experience accumulates with the other agents.

At present clinical trials (phases I to III) are in progress with G-CSF, GM-CSF, and IL-3. GM-CSF is being studied to treat the leukopenia associated with human immunodeficiency virus-1 infection (35), aplastic anemia (1,20,105), myelodysplastic syndrome (33,69,106), cytotoxic chemotherapy (2,107), and in the setting of bone marrow transplantation (8,13,70,71). G-CSF is primarily under study for the treatment of neutropenia following cytotoxic chemotherapy (15,30,65) and for cases of idiopathic neutropenia (43), cyclic neutropenia (37), and congenital neutropenia (10). More recently, G-CSF has been used to treat the myelosuppression of remission induction chemotherapy for acute myelogenous leukemia (79) and the neutropenia associated with myelodysplastic syndrome (68).

COMPARISONS OF CYTOKINE TOXICITIES IN CLINICAL TRIALS

One general and striking observation based on the expanding number of reported trials is that many of the toxicities observed with one cytokine are often seen with others (Table 1). As an example, one of the most common and problematic side effects of intensive therapy with IL-2 has been a vascular leak syndrome characterized by peripheral and pulmonary edema and occasional ascites and/or pleural effusions, and often complicated by hypotension, oliguria, and sometimes respiratory failure (90). GM-CSF has caused a somewhat similar syndrome with pleuro-pericardial effusions and edema, although it is generally much less severe than is the case with IL-2. This particular side effect of GM-CSF was unanticipated because it had not developed during preclinical animal studies and its pathogenesis remains of considerable practical and theoretical interest (2,13,20,51).

TABLE 1. *Frequent clinical toxicities of some cytokines*[a]

Symptoms	G-CSF	GM-CSF	IL-2	Interferon-alpha	Tumor necrosis factor
Fever	—	+ + +	+ + +	+ + +	+ + +
Malaise	—	+ + +	+ + +	+ + +	+ + +
Skin reactions	—	+ + +	+ + +	+ + +	+ + +
Chills	—	+ + +	+ + +	+ +	+ +
Fatigue	—	+ + +	+ +	+ + +	+ + +
Myalgias, arthralgias	—	+ + +	+ +	+ + +	+ +
Anorexia	—	+ + +	+ +	+ + +	+ +
Diarrhea	—	+	+ + +	+ +	+
Dyspnea	—	+	+ + +	+	+ + +
Headache	—	+	+ + +	+ + +	+ + +
Bone pain	+ + +	+ + +	—	—	—
Nausea/vomiting	—	—	+ +	+ +	+ +
Mood changes	—	—	+ +	+ +	—
Signs					
Vascular leak syndrome	—	+ + +	+ + +	—	+ +
Weight gain	—	+ +	+ + +	—	—
Pulmonary edema	—	+ + +	+ + +	—	+ + +
Hepatotoxicity	—	+	+ + +	+	+ +
Nephrotoxicity	—	+	+ + +	+	+ +
Hypotension	—	+ + +	+ + +	+ +	+ + +
Tachycardia	—	—	+ + +	+ +	+ + +
Arrhythmias	—	—	+ +	—	+
Confusion/disorientation	—	—	+ +	+	—
Lymphopenia	—	—	+ + +	+ +	+ +
Neutropenia	—	—	+ +	+ + +	+ + +
Thrombocytopenia	—	+	+ +	+ + +	+ +
Anemia	—	—	+ + +	+ +	+
Eosinophilia	—	+	+ + +	—	+

[a]Toxicities have been grouped according to symptoms (noted or experienced by patients) and signs (noted by health care personnel or documented by laboratory abnormalities). 3 +, noted frequently; 2 +, noted on occasion; 1 +, noted infrequently; —, not noted. Data were compiled from the clinical studies referred to in the text and from the table presented in Fent and Zbinden, ref. 29.

Many of the side effects seen with IL-2 in patients are similar to those that have been observed with interferon-alpha. Although neither cytokine is a direct pyrogen, IL-2, like interferon-alpha, frequently causes fever (62). Other influenza-like symptoms (e.g., malaise, myalgias, arthralgias, asthenia), along with nausea, vomiting, diarrhea, and headache, are not uncommon (53a). As with interferon-alpha, dermatological complications are also common with IL-2 and include macular erythema with pruritus, sometimes leading to generalized erythroderma (34). Stomatitis (23) and exacerbation of psoriasis have also been reported (49). Hematological effects of IL-2 are common and include lymphopenia, thrombocytopenia, neutropenia, and anemia as in the interferon-alpha studies, but also lymphocytosis and eosinophilia (101). Although no endocrinological effects of either interferon-alpha or IL-2 were anticipated, interferon-alpha has significant effects on reproductive endocrinology, and IL-2 may cause hypothyroidism and elevations of adrenocorticotropic hormone and cortisol levels (3,108). Cardiac toxicities, including a cardiomyopathy in patients with human immunodeficiency virus that is clearly independent of febrile tachycardia (24), have been reported with interferon-alpha but have been even more of a problem with high-dose IL-2 and include arrhythmias, hypocontractility, myocarditis, ischemia, and infarction (50,75,78). Unexpectedly, central nervous system toxicity has been a dose-limiting toxicity in intensive regimens of both interferon-alpha and IL-2, with depression and confusion occurring with the former and agitation and confusion more common with the latter (95,96). Both cytokines often cause asymptomatic and reversible abnormalities in liver function tests, although enzyme elevations generally predominate with interferon-alpha, whereas bilirubin elevations are more common with IL-2 (90).

Some of the toxicities that are seen with IL-2 are less reminiscent of the experience with interferon-alpha. IL-2 has caused significant nephrotoxicity, apparently resulting from impaired renal perfusion and usually resolving when IL-2 is discontinued (98,104,111). There is also a high incidence of bacteremia in patients who receive IL-2 and lymphokine-activated killer cells. Although there are many predisposing factors to this complication, it is noteworthy that in one study of patients with acquired immunodeficiency syndrome treated with IL-2 (and no activated cells), the incidence of nonopportunistic bacterial infections was significantly higher than in a similar population treated with interferon-gamma at the same institution (67). Recently, IL-2 therapy has been shown to induce a reversible defect in neutrophil chemotaxis (41,44) and Fc receptor expression (41), which might account for the high number of staphylococcal bacteremias.

In general, when compared with IL-2 and interferon-alpha, the side effects of the CSFs have been less severe. But as was also the case with IL-2, their use in humans has revealed a new set of immune and nonimmune toxicities. The principal toxicity of G-CSF has been minor bone pain, which has been termed "medullary" based upon its distribution in the skeleton, the fact that it precedes the increase in white blood cells, and the belief that it is attributable to a rapid expansion of the myeloid compartment of the bone marrow. Minor, reversible elevations of alkaline phosphatase and lactic dehydrogenase enzymes have also been noted. There have also been exacerbations of neutrophilic dermatoses, particularly psoriasis.

Granulocyte-macrophage-colony stimulating factor has proved to be somewhat more toxic than G-CSF. It is again worth noting that many of its toxic effects, some of them potentially life-threatening, did not occur in animal studies even at very high doses of the drug (90–300 μg/kg/day) or with routes of administration that closely approximated the routes and schedules used in human trials (25,26). The most severe, dose-limiting toxicity of GM-CSF has been a clinical presentation with similarities to the capillary leak syndrome referred to above with IL-2, occurring at doses exceeding 30 μg/kg/day (2,13,20,35,51). Toxicity has been a particular problem in the elderly at higher doses (5). Pericardial effusions are common and are often associated with pericarditis. These effusions often, but not always, occur at sites of preexisting disease. Erythroderma (which was seen with IL-2) has been seen. Severe bone pain, leg pains, myalgias, and arthralgias have also been doselimiting (2,13,20,35,51,106–107). Other less severe dose-related abnormalities have included reversible rises in serum lactic dehydrogenase, transaminases, and alkaline phosphatase values (35,39,106,107).

Common and moderately severe clinical side effects of GM-CSF appear to be shared by therapy with all cytokines. These include fever, headache, myalgias of mild degree, nausea and vomiting, and influenza-like symptoms (chills, malaise, anorexia, asthenia) (20,35,105). Local erythema at sites of injection, along with macular rashes, pruritus, and occasional generalized maculopapular eruptions, have also been seen (13,51). Moderate weight gain, sometimes accompanied by edema of the wrists and ankles, may be a mild or early form of capillary leak syndrome (51,105).

Some additional toxicities have been noted with use of GM-CSF and may have a partial immune basis. These include phlebitis (also noted in animal studies) (26), thrombus formation at the tips of central venous catheters, and pulmonary emboli (1,20,33,35). In addition to the mild skin rashes noted above, rashes sometimes occur at subcutaneous injection sites and recur at previous injection sites when GM-CSF is readministered up to 1 week later (51). This particular side effect, although seemingly innocuous in the short term, could become a significant limitation to chronic therapy by the subcutaneous route. Granulocyte-macrophage-colony stimulating factor can also cause a first dose reaction of flushing, hypotension, tachycardia, and transient hypoxemia, which has been attributed to the sudden release of vasodilators causing pulmonary vascular shunts or to leukocyte margination in the lungs (39,51). Occasional side effects include thrombocytopenia (39,51) and a decrease in serum cholesterol level. The latter was noted in patients with aplastic anemia and has been attributed to macrophage activation (74). Since macrophages serve as a reservoir of human immunodeficiency virus-1 infection in patients with acquired immunodeficiency syndrome, concern has also been expressed that macrophage activation by GM-CSF could lead to enhanced viral replication. Initial studies did not show an increase in human immunodeficiency virus replication as detected by cell culture methods (35), but more recent data indicate that serum p24 levels rise in human immunodeficiency virus patients treated with GM-CSF, suggesting that viral replication is indeed enhanced by the drug (85). Unlike the interferons and IL-2, GM-CSF has not been associated with significant nephro- or neurotoxicity.

Early results with IL-3 indicate that fever and local erythema at injection sites are common. Lymphocytosis with elevations of IgA and IgM levels has been seen, along with stimulation of malignant B-cell tumors. Bone marrow fibrosis has been noted. The most unusual side effects of IL-3 have been headache and neck stiffness at higher doses. Finally, facial flushing has been noted, perhaps owing to the elevation of circulating basophils with resultant increases in histamine levels (31,32).

In addition to the immune toxicities that have actually occurred during animal studies and human trials, there are a number of potential toxicities for which we will need to monitor patients. Although formation of neutralizing antibodies has not been a major problem in human trials of CSFs, it has been a limiting factor in several animal studies and has occurred in humans with other cytokines (e.g., interferon-alpha). Granuloma formation at subcutaneous injection sites owing to chronic macrophage activation needs to be looked for in patients receiving CSFs. Tissue damage (particularly to the heart and lungs) resulting from eosinophilia may be another consequence of long-term use. Concern has been expressed that use of

CSFs in the setting of bone marrow transplantation could activate T cells, leading to an acceleration of graft versus host disease. In clinical trials to date, exacerbation of graft versus host disease in bone marrow transplant patients has not occurred, but the number of treated patients is still small (70). Potentiation of neoplastic cell growth in the settings of acute myelogenous leukemia (79,109), MDS (33), and postchemotherapy myelosuppression remains a concern, particularly since GM-CSF receptors are widely distributed on cells of many types, including non-hematopoietic cancer cells. In the case of small cell lung cancer cells *in vitro*, GM-CSF caused differentiation without proliferation (94), but various cytokines did stimulate proliferation of certain colon carcinoma cell lines (7). Some investigators are also concerned that long-term hematopoietic growth factor use could lead to eventual bone marrow failure because of stem cell "exhaustion." Reduced production of other hematopoietic lineages during therapy because of diversion of differentiation to a single lineage is another concern. It could be that the thrombocytopenia noted in some patients with use of G-CSF and GM-CSF is one clinical manifestation of this problem. Finally, as with any new therapeutic agent, long-term effects on fetal and childhood growth and development will require close monitoring, particularly now that the use of CSFs is being advocated for some of the congenital neutropenias and some cases of aplastic anemia. If the CSFs can also stimulate the production of other growth factors (for example, transforming growth factor-beta or fibroblast growth factor [FGF]), this will mean that the risks to childhood growth and fetal development will require particular scrutiny.

SOME MECHANISMS OF CYTOKINE TOXICITY

It is clear from the preceding overview that certain toxic side effects recur in clinical studies of the cytokines (see Table 1). One reason for this may be that all these agents can influence the expression of many other cytokines. A few examples of this phenomenon include the induction of tumor necrosis factor-alpha (18,19, 99,114), IL-1α and IL-1β (63,72,99), IL-2 (64), interferons (114), M-CSF (40), and perhaps transforming growth factor-beta, by GM-CSF. M-CSF stimulates tumor necrosis factor-alpha and IL-1 release from mature macrophages (55). Likewise, IL-2 can influence the expression of IL-1, interferon-gamma, and tumor necrosis factor-alpha (53). The networks of cytokine interactions with the immune system are quite extensive and involve multiple positive feedback loops, some of which are illustrated in Fig. 1. In the case of IL-2, there is some evidence suggesting that the pyrogenic effect (62), the eosinophilia and anemia (52), and perhaps the vascular leak syndrome (103) might be mediated in part by the release of soluble factors such as cytokines *in vivo*.

Although the exact cause of the vascular leak syndrome due to IL-2 is not known, it is believed to be mediated by competent immune cells, since nude or irradiated mice do not develop the syndrome (93), and administration of lymphokine-activated killer cells contributes to the IL-2–induced syndrome in mice (28). It is reasonable to postulate that GM-CSF, by virtue of its ability to stimulate production of cyto-

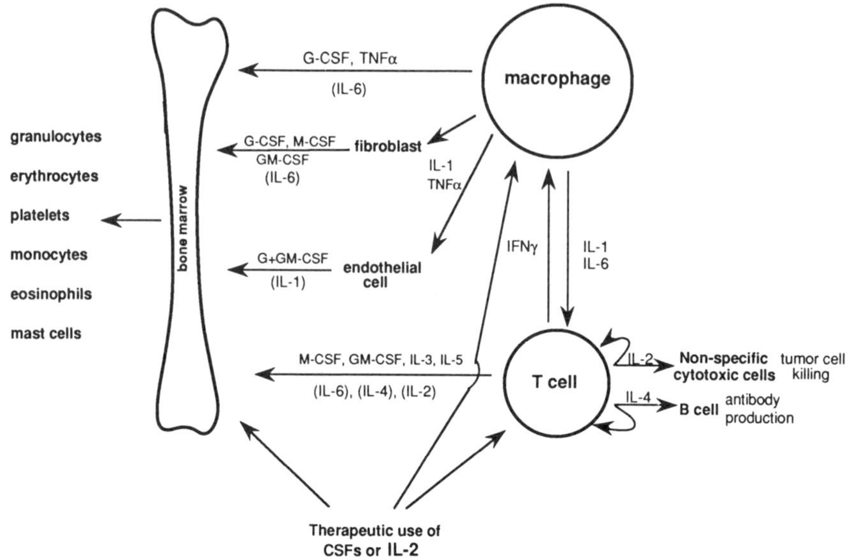

FIG. 1. Administration of CSFs and IL-2 to patients activates an elaborate network of immune effector cells and secondary cytokine secretion. ILs in parentheses affect hematopoiesis indirectly.

kines such as IL-1, IL-2, interferon-gamma and tumor necrosis factor-alpha, could activate many of the same immune effector networks, leading to similar patterns of tissue damage. Cytotoxicity may also result from the direct effects of CSF-stimulated leukocyte effector functions (reviewed in 93,102), such as the elaboration of prostaglandins and leukotrienes (46). These secondary mediators could, in turn, induce inflammation, modulate immune responses, and affect vascular tone and permeability. Granulocyte-macrophage-colony stimulating factor induces the expression of the CD11b surface antigen on granulocytes (100). This antigen is essential for adhesion-dependent granulocyte functions such as phagocytosis, aggregation, and chemotaxis. Enhanced neutrophil aggregation may be one of the mechanisms causing pulmonary sequestration of neutrophil aggregates that would help to explain the dyspnea and hypoxemia (and possibly, the adult respiratory distress syndrome) that are sometimes seen when CSFs are administered. The CSFs also stimulate respiratory burst activity, cytotoxicity, and antimicrobial activity in monocytes (112). M-CSF and GM-CSF also cause macrophage release of plasminogen activator (36). Involvement of cytokines in clotting mechanisms may be related to the phlebitis and thrombosed vascular catheters that have been noted on occasion. The CSFs may also stimulate the secretion of growth factors such as FGF and transformation growth factor-beta, which could lead to widespread effects on tissue repair and wound healing. It is easy therefore to imagine how these diverse interactions could contribute to an exuberant immune response at multiple levels, leading to extensive tissue damage.

ANIMAL MODELS

Animal studies of cytokines have been of variable value in predicting and assessing their toxicity in humans. As noted above, a vascular leak syndrome has been a common and problematic side effect of therapy with IL-2. Although this toxicity was not anticipated as a result of preclinical testing, it can be reproduced in animal models (93), and such models have been of considerable value in evaluating its mechanisms and designing strategies to avoid it.

Preclinical studies of human G-CSF in nonhuman primates showed hematopoietic effects but minimal toxicity regardless of route of administration or dose (113), and this relative lack of toxicity has been the rule in human trials performed to date with this agent. Preclinical studies of GM-CSF in nonhuman primates likewise have shown good hematopoietic effects, and toxic effects were observed only at very high doses administered as an intravenous bolus injection (90–300 µg/kg/day), and these were limited to slight decreases in red blood cell counts, eosinophilia, phlebitis, fever, weight loss, and skin rashes (26). It turns out that the animal studies failed to predict the full range of toxic effects that were eventually observed in human studies. Preclinical testing of IL-3 and M-CSF continues, and thus far these CSFs in animal studies appear to have less effect on levels of circulating cells compared with G-CSF and GM-CSF, and there are also preliminary indications that they may promote a shift in hematopoiesis to the spleen (61).

The failure of animal models to express the full range of toxic effects observed with some cytokines (e.g., GM-CSF) in humans may reflect the inherent limitations of testing human proteins in animals when there is a high degree of species specificity to the protein's receptor binding and bioactivity. Indeed, of the cytokines discussed, those for which animal models proved most accurate, namely, IL-2 and G-CSF, are cytokines for which the human molecule is active in many mammalian species. Given the fact that many cytokines are quite species-specific, it will be critical to validate animal models by quantitating the extent of species specificity in order to extrapolate reliably the findings to humans. Data of this type could be obtained by comparing cells of human and test animal origin with respect to the affinities of the cytokine for its receptors, the biological effects of the cytokine, and the concentrations required to achieve those effects.

One solution to developing animal models that are more sensitive to cytokine toxicities would be to test the homologous cytokine in the homologous species. This approach might also limit antibody formation, which has made longer term animal studies of GM-CSF, for example, difficult to perform and interpret. A more complex approach to the study of long-term *in vivo* side effects of cytokines would be to create transgenic mouse models of cytokine expression and overproduction. In the two published examples of transgenic mice expressing GM-CSF, unregulated expression of the cytokine in multiple organs or in the bone marrow has led to a myeloproliferative syndrome (42,47). These transgenic mouse studies have been very useful in pointing out some of the toxic side effects of constitutive cytokine overexpression; the infiltrates of activated macrophages in many tissues, for example, indicate a new set of potential toxicities caused by GM-CSF that were not detected either in preclinical animal studies or in human trials; these toxicities will therefore require our vigilance in the future. There are several problems with the current transgenic modeling as applied to the CSFs. First, unlike potential human trial subjects, the mice expressing the factor are not sick to start with and do not have a hematopoietic cellular lineage deficiency for which they are being treated. Second, their "treatment" begins *in utero*. Third, the constitutive overproduction of any protein may ultimately be toxic to a variety of organs independently of its biological specificity. Fourth, at present there is no means to turn off cytokine production. As the normal regulation of cytokine gene expression becomes better understood, it should be possible to improve the transgenic model so that tissue-specific regulated expression occurs, as has been achieved with the globin proteins (6).

COMBINATION THERAPY WITH CYTOKINES

Many of the lymphokines are currently being tested in various combinations, and a similar trend is certain to emerge in the clinical use of CSFs. There is substantial *in vitro* (21,82) and preclinical evidence for synergy in cytokine action, and these synergistic effects might allow lower doses of cytokines to be given (25,54,97). At lower doses, the actions of two cytokines given together might be predominantly on proliferation and differentiation without effects on immune effector networks, thereby leading to less toxicity. A variety of combinations have been proposed based on animal studies, and these include IL-1 + M-CSF, IL-1 + GM-CSF, GM-CSF + G-CSF, M-CSF + G-CSF, and IL-3 + G-CSF (14). Of course, where there is a possibility of synergy of therapeutic effects, there is also a possibility of synergy of undesired effects (88). For this reason, it may be advisable to employ some of the techniques used in the development of a new cytokine (e.g., preclinical studies, dose escalation studies) in the clinical development of new cytokine combinations.

APPROACHES TO MINIMIZING TOXICITY

It is of particular interest that in the case of GM-CSF, nonhuman primate testing was more efficient in modeling the desired effects than the undesired side effects. Two plausible explanations of this phenomenon have interesting implications. One is that the proliferative and differentiating effects of the CSF may be the result of high-affinity receptor-ligand interactions, whereas the secondary immune toxicities may be attributable to low-affinity interactions. Since it is likely that the affinity for heterologous receptors would be lower than for homologous receptors, cytokine concentrations might be insufficient to interact effectively with the animal's low affinity receptors. Hence, the animal model may predominantly reflect the effects caused by interactions with the high-affinity receptor, whereas in clinical trials in the homologous species (i.e., humans), both sets of effects will be seen. If this interpretation is correct, it implies that high- and low-affinity receptor-dependent events might be distinguishable and ultimately separable at the molecular level. A redesigned cytokine without effects on tumor necrosis factor-alpha, IL-1, and the other secondary immune mediators would represent a therapeutic breakthrough. An alternative possibilility is that both the desired and undesired effects are mediated by the same receptor but in different tissues. Again, if differential affinity for the heterologous and homologous receptors is postulated, it is possible that cytokine concentrations achieved in the therapeutic target tissue (perhaps blood or bone marrow) are sufficient for bioactivity in both the animal model and clinical studies but that concentrations achieved at the toxicity target tissue are sufficient to bind and activate only the homologous human receptors. Either of these possibilities raises the prospect that an appropriate dose, route, and schedule of administration in humans might minimize undesired effects.

Pharmacological efforts that have been applied to the toxicity of IL-2 therapy might also be directed toward therapy of cytokine toxicity. Use of prophylactic antibiotics has been reported to markedly decrease the incidence of sepsis in patients undergoing IL-2 therapy (9,38). However, since sepsis (and some antibiotics) will modulate immune responses, it remains to be demonstrated whether such use alters clinical efficacy. Nonsteroidal antiinflammatory agents are effective at relieving fever produced by IL-2, but at the cost of increased nephrotoxicity (62,84). Glucocorticoids can eliminate IL-2 therapy toxicity (and perhaps its efficacy as well) (110), but they also have their own immune toxicities, particularly in the immunocompromised hosts who are candidates for CSF therapy. It is of interest to note that in animal models, IL-1 has been shown to decrease IL-2-as well as IL-2- and interferon-alpha–induced vascular leak syndrome in mice (89).

In the long term, several approaches to alleviating cytokine toxicity might be considered. When structural-functional relationships between receptor and ligand are clarified, it might be possible, as noted above, to redesign the cytokine and molecularly dissociate its therapeutic and toxic effects. It is also possible that temporary administration of monoclonal antibodies directed at some of the putative effectors of immune toxicities (e.g., IL-1 and tumor-necrosis factor-alpha) could eventually be employed. For some of the chronic cytopenias in which long-term cytokine expression is desired, these patients would seem to be excellent candidates for gene therapy in which the cytokine could be expressed locally in the bone marrow at physiological concentrations.

In conclusion, we are now approaching the end of the first decade of administration of highly purified recombinant cytokines to animals and humans. Careful study of the considerable accumulated data can lead to generalizations that may prove to be very useful in the prediction, evaluation, treatment, and avoidance of cytokine toxicities in the future.

REFERENCES

1. Antin, J. H., Smith, B. R., Holmes, W. and Rosenthal, D. S. (1988): Phase I/II study of recombinant granulocyte-macrophage colony stimulating factor in aplastic anemia and myelodysplastic syndrome. *Blood*, 72:705–713.
2. Antman, K. S., Griffin, J. D. Elias, A. et al. (1988): Effect of recombinant human granulocyte-macrophage colony stimulating factor on chemotherapy induced myelosuppression. *N. Engl. J. Med.*, 319:593–595.
3. Atkins, M. B., Mier, J. W., Parkinson, D. R. et al. (1988): Hypothyroidism after treatment with IL-2 and lymphokine activated killer cells. *N. Engl. J. Med.*, 318:1557–1563.
4. Balkwill, F. R. (1989): Interferons. *Lancet*, 1:1060–1063.
5. Barlogie, B., Jagannath, S., Dixon, D. O. et al. (1990): High dose melphalan and GM-CSF for refractory multiple myeloma. *Blood*, 76:677–680.
6. Behringer, R. R., Ryan, T. M., Reilly, M. P. et al. (1989): Synthesis of functional human hemoglobin in transgenic mice. *Science*, 245:971–973.
7. Berdel, W. E., Danhauser-Riedl, S., Steinhauser, G. et al. (1989): Various human hematopoietic growth factors (IL3, GM-CSF, G-CSF) stimulate clonal growth of non-hematopoietic tumor cells. *Blood*, 73:80–83.
8. Blazar, B. R., Kersey, J. H., McGlave, P. B. et al. (1989): *In vivo* administration of recombinant human granulocyte macrophage colony stimulating factor in acute lymphoblastic leukemia patients receiving purged autografts. *Blood*, 73:849–857.
9. Bock, S. N., Lee, R. E., Fisher, B. et al. (1990): A prospective randomized trial evaluating prophylactic antibiotics to prevent triple lumen catheter related sepsis in patients treated with immunotherapy. *J. Clin. Oncol.*, 8:161–169.
10. Bonilla, M. A., Gillio, A. P., Ruggiero, M. et al. (1989): Effects of recombinant human granulocyte colony stimulating factor on neutropenia in patients with congenital granulocytopenia. *N. Engl. J. Med.*, 320:1574–1580.
11. Bonnem, E. M. and Morstyn, G. (1988): GM-CSF current status and future development. *Semin. Oncol.*, 15:46–51.
12. Bradley, T. R. and Metcalf, D. (1986): The growth of mouse bone marrow cell in vitro. *Austr. J. Exp. Biol. Med.*, 44:287–300.
13. Brandt, S. J., Peters, W. P., Atwater, S. K. et al. (1988): Effect of recombinant granulocyte macrophage colony stimulating factor on hematopoietic reconstitution after high dose chemotherapy and autologous bone marrow transplantation. *N. Engl. J. Med.*, 318:869–876.
14. Bronchud, M. H. and Dexter, T. M. (1989): Clinical use of hematopoietic growth factors. *Blood Reviews*, 3:66–70.
15. Bronchud, M. H., Scarffe, J. H., Thatcher, N. et al. (1987): Phase I/II study of recombinant human granulocyte colony stimulating factor in patients receiving intensive chemotherapy for small cell lung cancer. *Br. J. Cancer*, 56:809–813.
16. Bussolino, F., Wang, J. M., Defilippi, P. et al. (1989): G- and GM-CSF induce human endothelial cells to migrate and proliferate. *Nature*, 337:471–473.
17. Cannistra, S. A. and Griffin, J. D. (1988): Regulation of the production and function of granulocytes and monocytes. *Semin. Hematol.*, 25:173–188.
18. Cannistra, S. A., Rambaldi, A., Spriggs, D. R. et al. (1987): Human GM-CSF induces expression of the TNF gene by the U937 cell line and by normal human monocytes. *J. Clin. Invest.*, 79:1720–1728.
19. Cannistra, S. A., Vellenga, E., Groshek, P., et al. (1988): Human GM-CSF and IL-3 stimulate monocyte cytotoxicity through a tumor necrosis factor-dependent mechanism. *Blood*, 71:672–676.
20. Champlin, R. E., Nimer, S. D., Ireland, P. et al. (1989): Treatment of refractory aplastic anemia with recombinant human granulocyte macrophage colony stimulating factor. *Blood*, 73:694–699.
21. Chen, B. D.-M., Clark, C. R. and Chou, T.-H. (1988): Interleukin 3 (IL-3) regulates the *in vitro* proliferation of both blood monocytes and peritoneal exudate macrophages: Synergism between a macrophage lineage specific colony stimulating factor and IL-3. *Blood*, 71:997–1002.
22. Clarke, S. C. and Kamen, R. (1987): The human hematopoietic colony stimulating factors. *Science*, 236:1229–1237.
23. Creekmore, S. P., Harris, J. E., Ellis, T. M. et al. (1989): A phase I trial of recombinant IL-2 by periodic 24 hour intravenous infusion. *J. Clin. Oncol.*, 7:276–284.

24. Deyton, L. R., Walker, R. E., Kovacs, J. A. et al. (1989): Reversible cardiac dysfunction associated with interferon alpha therapy in AIDS patients with Kaposi's sarcoma. *N. Engl. J. Med.*,
321:1246–1249.
25. Donahue, R. E., Seehra, J., Metzger, M., et al. (1988): Human IL-3 and GM-CSF act synergistically in stimulating hematopoiesis in primates. *Science*, 241:1820–1823.
26. Donahue, R. E., Wang, E. A., Stone, D. K., et al. (1986): Stimulation of hematopoiesis in
primates by continuous infusion of recombinant human GM-CSF. *Nature London*, 321:872–875.
27. Eschbach, J. W., Egrie, J. C., Downing, M. R., et al. (1987): Correction of the anemia of end-
stage renal disease with recombinant human erythropoietin: Results of a phase I and II clinical trial.
N. Engl. J. Med., 316:73–78.
28. Ettinghausen, S. E., Puri, R. K. and Rosenberg, S. A. (1988): Increased vascular permeability in
organs mediated by the systemic administration of lymphokine activated killer cells and recombinant IL-2 in mice. *J. Natl. Cancer Inst.*, 80:177–188.
29. Fent, K. and Zbinden, G. (1987): Toxicity of interferon and interleukin. *Trends in Pharmacological Science*, 8:100–105.
30. Gabrilove, J., Jakubowski, A., Scher, H., et al (1988): Effect of granulocyte colony stimulating
factor on neutropenia and associated morbidity due to chemotherapy for transitional cell carcinoma
of the urothelium. *N. Engl. J. Med.*, 318:1414–1422.
31. Ganser, A., Lindemann, A., Seipelt, G., et al. (1990): Effects of recombinant human IL-3 in
patients with normal hematopoiesis and in patients with bone marrow failure. *Blood*, 76:666–676.
32. Ganser, A., Seipelt, G., Lindemann, A. et al. (1990): Effects of recombinant human IL-3 in
patients with myelodysplastic syndromes. *Blood*, 76:455–462.
33. Ganser, A., Volkers, B., Greher, J. et al. (1989): Recombinant human GM-CSF in patients with
myelodysplastic syndromes- a phase I/II trial. *Blood*, 73:31–37.
34. Gaspari, A. A., Lotze, M. T., Rosenberg, S. A., et al. (1987): Dermatologic changes associated
with IL-2 administration. J.A.M.A., 258:1624–1629.
35. Groopman, J. E., Mitsuyasu, R. T., DeLeo, M. J., Oette, D. H. and Golde, D. W. (1987): Effect
of recombinant human granulocyte macrophage colony stimulating factor on myelopoiesis in the
acquired immunodeficiency syndrome. *N. Engl. J. Med.*, 317:593–598.
36. Hamilton, J. A., Stanley, E. R., Burgess, A. W. and Shadduck, R. K. (1980): Stimulation of
macrophage plasminogen activator activity by CSFs. *J. Cell Physiol.*, 103:435–445.
37. Hammond, W. P., Price, T. H., Souza, L. M. and Dale, D. C. (1989): Treatment of cyclic
neutropenia with granulocyte colony stimulating factor. *N. Engl. J. Med.*, 320:1306–1311.
38. Hartmann, L. C., Urba, W. J., Steis, R. G. et al. (1989): Use of prophylactic antibiotics for
prevention of intravascular catheter related infections in IL-2 treated patients. *J. Natl. Cancer Inst.*,
81:1190–1193.
39. Herrmann, F., Schulz, G., Lindemann, A. et al. (1989): Hematopoietic responses in patients with
advanced malignancy treated with recombinant human GM-CSF. *J. Clin. Oncol.*, 7:159–167.
40. Horiguchi, J., Warren, M. K. and Kufe, D. (1987): Expression of the macrophage specific colony
stimulating factor in human monocytes treated with GM-CSF. *Blood*, 69:1259–1261.
41. Jablons, D., Bolton, E., Mertins, S. et al. (1990): IL-2 based immunotherapy alters circulating
neutrophil Fc receptor expression and chemotaxis. *J. Immunol.*, 144:3630–3636.
42. Johnson, G. R., Gonda, T. J., Metcalf, D. et al. (1988): A lethal myeloproliferative syndrome in
mice transplanted with bone marrow cells infected with a retrovirus expressing GM-CSF. *EMBO J*,
8:441–448.
43. Jakubowski, A. A., Souza, L. M., Kelly, F. et al. (1989): Effects of human granulocyte colony
stimulating factor in a patient with idiopathic neutropenia. *N. Engl. J. Med.*, 320:38–42.
44. Klempner, A. S., Noring, R., Mier, J. W. et al. (1990): An acquired chemotactic defect in neutrophils from patients receiving IL-2 immunotherapy. *N. Engl. J. Med.*, 322:959.
45. Komiyama, A., Ishiguro, A., Kubo, T. et al. (1988): Increases in neutrophil counts by purified
human urinary colony stimulating factor in chronic neutropenia of childhood. *Blood*, 71:41–45.
46. Kurland, J. I., Pelus, L. M., Ralph, P. et al. (1979): Induction of prostaglandin E synthesis in
normal and neoplastic macrophages: Role for CSF(s) distinct from effects on myeloid progenitor
cell proliferation. *Proc. Natl. Acad. Sci. U.S.A.*, 76:2326–2330.
47. Lang, R. A., Metcalf, D., Cuthbertson, R. A. et al. (1987): Transgenic mice expressing a hemopoietic growth factor gene (GM-CSF) develop accumulations of macrophages, blindness, and a
fatal syndrome of tissue damage. *Cell*, 51:675–686.
48. LeBeau, M. M., Lemons, R. S., Espinosa, R. et al. (1989): IL-4 and IL-5 map to human chromo-

some 5 in a region encoding growth factors and receptors and are deleted in myeloid leukemia with a del(5q). *Blood*, 73:647–650.

49. Lee, R. E., Gaspari, A. A., Lotze, M. T., et al. (1988): IL-2 and psoriasis. *Arch. Dermatol.*, 124: 1811–1815.

50. Lee, R. E., Lotze, M. T., Skibber, J. M. et al. (1989): Cardiorespiratory effects of immunotherapy with IL-2. *J. Clin. Oncol.*, 7:7–20.

51. Lieschke, G., Maher, D., Cebon, J. et al. (1989): Effects of bacterially synthesized recombinant human granulocyte macrophage colony stimulating factor in patients with advanced malignancy. *Ann. Intern. Med.*, 110:357–364.

52. Liu, S. J., Ascensao, J. L., Podack, E. et al. (1987): Cellular interactions in hematopoiesis. *Blood Cells*, 13:101–110.

53. Lotze, M. T., Matory, Y. L., Ettinghausen, S. E. et al. (1985): *In vivo* administration of purified human IL-2. II: Half-life, immunologic effects, and expansion of peripheral lymphoid cells *in vivo* with recombinant IL-2. *J. Immunol.*, 135:2865–2873.

53a. Lotze, M.T., Matory, Y. L, Rayner, A. A. et al (1986): Clinical effects and toxicity of IL-2 in patients with cancer. *Cancer*, 58:2764–2772.

54. McNiece, I. K., Andrews, R. G., Stewart, F. M. and Quesenberry, P. J. (1988): Synergistic interactions of human growth factors in *in vitro* cultures of human bone marrow cells. *Blood*, 72(Suppl.):410a.

55. Metcalf, D. (1984): The Hemopoietic Colony Stimulating Factors. Elsevier Science, Amsterdam.

56. Metcalf, D. (1985): The granulocyte-macrophage colony stimulating factors. *Science*, 229:16–22.

57. Metcalf, D. (1986): The molecular biology and functions of the granulocyte macrophage colony stimulating factors. *Blood*, 67:257–267.

58. Metcalf, D. (1989): Haemopoietic growth factors 1. *Lancet*, 1:825–827.

59. Metcalf, D. (1989): Haemopoietic growth factors 2: Clinical applications. *Lancet*, 1:885–887.

60. Metcalf, D. (1989): The molecular control of cell division, differentiation commitment and maturation in hemopoietic cells. *Nature London*, 339:27–30.

61. Metcalf, D., Begley, C. G., Johnson, G. R., et al (1986): Effects of purified bacterially synthesized murine multi-CSF (IL-3) on hematopoiesis in normal adult mice. *Blood*, 68:46–57.

62. Michie, H. R., Eberlein, T. J., Spriggs, D. R., et al. (1988): IL-2 initiates metabolic responses associated with critical illness in humans. *Ann. Surg.*, 208:493–503.

63. Moore, R. N., Oppenheim, J. J., Farrar, J. J. et al. (1980): Production of lymphocyte-activating factor (IL-1) by macrophages activated with CSFs. *J. Immunol.*, 125:1302.

64. Morrissey, P. J., Bressler, L., Park, L. S., Alpert, A. and Gillis, S. (1987): GM-CSF augments the primary antibody response by enhancing the function of antigen presenting cells. *J. Immunol.*, 139: 1113–1119.

65. Morstyn, G., Souza, L. M., Keech, J., et al. (1988): Effect of granulocyte colony stimulating factor on neutropenia induced by cytotoxic chemotherapy. *Lancet*, 1:667–672.

66. Motoyoshi, K., Takaku, F., Maekawa, T. et al. (1986): Protective effect of partially purified human urinary colony stimulating factor on granulocytopenia after antitumor chemotherapy. *Exp. Hematol.*, 14:1069–1075.

67. Murphy, P. M., Lane, H. C., Gallin, J. I. and Fauci, A. S. (1988): Marked disparity in incidence of bacterial infections in patients with AIDS receiving IL-2 or interferon-gamma. *Ann. Intern. Med.*, 108:36–41.

68. Negrin, R. S., Haeuber, D. H., Nagler, A. et al. (1990): Maintenance treatment of patients with myelodysplastic syndromes using recombinant human G-CSF. *Blood*, 76:36–43.

69. Negrin, R. S., Haeuber, D. H., Nagler, A., Olds, L. C., Donlon, T., Souza, L. M. and Greenberg, P. L. (1989): Treatment of myelodysplastic syndromes with recombinant human granulocyte colony stimulating factor: A phase I-II trial. *Ann. Intern. Med.*, 110:976–984.

70. Nemunaitis, J., Singer, J., Buckner, C. D. (1990): The use of recombinant human granulocyte macrophage colony stimulating factor for graft failure in patients after bone marrow transplantation. *Blood*, 76:245–253.

71. Nemunaitis, J., Singer, J. W., Buckner, C. D., et al. (1988): Use of recombinant human granulocyte macrophage colony stimulating factor in autologous bone marrow transplantation for lymphoid malignancies. *Blood*, 72:834–836.

72. Neta, R., Douches, S. and Oppenheim, J. J. (1986): Interleukin I is a radioprotector. *J. Immunol.*, 136:2483.

73. Nicola, N. A. (1989): Hemopoietic cell growth factors and their receptors. *Annu. Rev. Biochem.*, 58:45–77.

74. Nimer, S. D., Champlin, R. E. and Golde, D. W. (1988): Serum cholesterol lowering activity of granulocyte macrophage colony stimulating factor. *J.A.M.A.*, 260:3297.
75. Nora, R., Abrams, J. S., Tait, N. S. et al. (1989): Myocardial toxic effects during recombinant IL-2 therapy. *J. Natl. Cancer Inst.*, 81:59–63.
76. O'Garra, A. (1989): Interleukins and the immune system 1. *Lancet*, 1:943–947.
77. O'Garra, A. (1989): Interleukins and the immune system 2. *Lancet*, 1:1003–1005.
78. Ognibene, F. P., Rosenberg, S. A., Lotze, M. T. et al. (1988): IL-2 administration causes reversible hemodynamic changes and left ventricular dysfunction similar to those seen in septic shock. *Chest*, 94:750–754.
79. Ohno, R., Tomonaga, M., Kobayashi, T. et al. (1990): Effect of G-CSF after intensive induction therapy in relapsed or refractory acute leukemia. *N. Engl. J. Med.*, 323:871–877.
80. Oliff, A. (1988): The role of tumor necrosis factor (cachectin) in cachexia. *Cell*, 54:141–142.
82. Paquette, R. L., Zhou, J.-Y., Yang, Y.-C., et al. (1988): Recombinant gibbon IL-3 acts synergistically with recombinant human G-CSF and GM-CSF *in vitro*. *Blood*, 71:1596–1600.
83. Pestka, S., Langer, J. A., Zoon, K. C. and Samuel, C. E. (1987): Interferons and their actions. *Annu. Rev. Biochem.*, 56:727–777.
84. Peters, W. P., Shogen, J., Shpall, E. J., Jones, R. B. and Kim, C. S. (1988): Recombinant human GM-CSF produces fever. [Letter] *Lancet*, 1:950.
85. Pluda, J. M., Yarchoan, R., Smith, P. D. et al. (1990): Subcutaneous recombinant granulocyte macrophage colony stimulating factor used as a single agent and in an alternating regimen with azidothymidine in leukopenic patients with severe human immunodeficiency virus infection. *Blood*, 76:463–472.
86. Pluznik, H. D. and Sachs, L. (1965): The cloning of normal "mast" cells in tissue culture. *J. Cell Comp. Physiol.*, 66:319–324.
87. Pluznik, H. D. and Sachs, L. (1966): The induction of clones of normal "mast" cells by a substance from conditioned medium. *Exp. Cell Res.*, 43:553–561.
88. Puri, R. K. and Rosenberg, S. A. (1989): Combined effects of interferon alpha and IL-2 on the induction of a vascular leak syndrome in mice. *Cancer Immunol. and Immunother.*, 28:267–274.
89. Puri, R. K., Travis, W. T. and Rosenberg, S. A. (1989): Decrease in IL-2 induced vascular leakage in the lungs of mice by administration of recombinant IL-1 alpha *in vivo*. *Cancer Res.*, 49:969–976.
90. Rosenberg, S. A., Lotze, M. T., Muul, L. M. et al. (1987): A progress report on the treatment of 157 patients with advanced cancer using lymphokine activated killer cells and IL-2 or high dose IL-2 alone. *N. Engl. J. Med.*, 316:889–897.
91. Rosenberg, S. A., Lotze, M. T. and Mule, J. J. (1988): New approaches to the immunotherapy of cancer using IL-2. *Ann. Intern Med.*, 108:853–864.
92. Rosenberg, S. A., Packard, B. S., Aebersold, P. M., et al. (1988): Use of tumor infiltrating lymphocytes and IL-2 in the immunotherapy of patients with metastatic melanoma. *N. Engl. J. Med.*, 319:1676–1680.
93. Rosenstein, M., Ettinghausen, S. E. and Rosenberg, S. A. (1986): Extravasation of intravascular fluid mediated by the systemic administration of recombinant IL-2. *J. Immunol.*, 137:1735–1742.
94. Ruff, M. R., Farrar, W. I. and Pert, C. (1986). Interferon gamma and GM-CSF inhibit growth and induce antigens characteristic of myeloid differentiation in small-cell lung cancer cell lines. *Proc. Natl. Acad. Sci. U.S.A.*, 83:6613–6617.
95. Sarna, G. P., Figlin, R. A., Pertchek, M. et al. (1989): Systemic administration of recombinant methionyl human IL-2 (ala 125) to cancer patients; clinical results. *J. Biol. Response Mod.*, 8:16–24.
96. Sculier, J. P., Bron, D., Verboven, N. and Klastersky, J. (1988): Multiple organ failure during IL-2 administration and LAK cells infusion. *Intensive Care Med.*, 14:666–667.
97. Sieff, C. A. and Ekern, S. (1988): IL-3 and GM-CSF are synergistic and act independently. *Blood*, 72(Suppl.):447a.
98. Simpson, C., Seipp, C. A. and Rosenberg, S. A. (1988): The current status and future applications of IL-2 and adoptive immunotherapy in cancer treatment. *Semin. Oncol. Nurs.*, 4:132–141.
99. Sisson, S. D. and Dinarello, C. A. (1988): Production of interleukin-1 alpha, interleukin-1 beta and tumor necrosis factor by human mononuclear cells stimulated with granulocyte macrophage colony stimulating factor. *Blood*, 72:1368–1374.
100. Socinski, M. A., Cannistra, S. A., Sullivan, R. et al. (1988): GM-CSF induces the expression of the CD11b surface adhesion molecule on human granulocytes *in vitro*. *Blood*, 72:691–697.
101. Sosman, J. A., Kohler, P. C., Hank, J. A., et al. (1988): Repetitive weekly cycles of IL-2. II.

Clinical and immunologic effects of dose, schedule, and addition of indomethacin. *J. Natl. Cancer Inst.*, 80:1451–1461.

102. Steward, W. P. and Scarffe, J. H. (1989): Clinical trials with hemopoietic growth factors. *Prog. Growth Factor Res.*, 1:1–12.

103. Stolpen, A. H., Guinan, E. C., Fiers, W. and Pober, J. S. (1986): Recombinant TNF and immune interferon act singly and in combination to reorganize human vascular endothelial cell monolayers. *Am. J. Pathol.*, 123:16–24.

104. Textor, S. C., Margolin, K., Blayney, D. et al. (1987): Renal, volume, and hormonal changes during therapeutic administration of recombinant IL-2 in man. *Am. J. Med.*, 83:1055–1061.

105. Vadhan-Raj, S., Buescher, S., Broxmeyer, H. E. et al. (1988): Stimulation of myelopoiesis in patients with aplastic anemia by recombinant human granulocyte macrophage colony stimulating factor. *N. Engl. J. Med.*, 319:1628–1634.

106. Vadhan-Raj, S., Buescher, S., LeMaistre, A. et al. (1988): Stimulation of hematopoiesis in patients with bone marrow failure and in patients with malignancy by recombinant human granulocyte macrophage colony stimulating factor. *Blood*, 72:134–141.

107. Vadhan-Raj, S., Keating, M., LeMaistre, A. et al. (1987): Effects of recombinant human granulocyte macrophage colony stimulating factor in patients with myelodysplastic syndromes. *N. Engl. J. Med.*, 317:1545–1552.

108. Van Liessum, P. A., de Mulder, P. H., Mattijssen, E. J. and Corstens, F. H. (1989): Hypothyroidism and goiter during IL-2 therapy without LAK cells. [Letter] *Lancet*, 1:224.

109. Vellenga, E., Ostapovicz, D., O'Rourke, B. and Griffin, J. D. (1987): Effects of recombinant IL-3, GM-CSF, and G-CSF on proliferation of leukemic clonogenic cells in short-term and long-term cultures. *Leukemia*, 1:584–589.

110. Vetto, J. T., Papa, M. Z., Chang, A. E. and Rosenberg, S. A. (1987): Reduction of toxicity of IL-2 and lymphokine activated killer cells in humans by administration of corticosteroids. *J. Clin. Oncol.*, 5:496–503.

111. Webb, D. E., Austin, H. A., Belldegrun, A. et al. (1988): Metabolic and renal effects of IL-2 immunotherapy for metastatic cancer. *Clin. Nephrol.*, 30:141–145.

112. Weisbart, R. H., Kwan, L., Golde, D. W. and Gasson, J. (1987): Human GM-CSF primes neutrophils for enhanced oxidative metabolism in response to the major physiologic chemoattractants. *Blood*, 69:18–21.

113. Welte, K., Bonilla, M., Gillio, A. P. et al. (1987): Effects on hematopoiesis in normal and cyclophosphamide treated primates. *J. Exp. Med.*, 165:941–948.

114. Wing, E. J., Magee, D. M., Whiteside, T. L., Kaplan, S. S. and Shadduck, R. K. (1989): Recombinant human granulocyte macrophage colony stimulating factor enhances monocyte cytotoxicity and secretion of tumor necrosis factor alpha and interferon in cancer patients. *Blood*, 73:643–646.

115. Yang, Y-C, Kovacic, S., Kriz, R. et al (1988): The human genes for GM-CSF and IL-3 are closely linked in tandem on chromosome 5. *Blood*, 71:958–961.

Clinical Immunotoxicology, edited by
D. S. Newcombe, N. R. Rose, and J. C. Bloom.
Raven Press, Ltd., New York © 1992.

8

Immunopathogenesis of the Acquired Immune Deficiency Syndrome: Relevance to Immunotoxicity

Joseph B. Margolick

Department of Environmental Health Sciences, Johns Hopkins University, School of Hygiene and Public Health, 615 N. Wolfe Street, Room 7032, Baltimore, MD 21205

Since its recognition as a distinct clinical entity in 1981 (1,2), the acquired immune deficiency syndrome (AIDS) has become a classic example of cellular immune deficiency (3–5). However, AIDS is also characterized by increased incidence of hypersensitivity and autoimmune reactions, phenomena which, together with immunosuppression, constitute the full spectrum of immunotoxicity (6). This conceptual link between AIDS and immunotoxicity suggests that an understanding of the pathogenesis and manifestations of AIDS may hold important lessons for our understanding of the mechanisms by which toxic substances injure the immune system. Of equal importance, AIDS has provided both an opportunity and an impetus to develop new methods by which injury to the immune system can be detected and assessed quantitatively. This chapter reviews current knowledge regarding immunopathogenesis of AIDS and discusses its implications for mechanisms of immune deficiency and the field of immunotoxicity.

DEFINITION OF THE ACQUIRED IMMUNE DEFICIENCY SYNDROME

The definition of AIDS has been revised several times since 1981, but it is still fundamentally a clinical definition (7). In most cases, to be diagnosed as having AIDS a patient must have (a) a reliably diagnosed disease that is indicative of an underlying cellular immune deficiency, and (b) evidence of infection with human immune deficiency virus, type 1 (HIV-1). In the United States, the most common diseases indicating cellular immune deficiency are Kaposi's sarcoma and pneumonia caused by the protozoan *Pneumocystis carinii*. Recently the spectrum of illnesses diagnostic of AIDS has been extended to include dementia and cachexia for which no other cause can be found (7).

Before the identification of HIV-1 as the etiological agent for AIDS (8–10), the diagnosis of AIDS required the patient to be under 60 years of age and also past childhood, so that congenital and age-related immune deficiencies were excluded, and to be without evidence of any other cause of underlying immune deficiency such as immunosuppressive therapy or malignancy of the lymphoreticular system. However, these requirements have been superseded by the ability to identify individuals who are infected with HIV-1; they now apply primarily to cases in which the patient cannot be tested for infection with HIV-1 or the test is inconclusive. In addition, individuals who test negative for HIV-1 can still be diagnosed as having AIDS if they have a marker illness such as *Pneumocystis* pneumonia and fewer than 400 circulating helper-inducer (T4 or CD4) T lymphocytes per cubic millimeter *and* if the causes of secondary immune deficiency mentioned above have been excluded (7).

The essential point is that the definition of AIDS depends on clinical diagnoses. In particular, there is no laboratory test that is diagnostic of AIDS. Although a host of immune abnormalities are present in patients with AIDS, many of these same abnormalities are also seen in other stages of HIV-1 infection, other types of immune deficiencies, and, in some cases, immunologically normal individuals.

A discussion of the opportunistic infections and neoplasms that occur in AIDS is beyond the scope of this chapter and is available elsewhere (11–13). Suffice it to say that the infections seen in AIDS tend not to be caused by the common pyogenic organisms, as is common in patients with humoral immune deficiency. Rather, they are produced by viral, parasitic, fungal, and other intracellular organisms against which the primary host defense mechanisms depend on cellular immunity.

PATHOGENESIS OF ACQUIRED IMMUNE DEFICIENCY SYNDROME: CRITICAL ROLE OF THE CD4 LYMPHOCYTE

AIDS is characterized by decreased numbers of CD4 lymphocytes. The main cell that is affected in the pathogenesis of AIDS is the CD4 (T4)-positive T lymphocyte. Numbers of circulating CD4 lymphocytes are generally dramatically reduced in patients with AIDS, as compared with immunologically healthy individuals (3,5, 11, 14). The normal number is approximately 800 to 1,200/mm^3. Patients with AIDS usually have less than 200 (15,16), although some have 200 to 400 CD4 lymphocytes and a few have more than 400 (17). Infection with HIV-1 may not be followed by immune deficiency for many years, but it is associated with an initial decrease in the number of circulating CD4 lymphocytes, which may then stabilize, decline slowly, or decline rapidly (18,19). The reasons for the decline in CD4 numbers after infection with HIV-1 and for the highly variable rate of this decline are not known. Numbers of CD8 (T8)-positive lymphocytes, or suppressor-cytotoxic lymphocytes, are generally normal or elevated in HIV-1-infected individuals, including most patients with AIDS (18). Thus, the lymphopenia that occurs in AIDS is caused almost entirely by a drop in the number of CD4 lymphocytes, at least in the early stages of the disease. Later on, in the advanced stages of AIDS, there may be a loss of CD8 lymphocytes also. Similarly, the reversal of the CD4/CD8 (T4/T8) ratio that is seen in AIDS is primarily attributable to a drop in the number of CD4 lymphocytes.

It is important to distinguish between the reduced or reversed T4/T8 ratio seen in AIDS and that seen in a number of other viral diseases, the most common of which is infectious mononucleosis. These other viral diseases are characterized by a temporary increase in the number of CD8-positive lymphocytes, reducing or reversing the normal CD4/CD8 (T4/T8) ratio (20,21). However, this reduction is transient and is produced by an increase in CD8 lymphocytes as opposed to the reversal seen in AIDS, which is protracted and due to a loss of CD4 lymphocytes. Reversed CD4/CD8 (T4/T8) ratios are not uncommon among asymptomatic HIV-1-negative individuals, and a reversed ratio on one specimen does not imply abnormal cellular immune function.

The mechanism of depletion of CD4 cells in AIDS is not known, but several possibilities have been proposed (Table 1A). The depletion of CD4 lymphocytes could be the *in vivo* correlate of the direct cytopathic effect of HIV-1 on CD4-positive T lymphocytes that occurs *in vitro* (9,22), but there is still no direct proof of this. Using the most sensitive techniques available, active infection with HIV-1 can be demonstrated in no more than 1 in 1,000 or as few as 1 in 10^5 lymphocytes freshly obtained from the peripheral blood of infected individuals (23,24). Whether the rather low level of destruction of CD4 cells that could be explained by lytic infection of these cells at a given time could account for the profound depletion of these cells that occurs over many years is not known. This question thus exposes a fundamental gap in our understanding of the normal biology of the immune system.

More recent studies have suggested that the proportion of CD4 lymphocytes latently infected with HIV-1 may be much higher than the proportion that is actively replicating HIV-1 (25–28). These data suggest that the reservoir for direct lysis of CD4 cells may be as large as one CD4 cell in 100 at a given time in persons with AIDS (25).

CD4 cells infected with HIV-1 expressing viral antigens on their surface can fuse

TABLE 1. *Possible mechanisms of deficient antigen-induced immunity in acquired immune deficiency syndrome*

A. Death and depletion of CD4 lymphocytes
    Direct cytopathic effect of HIV-1 on CD4 cells
    Fusion of infected CD4 cells with uninfected CD4 cells
    "Autoimmune" destruction of uninfected CD4 cells
    Decreased production of CD4 lymphocytes
B. Decreased clonal expansion of CD4 lymphocytes
C. Functional inhibition of CD4 lymphocytes
    Production of soluble suppressor factors
    Binding of HIV-1 or viral proteins (gp 120 env) to CD4
    Binding of HIV-1 or viral proteins to other surface molecules
D. Functional inhibition of mononuclear phagocytes

with uninfected CD4 cells *in vitro* (29). This fusion is mediated by the HIV-1 envelope protein gp 120, which binds to the CD4 molecule, the receptor for the virus on the lymphocyte surface membrane (22,30–32). It has been reported that gp 120 on the surface of infected cells can bind to CD4 on uninfected cells, leading to the fusion of the infected and uninfected cells and the formation of a syncytial giant cell, which then dies. By this mechanism, infection of one lymphocyte could lead to the death of many uninfected lymphocytes. However, fusion of CD4-positive cells does not appear to be required for the cytopathic effect of HIV-1 on these cells (33), although CD4 is required. Binding of gp 120 to surface CD4 of uninfected T cells could also lead to destruction of these cells by immunological mechanisms directed at gp 120 (see below).

AIDS is characterized by decreased function of CD4 lymphocytes. In some patients with AIDS, as mentioned above, the reduction in numbers of CD4 lymphocytes is less dramatic than the profound loss of cellular immune function. This finding raised the possibility that intrinsic abnormalities of CD4 lymphocyte *function*, as well as *number*, might also be present and contributing to the immune deficiency. Several studies have suggested that such abnormalities might be important. Patients with AIDS generally exhibited reduced proliferation of peripheral blood lymphocytes, as measured by incorporation of tritiated thymidine, in response to both mitogens and soluble antigens such as tetanus toxoid. However, if CD4 cells from the AIDS patients were purified and added back to the cultures, most of the decrease was reversed for mitogen-induced but not tetanus toxoid–induced proliferation (34). Similarly, when purified CD4 cells and CD8 cells from patients with AIDS and from healthy individuals were added to B cells from a healthy individual and pokeweed mitogen–induced immunoglobulin production was measured, the AIDS CD4 cells but not the AIDS CD8 cells functioned abnormally (35). These findings suggest that depletion of CD4 lymphocytes is not the only defect in CD4 lymphocyte function, at least in these *in vitro* systems.

The defect in T-cell responses to soluble antigen, together with the depletion of the CD4 lymphocyte that represents the principal mediator of antigen-induced responses (36), suggests that loss of antigen-induced CD4 cell function is one of the hallmarks that leads to the development of clinical AIDS. In support of this conclusion, most if not all of the myriad immunological functions that are abnormal in patients with AIDS require induction of precursor or inactive cells to an active state, and this induction is dependent on the production of lymphokines or other helper T-cell–mediated mechanisms. For example, cytotoxic function of natural killer cells from patients with AIDS, although highly deficient compared with cells from healthy donors, could be augmented to virtually normal levels by culturing the cells from the donors with AIDS in the presence of interleukin-2 (IL-2) for 1 to 72 hours (37). Similar results were observed with respect to T-cell–mediated cytotoxicity against target cells infected with cytomegalovirus (37). Thus, at least some of the cells that are needed to perform immunological functions such as cytotoxicity are present in patients with AIDS but are in "immunologic neutral" because they do not receive the necessary activation signals to "shift into gear." In addition, lack of antigen-induced lymphokine production has been documented in persons with AIDS (38) as well as persons with AIDS-related complex (39), in whom lack of lymphokine production was strongly correlated with subsequent development of AIDS.

Many mechanisms could be envisioned to account for this deficient antigen-induced T-helper cell function (see Table 1). Depletion of CD4 cells has been discussed above. Depletion of a specific subpopulation of CD4 cells that is responsible for antigen-induced function has also been reported to be present early, although not later on, in the course of HIV-1 infection (40,41). The ability of immune cells to proliferate normally in response to a soluble antigen may also be directly impaired by HIV-1. In our experiments (42), cells exposed to tetanus toxoid on day 0 and then HIV-1 on day 3 were maintained in culture for 21 days and then reexposed to the same antigen (Table 2). Whereas cells that were not exposed to virus on day 3 gave a normal proliferative response, cells that had been exposed to a 10^{-4} dilution of virus exhibited virtually no antigen-induced proliferation. For cells exposed to a 10^{-5} dilution on day 3, the proliferative response 18 days later was only half the control value. Whether this HIV-1-induced inhibition of antigen-induced reactivity has to do with destruction of specific cell populations or with the effects of viral proteins on normal cell populations is not yet known. However, in our experiments, virus that had been heated to 56°C for 30 minutes also did not cause subsequent loss of lymphoproliferative responses, and Pahwa and coworkers (43,44) have reported a direct inhibition of both antigen- and mitogen-induced lymphoproliferative responses by banded, noninfectious HIV-1 preparations.

Another mechanism by which HIV-1 may functionally inhibit lymphocytes without actually killing them is through the production of soluble suppressor factors (45). These may actually be normal factors produced in abnormal quantities. In addition, HIV-1 proteins such as the envelope protein gp 120 can bind to CD4, as mentioned above, and binding of other ligands to CD4 has been reported to be immunosuppressive in and of itself (46). Finally, HIV-1 has been shown to have significant homology at the genomic and protein levels with certain immunoregulatory molecules such as neuroleukins (47,48). One could speculate that binding of these proteins to receptors on lymphocytes could disrupt the normal functions of these cells. (Binding of HIV-1 proteins to neurons, competitively inhibiting the binding of nerve growth factors, has been proposed to contribute to the pathogenesis of AIDS dementia [49].)

Mononuclear phagocytes express CD4 and can be infected with HIV-1 *in vivo* and *in vitro* (50,51). Unlike T cells, however, they are not killed by HIV-1 and therefore may produce HIV-1 for much longer than T cells and at higher levels (51). Thus, the possibility exists that HIV-1 may impair one or more of the critical functions of mononuclear phagocytes in induction of antigen-specific immune responses, such as antigen processing, antigen presentation, or IL-1 production. Indeed, abnormalities of monocyte function have been reported in AIDS: decreased intracellular killing (38), decreased chemotactic responses (52), and increased spontaneous IL-1 production (52). Again, most or all of these abnormalities may be due

TABLE 2. *Inhibition of proliferative responses of peripheral blood mononuclear cells[a] by prior exposure to human immunodeficiency virus*

1° Stimulus (day 0) 2° Stimulus (days 17–21) Virus (day 3)	Experiment 1							Experiment 2	Experiment 3
	KLH		TT		No antigen			No antigen	No antigen
	PHA	KLH	PHA	TT	PHA	TT	KLH	PHA	PHA
0	51,182[b]	29,349	52,449	19,126	23,447	12,700	6,712	36,918	77,255
10^{-4}	8,767	392	6,598	341	7,815	97	0	8,751	35,215
10^{-5}	27,979	14,804	24,101	10,959	30,409	2,863	2,436	36,389	49,416

[a]Peripheral blood mononuclear cells were incubated with the 1° stimulus, either antigen (TT, tetanus toxoid at 10 μg/ml; KLH, keyhole limpet hemocyanin at 100 μg/ml); PHA, phytohemagglutinin or medium alone, on day 0, exposed to live virus on day 3, and maintained in the culture until restimulation with the 2° stimulus on days 17 to 21 as described by Margolick and coworkers (ref. 42).

[b]Data are presented as change in counts per minute compared with cells restimulated with medium (including irradiated autologous peripheral blood mononuclear cells) alone.

to or exacerbated by the lack of normal regulatory or inducing influences exerted by CD4 cells, such as secretion of interferon-gamma. Although overproduction of cytokines (e.g., tumor necrosis factor) may contribute to the cachexia of AIDS and/or to the activation of latent HIV-1 infection in some cells (53,54), the role of altered mononuclear phagocyte function in the pathogenesis of deficient antigen-induced CD4 cell function in AIDS has not been established. At least some evidence indicates that the monocyte-dependent aspects of this function are not necessarily impaired in the presence of HIV-1 infection, even in patients with AIDS (55,56).

Finally, there may be defects in responsiveness of individual T cells for unexplained reasons. In another study (57), we measured the cloning efficiency of purified T4 cells and T8 cells from patients with AIDS and from healthy individuals. In this assay, cells are plated in round bottomed tissue culture plates under conditions that allow individual T cells to proliferate and form colonies; the proportion of viable cells forming colonies represents the cloning efficiency of the cells. Reduction in cloning efficiency may be a defect that viable cells manifest only when they are required to undergo several rounds of proliferation. Therefore, we hypothesized that measurement of cloning efficiencies of T-cell populations could provide a more sensitive method for detecting injury to T lymphocytes than measuring numbers of cells or the functioning of bulk cell populations. In eight experiments, we found that both CD4 and CD8 lymphocytes from patients with AIDS had greatly reduced cloning efficiencies compared with cells from healthy individuals, indicating a T-cell defect at the level of the individual cell. The basis for this defect, as well as its possible role in the pathogenesis of immune deficiency, remains to be established. This defect may be a result of an increase in normal cells that do not have the ability to expand clonally or it may be attributable to a true abnormality in the T cells. According to Pantaleo and colleagues, at least some of the reduced cloning efficiency of CD8 cells is caused by an increase in cells expressing HLA-DR; these cells have a reduced cloning efficiency compared with CD8 cells lacking HLA-DR (58). This finding illustrates the importance of knowing the types of lymphocytes present and their characteristics before attributing defects to the cells.

Whatever the mechanism for the loss of CD4 lymphocyte function in AIDS, the severe immune suppression that characterizes this disease provides a graphic example of the dramatic consequences that can follow loss of a critical immune function and of how such an effect can result from an injury to a specific population of cells. The fact that CD4 numbers generally decline to less than $200/mm^3$ illustrates the degree of depletion associated with clinically important immune suppression caused by HIV-1. Conversely, the fact that some lymphocyte proliferative responses may be within the normal range in persons with AIDS illustrates the need for caution in interpreting such tests.

IMMUNE ACTIVATION AS A COFACTOR FOR SUSCEPTIBILITY TO IMMUNOTOXIC EFFECTS

Mitogen-induced activation of T cells has long been known to favor the replication of the AIDS retrovirus, and in fact that is how the virus was first propagated

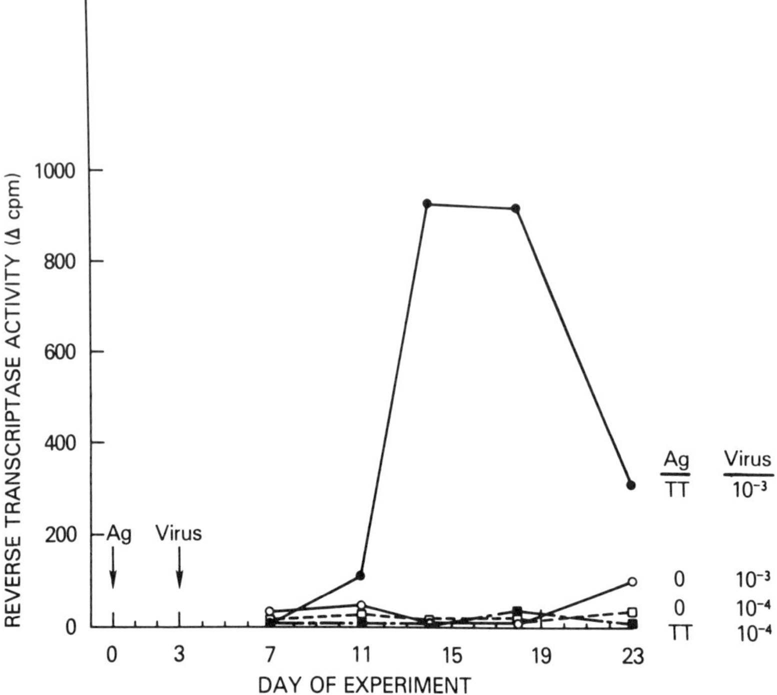

FIG. 1. The production of reverse transcriptase by normal human peripheral blood mononuclear cells exposed to a 10^3 dilution of stock HIV-1 if previously cultured with tetanus toxoid (TT) but not if cultured with medium alone. Cells exposed to a 10^4 dilution of HIV-1 did not produce detectable reverse transcriptase, whether cultured with TT or with medium alone. Reprinted with permission from Margolick et al., (42).

and identified (59). Since antigen-induced activation occurs by different mechanisms at the cellular level and certainly involves proportionately many fewer cells than mitogen-induced activation (60), we studied the role of antigen-induced T cell activation in the regulation of susceptibility of CD4 lymphocytes to infection with HIV-1 (42). In these experiments, peripheral blood monocytes from an immunologically normal donor were exposed to a soluble antigen such as tetanus toxoid or to medium alone on day 0, exposed to HIV-1 on day 3, washed free of antigen and virus, and maintained in culture for up to a total of 24 days. Supernatants from the cells were sampled twice a week for evidence of viral replication, e.g., production of reverse transcriptase or HIV-1 genomic products. As shown in Fig. 1, if cells cultured with tetanus toxoid were exposed to a 10^{-3} dilution of HIV-1, reverse transcriptase was produced. If the cells were exposed to the same concentration of virus without prior exposure to tetanus toxoid, no reverse transcriptase production was detectable. If the cells were exposed to a lower dilution of virus—10^{-4} instead of 10^{-3}—there was no reverse transcriptase produced even after culture with tetanus toxoid. Because relatively little antigen-induced proliferation actually occurred by day 3, these results indicate that the activation state of the lymphocytes is very important in determining the susceptibility of the cells to productive infection with HIV-1.

These experiments were done in cultures of 100,000 cells per well. Although we did not directly measure the number of cells that were activated by exposure to tetanus toxoid, in one published study the precursor frequency of such cells ranged from 1 in 750 to 1 in 11,500 (60). Thus, the number of cells actually activated by the antigenic stimulus in these experiments was probably less than 150 and may have been as low as less than 10, but this was still sufficient to provide the observed amplification of at least 30- to 40-fold (42).

In summary, these studies strongly suggest that the susceptibility of the immune system to toxic stimuli may depend very much on its state of activation. Thus, chemicals or other factors that impinge on T-cell activation play a critical role in determining the magnitude of toxic effects on these cells and immune function in general. One important possibility is that activation of T cells, which leads to several rounds of cell division, may permit replication of viruses that are latent in the cellular genome, thereby initiating an immunotoxic effect (61). Phorbol myristate acetate, which can serve as an activating signal for T cells and is also a tumor promoter, has been reported to increase HIV-1 replication in susceptible cells (62). Another possible mechanism for T-cell activation owing to exogenous agents is stimulation of mononuclear phagocytes to release the T-cell activating factor, IL-1 (63). As mentioned above, release of tumor necrosis factor by activated monocytes may also activate latent HIV-1 provirus (53,54). Of note is that tumor necrosis factor production by activated mononuclear phagocytes may play an important role in silica-induced pulmonary fibrosis (64).

B-CELL HYPERFUNCTION IN ACQUIRED IMMUNE DEFICIENCY SYNDROME: IMPLICATIONS FOR AUTOIMMUNITY

As a general rule, patients with AIDS have increased rather than reduced levels of circulating immunoglobulins. This fact, along with the clinical occurrence of illnesses that typify cellular rather than humoral immune deficiency, delayed the recognition of abnormalities in B-cell function in AIDS. However, it has been demonstrated that patients with AIDS, if immunized with a neoantigen such as keyhole limpet hemocyanin, failed to respond with the production of specific anti–keyhole limpet hemocyanin antibody (35). This indicated a failure of T-cell function, or B-cell function, or both. It was also demonstrated that the elevated levels of serum immunoglobulins were not a physiological response to immunological stimuli but rather were due to a polyclonal B cell activation similar in scope to that seen in systemic lupus erythematosus (35). The antibodies that are produced are believed to represent the entire repertoire of the host and are normal antibodies that confer protection against the standard pyogenic bacterial diseases such as pneumococcal pneumonia.

It is noteworthy that systemic lupus erythematosus is the prototypical autoimmune disease, characterized by the occurrence of autoantibodies and circulating immune complexes. These also occur in patients with AIDS (65,66) and may be important in the pathogenesis of thrombocytopenia and neutropenia owing to HIV-1 infection (67,68). Other autoantibodies were produced by individuals infected with HIV-1 (reviewed in [69]) as well as individuals at high risk for infection with HIV-1, and a correlation between stage of HIV-1 infection and autoantibody titer was suggested (66). Patients with AIDS have also been reported to have an increased incidence of oligoclonal immunoglobulins (70). These abnormalities may be related to an increased proportion of circulating B cells that are activated or immature (71).

The occurrence of these autoimmune phenomena in AIDS suggests that the mechanism for this polyclonal B-cell hypergammaglobulinemia may be important in understanding autoimmune manifestations of AIDS and other diseases. Several different mechanisms have been proposed (Table 3). One is a dysregulation such that normal T-cell suppressive influences are lacking. Another is that B cells may be transformed with Epstein-Barr virus, which can lead to immortalization and clonal expansion of antibody-producing cells (72,73). A third is that there is direct infection of B cells by HIV-1; this has been demonstrated to occur in B cells infected with Epstein-Barr virus *in vitro* (74) as well as *in vivo* (75), although such occurrences have been relatively uncommon. A fourth possibility is a direct action of HIV-1 on B cells, as distinct from infection of the cells with HIV-1 (76). However, most studies have suggested that the latter effect may have been the result of residual non–B cells in the B cells analyzed (44). Recent evidence indicates that elevated serum levels of IL-6 (77,78), possibly derived from monocytes (78), may contribute to this polyclonal B-cell activation and perhaps to the high incidence of B-cell lymphomas in HIV-1 infected individuals. Finally, the role of additional viruses that can infect B lymphocytes such as human herpesvirus type 6 (79) and cytomegalovirus (80) in the pathogenesis of polyclonal B cell activation in AIDS is not known.

Autoimmunity directed at T lymphocytes has been proposed as a mechanism of the profound T–helper cell depletion that occurs in AIDS (81,82). At least two mechanisms might account for this. First, viral envelope proteins attached to CD4 might provoke an immune response directed against CD4 cells carrying gp 120 or other viral antigens, or against CD4 itself. As mentioned above, CD4 cells do not

TABLE 3. *Possible mechanisms for B-lymphocyte hyperfunction in acquired immune deficiency syndrome*

Loss of T-cell regulation (suppression)
Transformation of B cells with Epstein-Barr virus
Infection of Epstein-Barr virus–transformed B cells with HIV-1
Direct effect of HIV-1 or HIV-1 components on B cells without infection
Effect of other viruses (cytomegalovirus, human herpesvirus type-6)
Elevated secretion of B-cell stimulating cytokines (IL-6)

have to be infected with HIV-1 for this to occur. Second, the polyclonal B-cell activation might stimulate the production of antibodies reacting with normal T-cell antigens. There is no definitive evidence for these mechanisms of destruction of CD4 cells at the present time, although antilymphocyte antibodies have been demonstrated in patients with AIDS (82–85).

ALTERED HYPERSENSITIVITY RESPONSES IN ACQUIRED IMMUNE DEFICIENCY SYNDROME

Patients with AIDS manifest abnormal reactivity to certain drugs, the most well-known example of which is the high incidence of adverse reactions in patients given sulfamethoxazole-trimethoprim for treatment of *Pneumocystis carinii* pneumonia. In other patients this drug combination has a very low incidence of such effects, but in AIDS many and even most patients develop unexplained maculopapular rashes, fever, and/or cytopenias after a week of therapy (86–88). The incidence of these reactions may be as high as 80%, and they frequently necessitate a change in drug therapy. The onset of AIDS has also been reported to be associated with the exacerbation or recurrence of quiescent atopic disease (89).

The mechanism for the increase in these adverse reactions in patients with AIDS is not understood. Elevated levels of circulating immunoglobulins caused by the polyclonal B cell activation may be implicated—either IgG, which is most commonly increased, or possibly IgE, which has been reported to be elevated in some patients with AIDS (90,91). Of note, an increase in cutaneous and other reactions to drugs has been observed in immunologically normal patients with infectious mononucleosis (92,93). Therefore, it is possible that Epstein-Barr virus, cytomegalovirus, or HIV-1 itself could play a role in the pathogenesis of drug reactions and other hypersensitivity responses in patients with AIDS. In this connection, elevated production of IgE binding factor by HIV-1 infected individuals has been demonstrated (94), suggesting dysregulation of IgE in all stages of HIV-1 infection.

Many patients with AIDS exhibit a relative or absolute eosinophilia. The mechanism and significance of this finding are also unknown.

CONCLUSION

In summary, AIDS is characterized by diverse disturbances in cellular and humoral immune function that are related to the depletion of CD4-positive lymphocytes and to impairments in the regulatory functions that these cells normally subserve, both in activating and in suppressing immune responses. The potential role of specific T-cell subsets, e.g., CD4 cells that have been activated, as targets for HIV-1 is underlined and provides a model for investigating susceptibility of these cells to other potentially toxic influences. In addition, the study of the pathogenesis of AIDS provides a model for the study of immunoregulation in the pathogenesis of autoimmunity and hypersensitivity. Finally, the study of AIDS reminds us that there are still many aspects of the disease that we do not fully understand, for example, the mechanisms for such common symptoms as cachexia, dementia, or chronic diarrhea. The possibility should be kept in mind that these symptoms may have an immunological basis, perhaps in the production of cytokines such as tumor necrosis factor, which can have diverse effects throughout the body (95). Thus, the occurrence of AIDS continues to broaden our concept of the scope of the human immune system as a target organ for toxic damage.

REFERENCES

1. Centers for Disease Control (1981): *Pneumocystis* pneumonia—Los Angeles. *M.M.W.R.*, 20:250–252.
2. Centers for Disease Control (1981): Kaposi's sarcoma and *Pneumocystis* pneumonia among homosexual men—New York City and California. *M.M.W.R.*, 25:305–328.
3. Gottlieb, M. S., Schroff, R., Schander, H. M., Weisman, D. O., Fan, P. T., Wolf, R. A., and Saxon, A. (1981): *Pneumocystis carinii* pneumonia and mucosal candidiasis in previously healthy homosexual men: Evidence for a new acquired cellular immunodeficiency. *N. Engl. J. Med.*, 305:1425–1431.
4. Masur, H., Michelis, M. A., Greene, J. B., Onorato, I., Vande Stouwe, R. A., Holzman, R. S., Wormser, G., Brettman, L., Lange, M., Murray, H. W., and Cunningham-Rundles, S. (1981): An outbreak of community-acquired *P. carinii* pneumonia: Initial manifestation of cellular immune dysfunction. *N. Engl. J. Med.*, 305:1411–1438.
5. Siegal, F. P., Lopez, E., Hammer, G. S., Brown, A. E., Kornfeld, S. J., Gold, J., Haset, J., Hirschman, S. Z., Cunningham-Rundles, C., Adelsberg, B. R., Parham, D. M., Siegal, M., Cunningham-Rundles, S., and Armstrong, D. (1981): Severe acquired immunodeficiency in male homosexuals manifested by chronic perianal ulcerative herpes simplex lesions. *N. Engl. J. Med.*, 305:1439–1444.
6. Dean, J. H., Murray, M. J., and Ward, E. C. (1986): In Toxicology the Basic Science of Poisons, edited by C. D. Klaassen, M. O. Amdur, and J. Doull, p. 245. Macmillan, New York.
7. Centers for Disease Control (1987): Revision of CDC surveillance case definition for acquired immunodeficiency syndrome. *M.M.W.R.*, 36:522–527.
8. Popovic, M., Read-Connole, E., and Gallo, R. C. (1984): T4 positive human neoplastic cell lines susceptible to and permissive for HTLV-III. *Lancet*, 2:1472–1473.
9. Gallo, R. C., Salahuddin, S. Z., Popovic, M., Shearer, G. M., Kaplan, M., Haynes, B. F., Palker T. J., Redfield, R., Oleske, J., Safai, B., White, G., Foster, P., and Markham, P. D. (1984): Frequent detection and isolation of cytopathic retroviruses (HTLV-III) from patients with AIDS and at risk for AIDS. *Science*, 224:500–503.
10. Schupbach Popovic, M. J., Gilden, R. V., Gonda, M. A., Sarngadharan, M. G., and Gallo, R. C. (1984): Serological analysis of a subgroup of human T-lymphotropic retroviruses (HTLV-III) associated with AIDS. *Science*, 224:503–505.
11. Fauci, A. S., Macher, A. M., Longo, D. L., Lane, H. C., Rook, A. H., Masur, H., and Gelmann, E. P. (1984): Acquired immunodeficiency syndrome: Epidemiologic clinical immunologic and therapeutic considerations. *Ann. Intern. Med.*, 100:92–106.
12. Fauci, A. S., Masur, H., Gelmann, E. P., Markham, P. D., Hahn, B. H., and Lane, H. C. (1985): The acquired immunodeficiency syndrome: An update. *Ann. Intern. Med.*, 102:800–813.
13. Levy, J. A. (1989): AIDS Pathogenesis and Treatment. Marcel Dekker, New York.
14. Mildvan, D., Mathur, U., Enlow, R. W., Roman, P. L., Winchester, R. J., Cop, C., Singman, H., Adelsberg, B. R., and Springland, I. (1982): Opportunistic infections and immunodeficiency in homosexual men. *Ann. Intern. Med.*, 96:700–704.
15. Phair, J., Munoz, A., Detels, R., Kaslow, R., Rinaldo, C., Saah, A., and the Multicenter AIDS Cohort Study Group (1990): The risk of *Pneumocystis carinii* pneumonia among men infected with human immunodeficiency virus type 1. *N. Engl. J. Med.*, 322:161–165.
16. Masur, H., Ognibene, F. P., Yarchoan, R., Shelhamer, J. H., Baird, B. F., Travis, W., Suffredini, A. F., Deyton, L., Kovacs, J. A., Falloon, J., Davey, R., Polis, M., Metcalf, J., Baseler, M., Wesley, R., Gill, V. J., Fauci, A. S., and Lane, H. C. (1989): CD4 counts as predictors of

opportunistic pneumonias in human immunodeficiency virus (HIV) infection. *Ann. Intern. Med.*, 111:223–231.

17. Lane, H. C., Masur, H., Gelmann, E. P., Longo, D. L., Steis, R. G., Chused, T., Whalen, G., Edgar, L. C., and Fauci, A. S. (1985): Correlation between immunologic function and clinical subpopulations of patients with the acquired immune deficiency syndrome. *Am. J. Med.*, 78:417–422.

18. Giorgi, J. V., Fahey, J. L., Smith, D. C., Hultin, L. E., Cheng, H., Mitsuyasu, R. T., and Detels, R. (1987): Early effects of HIV on CD4 lymphocytes *in vivo. J. Immunol.*, 138:3725–3730.

19. Eyster, M. E., Gail, M. H., Ballard, J. O., Al-Mondhiry, H., and Goedert, J. J. (1987): Natural history of human immunodeficiency virus infections in hemophiliacs: Effects of T-cell subsets platelet counts and age. *Ann. Intern. Med.*, 107:1–6.

20. Carney, W. P., Rubin, R. H., Hoffman, R. A., Hansen, W. P., Healey, K., and Hirsch, M. S. (1981): Analysis of T lymphocytes subsets in cytomegalovirus mononucleosis. *J. Immunol.*, 126:2114–2116.

21. Reinherz, E. L., O'Brien, C., Rosenthal, P., and Schlossman, S. F. (1980): The cellular basis for viral-induced immunodeficiency: Analysis by monoclonal antibodies. *J. Immunol.* 125:1269–1276.

22. Klatzmann, D., Barre-Sinoussi, F., Nugeyre, M. T., Dauguet, C., Vilmer, E., Griscelli, C., Brun-Vezinet, F., Rouzioux, C., Gluckman, J. C., Chermann, J. C., and Montagnier, L. (1984): Selective tropism of lymphadenopathy associated virus for helper-inducer T lymphocytes. *Science* 225:59–63.

23. Shaw, G. M., Hahn, B. H., Arya, S. K., Groopman, J. E., Gallo, R. C., and Wong-Staal, F. (1984): Molecular characterization of human T cell leukemia (lymphotropic) virus type III in the acquired immune deficiency syndrome. *Science*, 226:1165–1171.

24. Harper, M. E., Marselle, L. M., Gallo, R. C., and Wong-Staal, F. (1986): Detection of lymphocytes expressing human T-lymphotropic virus type III in lymph nodes and peripheral blood from infected individuals by in situ hybridization. *Proc. Natl. Acad. Sci. U.S.A.*, 83:772–776.

25. Schnittman, S. M., Psallidopoulos, M. C., Lane, H. C., Thompson, L., Baseler, M., Massari, F., Fox, C. H., Salzman, N. P., and Fauci, A. S. (1989): The reservoir for HIV-1 in human peripheral blood is a T cell that maintains expression of CD4. *Science*, 245:305–308.

26. Schnittman, S. M., Greenhouse, J. J., Psallidopoulos, M. C., Baseler, M., Salzman, N. P., Fauci, A. S., and Lane, H. C. (1990): Increasing viral burden in CD4+ T cells from patients with human immunodeficiency virus (HIV) infection reflects rapidly progressive immunosuppression and clinical disease. *Ann. Intern. Med.*, 113:438–443.

27. Ho, D. D., Moudgil, T., and Alam, M. (1989): Quantitation of human immunodeficiency virus type 1 in the blood of infected persons. *N. Engl. J. Med.*, 321:1621–1625.

28. Coombs, R. W., Collier, A. C., Allain, J-P., Nikora, B., Leuther, M., Gjerset, G. F., and Corey, L. (1989): Plasma viremia in human immunodeficiency virus infection. *N. Engl. J. Med.*, 321:1626–1631.

29. Lifson, J. D., Feinberg, M. B., Reyes, G. R., Rabin, L., Banapour, B., Chakrabarti, S., Moss, B., Wong-Staal, F., Steimer, K. S., and Engleman, E. G. (1986): Induction of CD4-dependent cell fusion by the HTLV-III/LAV envelope glycoprotein. *Nature*, 323:725–728.

30. Dalgleish, A. G., Beverly, P. C. L., Clapham, P. R., Crawford, D. H., Greaves, M. F., and Weiss, R. A. (1984): The CD4 (T4) antigen is an essential component of the receptor for the AIDS retrovirus. *Nature*, 312:763–767.

31. Klatzmann, D., Champagne, E., Chamanet, E., Gruest, J., Guetard, D., Hercend, T., Gluckman, J. C., and Montagnier, L. (1984): T-lymphocyte T4 molecule behaves as the receptor for human retrovirus LAV. *Nature*, 312:767–768.

32. McDougal, J. S., Mawle, A., Cort, S. P., Nicholson, J. K. A., Cross, G. D., Scheppler-Campbell, J. A., Hicks, D., and Sligh, J. (1985): Cellular tropism of the human retrovirus HTLV-III/LAV. I. Role of T cell activation and expression of the T4 antigen. *J. Immunol.*, 135:3151–3162.

33. Somasundaran, M., and Robinson, H. L. (1987): A major mechanism of human immunodeficiency virus-induced cell killing does not involve cell fusion. *J. Virol.* 61:3114–3119.

34. Lane, H. C., Depper, J. M., Greene, W. S, Whalen, G., Waldemann, T. A., and Fauci, A. S. (1985): Qualitative analysis of immune function in patients with the acquired immunodeficiency syndrome: Evidence for a selective defect in soluble antigen recognition. *N. Engl. J. Med.*, 79–84.

35. Lane, H. C., Masur, H., Edgar, L. C., Whalen G., Rook, A. H., and Fauci, A. S. (1983): Abnormalities of B lymphocyte activation and immunoregulation in patients with the acquired immunodeficiency syndrome. *N. Engl. J. Med.*, 309:453–458.

36. Reinherz, E. L., Kung, P. C., Goldstein, G., and Schlossman, S. F. (1979): Separation of functional subsets of human T cells by a monoclonal antibody. *Proc. Natl. Acad. Sci. U.S.A.*, 76:4061–4065.
37. Rook, A. H., Masur, H., Lane, H. C., Frederick, W., Kasahara, T., Macher, A. M., Djeu, J. Y., Manischewitz, J. F., Jackson, L., Fauci, A. S., and Quinnan, G. V. (1983): Interleukin-2 enhances the depressed natural killer and cytomegalovirus-specific cytotoxic activities of lymphocytes from patients with the acquired immune deficiency syndrome. *J. Clin. Invest.*, 72:398–403.
38. Murray, H. W., Rubin, B. Y., Masur, H., and Roberts, R. B. (1984): Impaired production of lymphokines and immune (gamma) interferon in the acquired immunodeficiency syndrome. *N. Engl. J. Med.*, 310:883–889.
39. Murray, H. W., Hillman, J. K., Rubin, B. Y., Kelly, C. D., Jacobs, J. L., Tyler, L. W., Donnelly, D. M., Carriero, S. M., Godbold, J. H., and Roberts, R. B. (1985): Patients at risk for AIDS-related opportunistic infections: Clinical manifestations and impaired gamma interferon production. *N. Engl. J. Med.*, 313:1504–1510.
40. Vuillier, F., Lapresle, C., and Dighiero, G. (1988): Comparative analysis of CD4-4B4 and CD4-2H4 lymphocyte subpopulations in HIV negative homosexual, HIV seropositive and healthy subjects. *Clin. Exp. Immunol.*, 71:8–12.
41. Gruters, R. A., Terpstra, F. G., Jong, R. D., Van Noesel, C. J. M., Van Lier, R. A. W., and Miedema, F. (1990): Selective loss of T cell functions in different stages of HIV infection. *Eur. J. Immunol.*, 20:1039–1044.
42. Margolick, J. B., Volkman, D. J., Folks, T., and Fauci, A. S. (1987): Amplification of HTLV-III/LAV infection by antigen-induced activation of T cells and direct suppression by virus of lymphocyte blastogenic responses. *J. Immunol.*, 138:1719–1723.
43. Pahwa, S., Pahwa, R., Saxinger, C., Gallo, R. C., and Good, R. A. (1985): Influence of the human T-lymphotropic virus/lymphadenopathy-associated virus on functions of human lymphocytes: Evidence for immunosuppressive effects and polyclonal B cell activation by banded viral preparations. *Proc. Natl. Acad. Sci. U.S.A.*, 82:8198–8202.
44. Pahwa, S., Pahwa, R., Good, R. A., Gallo, R. C., and Saxinger, C. (1986): Stimulatory and inhibitory influences of human immunodeficiency virus on normal B lymphocytes. *Proc. Natl. Acad. Sci. U.S.A.*, 83:9124–9128.
45. Laurence, J., and Mayer, L. (1984): Immunoregulatory lymphokines of T hybridomas from AIDS patients: Constitutive and inducible suppressor factors. *Science*, 225:66–69.
46. Bank, I., and Chess, L. (1985): Perturbation of the T4 molecule transmits a negative signal to T cells. *J. Exp. Med.*, 162:1294–1303.
47. Gurney, M. E., Apatoff, B. R., Spear, G. T., Baumel, M. J., Antel, J. P., Bania, M. B., and Reder, A. T. (1986): Neuroleukin: A lymphokine product of lectin-stimulated T cells. *Science*, 234:574–581.
48. Gurney, M. E., Heinrich, S. P., Lee, M. R., and Yin, H. S. (1986): Molecular cloning and expression of neuroleukin, a neurotrophic factor for spinal and sensory neurons. *Science*, 234:566–574.
49. Lee, M. R., Ho, D. D., and Gurney, M. E. (1987): Functional interaction and partial homology between human immunodeficiency virus and neuroleukin. *Science*, 237:1047–1051.
50. Ho, D. D., Rota, T. R., and Hirsch, M. S. (1986): Infection of monocyte/macrophages by human T lymphotropic virus type III. *J. Clin. Invest.*, 77:1712–1715.
51. Gartner, S., Markovits, P. Markovitz, D. M., Kaplan, M. H., Gallo, R. C., and Popovic, M. (1986): The role of mononuclear phagocytes in HTLV-III/LAV infection. *Science*, 233:215–220.
52. Smith, P. S., Ohura, I., Masur, H., Lane, H. C., Fauci, A. S., and Wahl, S. M. (1984): Monocyte function in the acquired immune deficiency syndrome: Defective chemotaxis. *J. Clin. Invest.*, 74:2121–2128.
53. Clouse, K. A., Powell, D., Washington, I., Poli, G., Strebel, K., Farrar, W., Varstad, P., Kovacs, J., Fauci, A. S., and Folks, T. M. (1989): Monokine regulation of human immunodeficiency virus-1 expression in a chronically infected human T cell clone. *J. Immunol.*, 142:431–438.
54. Poli, G., Kinter, A., Justement, J. S., Kehrl, J. H., Bressler, P., Stanley, S., and Fauci, A. S. (1990): Tumor necrosis factor alpha functions in an autocrine manner in the induction of human immunodeficiency virus expression. *Proc. Natl. Acad. Sci. U.S.A.*, 87:782–785.
55. Murray, H. W., Jacobs J. L., and Bovabjerg, D. H. (1987): Accessory cell function of AIDS monocytes. *J. Infect. Dis.*, 156:696.
56. Hofmann, B., Odum, N., Jakosbsen, B. K., Plaatz, P., Ryder, L. P., Nielsen, J. O., Gerstoft, J., and Svejgaard, A. (1986): Immunological studies in the acquired immunodeficiency syndrome: II

Active suppression or intrinsic defect-investigated by mixing AIDS cells with HLA-DR identical normal cells. *Scand. J. Immunol.*, 23:669–678.

57. Margolick, J. B., Volkman, D. J., Lane, H. C., and Fauci, A. S. (1985): Clonal analysis of T lymphocytes in the acquired immunodeficiency syndrome: Evidence for an abnormality affecting individual helper and suppressor T cells. *J. Clin. Invest.*, 76:709–715.

58. Pantaleo, G., Koenig, S., Baseler, M., Lane, H. C., and Fauci, A. S. (1990): Defective clonogenic potential of CD8 + T lymphocytes in patients with AIDS. *J. Immunol.*, 144:1696–1704.

59. Montagnier, L., Chermann, J. C., Barre-Sinoussi, F., Chamaret, S., Gruest, J., Nugeyre, M. T., Rey, F., Dauguet, C., Axler-Blin, C., Vezinet-Brun, F., Rouzioux, C., Saimot, G-A., Rozenbaum, W., Gluckman, J. C., Klatzmann, D., Vilmer, E., Griscelli, C., Foyer-Gazengel, C., and Brunet, J. B. (1990): In Human T Leukemia Lymphoma Viruses, edited by R. C. Gallo, M. E. Essex, and L. Gross, Cold Spring Harbor Press, Cold Spring Harbor, NY. p. 363.

60. Van Oers, M. H. J., Pinkster, J., and Zeiilemaker, W. P. (1978): Quantification of antigen-reactive cells among human T lymphocytes. *Eur. J. Immunol.*, 8:477–484.

61. Zagury, D., Bernard, J., Leonard, R., Cheynier, R., Feldman, M., Sarin, P. S., and Gallo, R. C. (1986): Long-term cultures of HTLV-III-infected T cells: A model of cytopathology of T-cell depletion in AIDS. *Science*, 231:850–853.

62. Harada, S., Koyanagi, Y., Nakashima, H., Kobayashi, N., and Yamamoto, N. (1986): Tumor promoter TPA enhances replication of HTLV-III/LAV. *Virology*, 154:249–250.

63. Kampschmidt, R. F., Worthington, M. L., III, and Mesecher, M. I. (1986): Release of interleukin-1 (IL-1) and IL-1-like factors from rabbit macrophages with silica. *J. Leuk. Biol.*, 39:123–132.

64. Piguet, P. F., Collart, M. A., Grau, G. E., Sappino, A. P., and Vassalli, P. (1990): Requirement of tumour necrosis factor for development of silica-induced pulmonary fibrosis. *Nature*, 15:245–247.

65. Mcdougal, J. S., Hubbard, M., Nicholson, J. K. A., Jones, B. M., Holman, R. C., Roberts, J., Fishbein, D. B., Jaffe, H. W., Kaplan, J. E., Spira, T. J., and Evatt, B. L. (1985): Immune complexes in the acquired immunodeficiency syndrome (AIDS): Relationship to disease manifestation risk group and immunologic deficit. *J. Clin. Immunol.*, 5:130–138.

66. Matsiota, P., Chamaret, S., Montagnier, L., and Avrameas, S. (1987): Detection of natural autoantibodies in the serum of anti-HIV-positive individuals. *Ann. Inst. Pasteur Immunol.*, 138:223–233.

67. Walsh, C. M., Nardi, M. A., and Karpatkin, S. (1984): On the mechanism of thrombocytopenia in sexually active homosexual men. *N. Engl. J. Med.*, 311:635–639.

68. Murphy, M. F., Metcalfe, P., Waters, A. H., Carne, C. A., Weller, I. V. D., Linch, D. C., and Smith, A. (1987): Incidence and mechanism of neutropenia and thrombocytopenia in patients with human immunodeficiency virus infection. *Br. J. Haematol.*, 66:337–340.

69. Kopelman, R. G., and Zolla-Pazner, S. (1988): Association of human immunodeficiency virus infection and autoimmune phenomena. *Am. J. Med.*, 84:82–88.

70. Papadopoulos, N. M., Lane, H. C., Costello, R., Moutsopoulos, H. M., Masur, H., Gelmann, E. P., and Fauci, A. S. (1985): Oligoclonal immunoglobulins in patients with the acquired immunodeficiency syndrome. *Clin. Immunol. Immunopathol.*, 35:43–46.

71. Martinez-Maza, O., Crabb, E., Mitsuyasu, R. T., Fahey, J. L., and Giorgi, J. V. (1987): Infection with the human immunodeficiency virus (HIV) is associated with an in vivo increase in B lymphocyte activation and immaturity. *J. Immunol.*, 138:3720–3724.

72. Birx, D. L., Redfield, R. R., and Tosato, G. (1986): Defective regulation of Epstein-Barr virus infection in patients with acquired immunodeficiency syndrome (AIDS) or AIDS-related disorders. *N. Engl. J. Med.*, 314:874–879.

73. Yarchoan, R., Redfield, R. R., and Broder, S. (1986): Mechanisms of B cell activation in patients with acquired immunodeficiency syndrome and related disorders. *J. Clin. Invest.*, 78:439–447.

74. Montagnier, L., Gruest, J., Chamaret, S., Dauguet, C., Axler, C., Guetard, D., Nugeyre, M. T., Barre-Sinoussi, F., Chermann, J.-C., Brunet, J. B., Klatzmann, D., and Gluckman, J. C. (1984): Adaptation of lymphadenopathy associated virus (LAV) to replication in EBV-transformed B lymphoblastoid cell lines. *Science*, 225:63–66.

75. Casareale, D., Sinangil, F., Hedeskog, M., Ward, W., Volsky, D. J., and Sonnabend, J. (1984): Establishment of retrovirus-Epstein-Barr virus-positive B-lymphoblastoid cell lines from individuals at risk for acquired immune deficiency syndrome (AIDS). *AIDS Res.*, 1:253–270.

76. Schnittman, S., Lane, H. C., Higgins, S. E., Folks, T., and Fauci, A. S. (1986): Direct polyclonal

activation of human B lymphocytes by the acquired immunodeficiency syndrome virus. *Science*, 223:1084–1086.

77. Breen, E. C., Rezai, A. R., Nakajima, K., Beall, G. N., Mitsuyasu, R. T., Hirano, T., Kishimoto, T., and Martinez-Maza, O. (1990): Infection with HIV is associated with elevated IL-6 levels and production. *J. Immunol.*, 144:480–484.

78. Nakajima, K., Martinez-Maza, O., Hirano, T., Breen, E. C., Nishanian, P. G., Salazar-Gonzalex, J. R., Fahey, J. L., and Kishimoto, T. (1989): Induction of IL-6 (B cell stimulatory factor-2/IFN-B2) production by HIV. *J. Immunol.*, 142:531–536.

79. Lusso, P., Salahuddin, S. Z., Ablashi, D. V., Gallo, R. C., Veronese, F. diM., and Markham, P. D. (1987): Diverse tropism of human B-lymphotropic virus (human herpesvirus 6). *Lancet*, 2 743–744.

80. Yachie, A., Tosato, G., Straus, S. E., and Blaese, R. M. (1985): Immunostimulation by cyto-megalovirus (CMV); helper T cell-dependent activation of immunoglobulin production in vitro by lymphocytes from CMV-immune donors. *J. Immunol.*, 135:1395–1400.

81. Klatzmann, D., and Montagnier, L. (1986): Approaches to AIDS therapy. *Nature*, 319:10–11.

82. Stricker, R. B., McHugh, M., Moody, D. J., Morrow, W. J. W., Stites, D. P., Shuman, M. A., and Levy, J. A. (1987): An AIDS-related cytotoxic autoantibody reacts with a specific antigen on stimulated CD4 + T cells. *Nature*, 327:710–711.

83. Williams, R. C., Masur, H., and Spira, T. J. (1984): Lymphocyte-reactive antibodies in acquired immune deficiency syndrome. *J. Clin. Immunol.*, 4:118–127.

84. Tomar, R. H., John, P. A., Hennig, A. K., and Kloster, B. (1985): Cellular targets of anti-lymphocyte antibodies in AIDS and LAS. *Clin. Immunol. Immunopathol.*, 37:37–47.

85. Ardman, B., Mayer, K., Bristol, J., Ryan, M., Settles, M., and Levy, E. (1990): Surface immu-noglobulin-positive T lymphocytes in HIV-1 infection: Relationship to CD4 + lymphocyte deple-tion. *Clin. Immunol. Immunopathol.*, 56:249–258.

86. Jaffe, H. S., Abrams, D. I., Amran, A. J., Lewis, B. J., and Golden, J. A. (1983): Complica-tions of co-trimoxazole in treatment of AIDS-associated *Pneumocystis carinii* pneumonia in homo-sexual men. *Lancet*, 2 1109–1111.

87. Mitsuyasu, R., Groopman, J., and Volberding, P. (1983): Cutaneous reaction to trimethoprim-sulfamethoxazole in patients with AIDS and Kaposi's sarcoma. *N. Engl. J. Med.*, 308:1535–1536.

88. Gordin, F. M., Simon, G. L., Wofsy, C. B., and Mills, J. (1984): Adverse reactions to tri-methoprim-sulfamethoxazole in patients with acquired immunodeficiency syndrome. *Ann. Intern. Med.*, 100:495–499.

89. Parkin, J. M., Eales, L. J., Galazka, A. R., and Pinching, A. J. (1987): Atopic manifestations in the acquired immunodeficiency syndrome: Response to recombinant interferon gamma. *Br. Med. J.*, 294:1185–1186.

90. Amman, A. J., Abrams, D., Conant, M., Dhudwin, D., Cowan, M., Volberding, P., Lewis, B., and Casavant, C. (1983): Acquired immune dysfunction in homosexual men: Immunologic profiles. *Clin. Immunol. Immunopathol.*, 127:315–325.

91. Ring, J., Froschl, M., Brunner, R., and Braun-Falco, O. (1986): LAV/HTLV-III infection and atopy; serum IgE and specific IgE antibodies to environmental allergens. *Acta Derm. Venereol.* 66: 530–532.

92. Pullen, H., Wright, N., and Murdoch, J. M. (1967): Hypersensitivity reactions to antibacterial drugs in infectious mononucleosis. *Lancet*, 2:1176–1178.

93. Klemola, E. (1970): Hypersensitivity reactions to ampicillin in cytomegalovirus mononucleosis. *Scand. J. Infect. Dis.*, 2:29–31.

94. Carini, C., Margolick, J. B., Yodoi, J., and Ishizaka, K. (1989): Formation of IgE-binding factors by T cells of HIV-1 infected patients. *Proc. Natl. Acad. Sci. U.S.A.*, 88:9214–9218.

95. Torti, F. M., Dieckmann, B., Beutler, B., Cerami, A., and Ringold, G. M. (1985): A macrophage factor inhibits adipocyte gene expression: An in vitro model of cachexia. *Science*, 229:867–872.

Clinical Immunotoxicology, edited by
D. S. Newcombe, N. R. Rose, and J. C. Bloom.
Raven Press, Ltd., New York © 1992.

9

Cyclosporine: Lessons from a Useful Immunosuppressant

Ahmed H. Esa and Allan D. Hess

*Bone Marrow Transplantation Unit, Oncology Center,
Johns Hopkins University, School of Medicine, Baltimore, MD*

Cyclosporine (CsA) was isolated from the soil fungi *Cylindrocarpon lucidium Booth* and *Tolypocladium inflatum Gams* and initially described as an antifungal metabolite. It is a cyclic endecapeptide with a characteristic unsaturated C-9 amino acid (the structure of CsA is illustrated in Fig. 1). CsA has proved to be a panacea for solid organ transplantation and very useful for the prevention of graft-versus-host disease (1,2). Several centers are now investigating its efficacy in the treatment of selected autoimmune diseases (3). Although CsA does not qualify as a *bona fide* immunotoxic agent, the experience gained from the extensive research and use of this immunosuppressive agent serves us well in considering general principles and in establishing useful methodological assays in the identification of agents that may adversely affect the immune system.

INITIAL STUDIES

The initial studies into the immunosuppressive potential and mechanism of action of CsA have recently been reviewed (4,5). Despite its potent immunosuppressive properties, CsA is not myelotoxic or cytotoxic for peripheral blood mononuclear cells. In these early studies, CsA was shown to inhibit antibody formation to T-dependent antigens, to prolong graft survival, and to suppress delayed type hypersensitivity. In *in vitro* experiments, CsA inhibited, in a dose-dependent manner, lymphocyte proliferative responses to mitogens and alloantigens, with an apparent selection toward T-cell responses. Secondary responses were more resistant to CsA than primary responses, and as discussed later, B-lymphocyte responses to polyclonal activators were found to have variable sensitivity to CsA. *In vivo* CsA facilitated the induction of transplantation tolerance across major histocompatibility complex (MHC) barriers with limited postgrafting immunosuppression. Orthotopic and cardiac allografts from MHC-mismatched donors were retained indefinitely (6).

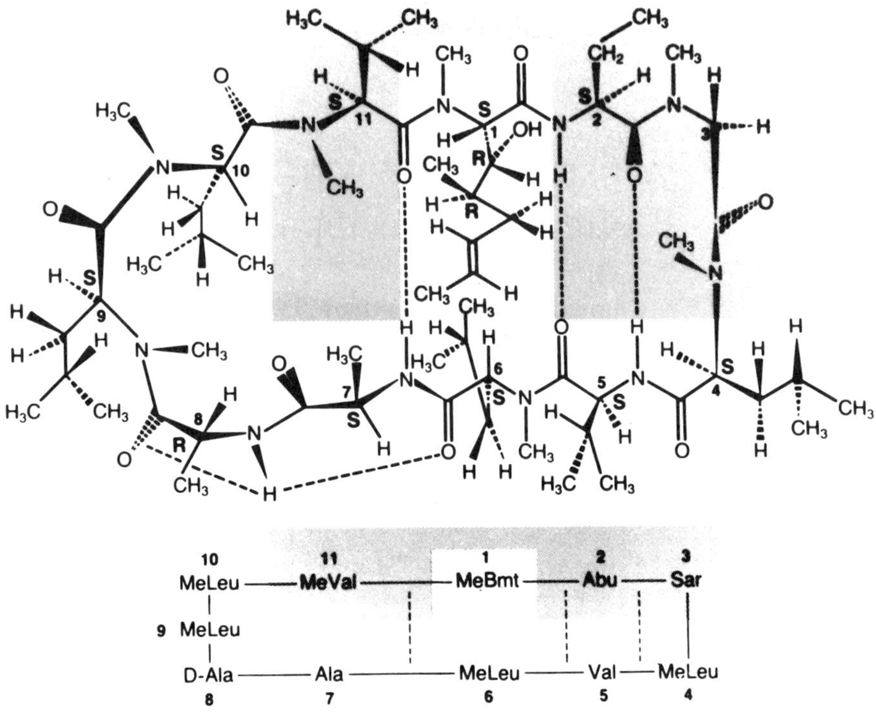

FIG. 1. Structure of CsA.

Similarly, in a rat bone marrow transplantation model, CsA was shown to prevent graft-versus-host disease (7). Unfortunately, in spite of the success in these animal systems, CsA does not lead to permanent tolerance in humans, and continued immunosuppression is necessary for the prevention of rejection and graft-versus-host disease.

During these initial studies it became clear that CsA has a very narrow time window for the expression of its full activity. To effectively inhibit T-cell proliferative responses, CsA must be present during the early stages of culture initiation. Delay in the addition of CsA to mitogen-stimulated cultures by as little as 1 to 2 hours resulted in a significant reduction in the efficacy of CsA to suppress lymphocyte proliferative responses. This narrow time frame for the effectiveness of CsA suggested that it interfered with an early event or events in T-cell activation prior to DNA synthesis and cell division. Inhibition of lymphocyte proliferative responses is, however, only a simple measure of the efficacy of this immunosuppressive agent and offers little insight into the effect of CsA on the requisite cell-to-cell collaboration necessary for a competent allograft response. In particular, these studies could not explain the ability of CsA to facilitate prolonged graft survival and induce transplantation tolerance after discontinuation of CsA treatment or reduction of dose (6).

EFFECTS OF CYCLOSPORINE ON CELLS OF THE IMMUNE SYSTEM

Effects of Cyclosporine on T-Lymphocyte Subpopulations

The mixed lymphocyte reaction is used as an *in vitro* model of the complex cellular and humoral processes involved in graft rejection and graft-versus-host disease. This *in vitro* model measures the response of immunocompetent cells from one individual to the alloantigens of another. Thus it approximates the situation in transplantation where foreign antigens from a donor are transferred to a recipient host. The mixed lymphocyte reaction as it occurs *in vitro* involves a complex set of events and cell-cell cooperation: (a) accessory cells that process and present antigens to immunocompetent lymphocytes and also elaborate interleukin-1 (IL-1) and other immunomodulating monokines, (b) precursor cytotoxic T lymphocytes that are activated to acquire a receptor for interleukin-2 (IL-2), (c) T-helper lymphocytes that synthesize and release IL-2 (the production of IL-2 is accentuated by IL-1) after activation, (d) the clonal amplification of activated cytotoxic T lymphocytes by IL-2, and (e) suppressor T lymphocytes that down-regulate or control this response.

Much of the data relating to the cellular effects of CsA has been derived from experiments designed to assess its effects on the various components of the mixed lymphocyte reaction, and the results have revealed important clues about the nature and sites of action of this agent. The series of investigations has been reviewed elsewhere (4,5); the pertinent conclusions are outlined as follows:

1. Cyclosporine inhibits the production of IL-2 and other lymphokines; CsA also down-regulates lymphokine mRNA transcription, presumably by blocking the activation signal. There is also some evidence that IL-2 receptor formation may be inhibited by CsA. This later effect of CsA may be stimulus-dependent; IL-2 receptor induction by alloantigen stimulation is apparently more sensitive to CsA than to mitogen stimulation. Down-regulation of the IL-2 receptor may be secondary to diminished IL-2.
2. Cyclosporine does not inhibit the clonal expansion of activated cells expressing the IL-2 receptor in response to exogenous IL-2.
3. Cyclosporine inhibits the precursor cytotoxic T cell from acquiring functional responsiveness to IL-2, which may be mediated via inhibition of IL-2 receptor formation.
4. Cyclosporine inhibits the activation of cytotoxic T lymphocytes but permits the activation and amplification of suppressor T lymphocytes, creating a disequilibrium that favors the induction of specific immunological unresponsiveness to the stimulating alloantigen *in vitro*.
5. Addition of exogenous IL-1 or IL-2 does not entirely overcome the immunosuppressive effects of CsA. At doses higher than 100 ng/ml of CsA, some restoration of proliferation but not of cytotoxic T-lymphocyte activity can be observed.
6. Cyclosporine appears to inhibit monocyte/macrophage accessory functions by inhibiting antigen presentation. Other effects of CsA on monocytes may include

modulation of arachidonic acid metabolism, which may influence lymphocyte function and magnify the effects of CsA (8). CsA may alter IL-1 production, but this appears to be dose- and stimulus-dependent (9–11), and finally CsA may also down-regulate IL-1 receptors on T-helper cells (11).

As summarized in Table 1, these effects of CsA are variable and dose-dependent. Interleukin-2 production is more sensitive than IL-2 receptor formation, whereas monocyte functions are generally less sensitive than both. In contrast, inhibition of suppressor T-cell activation and IL-2–dependent growth is relatively resistant to CsA. Cyclosporine, therefore, appears to prevent graft rejection mainly by inhibiting the ability of the precursor cytotoxic T lymphocyte to develop IL-2 responsiveness. However, maintenance doses of CsA are designed to produce serum through levels that are sufficient to inhibit the spectrum of lymphocyte responses described above (12).

The data summarized above would suggest that helper T cells are the primary target for CsA immunosuppression. Subsequent to inhibition of helper T-cell production of IL-2, precursor cytotoxic T-lymphocyte cells are prevented from acquiring responsiveness to IL-2. More recent studies have focused on IL-2 receptor expression, and although the data are not always consistent, it appears that IL-2 receptors for some stimuli are inhibited (13). In contrast, in a variety of systems, CsA was shown not to affect the activation of suppressor cells. First, using a colony-forming assay, Gordon and Singer (14) showed that CsA did not inhibit the clonal expansion of cells with suppressor T-cell characteristics. Similarly, Hess and Tuschka (15), using the human mixed lymphocyte reaction, showed that functional suppressor cell activity was spared, whereas cytotoxic T-cell activation was abrogated by CsA. The results of these *in vitro* studies lead to the postulate, advanced by Hess and coworkers (16), that CsA induces functional tolerance by creating a helper/suppressor T-cell disequilibrium in favor of suppressor T cells. This sugges-

TABLE 1. *Relative sensitivity of various T-lymphocyte functions to cyclosporine*

	IC_{50} of CsA in ng/ml
Very Sensitive	
Proliferation (mitogen or antigen)	20–50
IL-2 production	10–20
Induction of cytotoxic T lymphocytes	20–50
Moderately Sensitive	
IL-2 induction with mixed lymphocyte reaction	100–200
with ConA	200–500
with PHA	500–1,000
Resistant	
IL-2–dependent proliferation	Over 1,000
Suppressor T-cell activation	Over 1,000
Cell-mediated lympholysis	Over 1,000

Refs 4 and 5.

tion was subsequently confirmed in many *in vitro* systems and, *in vivo*, in some animal model systems (4,5). These regulatory cells have been implicated in the induction and maintenance of allograft specific tolerance (17), and therefore an imbalance between suppressor T cell and T-helper and/or cytotoxic T cells may lead to tolerance induction and graft prolongation. Confirmation of this hypothesis in humans has proved elusive, since tolerance induction is not readily demonstrable in humans or in some animal systems. However, recent studies show that in human renal transplant recipients, the presence of donor-specific suppressor T cells correlates with a low incidence of graft rejection (19).

Effects on Accessory Cells

Accessory cells, or antigen-presenting cells, constitute a heterogeneous cell population, including peripheral blood monocytes, tissue macrophages, dendritic, Langerhans', and vascular endothelial cells. In addition to presenting antigens to competent lymphocytes, accessory cells, particularly monocytes and macrophages, synthesize and release many essential humoral mediators. Because of the critical importance of accessory cells during the inductive phase of immunological responsiveness, when CsA is most effective, a number of laboratories have sought to evaluate the effects of CsA on accessory cells. Monocytes and macrophages bind and internalize large amounts of CsA (19), and this may disrupt the cascade of events that leads to successful processing and presentation of antigens. In general, the data suggest that *in vitro*, CsA inhibits antigen presentation (20–23). Typically, these studies used a protocol in which monocytes were treated *in vitro* with antigen and CsA and washed to remove excess antigen and residual CsA; then their ability to induce proliferation or IL-2 production was examined. The doses of CsA required to produce significant suppression of antigen presentation in these experiments are usually on the order of 1 μg/mL and much higher than those reported to inhibit IL-2 production. The mechanism of CsA-induced inhibition of antigen presentation and the role this may play in the immunosuppressive activity of CsA are unclear. Major histocompatibility complex class II determinants are known to be essential for effective antigen presentation, and perturbations in the expression of these determinants would be expected to modulate antigen presentation. Unfortunately, conflicting reports about the effects of CsA on Ia antigen expression make an evaluation of the role of Ia antigen in CsA-induced immunosuppression difficult. Two recent studies by Snyder and colleagues (22) and Palay and coworkers (23) indicate that CsA-treated accessory cells were impaired in their ability to present antigens but could not demonstrate any significant depression in HLA-DR expression. In contrast, a number of earlier studies found that CsA inhibited the expression of Ia antigen on Ia–antigen expressing cells (24,25). Likewise, the data with respect to the effects of CsA on IL-1 production are largely inconclusive. Bendzten and associates (26) reported data suggesting that CsA interfered with IL-1-dependent functions either by inhibiting its synthesis or by inhibiting the induction of IL-1 receptors on T cells.

However, exogenous IL-1 is incapable of restoring monocyte antigen presentation functions after these cells have been treated with CsA (20). Similarly, CsA-treated primary mixed lymphocyte reaction cultures remain unresponsive to exogenous IL-1, and IL-2-producing cells treated with CsA are also refractory to additional IL-1 (27,28).

A number of laboratories provide evidence that CsA enhances the synthesis of some arachidonic acid metabolites, particularly prostaglandin E_2 (PGE_2) and thromboxane (29,30). Prostaglandin E_2 is a powerful mediator with functions that could potentially underlie many of the suppressive properties known to be affected by CsA. Prostaglandin E_2 inhibits IL-2 production, is thought to diminish Ia antigen expression, and facilitates the activation of T-suppressor cells (31–33). As discussed earlier, CsA appears to spare suppressor T-cell activation. Moreover, PGE_2 leads to an elevation of cyclic adenosine monophosphate and thereby could inhibit ornithine decarboxylase. Ornithine decarboxylase is necessary for the conversion of ornithine to polyamines (spermine and spermidine), a step required for DNA synthesis. Interestingly, evidence that CsA inhibits ornithine decarboxylase has been reported (34). At present, the role of PGE_2 in CsA-induced inhibition of antigen presentation is to be regarded as unresolved, as some investigators could not discern a direct role for reduced PGE_2 (22,23).

Other circumstantial observations support the contention that CsA may, at least in part, mediate immunosuppression by inhibiting monocyte antigen presentation. Cyclosporine, like chloroquine—a known inhibitor of antigen presentation—may be lysosomotropic as reported by Koponen and coworkers (35). Moreover, CsA has been shown to reverse multidrug resistance in some tumor cells, another similarity it seems to share with chloroquine (36). Gupta and colleagues also report that macrophages isolated from CsA-treated animals lacked characteristic rough endoplasmic reticulum and contained incompletely digested Bacillus Calmette-Guérin (37).

Another arachidonate metabolite, thromboxane, has also been found to be elevated by CsA. Thromboxane is a vasoconstrictor and a promoter of platelet aggregation. Earlier initial reports also indicated that prostacyclin, which counteracts the actions of thromboxane, was inhibited by CsA. Thus it is possible that an imbalance between the synthesis of thromboxane and prostacyclin could underlie CsA nephrotoxicity. The role of thromboxane in CsA kidney toxicity is supported by a number of animal studies indicating that prostaglandin analogues or thromboxane synthetase inhibitors ameliorate CsA-caused renal disease (38). In a most recent study, Rogers and colleagues (39) indicated that diets low in fat that diminish cyclooxygenase metabolites counteract CsA-induced renal damage. However, at present the data about the role of CsA metabolites in renal dysfunction must be regarded as still incomplete, and other possibilities, particularly the role of CsA metabolites in CsA nephrotoxicity, must be evaluated.

Recent studies indicate that peripheral blood monocytes may be functionally heterogeneous (8,40–42). In our laboratory we have identified two subsets that preferentially induce immunosuppression or stimulation. These subsets, which can be separated on the basis of size and density differences, are both esterase-positive and share most monocyte phenotypic markers with the exception of leu-10 (HLA-DQ), which is expressed mainly by the suppressor-inducer subset. Functionally, large monocytes present antigens poorly but are more effective in the activation of suppressor cells, whereas small monocytes present antigens efficiently. These results suggest that immunoregulation may begin at the level of antigen presentation. As discussed previously, CsA appears to spare the activation of suppressor T cells. Thus it was of interest to examine whether the suppressor-inducer and the antigen-presenting monocyte subset differed in their sensitivity to CsA. Out results showed that although the suppressor-inducer large monocyte subset stains strongly with dan-CsA, it appears to be more resistant to CsA than the antigen-presenting small monocyte subset that binds relatively less dan-CsA. Small monocytes exposed to CsA released significantly more arachidonate metabolites, particularly PGE_2 and thromboxane, than large monocytes. However, the ability of both monocyte subsets to present antigens was inhibited by CsA, although inhibition by CsA of small monocyte antigen presentation was partially sensitive to cyclooxygenase blockade with indomethacin. In contrast to the small monocytes, however, large monocytes exposed to CsA were not responsive to indomethacin. These results would seem to indicate that CsA inhibits antigen presentation at more than one step (8).

Effect on B-Lymphocyte Responses

The effects of CsA on B-lymphocyte responses is summarized in Table 3. Cyclosporine inhibits antibody responses to T-dependent antigens, primarily by interfering with necessary helper T-cell functions (4,5,43). Initially CsA was thought not to directly affect B-cell responses to T-independent antigens, such as anti-immunoglobulin, bacterial lipopolysaccharide, and Epstein-Barr virus (EBV) (44,45). It now appears that CsA can also selectively inhibit some T-independent B-cell responses. In a number of studies, the antibody response to type 2 T-independent antigens such as dinitrophenyl conjugates of Ficoll and dextran was found to be inhibited by CsA. B-lymphocyte responses to type 1 T-independent antigens (hapten conjugates of lipopolysaccharide), however, appear to be resistant to CsA

TABLE 2. *Effects of cyclosporine on monocytes and macrophages*

Function	Cyclosporine effect
Antigen presentation	Inhibited (refs. 8,20–23)
Ia antigen expression	Variable (refs. 22,23,25,26)
Arachidonate metabolism	
Prostacyclin	Inhibited (ref. 39)
PGE_2	Enhanced *in vitro* (refs. 8,25,26), largely unaffected *in vivo* (ref. 38)
Thromboxane	Enhanced *in vivo* and *in vitro* (refs. 25, 26,38,39)
LTB_4	Enhanced *in vitro* (refs. 25,26)

Reprinted from Hess et al., ref 5, by permission.

TABLE 3. *Effect of cyclosporine on B-lymphocyte responses*

B-lymphocyte function	Response to CsA
In vivo	
T-dependent antibody production	Sensitive
Type 1 T-independent antibody production	Sensitive
Type 2 (hapten-lipopolysaccharide) antibody production	Resistant
In vitro	
Anti-Ig-, ConA- or calcium ionophore-induced proliferation	Sensitive (IC$_{50}$ 5–15 ng/ml)
Lipopolysaccharide-, phorbol ester– or IL-4–induced proliferation	Resistant (IC$_{50}$ 100 ng/ml)

Data from refs. 4, 5, and 43–47.

(43,46,47). Cyclosporine did not adversely affect the primary or secondary response to trinitrophenyl-lipopolysaccharide (TNP-LPS) but inhibited the triggering of virgin B lymphocytes and TNP-LPS–induced memory cells by dinitrophenyl-Ficoll. These studies suggested the existence of two broad compartments of B cells that differed in their sensitivity to CsA: a CsA-sensitive cell responding to type 2 T-independent antigens and a CsA-resistant compartment responsive to type I T-independent antigens. Further analysis utilizing a variety of mitogenic and non-mitogenic polyclonal B cell activators suggested distinct activation pathways for CsA-resistant and CsA-sensitive responses. Responses of B cells to antiim-munoglobulin, ConA, or Ca^{2+} ionophores were remarkably sensitive, whereas B lymphocyte responses to lipopolysaccharide, phorbol esters, or IL-4 were found to be resistant (47). The mechanism by which some B-cell responses are sensitive to CsA and whether these responses reflect distinct properties of each B cell remain to be elucidated. In B cells, CsA does not inhibit antigen recognition or antiim-munoglobulin-stimulated phosphoinositol breakdown (48) but interferes with a calcium-dependent step as indicated in the mitogen studies above. The CsA-resistant responses appeared to be activated by an alternative, calcium-independent pathway. This finding is remarkably similar to that described for T lymphocytes, as is discussed in the following section.

EFFECT ON SUBCELLULAR EVENTS IN T-CELL ACTIVATION

Effect of Cyclosporine on the Activation Cascade

Activation of T lymphocyte by antigen triggers a complex cascade of ionic and enzymatic events that lead to DNA synthesis and replication, cell division and maturation, and the acquisition of specific effector functions. The precise sequence of events from membrane to nucleus has not been clearly delineated, but a framework has been proposed for these events.

Mitogens or antigens bind to the T-cell receptor in association with macrophage class II antigen (HLA-DR). This interaction is accompanied by a rise in intracellular calcium (49). The rise in intracellular calcium activates or facilitates the activities of a number of cell proteins or enzymes, including calmodulin, phospholipase A_2, and phospholipase C. Each of these proteins is thought to play a central role in cell activation and to regulate various cell activities through second messenger systems: cyclic nucleotides (calmodulin); arachidonic acid turnover prostaglandins/leukotrienes (phospholipase A_2), and diacylglycerol/inositol triphosphate (phospholipase C) (50,51). Inositol triphosphate further alters intracellular calcium levels by promoting the release of intracellular calcium stores. The relative importance of each of these calcium-dependent proteins for T-lymphocyte activation is currently under investigation. Activation of another enzyme, protein kinase C, by diacylglycerol, phospholipids, and calcium appears to be a second important step in T-lymphocyte activation (52). Lymphokines such as interleukin-1 and interleukin-2 may provide the necessary second signal for full T-cell activation through protein kinase C (53). Protein kinase C phosphorylates a number of enzymes, which results in the activation and/or enhancement of their enzymatic activity. Phorbol esters, which appear to directly activate protein kinase C, may substitute for these lymphokines during T-lymphocyte activation and also promote IL-2 receptor formation (53).

Following the cytoplasmic activation of calmodulin-dependent protein kinase cyclic adenosine monophosphate-dependent protein kinase, and phospholipid-dependent protein kinase C, the T-lymphocyte activation sequence progresses to nuclear induction of ornithine decarboxylase, which converts ornithine to the polyamines necessary for gene activation and expression, mRNA and DNA synthesis, and cell division.

To cause maximum *in vitro* immunosuppression, CsA must be added within 2 to 4 hours after stimulation of lymphocytes. If added within the first 4 hours, CsA prevents cells from proceeding to the S phase of the cell cycle and inhibits the synthesis of mRNA and new protein synthesis and the induction of ornithine decarboxylase (54). Cyclosporine was also found to inhibit mitogenesis by calcium ionophores, which trigger the calcium-dependent pathway, but not to inhibit the rise in intracellular calcium (55,56). On the other hand, stimulation by phorbol esters—which directly stimulate protein kinase C and induce IL-2 receptor formation—is relatively resistant to the effects of CsA (57). In addition, stimulation of lymphocytes with submitogenic doses of phorbol esters and calcium ionophore results in vigorous proliferative responses. These studies suggested that the primary effect of CsA was on the calcium-dependent pathway. Further evidence that CsA may act along this calcium-dependent pathway is derived from a number of other studies. First, CsA-sensitive T-lymphocyte proliferation requires a rise in intracellular calcium, whereas some CsA-resistant B-lymphocyte proliferative responses appear to be calcium-independent (48,58). Second, lymphokine production (CsA-sensitive) by the T-helper cell is calcium-dependent, whereas expression of IL-2 receptors (less sensitive to CsA) may be calcium-independent (59). It also appears that the ablation of the calcium-dependent signal accounts for the down-regulation of active lymphokine mRNA transcription. Third, the inhibitory effect of CsA on T-lymphocyte proliferation appears to be potentiated by calcium channel blockers (60,61).

Taken together, the evidence is consistent with the hypothesis that CsA primarily blocks the rise in intracellular calcium and inhibits a calcium-dependent activation pathway of both T and B lymphocytes. On the other hand, the activation signal mediated by protein kinase C is relatively CsA-resistant.

Intracellular Receptors

The preceding discussion indicates that CsA affects T and B lymphocytes at a point distal to antigen or mitogen binding and raises the possibility of the existence of intracellular target proteins. A number of cytoplasmic proteins that bind CsA have now been identified (62). Two of these proteins are cyclophilin, a novel 17 kDa basic protein, and the ubiquitous calmodulin, a 19 kDa acidic protein (63,64). Other CsA binding proteins have been identified but their functions are unknown and they appear to be present in minute quantities (65).

Cyclophilin was isolated in 1984 from bovine brain preparation (63). Its function remains unclear, but recent evidence suggests that it has a kinase activity (66). Cyclophilin has a high affinity for CsA (10^{-8}kDa) and exhibits a strong stereospecificity for active CsA derivatives. Calmodulin has a wide cellular distribution and is crucial to many cellular functions (67). The activation of calmodulin secondary to the rise in intracellular calcium results in the activation of calmodulin-dependent protein kinase, phosphorylases, phosphatases, and enzymes involved in glucose metabolism and energy production. Calmodulin is also involved in cell cycle progression and gene expression and may also may play a regulatory role in cyclic nucleotide levels and prostaglandin synthesis and metabolism. Cyclosporine has been shown to bind calmodulin and to inhibit the activation of cyclic nucleotide phosphodiesterase and calmodulin-dependent protein kinase (64,68). A number of known calmodulin antagonists compete with fluorescent CsA for binding to intact T cells. Although the reported affinity of CsA binding to calmodulin (kDa 10^{-7}M) is lower than that of cyclophilin, the functional studies described above provide strong evidence that binding to calmodulin may be a central mechanism for the immunosuppressive effects of CsA. Enthusiasm for this postulate has been tempered somewhat by the demonstration that calmodulin can also bind the inactive derivative CsH (68). It appears, however, that this inactive derivative does not partition into the cell membrane effectively, which may account for its inactivity (69). More recently, Wells and coworkers (70) demonstrated the difficulty of assessing CsA-calmodulin interactions and also found variations in the ability of CsA to compete for the binding of distinct calmodulin receptors, indicating that CsA may not inhibit all calmodulin functions equally. These findings, and the uncertainty about the role of calmodulin in T-cell activation, make it difficult to·arrive at definite conclusions about the central role of calmodulin in the mechanism of action of CsA. However, there are a number of parallels between classic calmodulin inhibitors and CsA that provide indirect evidence that CsA may be acting through calmodulin inhibition. Like CsA, these calmodulin inhibitors interrupt the cell cycle at the G_1-S interface (34,71); create nuclear lobulation of lymphocytes, presumably by disrupting the microtubular or microfilament cytoskeleton of the cells (72); and cause renin release from the kidney and prolactin release from the posterior pituitary (73,74). Cyclosporine, the classic calmodulin inhibitors, and the calcium channel blockers all overcome the resistance of certain leukemia cell lines to vincristine, perhaps by blocking calcium, calmodulin-dependent adenosine triphosphatase, and drug efflux (36).

The classic calmodulin antagonists also inhibit lymphocyte proliferation in a dose-dependent fashion, without cytotoxicity. In drug combination studies, these agents antagonize the immunosuppressive effect of CsA, indicating similar sites of action (75). Recent studies have shown that the calmodulin inhibitor, W-7, much like CsA, inhibits IL-2 production, but the antiproliferative effects may be overcome with exogenous IL-2 (76).

The role of the two intracellular receptors is further complicated by the observation that resistance and sensitivity to CsA are inversely correlated with binding of fluorescent or native CsA or both to intact T lymphocytes (72). The subset demonstrating the greatest uptake of a fluorescent derivative of CsA included antigen-specific suppressor T cells that were less affected by CsA. On the other hand, the cell subset demonstrating the least uptake of CsA, which contained precursor cytotoxic T lymphocytes and IL-2 producing helper cells, was exquisitely sensitive to inhibition by CsA. More important, calmodulin content of the two subsets was nearly identical, whereas cyclophilin content as determined by the LH-20 column assay was increased eight-fold in the resistant subset. Other CsA-resistant cells also express a relatively high content of cyclophilin (77). In fact, the fluorescent derivative distinguishes several discrete populations of lymphocytes (B and T) and monocytes based on binding and flow cytometric analysis, each with apparent distinct functions. These paradoxical data cannot be fully explained. There are several possibilities that can account for these data: (a) cyclophilin may have a negative regulatory influence on the immunosuppressive activity of CsA, (b) cyclophilin and calmodulin may work in concert to mediate CsA immunosuppression, and (c) cyclophilin and calmodulin may be affected by CsA at different points in the activation cascade and therefore mediate different dose-dependent effects on the immune system.

SUMMARY

Much has been learned about CsA, but in spite of these extensive studies, the precise mechanism of this immunosuppressive agent remains to be defined. Cyclosporine does not inhibit the ability of antigens to bind to its T-cell receptor and does not prevent the subsequent rise in intracellular calcium levels. Cyclosporine also does not inhibit protein kinase C activation. It appears to inhibit a calcium-dependent pathway that may be central to the synthesis and production of IL-2. Functionally, the data suggest that CsA causes immunosuppression by sparing the activation of suppressor T cells while interfering with the generation of cytotoxic T lymphocytes, thereby creating an immunological disequilibrium that favors tolerance.

For the immunotoxicologist, the complete evaluation of the immunotoxic potential of agents such as CsA that show no myelotoxicity or peripheral cytotoxicity presents a formidable challenge. As the preceding discussion illustrates, the susceptible target sites for these agents are many, and the possible immunological changes are often subtle. Moreover, changes in any immunological parameter(s) may not always be associated with risks for the host, and parallel risk-assessment studies are necessary. The effects of toxicants are likely to depend on the exposure level, and different target sites may be affected as the exposure levels vary. Most important, because of the interactive nature of the immune system, even slight or subtle changes may have both profound implications and easy to evaluate overt manifestations.

ACKNOWLEDGMENTS

Supported by Grants CA15396 and AI24682 from the National Institutes of Health, Grant IM398 from the American Cancer Society, and a gift from the Harley W. Howell Foundation.

REFERENCES

1. Morris, P. J. (1981): Cyclosporine A. *Transplantation*, 32:349.
2. Cohen, D. J., Loertscher, R., Rubin, M., Tilney, N. L., Carpenter, C. B., and Strom, T. B. (1984): Cyclosporine: A new immunosuppressive agent for organ transplantation. *Ann. Intern. Med.*, 101:667.
3. VonGreffenreid, B. (1986): Cyclosporin in auto-immune diseases. *Progress. Allerg.*, 38:432.
4. Shevach, E. (1985): The effects of cyclosporin A on the immune system. *Ann. Rev. Immunol.*, 3:397.
5. Hess, A. D., Colombani, P. M. and Esa, A. H. (1986): Cyclosporine and the immune response: Basic aspects. *Crit. Rev. Immunol.*, 6:123.
6. Green, G. I. and Allison, A. C. (1978): Extensive prolongation of rabbit kidney allograft survival after short-term cyclosporin A treatment. *Lancet* 1:1182.
7. Tutschka, P. K., Beschorner, W. E., Allison, A. C., Burns, W. H. and Santos, G. W. (1979): Use of cyclosporine A in allogeneic bone marrow transplantation (BMT) in the rat. *Nature* 280:5718.
8. Esa, A. H., Paxman, D. G., Noga, S. J. and Hess, A. D. (1988): Sensitivity of monocyte subpopulations to cyclosporine arachidonate metabolism and *in vitro* antigen presentation. *Trans. Proc.*, XX:80–86.
9. Lafferty, K. J., Borel, J. F., and Hodgkins, F. (1983): Cyclosporine-A (CsA): Models for the mechanism of action. *Transplant. Proc.*, 15:2242.
10. Granelli-Piperno, A., Keene, M. and Steinman, R. (1987): Evidence that cyclosporine inhibits all-mediated immunity primarily at the level of the T lymphocyte rather than accessory cell. *Transplantation* 46:535.
11. Bunjes, D., Hardt, C, Rollinghoff, M., and Wagner, H. (1981): Cyclosporin A mediates immunosuppression of primary cytotoxic T cell responses by impairing the release of interleukin 1 and interleukin 2. *Eur. J. Immunol.*, 8:657.

12. White, D. J. G. (1982): Cyclosporin A: Clinical pharmacology and therapeutic potential. *Drugs*, 24:322.

13. Dos Reis, G. A. and Shevach, E. M. (1983): Cyclosporin A treated guinea pigs responder cells secrete a genetically restricted factor that suppresses the mixed leukocyte reaction. *J. Clin. Invest.*, 71:165.

14. Gordon, M. Y., and Singer, J. W. (1979): Selective effects of cyclosporin A on colony-forming lymphoid and myeloid cells in man. *Nature*, 279:433.

15. Hess, A. D. and Tutschka, P. J. (1980): Effects of cyclosporine A on human lymphocyte responses *in vitro*. I. CsA allows for the expression of alloantigen-activated suppressor cells while preferentially inhibiting the induction of cytolytic effector lymphocytes in MLR. *J. Immunol.*, 124:2601.

16. Hess, A. D. and Tutschka, P. J. and Santos, G. W. (1981): Effect of cyclosporin A on human lymphocyte responses *in vitro*. II. Induction of specific alloantigen unresponsiveness mediated by a nylon wool adherent suppressor cell. *J. Immunol.*, 126:961.

17. Kupiec-Weglinski, J. W., Filho, M. A., Strom, T. B. and Tilney, N. L. (1984): Sparing of suppressor cells: A critical action of cyclosporine. *Transplantation*, 38:97.

18. Kerman, R. H., Fleckner, J. M., VanBuren, C. T., Lorber, M. I. and Kahan, B. D. (1987): Immunoregulatory mechanisms in cyclosporin-treated renal allograft recipients. *Transplantation*, 43:205.

19. Ryffel, B., Willard-Gallo, K. E., Tammi, K., and Loken, M. R. (1984): Quantitative fluorescent analysis of cyclosporine binding to human leukocytes. *Transplantation*, 37:276.

20. Esa, H. H., Converse, P. J. and Hess, A. D. (1987): Cyclosporine inhibits soluble antigen and alloantigen presentation by human monocytes *in vitro*. *Int. J. Immunopharmacol*, 9:893.

21. Kunkl, A., Manca, F., and Celada, F. (1985): Inhibition of accessory function of murine macrophages *in vitro* by cyclosporine. *Transplantation*, 39:644.

22. Snyder, D. S., Wright, C. L. and Tiong, C. (1986): Inhibition of human monocyte antigen presentation, but not HLA-DR, by cyclosporine. *Transplantation*, 44:407.

23. Palay, D. A., Cluff, C. W., Wentworth, P. A. and Ziegler, H. K. (1986): Cyclosporine inhibits macrophage mediated antigen presentation. *J. Immunol.*, 136:4348.

24. Groeniwegen, G., Buurman, W. S., Jeanhomme, G. M. A. et al (1985): Effects of cyclosporine on MAC II antigen expression on arterial and venous endothelium *in vitro*. *Transplantation*, 40:21.

25. Whistler, R. L., Lindsey, J. A., Proctor, K. V. W., Morisaki, N., and Cornwell, D. G. (1984): Characteristics of cyclosporine induction of increased prostaglandin levels from human peripheral blood monocytes. *Transplantation*, 38:377.

26. Bendzten, K., and Dinarello, C. A. (1984): Mechanism of action of cyclosporin A: Effect on T-cell binding of interleukin 1 and antagonizing effect of insulin. *Scan. J. Immunol.*, 20:43.

27. Palacios, R., and Moller, G. (1981): Cyclosporin A blocks receptors for HLA-DR antigens on T cells. *Nature*, 290:792.

28. Hess, A. D., Tutschka, P. J. and Santos, G. W. (1983): Effect of cyclosporine on the induction of cytotoxic T lymphocytes: Role of interleukin 1 and interleukin 2. *Transplant. Proc.*, 15:2248.

29. Whistler, R. L., Lindsey, J. A., Procter, K. V. W., Morisaki, N., and Cornwell, D. G. (1985): The impaired ability of human monocytes to stimulate autologous allogeneic mixed lymphocyte reactives after exposure to cyclosporine associated alterations of HLA-DR expression and physical characteristics of monocytes. *Transplantation*, 40:57.

30. Schultz, G., Stahl, P., Nigam, S., Sieber, G., Offermann, G., and Moltzhan, M. (1984): Effect of cyclosporine on the generation of prostanoids by cultured peripheral lymphocyte. *Transplant. Proc.*, 14:1214.

31. Rappaport, R. S., and Dodge, G. R. (1982): Prostaglandin E inhibits the production of human interleukin 2. *J. Exp. Med.*, 155:943.

32. Snyder, D. S., Beller, D. J., and Unanus, E. R. (1985): Prostaglandins modulate macrophage Ia expression. *Nature*, 299:163.

33. Makoul, G. T., Robinson, D. R., Bhalla, A. K. and Glimcher, L. H. (1985): Prostaglandin E_2 inhibits the activation of cloned T cell Hybridomas. *J. Immunol.*, 134:2645.

34. Fidelus, R. K., Laughler, A. H., Towney, J. J., et al (1984): The effect of cyclosporine on ornithine decarboxylase induction with mitogens, antigens and lymphokines. *Transplantation*, 37:383.

35. Koponen, M., Grieder, A., Hauser, R. and Loor, F. (1985): Interference of cyclosporine with lymphocyte proliferation: Effects on mitochondria and lysosomes of cyclosporine-sensitive or resistant cell clones. *Cell Immunol.*, 134:2645.

36. Slater, L. M., Sweet, P., Stupecky, M., and Gupta, S. (1986): Cyclosporine A reverses vincristine and daurubicin resistance in acute lymphocytic leukemia *in vitro*. *Clin. Invest.*, 77:1405.

37. Gupta, S. K., Curtis, J., and Turk, J. L. (1985): The effect of hydrocortisone and cyclosporine A on Bacillus Calmette Guerin Epitheliod. *Cell Immunol.*, 93:481.
38. Perico, N., Benigni, A., Zoja, C., Delaini, F., and Remuzzi, G. (1986): Functional significance of exaggerated renal thromboxane A^2 synthesis induced by cyclosporine A. *Am. J. Physiol.*, 251:F581.
39. Rogers, T. S., Elzinga, L. E., Bennett, W. M., and Kelly, V. E. (1988): Selective enhancement of thromboxane in macrophages and kidneys in cyclosporine-induced nephrotoxicity. Dietary protection of fish oil. *Transplantation*, 45:153.
40. Esa, A. H., Noga, S. J., Donnenberg, A. D., and Hess, A. D. (1985): Immunologic heterogeneity of human monocyte subsets prepared by counterflow centrifugation elutriation. *Immunology*, 59:95.
41. Rosensen-Schloss, R. and Reinisch, C. (1985): Selective activation of immunoregulatory T-cell circuits by an Ig + antigen presenting cell line. *Cell Immunol.*, 93:475.
42. Gulberg, M., and Smith, K. A. (1986): Regulation of T cell autocrine growth $T4^+$ cells become refractory to interleukin 2. *J. Exp. Med.*, 163:270.
43. Borel, J. F., Feuer, C., Magnee, C., and Stahelin, H. (1977): Effects of the new anti-lymphocyte peptide cyclosporin A in animals. *Immunology*, 32:1017.
44. Burkhardt, J. J. and Guggenheim, B. (1979): *In vivo* and *in vitro* suppression of rat T-lymphocyte function. *Immunology*, 36:753.
45. Tosato, G., Pike, S. E., Koski, I. R., and Blaese, R. M. (1982): Selective inhibition of immunoregulatory cell functions by cyclosporin A. *J. Immunol.*, 128:1986.
46. Kunkl, A., and Klaus, G. G. B. (1980): Selective effects of cyclosporine A on functional B cell subsets in the mouse. *J. Immunol.*, 125:2526.
47. Dongworth, A. W. and Klaus, G. G. B. (1982): Effects of cyclosporin on the immune system of the mouse. I. Evidence for a direct selective effect of cyclosporin A on B cells responding to anti-immunoglobulin antibodies. *Eur. J. Immunol.* 12:1018,1982.
48. Bijsterbosch, M. K., and Klaus, G. G. B (1985): Cyclosporine does not inhibit mitogen-induced inositol phospholipid degradation in mouse lymphocytes. *Immunology*, 56:435.
49. Lichtman, A. H., Segal, G. B., and Lichtman, M. A. (1983): The role of calcium in lymphocyte proliferation (an interpretive review). *Blood*, 61:413.
50. Coffey, R. G., Hadden, E. M., and Hadden, J. W. (1977): Evidence for cyclic GMP and calcium mediation of lymphocyte activation by mitogens. *J. Immunol.*, 119:1387.
51. Nishizuka, Y. (1984): The role of protein kinase C in cell surface signal transduction and tumour promotion. *Nature London*, 308:693.
52. Hirano, T., Fujimoto, K., Teranishi, T., Nishino, N., Omoue, K., Maeda, S., and Shimada, K. (1984): Phorbol ester increases the level of interleukin-2 mRNA in mitogen-stimulated human lymphocytes. *J. Immunol.*, 132:2165.
53. Depper, J. M., Leonard, W. J., Kronke, M., Noguchi, P. D., Cunningham, R. E., Waldmann, T. A., and Greene, W. C. (1984): Regulation of interleukin-2 receptor expression: Effects of phorbol diester, phospholipase C and reexposure to lectin or antigen. *J. Immunol.*, 133:3054.
54. Kopenen, M., Grieder, A., and Loor, F. (1982): The effects of cyclosporine on the cell cycle of T-lymphocyte cell lines. *Exp. Cell Res.*, 140:237.
55. Kay, J. E., Benzie, C. R., and Borghetti, A. F. (1983): Effect of cyclosporin A on lymphocyte activation by the calcium ionophore A23187. *Immunology*, 50:441.
56. Metcalf, S. (1984): Cyclosporine does not prevent cytoplasmic calcium changes associated with lymphocyte activation. *Transplantation*, 38:161.
57. Kay, J. E. (1987): The cyclosporine-A-sensitive event in lymphocyte activation. *Ann. Inst. Pasteur. Immunol.*, 138:622.
58. Klaus, G. G. B. (1987): Cyclosporine A probe for different modes of lymphocyte activation. *Ann. Inst. Pasteur. Immunol.*, 138:626.
59. Gelfand, E. W., Cheung, R. K., Grinstein, S., and Mills, G. B. (1986): Characterization of the role for calcium influx in mitogen-induced triggering of human T cells. Identification of calcium-dependent and calcium independent signals. *Eur. J. Immunol.*, 16:907.
60. Tesi, R. J., Wait, R. B., Butt, K. M. H., Jaffee, B. M., and Memillan, M. A. (1985): Calcium antagonists potentiate cyclosporin effects on human lymphocytes. *Surg. Forum*, 36:339.
61. Palacios, R. (1982): Role and functional relationship of HLA-DR antigen and interleukins. *Immunol. Rev.*, 63:73.
62. Hess, A. D., Tuszynski, T., Engel, P., Colombani, P. M., Farrington, J., Wenger, R., and Ryffel, B. (1986): Intracellular and nuclear localization of cyclosporine in peripheral blood mononuclear cells. *Trans. Proc.*, 18:861–865.
63. Colombani, P. M., Robb, A. and Hess, A. D. (1985): Cyclosporine A binding to calmodulin: A possible site of action on T-lymphocytes. *Science*, 228:337.

64. Handschumacher, R. E., Harding, M. W., Rice, J., and Drugge, R. J. (1984): Cyclophilin: A specific cytosolic binding protein for cyclosporin A. *Science*, 226:544.
65. Hess, A. D. and Colombani, P. M. (1986): Mechanisms of action of cyclosporine: Role of calmodulin, cycophilin and other cyclosporine-binding proteins. *Trans. Proc.*, 18:219.
66. Harding, M. W., Gorelick, F. S. and Handschumacher, R. E. (1987): Cyclophilin represents a novel class of protein kinases. *Fed. Proc.*, 46:2162.
67. Means, A. R., Lagace, L., Guerrieo, B., and Chaffouleas, J. G. (1982): Calmodulin as a mediator of hormone action and cell regulation. *J. Cell Biochem.*, 20:317.
68. LeGrue, S. J., Turner, R., Weisbrodt, N., and Dedman, J. R. (1986): Does the binding of cyclosporin to calmodulin result in immunosuppression? *Science*, 234:68.
69. Colombani, P. M., Bright, E. C., and Hess, A. D. (1988): Comparison of binding of peripheral blood lymphocytes between active and inactive derivatives of cyclosporin. *Transplant. Proc.*, 20(2):46.
70. Wells, M. S., Vogelsang, G. B., Colombani, P. M., and Hess, A. D. (1989): Cyclosporine binding to Calmodulin. *Transpl. Proc.*, 121:850–852.
71. Ying, M. L. (1982): Calmodulin. *Mol. Cell Biochem.*, 45:101–112.
72. Simons, J. W., Noga, S. J.,. Colombani, P. M., Beschorner, W., Coffey, D. S. and Hess, A. D. (1986): Cyclosporine A, an *in vitro* Calmodulin antagonist, induces nuclear lobulations in human T cell lymphocytes and monocytes. *J. Cell Biol.*, 102:145–150.
73. Bantle, J. P., Nath, K. A., Sutherland, D. E. R., Najarian, J. S., and Ferris, T. F. (1985): Effects of cyclosporine on the renin-angiotensin-aldosterone system and potassium excretion in renal transplant recipients. *Arch. Intern. Med.*, 145:505.
74. Klee, C. B., and Vanaman, T. C. (1982): Calmodulin. *Adv. Protein Chem.*, 35:213.
75. Colombani, P. M., Bright, E. C., Monastyrskyj, O., and Hess, A. D. (1987): Subcellular action of CsA: Interaction between CsA and Calmodulin antagonists. *Transplant. Proc.*, 19:1171.
76. LeGrue, S. J. and Munn, C. G. (1987): Comparison of the immunosuppressive effects of cyclosporine, lipid-soluble anesthetics and Calmodulin antagonists. *Transplantation*, 42:679.
77. Koletsky, A. J., Harding, M. W. and Handschumacher, R. E. (1986): Cyclophilin: Distribution and variant properties in normal and neoplastic tissues. *J. Immunol.*, 137:1054.

Clinical Immunotoxicology, edited by
D. S. Newcombe, N. R. Rose, and J. C. Bloom.
Raven Press, Ltd., New York © 1992.

10

Drug-induced Immunological Disorders of the Blood

Kent Holland* and Jerry L. Spivak†

*Oncology Center, Johns Hopkins University, School of Medicine,
Baltimore, MD; †Division of Hematology, Department of Medicine,
Johns Hopkins University, School of Medicine, Baltimore, MD*

Adverse reactions to drugs are an unavoidable consequence of medical therapy, and the blood is frequently the target organ. Although pyrogenic and dermatological reactions and hepatic toxicity occur with a higher frequency than hematological toxicity, drug-induced damage to the blood usually has a greater impact with respect to morbidity and mortality (4,12). Adverse drug reactions may occur directly owing to chemical toxicity or indirectly through immunological mechanisms. In this chapter, we discuss drug-induced blood disorders resulting in abnormalities of hematopoiesis that are immunologically mediated.

The blood may serve as a target for drug-induced immune damage at many levels. Within the circulation, there may be damage and destruction of the various mature formed elements. Hemolytic anemia, agranulocytosis, and thrombocytopenia alone or together are the most commonly recognized consequences of immunological drug toxicity, and until recently they were the only types that could be evaluated on a quantitative as well as a qualitative basis. The production of antibodies to coagulation factors is a less common consequence of immunological drug toxicity. Immunological drug toxicity can also involve the immature hematopoietic precursor cells within the marrow, and on occasion both the circulating mature formed elements and the immature marrow precursor cells are involved.

Distinctions between the various levels of involvement can sometimes be made on morphological grounds alone, but more often sophisticated immunological and hematological analysis are required.

The development of clonal assays for hematopoietic progenitor cells has broadened our understanding of the mechanisms of hematopoiesis and has also permitted the detection of previously undefined mechanisms for drug-induced immunological hematopoietic toxicity. Using techniques of the experimental hematologist together with those of the immunologist, we can now identify the target cells involved in immunologically mediated drug toxicity in a manner not previously possible.

Figure 1 illustrates the central dogma of experimental hematology, that is, that

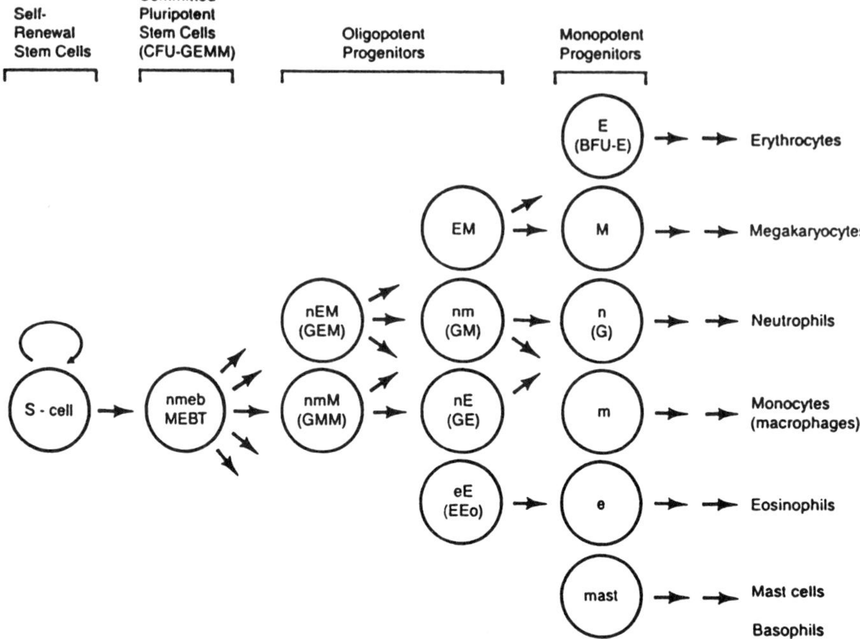

FIG. 1. A schematic representation of hematopoietic stem cell commitment as derived from *in vitro* clonal assays. Although not represented in this scheme, lymphocytes also arise from the pluripotent hematopoietic stem cell. (Adapted from Ogawa et al., ref. 44).

there is a pluripotent hematopoietic stem cell from which arise (presumably in a stochastic fashion) committed multipotent hematopoietic progenitor cells that become progressively restricted with respect to lineage development as they mature (44). The committed progenitor cells for erythroid, myeloid, and megakaryocyte cells can be grown *in vitro*, permitting the interaction of these cells with specific drugs or their metabolites to be measured quantitatively. The extent to which such cells possess receptors for specific growth factors is a reflection of their degree of lineage restriction (58). Commitment and maturation are also associated with the expression or modulation of specific cell surface antigens, and it is most likely these antigens that define the specificity of the particular drug-induced immunological hematopoietic toxicity. Although the nature of many of these antigens is undefined, examples of lineage-specific progenitor cell toxicity have been described, and this has added a new dimension to our knowledge of hematopoietic drug toxicity. Thus, drug toxicity may be manifested by destruction of one or more of the formed elements of the blood, by destruction of recognizable hematopoietic precursor cells in the marrow or both, or by destruction of or inhibition of the proliferation of the morphologically unrecognizable hematopoietic progenitor cells within the marrow.

In this chapter, we will describe examples of each form of immunologically mediated drug toxicity.

Understanding adverse hematological reactions to drugs is often hindered by the richness of our therapeutic options. For example, in a hospital setting, the average number of different drug exposures for an individual patient may be as high as ten for a stay of 2 to 3 weeks (12). Such polypharmacy, although often medically justifiable, makes it difficult to determine which drug might be the offender in an adverse drug reaction. However, the frequency with which certain drugs have been associated with specific adverse hematological reactions permits their indictment with some certainty. It should be emphasized that failure to implicate other drugs may relate to the frequency with which they are employed. Studies in Sweden, where medical demographics are excellent, have indicated that adverse drug reactions occur most often in older individuals and in women in particular (12). It should also be noted that failure to implicate a particular drug when conducting *in vitro* toxicological studies may be caused by failure to recognize that the offending agent is a metabolite of the drug and not the drug itself (51). In the sections that follow, we discuss drug-induced immunological peripheral blood toxicity and then document examples of newly recognized immunologically mediated, drug-induced marrow toxicity involving hematopoietic progenitor cells. As experience with clonal assays for hematopoietic progenitor cells accumulates and these assays become more widely available, the mechanism of drug-induced immunological hematopoietic toxicity will be better understood.

DRUG-INDUCED IMMUNE HEMOLYTIC ANEMIA

Three well-defined immunological mechanisms are responsible for drug-mediated immunological damage to erythrocytes. Each has a distinct drug-erythrocyte interaction and a distinct mechanism for red blood cell destruction. Drugs identified as causing immune-mediated hemolysis are listed in Table 1.

Hapten Hemolysis

The hapten mechanism is associated with the penicillin antibiotics. It was initially described in patients receiving high doses of penicillin (10 to 30 million U/day) (45,60). The associated hemolytic anemia was usually mild and resolved within days to weeks after discontinuation of the drug. Hemolysis was initially postulated to result from the drug combining with a serum macromolecule that stimulated IgG antibody production (the Miescher-Schulman theory) (41,54). According to this theory, a drug-antibody hapten complex was formed that bound to the red blood cell surface, resulting in destruction of the erythrocyte with or without complement activation. It has subsequently been shown that at high serum concentrations, penicillin coats the red blood cell surface, and this may be followed by production of IgG antibodies that bind to the red cell–penicillin complex (2). The direct Coombs

TABLE 1. *Drugs causing immune hemolysis*

Antibiotics:
  Cephalosporins
  Penicillin
  Para-aminosalicylic acid
Rifampin
  Stibophen
  Sulfonamides
Sulfonamide Derivatives:
  Chlorpropamide
  Tolbutamide
Phenothiazines
Thiazides
Analgesics:
  Acetaminophen
  Ibuprofen
  Phenacetin
Miscellaneous:
  Procainamide
  Methyldopa
  L-dopa
  Quinine, quinidine
  Hydralazine

test results are positive with this mechanism, and the indirect Coombs test shows that antibody from either the patient's serum or eluted from the patient's red blood cells reacts only with penicillin-coated erythrocytes. The IgG antibody is directed at either the benzylpenicillocyl or nonbenzylpenicilloyl determinant of the penicillin molecule (33,68). The resulting hemolysis occurs primarily from splenic sequestration of the antibody-coated erythrocytes as opposed to intravascular hemolysis, although the latter may on occasion occur owing to complement-mediated membrane damage in the absence of penicillin binding (21).

A similar hapten mechanism may be seen rarely in cephalosporins that have antigenic cross-reactivity with penicillin (23). Tetracycline has also been observed to cause a similar hemolytic process (66).

Immune Complexes

The immune complex mechanism has been associated not only with erythrocytic destruction but also with thrombocytopenia and neutropenia. Unlike what occurs in the hapten mechanism, only a small quantity of drug is needed to activate hemolysis. Ackroyd and Rook suggested that the drug forms an antigenic complex on the red blood cell surface, which when combined with an antibody promotes intravascular hemolysis in the presence of complement (2). Based on studies of drug-antibody and erythrocyte-drug affinities, Schulman proposed that the drug forms an immune complex (with either an IgM or IgG antibody) in the serum that can reversibly bind to the red blood cell surface (55). The immune complex remains intact after activating complement on the red cell surface and can proceed to hemolyze other red cells, thereby explaining the extensive hemolysis observed even when only small quantities of the drug are present.

The drug stibophen used in the treatment of schistosomiasis appears to cause hemolytic anemia by the immune complex mechanism (27). Hemolysis usually occurred after more than one exposure to the drug, and it demonstrated a serum antibody in the presence of stibophen agglutinated normal red blood cells. The drug-antibody immune complex became adsorbed onto the red blood cell surface, and in the presence of complement, an "innocent bystander" lysis resulted.

Quinidine-induced hemolytic anemia also appears to occur by a similar mechanism. Ballas and associates reported the presence of an IgG antibody to quinidine (6). *In vitro* studies confirmed immune complex formation and also showed that quinidine-coated red cells (hapten mechanism) did not promote agglutination with the IgG antibody. Quinidine-associated hemolysis has, however, been reported to occur by a hapten mechanism as well (7). 5-Fluorouracil (5-FU), a commonly used chemotherapeutic agent, was reported by Sandvei and coworkers to cause acute intravascular hemolysis (53). A drug-dependent complement-activating IgM antibody was detected in the patient's serum, presumably causing hemolysis by the immune complex mechanism.

Ackroyd and Rook postulated that hemolysis could also result from drug metabolites (2). Salama and colleagues recently reported 19 cases of acute intravascular hemolysis associated with the drug nomifensine, an antidepressant (51). Strong IgG and IgM antibody reactions were found against the metabolites of nomifensine, and only a minority of the antibodies were against the parent drug. The metabolite-associated immune complexes were able to activate complement.

Autoantibody Formation

Autoantibody production directly against red blood cells has been reported with alpha-methyldopa, L-dopa, procainamide, and mefenamic acid (31,56,61,69). Unlike what occurs in immune complex–mediated hemolysis, the drugs do not directly participate in red blood cell destruction. Hemolysis results from IgG antibodies that react directly with the red blood cell membrane, causing sequestration of the antibody-coated cells by the spleen. Hemolysis is usually mild to moderate and uncommon in occurrence.

Alpha-methyldopa was observed to produce a positive direct Coombs' test result after 3 months of use in 15% of patients (13). Only 1% of Coombs' positive-patients developed a hemolytic anemia, which did not appear to be related to the quantity of alpha-methyldopa ingested. The indirect Coombs test findings could also be positive, and the IgG antibodies had specificity for the red blood cell membrane Rh complex (35).

The drug cianidanol, a flavonoid used for treating hepatitis, has been associated with life-threatening hemolysis. Salama and coworkers reported that this drug caused hemolysis both by autoantibody promotion and by drug-dependent antibodies directed against the red blood cell (50). Six patients were reported with this problem. One patient developed an IgG autoantibody causing *in vitro* erythrocyte agglutination independent of the drug. Four patients demonstrated drug-dependent antibodies of the IgG and IgM class directed at the drug or its metabolites. This latter group demonstrated a hapten mechanism, i.e., tight binding of the drug to the cell membrane, which interacted with antibodies to form a drug-cell complex. A sixth patient showed both autoantibodies and a hapten-antibody interaction. These observations demonstrate that the same drug can cause immunologically mediated red blood cell damage by several different mechanisms.

DRUG-INDUCED IMMUNE THROMBOCYTOPENIA

Drug-induced immune thrombocytopenia is a frequent complication of a variety of medications. The thrombocytopenia results from the sequestration of antibody-coated platelets. Examination of the bone marrow usually reveals an increase in megakaryocyte number. Thrombocytopenic purpura was first associated with the drug quinine in 1865 by Vipan (65). It was subsequently demonstrated that when the serum of an affected patient was exposed to quinine, it was capable of causing platelet agglutination (24).

A vast number of drugs have been associated with immunological thrombocytopenia and are listed in Table 2. Quinidine and allylisopropylacetylurea (Sedormid) have been the most extensively studied and are the prototypes for the observed immune mechanism. Ackroyd showed that patients sensitive to Sedormid had a "plasma factor" that by itself did not cause platelet agglutination (1). However, when Sedormid was added to the plasma, platelet agglutination occurred. A similar reaction was noted with quinidine.

TABLE 2. *Drugs causing immune thrombocytopenia*

Antibiotics:	*Antihistamines*:
Cephalothin	Chlorpheniramine
Rifampin	Diphenyhydramine
Stibophen	*Miscellaneous*:
Sulfonamides	Gold salts
Sulfonamide Derivatives:	Heparin
Chlorpropamide	Digitoxin
Tolbutamide	Methyldopa
Acetazolamide	Phenytoin
Thiazides	Quinidine, quinine
Sedatives:	Ethanol
Ethchlorvynol	Carbamazepine
Barbiturates	
Analgesics:	
Acetylsalicylic acid	
Phenacetin	

Ackroyd postulated a hapten-like mechanism for the platelet agglutination, but subsequent studies supported an immune-complex mechanism (53). Platelets exposed to the drug and then subjected to a quick saline wash are incapable of antibody attachment in the absence of the drug. This supports the theory of a drug-antibody complex that is adsorbed by the platelet membrane (55). The immune complex forms a high affinity bond with the platelet surface, resulting in an innocent bystander lysis or agglutination of the platelet. Smith demonstrated that the Fab domain of the IgG molecule supported the attachment of the drug-induced antibody to the platelet surface (14). This explains the observation of little or no cross-reactivity with myeloid or erythroid elements. In this regard, it is also of interest that quinidine-induced thrombocytopenia is produced by an IgM antibody whereas quinidine-induced hemolytic anemia is due to an IgG antibody, and both may be present in the same patient (19). Furthermore, in most but not all patients, drug-induced antibodies appear to be stereospecific, and those induced by quinidine do not react with quinine. The target platelet antigen in some patients with drug-induced immunologically mediated thrombocytopenia appears to be platelet glycoprotein membrane Ib (18).

Heparin has been implicated as a frequent cause of drug-induced thrombocytopenia. The incidence is reported to be as high as 30% with beef-lung heparin extract but is lower with the porcine intestine preparation (8,9,37). Rhodes demonstrated a heparin-dependent antiplatelet antibody in studies of *in vitro* platelet aggregation and complement fixation studies (48). However, thrombocytopenia associated with heparin can occur without evidence of immunological mediation (8).

DRUG-INDUCED IMMUNE NEUTROPENIA

Drug-induced immune neutropenia can be a life-threatening condition, and symptomatic patients may succumb to bacterial infection within hours if not treated with antibiotics. The diagnosis of immune neutropenia is often difficult, since unlike in the hemolytic anemias, there are no characteristic morphological abnormalities on the blood smear. The immunological reaction causing the neutropenia can be directed at any stage of myeloid development from the circulating mature neutrophils to early progenitor cells in the bone marrow.

Multiple agents have been implicated in drug-induced immune neutropenia (Table 3). Aminopyrine, an analgesic, has a well-defined association with granulocytopenia and represents the classic drug-antibody–mediated mechanism for destruction of circulating neutrophils (36). Susceptible patients develop the complication within 7 to 10 days of drug administration. Readministration of even minute quantities of drug to a sensitized patient will result in a brisk and severe neutropenia owing to leukoagglutination and destruction of circulating granulocytes.

Antithyroid medications are a common cause of drug-induced immune neutropenia. Bilezikian and coworkers demonstrated the presence of circulating IgM

TABLE 3. *Drugs causing immune granulocytopenia*

Antibiotics:	*Antithyroid Drugs*:
Chloramphenicol	Propylthiouracil
Ampicillin	Methimazole
Carbenicillin	*Phenothiazines*
Cephalothin	*Thiazides*
Methicillin	*Miscellaneous*:
Nafcillin	Aprindine
Penicillin	Cimetidine
Oxacillin	Colchicine
Gentamicin	Penicillamine
Sulfonamides	Phenylbutazone
Trimethoprim-sulfamethoxazole	Phenytoin
Sulfonamide Derivatives:	Procainamide
Chlorpropamide	
Tolbutamide	
Acetazolamide	

antineutrophil antibodies in propylthiouracil-induced agranulocytosis that inhibited leukocyte metabolism but did not cause leukoagglutination (10). Weitzman and Stossel postulated neutrophil opsonization by a complement-dependent mechanism presumably involving an IgM antibody, with sequestration and phagocytosis of the opsonized granulocytes (67). This was also supported by Guffy and associates, who demonstrated that cytotoxicity was mediated by an IgM complement–dependent antibody (25).

Synthetic penicillins have been implicated in promoting neutropenia in a hapten-like mechanism, although the data remain limited (3,43). Stossel and Weitzman reported that a high concentration of these agents was required to cause an opsonizing reaction (67). Ahern observed the development of neutropenia in patients treated with high-dose intravenous oxacillin (3). Patients developed neutropenia after 2 weeks of therapy and had associated eosinophilia. Cephalosporin-induced immune neutropenia has been reported in two patients by in whom an IgG antibody was demonstrated by Murphy (43). In one patient, a hapten-antibody mechanism similar to that associated with penicillin-induced hemolytic anemia was observed. In the other, an immune complex mechanism was likely.

Antiarrhythmic drugs associated with neutropenia include lidocaine, quinidine, phenytoin, procainamide, and flecainide (26,29,40,52,57,67). Flecainide-induced immune neutropenia was described by Samlowski (57). The patients had an IgG antibody that bound to neutrophils in a hapten-like fashion. Kelton and coworkers described a patient taking quinidine sulfate who developed both myeloid and erythroid suppression (32). After exposure to quinidine, the patient's serum suppressed allogeneic granulocyte and erythroid precursors *in vitro* as well as the patient's own marrow precursor cells. These latter observations supported the presence of a drug-antibody immune complex mechanism for the suppression of granulopoiesis.

Leukoagglutinins have been described during acute phases of agranulocytosis attributed to sulfonamides. The presence of the drug was required to demonstrate antibody activity. The sulfonamides or their derivatives implicated include sulfapyridine, salicylazosulfapyridine, sulfamethoxypyridazine, and chlorpropamide (20,30,42). Other drugs that have shown *in vitro* leukoagglutination include phenothiazines, chloral hydrate, meprobamate, and barbiturates (46,59,62,63,67).

Although classic agranulocytosis was once considered to be caused by peripheral destruction of antibody-coated neutrophils, recent studies indicate that certain drug-related antibodies can cause severe neutropenia resulting from marrow cell toxicity. In addition to the observations of Kelton and coworkers (32) described above, Levitt reported a case of chlorpropamide-induced pure white blood cell aplasia (34). *In vitro* inhibition of autologous granulocyte progenitor cells (CFU-GM) was demonstrated in the presence of the patient's serum and chlorpropamide. There was minimal inhibition of erythroid or multipotent hematopoietic progenitor cells. These observations were duplicated with allogeneic marrow progenitor cells. No circulating antineutrophil antibody was detected in the patient's serum. In addition, in the absence of either drug or serum, there was no inhibition of colony promotion by CFU-GM.

Ascensao and coworkers reported a patient with quinidine-induced agranulocytosis (5). In *in vitro* autologous marrow cultures, the presence of the patient's serum and quinidine caused an inhibition of CFU-GM proliferation. Antineutrophil antibodies were not detected, and in the absence of quinidine, CFU-GM proliferation was not suppressed. Mamus and colleagues reported on a patient who developed ibuprofen-associated pure white blood cell aplasia (38). The patient's marrow was normocellular, with only rare granulocytic precursors present. Antineutrophil antibodies were absent, but there was marked inhibition of CFU-GM proliferation in the presence of the patient's serum, ibuprofen, and complement. Erythroid progenitor cell proliferation was not inhibited. However, pluripotent stem cell growth *in vitro* was suppressed by this drug-immune complex. As with the other examples, in the absence of either ibuprofen or the patient's serum, there was no *in vitro* suppression of myelopoiesis.

DRUG-INDUCED IMMUNE RED BLOOD CELL APLASIA

Pure red blood cell aplasia is a syndrome that occurs either as a primary hematological disorder or a secondary phenomenon owing to infection, neoplasia, collagen vascular diseases, hemolytic anemia, and renal disease. It has also been associated with drug exposure. The syndrome manifests as a severe normochromic, normocytic anemia with reticulocytopenia. The bone marrow shows profound erythroid hypoplasia with otherwise normal cellularity and abundant myeloid precursors and megakaryocytes (17).

Although many drugs have been implicated in causing pure red blood cell aplasia, an immunological mechanism has been established for only a few. Pure red blood cell aplasia induced by phenytoin has been demonstrated to be an immunologically mediated event caused by an IgG inhibitor. Dessypris and coworkers reported a patient whose serum IgG in the presence of phenytoin suppressed normal allogeneic marrow erythroid colony-forming (CFU-E and BFU-E) activity as well as autologous BFU-E proliferation (17). No suppression was seen in the absence of the drug, and there was no inhibition of CFU-GM proliferation *in vitro*. The authors also demonstrated that the serum and drug combination neither exerted a direct cytotoxic effect on immature marrow erythroblasts nor interfered with erythropoietin. It was postulated that the drug-antibody complex inhibited erythroid progenitors differentiating into erythroblasts. Similar mechanisms have also been postulated for isoniazid- and chlorpropamide-induced red blood cell aplasia (15,47).

DRUG-INDUCED LUPUS ERYTHEMATOSUS AND HEMATOPOIETIC TOXICITY

Drug-induced lupus erythematosus occurs in up to 29% of patients and is commonly associated with procainamide and hydralazine administration (28). The development of antinuclear antibodies occurs in 20% to 80% of patients taking these medications, a frequency that greatly exceeds the clinical development of lupus erythematosus (16,31). Associated blood dyscrasias are even less common and are often not associated with other overt symptoms of lupus erythematosus. Coombs'-positive anemia (11), thrombocytopenia (39), neutropenia (29,64) and pure red blood cell aplasia (22) have all been reported.

In patients with procainamide-induced lupus erythematosus, 23% had a positive Coombs test result with a reagent that detects complement, whereas 10% had detectable IgG on their red blood cell membranes (11). Up to 13% of the patients were anemic, but clinically overt hemolytic anemia was rare. Jones and colleagues demonstrated that procainamide, like alpha-methyldopa, could induce *in vitro* red blood cell agglutination by stimulating IgG antibodies directed against red blood cell Rh antigens without requiring a drug-antibody complex or hapten formation (31).

Thrombocytopenia is less common and has been reported in patients both with and without clinically overt symptoms of lupus erythematosus (16,39). Meisner and coworkers reported six cases of thrombocytopenia in patients taking procainamide (39). Only three had antinuclear antibodies and only one had clinical symptoms of

TABLE 4. *Drugs causing lupus erythematosus*

Procainamide	Phenytoin
Hydralazine	Carbamazepine
Isoniazid	Ethosuximide
Methyldopa	Propylthiouracil
Chlorpromazine	Penicillamine
Quinidine	Sulfasalazine
Lithium	Acebutolol

lupus erythematosus. Thrombocytopenia presumably resulted from peripheral destruction of platelets because megakaryocytes were present in the bone marrow. The thrombocytopenia resolved with discontinuation of the procainamide.

Procainamide-induced agranulocytosis is also an uncommon but well-documented event. Neutropenia usually begins 30 to 90 days after the institution of the drug, with recovery of granulocytes beginning 10 to 14 days after its discontinuation. Procainamide-induced agranulocytosis in patients is often associated with positive antinuclear antibody findings (49). The bone marrow shows absence of myeloid elements beyond the promyelocyte stage. *In vitro* autologous bone marrow cultures for CFU-GM have shown that procainamide inhibited myeloid proliferation in acute phase marrow cells but not with the recovery phase marrow cells.

Pure red blood cell aplasia has been reported with procainamide by Giannone and associates (22). A patient taking procainamide for over a year developed an antinuclear antibody titer of 1:320 but had no overt clinical symptoms. Subsequently, he developed anemia and reticulocytopenia, and there was an absence of erythroid precursor cells in the bone marrow. Discontinuation of the procainamide resulted in prompt reticulocytosis and resolution of the severe anemia. *In vitro* proliferation of allogeneic erythroid progenitor cells was normal in the presence of the patient's serum and procainamide; thus, the actual mechanism of pure red blood cell aplasia associated with drug-induced lupus erythematosus remains to be elucidated.

REFERENCES

1. Ackroyd, J. F. (1949): The pathogenesis of thrombocytopenic purpura due to hypersensitivity to Sedormid (allyl-isopropyl-acetyl-carbamide). *Clin. Sci.*, 7:249.
2. Ackroyd, J. F., and Rook, A. J. (1968): Allergic drug reactions. In Clinical Aspects of Immunology, edited by P. G. H. Gill and R. R. A. Coombs. Blackwell Scientific Publications, Oxford and Edinburgh.
3. Ahern, M. J., Hicks, J. L., and Andriols, V. T. (1976): Neutropenia during high dose intravenous oxacillin therapy. *Yale J. Biol. Med.*, 49:351.
4. Arneborn, P., and Palblad, J. (1979): Drug-induced neutropenias in the Stockholm region (1976–1977). *Acta Med. Scand.*, 206:241.
5. Ascensao et al. (1984): Quinidine-induced neutropenia. Report of a case with drug-dependent inhibition of granulocyte colony formation. *Acta Haematol.*, 72:349.
6. Ballas, S. K., Caro, J. F., and Miguel, O. (1978): Quinidine-induced hemolytic anemia: Immunohematologic characterization. *Transfusion*, 18:215.
7. Bell, I. A., Zwicker, H., Lee, S., and Alpern, H. (1973): Quinidine hemolytic anemia in the absence of thrombocytopenia in a patient with quinidine hemolytic anemia with hemoglobin D. *Transfusion*, 13:100.
8. Bell, W. R. (1976): Thrombocytopenia occurring during heparin therapy. *N. Engl. J. Med.*, 295:276.
9. Bell, W. R., et al. (1976): Thrombocytopenia during the administration of heparin: A prospective study of 52 patients. *Ann. Intern. Med.*, 85:155.
10. Bilezikian, S. B., Yahya, L., Tsan, M. E., Hodkinson, B. A., Ice, S., and McIntyre, P. A. (1976): Immunological Reactions involving leukocytes: III agranulocytosis induced by antithyroid drugs. *Johns Hopkins Med. J.* 138:124.
11. Blomgren, S. E., Condemi, J. J., and Vaugn, J. H. (1972): Procainamide-induced lupus erythematosus. *Am. J. Med.*, 52:338.
12. Bottiger, L. E., Furhoff, A. K., and Hollenberg, L. (1979): Drug induced blood dyscrasias. *Acta Med. Scand.*, 205:457.

13. Cantor, S., and Barnett, A. J. (1967): Haematological effects of methyldopa. *Lancet*, 1:625.
14. Christie, D. J., Mullen, P. C., and Aster, R. H. (1985): Fab-mediated binding of drug-dependent induced antibodies to platelets in quinidine and quinine induced thrombocytopenia. *J. Clin. Invest.*, 75:310.
15. Clairborne, R. A., and Dwit, A. K. (1985): Isoniazid-induced pure red cell aplasia. *Am. Rev. Respir. Dis.*, 131:947.
16. Cush, J. J., and Goldings, E. A. (1985): Southwestern Internal Medicine Conference. Drug-induced lupus: Clinical spectrum and pathogenesis. *Am. J. Med. Sci.*, 290:36.
17. Dessypris, E. N., et al. (1985): Diphenylhydantoin-induced pure red cell aplasia. *Blood*, 65:789.
18. Devine, D. U., Currie, M. S., Rosse, W. R., and Greenberg, C. S. (1987): Pseudo-Bernard-Soulier syndrome: Thrombocytopenia caused by autoantibody to platelet glycoprotein Ib. *Blood*, 70:428.
19. Eisner, E. V., Crowell, E. B. (1972): Quinine-induced thrombocytopenia purpura due to an IgM and IgG antibody. *Transfusion*, 12:317.
20. Evans, R. S., and Ford, W. (1958): Studies of the bone marrow in immunological granulocytopenia following administration of salicylazosulfapyridine. *Arch. Intern. Med.*, 101:244.
21. Fearon, D. T. (1980): Identification of the membrane glycoprotein that is the C3b receptor of the human erythrocyte, polymorphonuclear leukocyte, and B lymphocyte and monocyte. *J. Exp. Med.*, 152:20.
22. Giannone, L., Kugler, J. W., and Krantz, S. B. (1987): Pure red cell aplasia associated with administration of sustained-release procainamide. *Arch. Intern. Med.*, 147:1179.
23. Gralnick, H. R., McGinnis, M. H., Elton, W., and McCurdy, P. (1971): Hemolytic anemia associated with cephalothin. *J.A.M.A.*, 217:1193.
24. Grandjean, L. L. (1948): A case of purpura haemorrhagica after administration of quinine with specific thrombocytolysis demonstrated in vitro. *Acta Scand.*, 131:165.
25. Guffy, M. M., Goeken, N. E., and Burns, C. P. (1984): Granulocytotoxic antibodies in a patient with propylthiouracil-induced agranulocytosis. *Arch. Intern. Med.*, 144:1687.
26. Harmon, D. C., Weitzman, S. A., and Stossel, T. D. (1984): The severity of immune neutropenia correlates with maturational specificity of antineutrophil antibodies. *Br. J. Haematol.*, 58:209.
27. Harris, J. W. (1956): Studies on the mechanism of a drug-induced hemolytic anemia. *J. Lab. Clin. Med.*, 47:760.
28. Hess, E. V. (1981): Introduction to drug-related lupus. *Arthritis Rheum.*, 24:vi.
29. Inouye, M., Millar, J., and Townsend, J. H. (1957): Agranulocytosis followed by maintenance dosage of Pronestyl. Report of serum case with recovery. *J.A.M.A.*, 147:652.
30. Johnson, F. O., and Korst, D. R. (1961): Pancytopenia associated with sulfamethoxypyridazine administration, the occurrence of leukopenia suggests an accumulative effect: Constant awareness is essential to prevent serious marrow damage. *J.A.M.A.*, 175:967.
31. Jones, G. W., George, T. L., and Bradley, R. D. (1978): Procainamide-induced hemolytic anemia. *Transfusion*, 18:224.
32. Kelton, J. G., Huanj, A. T., Mold, N., Logue, G., and Rosse, W. F. (1979): The use of in vitro techniques to study drug-induced pancytopenia. *N. Engl. J. Med.*, 301:621.
33. Levine, B. B., and Redmond, A. P. (1967): Immune mechanisms of penicillin-induced Coombs' positivity in man (abstract). *J. Clin. Invest.*, 46:1085.
34. Levitt, L. J. (1987): Chlorpropamide-induced pure white cell aplasia. *Blood*, 69:294.
35. LaBuglio, A. F., and Jandl, J. H. (1967): The nature of alpha-methyldopa red cell antibody. *N. Engl. J. Med.*, 276:658.
36. Madison, F. W., and Squier, T. L. (1934): The etiology of primary granulocytopenia (agranulocytic angina). *J.A.M.A.*, 102:755.
37. Malcolm, I. D., and Wigmore, T. A. (1978): Thrombocytopenia induced by low-dose subcutaneous heparin. *Lancet*, 1:444.
38. Mamus, S. W., Burton, J. D., et al. (1986): Ibuprofen-associated pure white cell aplasia. *N. Engl. J. Med.*, 314:624.
39. Meisner, D. J., Raymond, J. C., and Gottleb, A. J. (1985): Thrombocytopenia following sustained released procainamide. *Arch. Intern. Med.*, 145:700.
40. Menitove, J. E., Rassiga, A. L., McLaren, G. D., Daniel, T. M., and Mahmoud, A. A. F. (1981): Antigranulocyte antibodies and deranged immune function associated with phenytoin-induced serum sickness. *Am. J. Hematol.*, 10:277.
41. Miescher, P., and Straessle, R. (1956): Experimentelle Studien uber den Mechanismus der Thrombocyten-Schädigung durch Antigen-antidorperreaktian. *Vox Sang.*, 1:83.
42. Moeschlin, S. (1953): Immunoleukopenias et immunoagranulocytosis. *Rev. Hematol.*, 8:249.

43. Murphy, M. F., Metcalfe, P., Grint, P. C. A., Green, A. R., Knowles, S., Amess, J. A. L., and Watts, A. H. (1985): Cephalosporin-induced immune neutropenia. *Br. J. Haematol.*, 59:9.
44. Ogawa, M., Porter, P. N., and Nakohata, T. (1983): Renewal and commitment to differentiation of hemapoietic stem cells (an interpretive review). *Blood*, 61:823.
45. Petz, L. D., and Fudenberg, H. H. (1966): Coombs-positive hemolytic anemia caused by penicillin administration. *N. Engl. J. Med.*, 274:171.
46. Piciotta, A. V., et al. (1958): Agranulocytosis following administration of phenothiazine derivatives. *Am. J. Med.*, 25:210.
47. Planas, A. T., Ramon, N. K., Soletsky, H. B., and Pezzimenti, J. F. (1980): Chlorpropamide-induced pure RBC aplasia. *Arch. Intern. Med.*, 140:707.
48. Rhodes, G. R., Dixon, R. H., and Silver, D. (1973): Heparin-induced thrombocytopenia with thrombotic and hemorrhagic manifestations. *Surg. Gynecol. Obstet.*, 136:409.
49. Rosenblum, D., Wessler, S., and Avioli, L. A., (1973): Drug-induced blood dyscrasias. *Arch. Intern. Med.*, 131:750.
50. Salama, A., and Mueller-Eckhardt, C. (1987): Cianidanol and its metabolites bind tightly to red cells and are responsible for the production of auto- and/or drug-dependent antibodies against these cells. *Br. J. Haematol.*, 66:263.
51. Salama, A., and Mueller-Eckhardt, C. (1987): The role of metabolite-specific antibodies in nomifensine dependent immune hemolytic anemia. *N. Engl. J. Med.*, 313:469.
52. Samlowski, W. E., Frame, R. N., and Logue, L. (1987): Flecainide-induced immune neutropenia. Documentation of a hapten-mediated mechanism of cell destruction. *Arch. Intern. Med.*, 147:383.
53. Sandvei, P., Nordhagen, R., Michaelson, T. R., and Wolthuis, K. (1987): Fluorouracil-(5FU) induced acute immune haemolytic anaemia. *Br. J. Haematol.*, 65:357.
54. Schulman, N. R. (1963): Mechanism of blood cell damage by absorption of antigen-antibody complexes. In Immunopathology, IIIrd International Symposium, La Jolla, California; January, 1963, Schwabe, Basel and Stuttgart.
55. Schulman, N. R. (1964): A mechanism of cell destruction in individuals sensitized to foreign antigens and its implications in autoimmunity. *Ann. Intern. Med.*, 60:506.
56. Scott, G. L., Myles, A. B., and Bacon, P. A. (1968): Autoimmune hemolytic anemia and mafenamic acid therapy. *Br. Med. J.*, 3:543.
57. Soff, G. A., and Kain, M. E. (1987): Tocainamide-induced reversible agranulocytosis and anemia. *Arch. Intern. Med.*, 147:598.
58. Spivak, J. L. (1986): The mechanism of action of erythropoietin. *Int. J. Cell Cloning*, 4:139.
59. Stein, J. H., Hamilton, H. E., and Sheets, R. F. (1964): Agranulocytosis caused by chlorpropamide. *Arch. Intern. Med.*, 113:186.
60. Swanson, M. H., Chanmougan, D., and Schwartz, R. S. (1966): Immunohemolytic anemia due to antipenicillin antibodies: Report of a case. *N. Engl. J. Med.*, 274:178.
61. Terizito, M. L., Peters, R. W., and Tanaka, R. R. Autoimmune hemolytic anemia due to levodopa therapy. *J.A.M.A.*, 226:1347.
62. Tullis, J. L. (1958): Prevalence, nature and identification of leukocyte antibodies. *N. Engl. J. Med.*, 258:569.
63. Tullis, J. L. (1961): The role of leukocyte and platelet antibody tests in management of diverse clinical disorders. *Ann. Intern. Med.*, 54:1165.
64. Van Beek, R. J. J., Bieger, R., and den Ottolander, G. J. (1978): Reversible, severe anemia and granulocytopenia caused by procainamide. *Scand. J. Haematol.*, 21:150.
65. Vipan, W. H. (1865): Quinine as a cause of purpura. *Lancet*, 2:57.
66. Weinz, B., Klein, R. L., and Lalezari, P. (1974): Tetracycline-induced immune hemolytic anemia. *Transfusion*, 14:265.
67. Weitzman, S. A., Stossel, T. P. (1978): Drug-induced immunological neutropenia. *Lancet*, 2:1068.
68. White, J. M., Brown, D. L., Hedner, G. W., and Wrolledge, S. M. (1968): Penicillin-induced hemolytic anemia. *Br. Med. J.*, 3:26.
69. Worlledge, S. M., Carstairs, K. C., Dacie, J. V. (1966): Autoimmune haemolytic anemia associated with alpha-methyl dopa therapy. *Lancet*, 2:135.

Clinical Immunotoxicology, edited by
D. S. Newcombe, N. R. Rose, and J. C. Bloom.
Raven Press, Ltd., New York © 1992.

11

Halothane Hepatitis: A Possible Immune-mediated Hepatitis

Jackie L. Martin

*Department of Anesthesiology and Critical Medicine, Johns Hopkins Hospital
Baltimore, MD*

HISTORICAL PERSPECTIVES

Volatile halogenated inhalation anesthetics have been associated with hepatotoxicity since the introduction of chloroform in humans in 1847. Chloroform as well as carbon tetrachloride and trichloroethylene were all abandoned as anesthetic agents because of the often observed intrinsic hepatotoxicity associated with their use. With the introduction of halothane into clinical practice in 1956, this compound quickly gained widespread acceptance and use. Halothane (2-bromo-2-chloro-1,-1,1-trifluoroethane) was the first of the fluorinated alkane anesthetics and represented a major advance in general anesthetics because it was safe, nonflammable, nonexplosive, and well tolerated by patients. However, within 2 years of its introduction, numerous reports of hepatotoxicity and massive and often fatal hepatic necrosis associated with its use appeared in the medical literature (1–5). As a result of continuing reports, a large retrospective analysis was undertaken, "The National Halothane Study," under the auspices of the Committee on Anesthesia of the National Academy of Sciences–National Research Council (6). The purpose of this study was to compare the mortality and the incidence of postoperative hepatic necrosis associated with halothane with that of other general anesthetics (ether, cyclopropane, and balanced anesthesia). The study reviewed 865,515 general anesthetics from 1959 to 1962 at 34 medical institutions, identifying 82 cases of fatal hepatic necrosis. Drug-induced hepatic injury was suggested in nine of these cases, and seven of the nine patients had received halothane. Furthermore, four of the seven patients had received halothane on more than one occasion during the preceding 6 weeks. The study concluded that the mortality associated with the use of halothane compared favorably with that of other general anesthetics in use at the time and estimated the incidence of fatal hepatic necrosis associated with halothane at 1 in

TABLE 1. *Clinical features of halothane hepatitis*

Mild form	Fulminant form
Incidence 1:5	1:6,000 to 1:35,000
Repeat exposure is not necessary	Multiple exposure
Minor liver dysfunction	Fatal liver failure
Mild elevation of alanine aminotransferase, aspartate aminotransferase	High elevation of alanine aminotransferase, aspartate aminotransferase
Focal necrosis	Massive hepatic necrosis
	Jaundice, fever, eosinophilia, LKM, LSP, and other autoantibodies
	Risk factors
	History of allergy or eczema
	Female sex
	Obesity
	Development of organ-specific autoantibody

Provided by L. R. Pohl.

10,000 halothane anesthetics. It was further concluded that "unexplained fever and jaundice in a specific patient following the use of halothane should serve as a warning sign to avoid its subsequent use in that patient" (7). These findings provided much of the impetus over the past 25 years for the many studies on the etiology of halothane-induced hepatotoxicity. Although the exact mechanism of halothane hepatitis remains unknown, hepatitis following halothane anesthesia is now accepted as a distinct clinical entity.

CURRENT PERSPECTIVES

Halothane Hepatotoxicity: Clinical Syndromes

Halothane produces two types of toxicity in susceptible patients (Table 1). The first is a mild postoperative hepatotoxicity seen in 20% to 25% of patients given the drug as a general anesthetic (8–10). The clinical features of the mild toxicity are lethargy, a mild postoperative fever, nausea, vomiting, and mild transient elevations in liver aminotransferase enzymes (alanine aminotransferase, aspartate aminotransferase). This syndrome is usually self-limited and without significant sequelae. In contrast, a fulminant hepatic necrosis (halothane hepatitis) occurs in 1 out of 10,000 to 1 out of 30,000 patients exposed to halothane (7). This clinical syndrome is characterized by markedly elevated serum transaminase values, hepatomegaly, hepatic encephalopathy, jaundice, and often death. Laboratory studies reveal an eosinophilia and significantly elevated alanine aminotransferase, aspartate aminotransferase, bilirubin, alkaline phosphatase, and cholesterol levels (11). The predominant feature observed at histological examination of the liver shows acute hepatitis with centrilobular necrosis (11).

Risk Factors for Halothane Hepatitis

The mortality associated with halothane hepatitis has been reported to range from 40% to 75% (12). A variety of risk factors have been identified that are commonly associated with this clinical syndrome (13) (Table 2). Numerous studies have demonstrated that the risk of halothane hepatitis is greatly increased with use of an increasing number of anesthetics over a short period of time (14–17). There may be several explanations for this finding. Isoniazid, ethanol, and acetone (18–22) induce cytochrome P-450j, which metabolizes halothane to reactive intermediates. Some evidence does exist that enzyme induction may play a role in the liver injury observed in halothane hepatitis patients. A retrospective analysis of 279 patients with normal preoperative serum transaminase levels undergoing brain surgery with halothane anesthesia was undertaken (23). One hundred of the patients had been taking phenobarbital, seven of whom suffered postoperative liver injury with two deaths. Of the 179 patients not taking phenobarbital, there was one case of liver injury and no deaths, suggesting that enzyme induction may play a role in the development of the patients' liver injury.

It has been observed that antipyrine clearance is increased in patients following halothane anesthesia; this suggests that halothane can induce drug metabolism (24). In addition, halothane has been demonstrated to induce its own metabolism in mice (25,26), and it has been suggested that chronic exposure of operating room personnel increases the rate of halothane metabolism among this group (27). With use of an increasing number of anesthetics, greater amounts of metabolites might be generated, leading to liver toxicity. In a study in which the production of a reductive halothane metabolite (2-chloro-1,1,1-trifluoroethane) was measured in children after repeat halothane exposure over short periods of time, there was no observed trend toward increased reductive metabolism (28). In addition, other agents can induce the metabolism of halothane. Phenobarbital has been demonstrated to induce both oxidative and reductive metabolism of halothane, whereas phenytoin has been shown to induce generation of reductive halothane metabolites (29).

Another possibility is that halothane may produce a mild hepatic injury with initial exposure, thus altering the injured liver's response to subsequent halothane exposure. For example, initial halothane exposure may produce areas of decreased

TABLE 2. *Potential risk factors for halothane hepatitis*

Repeat halothane exposure
Genetic predisposition
Female sex
Obesity
Middle age
Liver hypoxia
Enzyme induction

perfusion, resulting in regions of local tissue hypoxia. This could conceivably lead to an increase in toxic reductive intermediates and promote hepatocellular damage. Further exposure to halothane could then lead to hepatocellular death. There currently exists no evidence in humans, however, that hypoxia contributes to halothane hepatitis.

Halothane hepatitis may have a hereditary basis. For example, it has been reported in three pairs of closely related women, a mother and daughter, two sisters, and first cousins (30). Furthermore, it has been shown that lymphocytes from halothane hepatitis patients and some of their relatives are more susceptible to damage by phenytoin electrophilic intermediates than are lymphocytes from healthy controls (31). The low incidence of the disease and the decreasing use of halothane make the study of the genetic effects difficult and emphasize the importance of developing an animal model of this disease.

Several other associations exist for the development of this disease. There is a clear sex difference observed in halothane hepatitis patients. Approximately twice as many females as males develop the disease (17,32–35). The reason for this disparity is unclear at present. Also, the vast majority of cases of halothane hepatitis have occurred in middle-aged adults, with relatively few cases reported in prepubertal children (36,37). The disease is also more common in obese than in nonobese patients (17,32,38).

There is currently no evidence to suggest that the risk of halothane hepatitis is increased in patients with liver disease unrelated to prior halothane exposure. However, since halothane can cause direct hepatotoxicity and other alternatives exist for the provision of general anesthesia, it is prudent to avoid halothane as well as the other related fluorocarbon inhalation anesthetics in patients with preexisting hepatic dysfunction.

Evidence for an Immune Basis of Halothane Hepatitis

Current evidence suggests that halothane hepatitis is caused by a reaction against liver proteins altered by halothane metabolites (17,39–43). This disease has clinical features of an allergic reaction, such as multiple halothane administrations increasing the incidence of hepatitis (14–17), with fever, rash, arthralgias, and peripheral eosinophilia being often observed signs (42). A cell migration assay demonstrated that 8 out of 12 halothane hepatitis patients' sera were sensitized to a liver homogenate subfraction from halothane-treated rabbits (44). Also, antibodies from 9 out of 11 halothane hepatitis patients were shown by indirect immunofluorescence to react with the cell surface of hepatocytes from halothane-treated rabbits. The antibodies rendered the hepatocytes susceptible to antibody-dependent cell-mediated cytotoxicity (45). These antibodies were not present in the sera of patients with other types of liver disease or in patients exposed to halothane without liver injury (46).

Many halothane hepatitis patients have serum antibodies directed against liver, kidney, smooth muscle, thyroid, and nucleic acid tissues (17,43,47). The hallmark

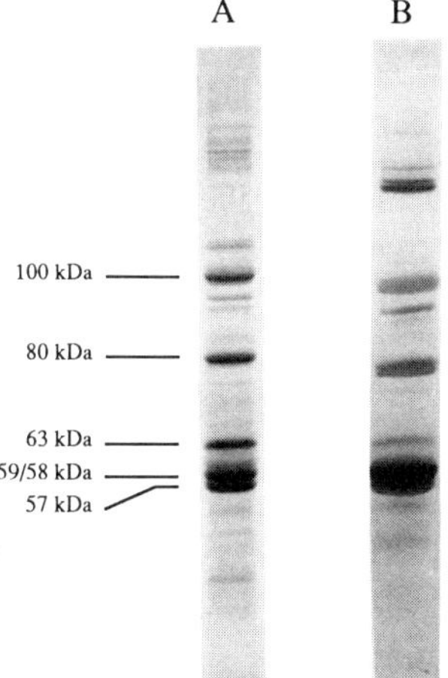

FIG. 1. **A:** Coomassie brilliant blue protein staining of 0.1% deoxycholate extracted liver microsomal neoantigens from halothane-treated rats, after sodium dodecyl sulfate polyacrylamide gel. The 54-kDa protein is not extractable under these conditions. **B:** Immunoblotting with hapten-specific anti-TFA antiserum demonstrates reactivity with each of the extracted proteins.

of the disease, however, is the presence of serum antibodies directed against halothane-induced protein neoantigens covalently modified by the reactive trifluoroacetyl chloride metabolite of halothane (TFA-Cl, TFA-X) (40). These neoantigens are of apparent monomeric molecular mass 100 kDa, 80 kDa, 63 kDa, 59 kDa, 58 kDa, 57 kDa, and 54 kDa (48) (Fig. 1). It has been previously shown that the patients' antibodies bind to epitopes consisting of the trifluoroacetyl (TFA) hapten and novel structural determinants of the carrier proteins (49,50).

The Hapten-Carrier Hypothesis

The immunogens involved in the generation of the halothane-mediated immune response are believed to be the halothane-induced metabolite neoantigens. The TFA groups on the neoantigens are thought to alter the antigenicity of liver cell constituents by serving as hapten (51). A hapten is a small functional group corresponding to a single antibody binding site or antigenic determinant. Immunization with free hapten generally does not elicit a humoral immune response. However, when hapten is covalently bound to a larger carrier protein molecule, immunogenicity may be achieved and an antibody response mounted against the hapten, the carrier protein, and new antigenic determinants may be created by conformational changes as the result of hapten-carrier conjugate binding. Thus, it is hypothesized that in halothane hepatitis, hepatocyte antigenicity is altered by the formation of hapten-carrier conjugates composed of reactive intermediates generated by halothane metabolism and native liver protein.

Laboratory studies seem to support this concept. For example, immunoblotting studies with sera from halothane hepatitis patients demonstrate that the patients' antibody response is not directed solely against the TFA-hapten but against portions of the native proteins as well (52). These results were confirmed by an enzyme-linked immunosorbent assay in which the halothane hepatitis patients' antibody response was tested for reactivity against the TFA group derived from halothane (49).

Halothane Metabolism

Approximately 20% of an administered dose of halothane is metabolized in humans via two primary metabolic pathways, both catalyzed by cytochrome P-450–dependent microsomal enzymes (Fig. 2). The major byproducts of the reductive pathway are inorganic bromide and fluoride and the volatile metabolites 2-chloro-1,1,1-trifluoroethane and 2-chloro-1,1-difluoroethylene (53,54). Oxidative metabolism results in the release of inorganic bromide and chloride and the formation of the TFA-Cl intermediate and trifluoroacetic acid (55–59). The consequence of the formation of reactive intermediates of halothane metabolism is that such metabolites may covalently bind to tissue macromolecules and produce toxicity. The products of both oxidative and reductive metabolism may bind to membrane phospholipids and microsomal proteins, whereas reductive metabolites may also bind to the acyl side chains of phosphatidylcholine and phosphatidylethanolamine (56). Current evidence suggests that it is the oxidative pathway of halothane metabolism that is responsible for the generation of immunogens implicated in the immune response leading to halothane hepatitis (39,60,61). Reductive metabolism has not been found to be involved in recognition of the halothane-induced metabolite neoantigens (61). Halothane metabolism is slow and continues for several days after discontinuation of the anesthetic because of halothane storage, primarily in fat tissues (62).

Identification of the Halothane-Induced Neoantigens

Recently the 100-kDa, 80-kDa, 63-kDa, 59-kDa, 58-kDa, and 57-kDa neoantigens have been purified and characterized (Table 3).

The 100-kDa protein has been identified as endoplasmin, an endoplasmic reticulum glycoprotein. Although the function of this protein is not known, it does bind calcium and may be involved in intracellular transport (63). It is believed to be localized in the lumen of the endoplasmic reticulum. This protein shows extensive homology with several proteins, including ERp99 (64), tumor rejection antigen, heat shock protein 108 (hsp 108), and glucose-regulated protein 94 (grp 94) (65). These proteins all appear to be products of a single gene (48,66).

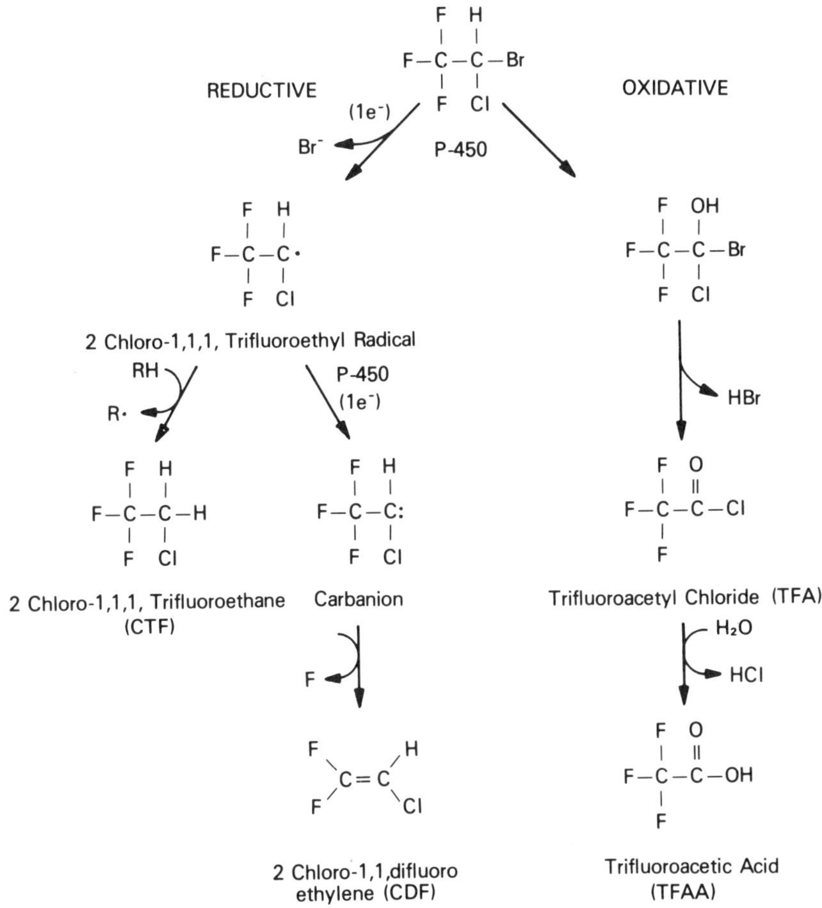

FIG. 2. The major byproducts of reductive and oxidative halothane metabolism are outlined. Both pathways are catalyzed by cytochrome P-450–dependent microsomal enzymes.

The 80-kDa protein shows high homology with ERp72 (48,67,68). ERp72 is a luminal endoplasmic reticulum protein with no known function. It contains three copies of the active site sequences of protein disulfide isomerase (69). In addition, a cDNA clone reported to be human deoxycytosine kinase is 85% homologous with ERp72 (70).

The 63-kDa protein is calreticulin (48,71). It is a calcium-binding protein that may participate in calcium homeostasis and in the maintenance of membrane integrity. This protein is present in the endoplasmic and sarcoplasmic reticulum and shows sequence homology with SLE/SS autoantigen (Ro/SS-A) (72).

TABLE 3. *Identification of the halothane-induced neoantigens*

Neoantigen	Identity	References
100 kDa	Endoplasmin	(48,66)
80 kDa	ERp72	(48,68)
63 kDa	Calreticulin	(48,71)
59 kDa	Carboxylesterase	(48,50,73)
58 kDa	Phosphoinositide	(48,74,75)
	Specific phospholipase C (?)	
57 kDa	Protein disulfide isomerase	(48,76)

The 59-kDa protein is a carboxylesterase enzyme (48,50,73). Carboxylesterases are found loosely associated with the lumen of the endoplasmic reticulum and are high mannose *N*-linked glycoproteins. Although the exact function of carboxylesterase enzymes is not understood, they are known to hydrolyze a variety of endogenous and exogenous substrates. The 59-kDa protein appears to be the most heavily trifluoroacetylated neoantigen (48).

The structure of the purified 58-kDa protein shows high homology to that reported as phosphoinositide-specific phospholipase-C form I (α) (PI-PLC) (48, 74,75), although it has not yet been shown to have this activity. This enzyme generates phosphoinositide-derived messenger molecules for the transmission of extracellular signals across cell membranes, thus functioning as an effective second messenger. This protein shows some homology with protein disulfide isomerase.

Protein disulfide isomerase was identified as the 57-kDa protein (48,76). Protein disulfide isomerase appears to be a multifunctional enzyme found in great abundance in the endoplasmic reticulum of cells active in the synthesis of secretory proteins. This enzyme catalyzes the posttranslational isomerization of disulfide bonds in a variety of protein substrates. It shows high sequence homology to several proteins, including thyroid hormone–binding protein (T_3BP) (77), thioredoxin (78,79), the β-subunit of prolyl-4 hydroxylase (80,81), idothyroxine 5′-monodeiodinase (82), glycosylation site binding protein (83), ERp 72 (67), form 1 of phosphoinositide-specific phospholipase-C (74), and microsomal triglyceride transfer protein complex (84).

The halothane-induced neoantigens belong to a class of proteins collectively known as reticuloplasmins, which also include BiP and RP60 (85,86). These are a family of abundant luminal endoplasmic reticulum proteins that are normally excluded from the cellular secretory pathway. A common characteristic of many reticuloplasmins is the presence of a tetrapeptide sequence KDEL or the related sequence KEEL, at the carboxy terminus, which functions to anchor the proteins within the endoplasmic reticulum. Studies indicate that reticuloplasmin secretion is induced by calcium perturbations and suppressed by the stress response (87).

It appears that the halothane-induced neoantigens represent major cellular proteins involved in a host of cellular functions and most probably represent the immunogens that elicit the patients' observed immune response.

Assays to Detect Sensitized Patients

The diagnosis of halothane hepatitis has always been one of exclusion, wherein other potential causes of liver injury such as hepatitis A, hepatitis B, cytomegalovirus, Epstein-Barr virus, hepatotoxic drugs, hypotension, or hypoxia were systemically ruled out as precipitating causes. One of the important goals of halothane hepatitis research is the development of an assay capable of detecting sensitized patients who may be at risk for developing a hypersensitivity response upon reexposure to halothane as well as detecting patients with the disease. The assays that have been developed measure serum antibodies in halothane hepatitis patients. Two general types of immunochemical assays have been reported for the detection of the patients' antibodies. The first method is immunoblotting. In this procedure, test antigens are microsomal proteins from halothane-treated rats or rabbits that have been separated into constituent polypeptides by sodium dodecyl sulfate polyacrylamide gel electrophoresis and transferred electrophoretically to the surface of nitrocellulose membranes. Using this technique, 42 of 68 (62%) patients with a clinical diagnosis of halothane hepatitis have been found to test positive for the halothane-induced antibodies (61). Although this approach provides important information about the apparent molecular mass of the neoantigens reacting with the patients' antibodies, it is laborious and time-consuming. It also has the potential disadvantage of being inherently less sensitive than other methods because it involves the protein denaturing conditions of dodecylsulfate polyacrylamide gel electrophoresis. This could lead to a decreased level of response if a patient's antibodies were directed against, at least in part, conformational epitopes of the TFA neoantigens (88).

The second immunochemical assay that has been employed for the detection of antibodies in the sera of patients with a clinical diagnosis of halothane hepatitis is based on the more rapid, facile, and potentially more sensitive enzyme-linked immunosorbent assay methodology in which test antigen is applied directly to the wells of a microtiter plate. One reported enzyme-linked immunosorbent assay procedure utilizes microsomes from halothane-treated rabbits as test antigen. Employing this approach, investigators have demonstrated the presence of the antibodies in the sera of 16 of 24 (67%) (89) and 28 of 39 (72%) (90) of the patients with a clinical diagnosis of halothane hepatitis. In another enzyme-linked immunosorbent assay that employs the TFA hapten as test antigen in the form of TFA–rabbit serum albumin, positive responses from patients with a clinical diagnosis of halothane hepatitis ranged from two of six (33%) patients (91) to five of six patients (83%) (92).

Recently the purified proteins from rat liver have been used as test antigen in the enzyme-linked immunosorbent assay. In a study employing three of the purified halothane-induced neoantigens (100 kDa, 80 kDa, and 57 kDa), 79% of a group of 24 halothane hepatitis patients tested positive by this assay (93). Future studies should prove that the best antigens for detection of sensitized patients are those derived from human liver.

CURRENT CONTROVERSIES

Enflurane Hepatitis

Enflurane (2-chloro-1,1,2-trifluoroethyl-difluoromethyl ether) is a stable non-flammable liquid, slightly less volatile than halothane; it was introduced into clinical practice as a general anesthetic agent in 1972. Reports have existed for a number of years concerning enflurane-induced hepatitis (94–96). A review of several of these cases revealed a pattern of hepatocellular damage with striking similarities to halothane-induced hepatic injury (22). In 67% of the cases there was a history of prior exposure to an inhalation anesthetic. Observed clinical signs included fever (79%), eosinophilia (29%), rash (13%), and renal failure (13%). The case fatality rate was found to be 21%. Histological examination of biopsy samples revealed varying degrees of centrilobular necrosis.

Studies in humans reveal that 2% of an administered dose of enflurane undergoes metabolism (97). Enflurane would be expected to yield oxidative reactive intermediates analogous to those of halothane (Fig. 3); thus the potential for cross-sensitization between halothane and enflurane exists. In fact, a recent report supports this concept. Liver microsomes from enflurane-treated rats were shown to react in an immunoblotting assay with antibodies in the serum of halothane hepatitis patients (98). This finding has important clinical implications. First, patients previously sensitized to halothane and subsequently exposed to enflurane could be at risk for the development of a hypersensitivity reaction. Conversely, patients sensitized to enflurane could be at risk upon being exposed to halothane. The existence of enflurane-induced hepatic injury remains the subject of ongoing debate. However, clinical and laboratory evidence strongly favors the existence of this clinical entity.

Isoflurane Hepatitis

Isoflurane (1-chloro-2,2,2-trifluoroethyl difluoromethyl ether) is an isomer of enflurane and was introduced into clinical practice as an inhalation anesthetic in 1980. Approximately 0.2% of an administered dose of isoflurane is metabolized in the body (99). Despite this low level of metabolism compared with halothane (20%) and enflurane (2%), there have been reports of hepatotoxicity, massive hepatic necrosis, and death following isoflurane anesthesia (100,101). In an examination of 45 cases of hepatic dysfunction following isoflurane anesthesia reported to the Food and Drug Administration between 1981 and 1984 by the Anesthetic and Life Support Advisory Committee of the Food and Drug Administration, it was concluded that "current evidence does not demonstrate a causal relationship between exposure to isoflurane and hepatic dysfunction" (102). Five years later this statement still appears to be true. As with enflurane, the potential for the formation of metabolic intermediates analogous to those produced by halothane exists (103). Unlike enflurane, however, reactivity of serum from halothane hepatitis patients with micro-

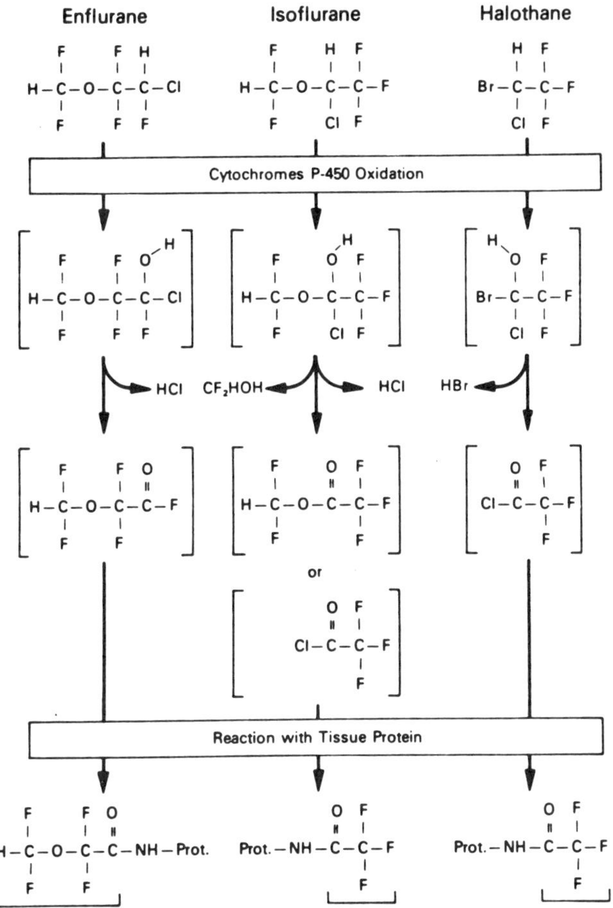

FIG. 3. Metabolic pathways for the possible formation of acylating intermediates from the oxidation of enflurane, isoflurane, and halothane. (Reproduced with permission from Christ, D. D., Satoh, H., Kenna, J. G., and Pohl, L. R. [1988], ref. 103.)

somes from isoflurane-treated rats has not been demonstrated. Although a theoretical molecular basis for isoflurane-induced hepatitis can be shown, at present there is no clinical evidence that this syndrome actually exists.

Halothane Hepatitis in Children

Barton reported the first case of halothane hepatitis in a child in 1959 (104). Since that time there have been numerous reports of hepatotoxicity and massive hepatic necrosis following halothane anesthesia in children (105–109). Two retrospective studies have examined the incidence of halothane-associated hepatotoxicity in children. The first study explored 165,400 halothane anesthetics in a children's hospital in the United Kingdom over the 23-year period from 1957 to 1979 and determined the incidence of halothane hepatitis in children to be 1 in 82,000 (36). The second study examined 200,311 cases conducted under halothane anesthesia between 1958 and 1983 in a United States children's hospital, finding one case, for an incidence of approximately 1 in 200,000 (37). In 1987, data were reported describing halothane hepatitis in seven children aged 11 months to 15 years, all of whom had received multiple halothane anesthetics (110). The diagnosis in this study was confirmed in all but one child by the presence of serum antibodies to halothane-altered hepatocyte antigens. There was one fatality in this group, and other causes of liver diseases were excluded by the investigators. This unequivocal report confirmed the finding that although it is much rarer than in adults, the clinical syndrome of halothane hepatitis does exist in prepubertal children. The reason for the difference in incidence of halothane hepatitis observed between adults and children is not clear at present because halothane has been found to be metabolized to a similar degree in both adults and children (111) and because immune competence is known to exist from birth (112).

Hydrochlorofluorocarbons

Chlorofluorocarbons (CFCs) were first identified as the compounds responsible for stratospheric ozone depletion in 1985 (113). CFC molecules emitted in the lower atmosphere may take up to seven years to diffuse upward into the stratosphere, where intense ultraviolet radiation liberates chlorine atoms that catalyze reactions that destroy ozone molecules. Once in place, these compounds may exist for 100 years or more. The depletion of stratospheric ozone may have adverse health effects worldwide, such as increases in the incidence of skin cancer and cataract formation. As a result, recommendations put forth by The Montreal Protocol on Substances That Deplete the Ozone Layer have been adopted by the Environmental Protection Agency in the United States and by several other countries (114). In short, these recommendations call for the total elimination of CFCs by the year 2000.

CFCs are widely employed throughout industry and have many uses, including as industrial refrigerants, foam blowing agents in the manufacture of plastics, aerosol propellants, food preservatives, and cleaning and sterilizing agents. The major source of CFC environmental contamination is the venting of automobile and truck air conditioning units into the atmosphere. CFCs are extremely stable, nontoxic, and nonflammable. The addition of hydrogen atoms into CFC molecules allows degradation of these compounds in the lower atmosphere with little effect on stratospheric ozone. 2,2-Dichloro-1,1,1-trifluoroethane (hydrochlorofluorocarbon-123) (HCFC-123) is a compound currently under investigation as a potential CFC replacement. At present a plant is being constructed by DuPont Chemical Company in Maitland, Ontario, Canada for the production of this compound in the fall of 1990. Because of the striking structural similarity between HCFC-123 and halothane (2-

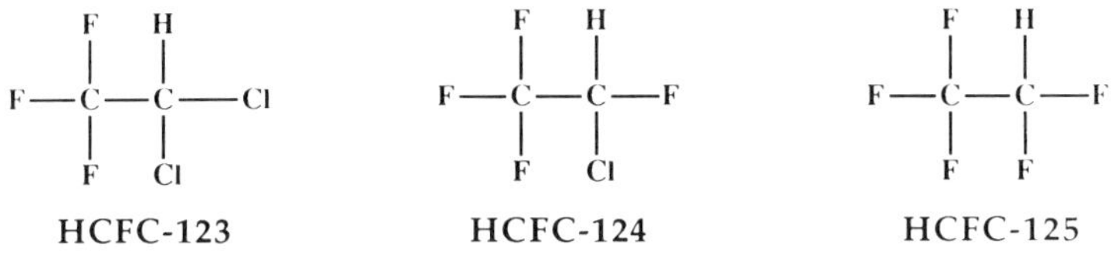

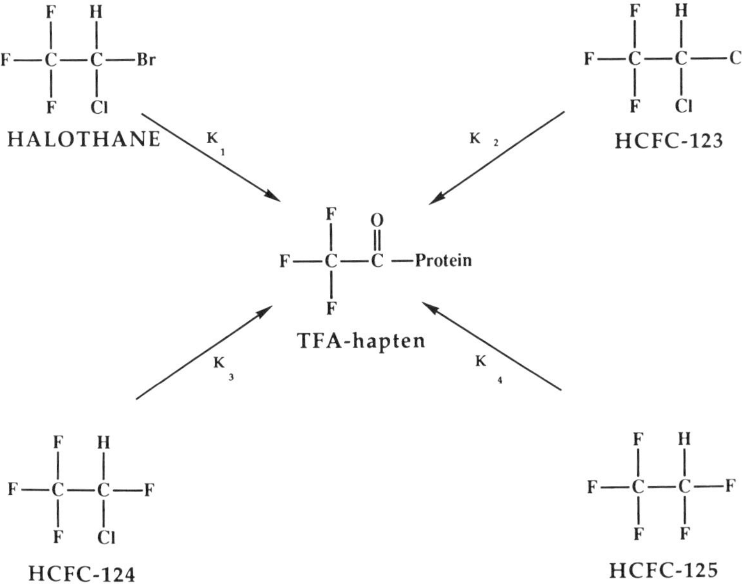

FIG. 4. The structures of halothane and the potential CFC replacements HCFC-123, HCFC-124, and HCFC-125.

bromo-2-chloro-1,1,1-trifluoroethane) (Fig. 4) and the problem of halothane hepatotoxicity, the metabolism of HCFC-123 was recently investigated.

In a recent report, rat liver microsomes from animals exposed to air, 1% halothane, or 1% or 0.5% HCFC-123 for 2 hours were probed with hapten-specific anti-TFA serum. Immunoblotting demonstrated that HCFC-123 and halothane are metabolized to trifluoroacetylated adducts with identical patterns of TFA labeling (115). These results are significant in light of what is known about halothane hepatitis. As noted previously, the hepatitis has all the signs of a drug-induced allergic or hypersensitivity response. The finding that HCFC-123 also leads to the formation of TFA-labeled proteins is not surprising, since it would be expected to undergo a similar cytochrome P-450 catalyzed oxidative dehydrohalogenation to TFA-Cl (Fig. 5). Since the level of TFA labeling of HCFC-123 was similar to that of halothane, this raises the possibility that susceptible individuals repeatedly exposed to this

FIG. 5. Halothane and the potential CFC replacements HCFC-123, HCFC-124, and HCFC-125 would all be expected to generate an identical reactive intermediate, although at different rates.

agent might become sensitized and develop hepatitis. It is also possible that individuals sensitized to HCFC-123 without hepatic injury might be at increased risk for hepatic damage following anesthesia with halothane or enflurane. It is unlikely that toxicity testing in animals will uncover hepatitis, since the drug-induced allergic response would be expected to be as rare in animals as in humans, unless by chance a genetically predisposed strain was used.

FUTURE PERSPECTIVES

Animal Model of Halothane Hepatitis

At the present time it is impossible to conclude whether the immune response produces the fulminant hepatotoxicity associated with halothane or occurs as a result of the liver damage. In order to convincingly demonstrate that halothane hepatitis has an immune basis, an animal model must be developed. Numerous attempts have been made over the past few years to develop an animal model of this disease. The first of these involved pretreatment of rats with aroclor 1254 (a combination of polychlorinated biphenyls) before halothane administration (116). Other attempts have included pretreatment of rats with triidothyronine without hypoxia or barbiturate pretreatment (117,118) and studies on rats treated with and without phenobarbital and exposed to hypoxic conditions (119). Guinea pig models have also been studied under normal and low oxygen tensions, and unlike the rat models, most of these animals develop hepatotoxicity without phenobarbital and/or hypoxia pretreatment (120,121). The pathology seen in these animals closely resembles the nonlethal form of halothane hepatitis seen in humans (122). More recently, pretreatment of rats with isoniazid under normoxic conditions has produced hepatic lesions in all exposed animals, suggesting that hepatic injury may be produced during enhanced oxidative metabolism of halothane (18). It has also been reported that the oxidative metabolism of halothane is increased in obese rats (123). This finding is significant because obesity has been implicated as a contributing factor in hepatotoxicity following halothane administration in humans (124). Furthermore, studies on obese animals (125) and patients (126–128) demonstrate enhanced serum metabolite concentrations compared with normal weight controls following the administration of inhalation agents. In a more recent attempt to develop an animal model of halothane hepatitis, rabbits were immunized with hepatocytes isolated from halothane-exposed litter mates, resulting in the formation of antibodies to native and halothane-altered liver proteins (129). Subsequent exposure of the immunized rabbits to halothane resulted in the disappearance of the antibodies. Although both rabbit and human lymphocytes were directly cytotoxic *in vitro* to the antibody-coated hepatocytes, no evidence of liver damage was seen. Other investigators have demonstrated a humoral immune response in rabbits directed against the TFA hapten of TFA-rabbit serum albumin after multiple halothane exposures under high oxygen tension (130,131).

Although hepatic necrosis has been observed in these animals, these are models of acute toxicity and do not parallel the fulminant hepatotoxicity observed in humans (132–134). Clearly, much work remains to be done in the development of an animal model of halothane hepatitis.

SUMMARY

Considerable clinical and experimental evidence suggests that halothane hepatitis is an immune-mediated toxicity (135,136). The often observed clinical features of halothane hepatitis include arthralgias, eosinophilia, fever, rash, and prior exposure to the anesthetic. These are all characteristics commonly associated with drug hypersensitivity reactions. Most important, the sera of many patients with a clinical diagnosis of halothane hepatitis have been found to contain specific antibodies that react with halothane-induced liver antigens (neoantigens), whereas the sera of patients with other forms of hepatitis do not contain antibodies of this specificity. It has recently been shown that the neoantigens are formed by the covalent interaction of the reactive oxidative TFA halide metabolite (CF_3COX, TFA-X) of halothane (49,50), with at least seven distinct classes of liver microsomal proteins (100 kDa, 80 kDa, 63 kDa, 59 kDa, 58 kDa, 57 kDa, and 54 kDa). These findings suggest that the TFA neoantigens represent the immunogens that have elicited the observed antibody responses and therefore may play an immunopathological role in the development of the liver injury associated with halothane hepatitis.

The degree of metabolism of halothane, enflurane, and isoflurane is thought to be related to their potential for causing hepatic injury. Both enflurane and isoflurane, although metabolized in the human body much less than halothane, have been associated with postoperative hepatotoxicity. There appears to be a distinct clinical entity of enflurane hepatitis, although no such syndrome is thought to exist for isoflurane. It is generally agreed that any patient exhibiting jaundice, fever, or malaise following halothane should not receive a repeat administration. In addition, because of the hepatotoxicity associated with halothane, it should not be used in adults unless a clear benefit can be derived. The record of halothane over the past 35 years warrants its continued use in children despite the very rare syndrome of halothane hepatitis in children.

A clear etiology of halothane hepatitis must await the development of an animal model of this disease that mirrors the clinical condition observed in humans. This should enable investigators to answer the question of whether the patient's antibodies incite the liver injury or occur as a consequence of the liver damage. An understanding of the contribution of humoral and cell-mediated immune responses may also be facilitated by this model.

The study of the mechanism of halothane hepatitis may serve as a useful model for the study of drug-induced hypersensitivity reactions and may provide a rational basis for the design of safer anesthetic agents as well as nonanesthetic drugs.

REFERENCES

1. Virtue, R. W., and Payne, K. W. (1958): Postoperative death after fluothane. *Anesthesiology*, 19:562–563.
2. Bunker, J. P., and Blumenfeld, C. M. (1963): Liver necrosis after halothane anesthesia, cause or coincidence? *N. Engl. J. Med.*, 268:531–534.
3. Brody, G. L., and Sweet, R. B. (1963): Halothane anesthesia as a possible cause of massive hepatic necrosis. *Anesthesiology*, 24:29–37.
4. Gall, E. A. (1968): Report of the pathology panel. National halothane study. *Anesthesiology*, 29:233–248.
5. Peters, R. L., Edmondson, H. A., Reynolds, T. B., Meister, J. C., and Curphey, T. J. (1969): Hepatic necrosis associated with halothane anesthesia. *Am. J. Med.*, 47:748–764.
6. Summary of the National Halothane Study (1966): *J.A.M.A.*, 197:157–158.
7. Bunker, J. P., Forrest, W. H., Mosteller, F., and Vandam, L. D. (eds.) (1969): The National Halothane Study, National Institutes of Health, National Institute of General Medical Sciences, Bethesda, Maryland.
8. Wright, R., Eade, O. E., Chilsom, M., Hawksley, M., Lloyd, B., Moles, T. M., Edwards, J. C., and Gardner, J. C. (1975): Controlled prospective study of the effect on liver function of multiple exposure to halothane. *Lancet*, 1:817.
9. Trowell, J., Peto, R., and Smith, A. C. (1975): Controlled trial of repeated halothane anesthetics in patients with carcinoma of the uterine cervix treated with radium. *Lancet*, 1:821.
10. Thompson, D. S., and Friday, C. D. (1978): Changes in liver enzyme values after halothane and enflurane for surgical anesthesia. *South. Med. J.*, 71:779–782.
11. Moult, P. J., and Sherlock, S. (1975): Halothane-related hepatitis. A clinical study of twenty-six cases. *Q. J. Med. (N. S.)*, 173:99–114.
12. Touloukian, J., and Kaplowitz, N. (1981): Halothane induced hepatic disease. *Semin. Liver Dis.* I:134–142.
13. Cousins, M. J., Plummer, J. L., and Hall, P. M. (1989): Risk factors for halothane hepatitis. *Aust. N.Z. J. Surg.*, 59:5–14.
14. Carey, R. M. T., and Van Dyke, R. A. (1972): Halothane hepatitis: A critical review. *Anesth. Analg.*, 51:135–160.
15. Klaiskin, G., and Smith, D. P. (1975): Halothane-induced hepatitis. In Drugs and the Liver, edited by W. Gerok and K. Sickinger, pp. 289–296. Schattauer-Verlag, New York.
16. Bottiger, L. E., Dalen, E., and Haller, B. (1976): Halothane induced liver damage: An analysis of the material reported to the Swedish Adverse Drug Reaction Committee 1966–1973. *Acta Anesthesiol. Scand.*, 20:40–46.
17. Walton, B., Simpson, B. R., Strunin, L., Doniach, D., Perrin, J., and Appleyard, A. J. (1976): Unexplained hepatitis following halothane. *Br. Med. J.*, 1:1171–1176.
18. Rice, S. A., Maze, M., Smith, C. M., Koesk, J. C., and Mazze, R. I. (1987): Halothane hepatotoxicity in Fischer 344 rats pretreated with isoniazid. *Toxicol. Appl. Pharmacol.*, 87:411–419.
19. Takagi, T., Ishii, H., and Takahashi, H. (1983): Potentiation of halothane hepatotoxicity by chronic ethanol administration in rat: An animal model of halothane hepatitis. *Pharmacol. Biochem. Behav.*, 28:461–465.
20. Ryan, D. E., Koop, D. R., Thomas, P. E., Coon, M. J., and Levin, W. (1966): Evidence that isoniazid and ethanol induce the same microsomal cytochrome P-450 in rat liver, an isozyme analogous to rabbit liver cytochrome P-450 isozyme 3a. *Arch. Biochem. Biophys.*, 246:633–644.
21. Thomas, P. E., Bandiera, S., Maines, S. L., Ryan, D. E., and Levin, W. (1987): Regulation of cytochrome P-450j, a high affinity N-nitrosodimethylamine demethylase, in rat hepatic microsomes. *Biochemistry*, 26:2280–2290.
22. Gruenke, L. D., Konopka, K., Koop, D. R., and Waskell, L. A. (1988): Characterization of halothane oxidation by hepatic microsomes and purified cytochrome P-450 using a gas chromatographic mass spectrometric assay. *J. Pharmacol. Exp. Ther.*, 246:454–459.
23. Nomura, F., Hatano, H., Ohnishi, K., Akikusa, B., and Okuda, K. (1986): Effects of anticonvulsant drugs on halothane-induced liver injury in human subjects and experimental animals. *Hepatology*, 6:952–956.
24. Nimmo, W. S., Thompson, P. G., and Prescott, L. F. (1981): Microsomal enzyme induction after halothane anesthesia. *Br. J. Clin. Pharmacol.*, 12:433–434.
25. Cohen, E. N., and Hood, N. (1969): Application of low-temperature autoradiography to studies of

the uptake and metabolism of volatile anesthetics in the mouse. III. *Halothane Anesthesiol.*, 31:553–559.

26. Cohen, E. N. (1971): Metabolism of the volatile anesthetics. *Anesthesiology*, 85:193–202.
27. Cascorbi, H. F., Vessel, E. S., Blake, D. A., and Helrich, M. (1971): Halothane biotransformation in man. *Ann. N.Y. Acad. Sci.*, 179:244–247.
28. Plummer, J. L., Steven, I. M., and Cousins, M. J. (1987): Metabolism of halothane in children having repeat anesthetics. *Anesth. Intensive Care*, 15:136–140.
29. Stenger, R. J., Johnson, E. A., and Rosenthal, W. S. (1972): Effects of phenobarbital pretreatment on the response of rat liver to halothane administration. *Proc. Soc. Exp. Biol. Med.*, 140:1319–1323.
30. Hoft, R. H., Bunker, J. P., Goodman, H. I., and Gregory, P. B. (1981): Halothane hepatitis in three pairs of closely related women. *N. Engl. J. Med.*, 304:1023–1024.
31. Farrell, G., Prendergast, D., and Murray, M. (1985): Halothane hepatitis. Detection of a constitutional susceptibility factor. *N. Engl. J. Med.*, 313:1310–1314.
32. Carney, F. M. T., and Van Dyke, R. A. (1972): Halothane hepatitis: A critical review. *Anesth. Analg.*, 51:135–160.
33. Inman, W. H. W., and Mushin, W. W. (1984): Jaundice after repeated exposure to halothane: An analysis of reports to the Committee on Safety of Medicines. *Br. Med. J.*, 1:5–10.
34. Klaiskin, G., and Smith, D. P. (1975): Halothane-induced hepatitis. In *Drugs and the Liver*, edited by W. Gerok and K. Sickinger, pp. 289–296. Schattauer-Verlag, New York.
35. Bottiger, L. E., Dalen, E., and Hallen, B. (1976): Halothane-induced liver damage: An analysis of the material reported to the Swedish Adverse Drug Reaction Committee, 1966–1973. *Acta Anaesthesiol. Scand.*, 20:40–46.
36. Wark, H. J. (1983): Postoperative jaundice in children. *Anesthesia*, 38:237–242.
37. Warner, L. O., Beach, T. J., Garvin, J. P., and Warner, E. J. (1984): Halothane and children: The first quarter century. *Anesth. Analg.*, 63:838–840.
38. Peters, R. L., Edmonson, H. A., Reynolds, T. B., Meister, J. C., and Curphey, T. J. (1969): Hepatic necrosis associated with halothane anesthesia. *Am. J. Med.*, 47:748–764.
39. Neuberger, J., Mieli-Vergani, G., Tredger, J. M., Davis, M., and Williams, R. (1981): Oxidative metabolism of halothane in the production of altered hepatocyte antigens in acute halothane-induced hepatic necrosis. *Gut*, 22:669–672.
40. Satoh, H., Fukuda, Y., Anderson, D. K., Ferrans, V. J., Gillette, J. R., and Pohl, L. R. (1985): Immunological studies on the mechanism of halothane-induced hepatotoxicity: Immunohistochemical evidence of trifluoroacetylated hepatotocytes. *J. Pharmacol. Exp. Ther.*, 223:857–862.
41. Inman, W. H. W., and Mushin, W. W. (1978): Jaundice after repeated exposure to halothane: A further analysis of reports to the committee on the safety of medicine. *Br. Med. J.*, 2:455–456.
42. Dienstg, J. L. (1980): Halothane hepatitis. Allergy or idiosyncrasy? *N. Engl. J. Med.*, 303:102–104.
43. Moult, P. J. A., and Sherlock, S. (1975): Halothane related hepatitis. A clinical study of 26 cases. *Q. J. Med.*, 44:99–114.
44. Vergani, D., Tsantoulas, D., Eddleston, A. L. W. F., Davis, M., and Williams, R. (1978): Sensitization to halothane-altered liver components in severe hepatic necrosis after halothane anesthesia. *Lancet*, 2:801–803.
45. Vergani, D., Mieli-Vergani, G., Alberti, A., Neuberger, J., Eddleston, A. L. W. F., Davis, M., and Williams, R. (1980): Antibodies to the surface of halothane-altered rabbit hepatocytes in patients with severe halothane-associated hepatitis. *N. Engl. J. Med.*, 303:66–71.
46. Neuberger, J., Gimson, A. E. S., Davis, M., and Williams, R. (1983): Specific serological markers in the diagnosis of fulminant hepatic failure associated with halothane anesthesia. *Br. J. Anaesth.*, 55:15–19.
47. Rodriguez, M., Paronetto, F., Schaffner, F., and Popper, H. (1969): Antimitochondrial antibodies in jaundice following drug administration. *J.A.M.A.*, 208:148–150.
48. Pohl, L. R., Thomassen, D., Pumford, N. R., Butler, L. E., Satoh, H., Ferrans, V. J., Perrone, A., Martin, B. M., and Martin, J. L. (1991): Hapten carrier conjugates associated with halothane hepatitis. *Adv. Exp. Med. Biol.*, 283.
49. Kenna, J. G., Satoh, H., Christ, D. D., and Pohl, L. R. (1988): Metabolic basis for a drug hypersensitivity: Antibodies in sera from patients with halothane hepatitis recognize liver neoantigens that contain the trifluoroacetyl group derived from halothane. *J. Pharmacol. Exp. Ther.*, 245:1103–1109.
50. Satoh, H., Martin, B. M., Schulick, A. H., Christ, D. D., Kenna, J. G., and Pohl, L. R. (1989):

Human anti-endoplasmic reticulum antibodies in sera of halothane hepatitis patients are directed against a trifluoroacetylated carboxylesterase. *Proc. Natl. Acad. Sci. U.S.A.*, 86:322–326.

51. Pohl, L. R., Kenna, J. G., Satoh, H., Christ, D. D., and Martin, J. L. (1989): Neoantigens associated with halothane hepatitis. *Drug Metab. Rev.*, 20:203–217.

52. Kenna, J. G., Neuberger, J., and Williams, R. (1987): Identification by immunoblotting of three halothane-induced liver microsomal polypeptide antigens recognized by antibodies in sera from patients with halothane-associated hepatitis. *J. Pharmacol. Exp. Ther.*, 242:733–740.

53. Mukai, S., Morio, M., Fujii, K., and Hanak, C. (1977): Volatile metabolites of halothane in the rabbit. *Anesthesiology*, 47:248–251.

54. Sharp, J. H., Trudell, J. R., and Cohen, E. N. (1979): Volatile metabolites and decomposition products of halothane in man. *Anesthesiology*, 50:2–8.

55. Gandolfi, A. J., White, R. D., Sipes, I. G., and Pohl, L. R. (1980): Bioactivation and covalent binding of halothane *in vitro*: Studies with (^{3}H) and (^{14}C)-halothane. *J. Pharmacol. Exp. Ther.*, 214:721.

56. Cohen, E. N., Trudell, J. R., Edmunds, H. D., and Watson, D. (1975): Urinary metabolites of halothane in man. *Anesthesiology*, 43:392–401.

57. Karashima D., Hirokata, Y., Shigematsu, A., and Furukawa, T. (1977): The *in-vivo* metabolism of halothane (2-bromo-2-chloro-1,1,1-trifluoroethane) by hepatic microsomal cytochrome P-450. *J. Pharmacol. Exp. Ther.*, 203:409.

58. McCarty, L. P., Malek, R. S., and Larsen, E. R. (1979): The effects of deuteration on the metabolism of halogenated anesthetics in the rat. *Anesthesiology*, 51:106.

59. Sipes, I. G., Gandolfi, A. J., Pohl, L. R., Krishna, G., and Brown, B. R. (1980): Comparison of the biotransformation and hepatotoxicity of halothane and deutrated halothane. *J. Pharmacol. Exp. Ther.*, 214:716.

60. Satoh, H., Gillette, J. R., Davies, H. W., Schulick, R. D., and Pohl, L. R. (1985): Immunochemical evidence of trifluoroacetylated cytochrome P-450 in liver of halothane treated rats. *Mol. Pharmacol.*, 28:468–474.

61. Kenna, J. G., Satoh, H., Christ, D. D., and Pohl, L. R.: Metabolic basis for a drug hypersensitivity: Antibodies in sera from patients with halothane hepatitis recognize liver neoantigens that contain the trifluoroacetyl group derived from halothane. *J. Pharmacol. Exp. Ther.*, 245:1103–1109.

62. Cousins, M. J. (1979): Halothane and the liver: "Firm ground at last?" *Anaesth. Intensive Care*, 7:5–8.

63. Welch, W. J., Garrels, J. I., Thomas, G. P., Lin, J. J. C., and Feramisco, J. R. (1983): Biochemical characterization of the mammalian stress proteins and identification of two stress proteins as glucose and Ca^{2+}-ionophore-regulated proteins. *J. Biol. Chem.*, 258:7102–7111.

64. Lee, A. S., Bell, J., and Ting, J. (1984): Biochemical characterization of the 94 and 78 kilodalton glucose regulated protein in hamster fibroblasts. *J. Biol. Chem.*, 260:3050–3057.

65. Koch, G. L. E., Macer, D. R. G., and Smith, M. J. (1987): Visualization of the intact endoplasmic reticulum by immunofluoresence with antibodies to the major endoplasmic reticulum glycoprotein, endoplasmin. *J. Cell Sci.*, 87:535–542.

66. Thomassen, D., Martin, B. M., Martin, J. L., Pumford, N. R., and Pohl, L. R. (1991): Characterization of a halothane induced trifluoroacetylated 100 kDa neoantigen that is related to a glucose regulated protein. *FASEB J.* 4:A599, 1990.

67. Mazzarella, R. A., Srinivasan, M., Hougejorden, S. M., and Green, M. (1990): ERp72, an abundant luminal endoplasmic reticulum protein contains three copies of the active site sequences of protein disulfide isomerase. *J. Biol. Chem.*, 265:1094–1101.

68. Pumford, N. R., Martin, B. M., Thomassen, D., Martin, J. L., and Pohl, L. R. (1990): Purification and partial characterization of a trifluoroacetylated (TFA) 80 kDa microsomal protein associated with halothane hepatotoxicity. *FASEB J.*, 4:A2101, AB# 2364.

69. Mazzarella, R. A., Srinivasan, M., Haugejorden, S. M., and Green, M. (1990): ERp72, an abundant luminal endoplasmic reticulum protein, contains three copies of the active site sequences of the protein disulfide isomerase. *J. Biol. Chem.*, 265:1094–1101.

70. Huang, S. H., Tomich, J. M., Wu, H., Jong, A., and Holenberg, J. (1989): Human deoxycytosine kinase. *J. Biol. Chem.*, 264:14762–14768.

71. Butler, L. E., Martin, J. L., Thomassen, D., Martin, B. M., and Pohl, L. R. (1990): Identification of calregulin as a neoantigen in halothane hepatitis. *FASEB J.*, 4:A2101, AB# 2362.

72. McCauliffe, D. P., Lux, F. A., Lieu, T. S, Sanz, I., Hanke, J., Newkirk, M. M., Bachinski,

L. L., Itoh, Y., Sicilaino, M. J., Reichlin, M., Sontheimer, R. D., and Capra, J. D. (1990): Molecular cloning, and chromosome 19 localization of a human Ro/SS-A autoantigen. *J. Clin. Invest.*, 85:1379–1391.

73. Long, R. M., Satoh, H., Martin, B. M., Kimura, S., Gonzalez, F., and Pohl, L. R. (1988): Rat liver carboxylesterase: cDNA cloning, sequencing and evidence for a multigene family. *BBRC*, 156:866–873.

74. Bennett, C. F., Balcarek, J. M., Varrichio, A., and Crooke, S. T. (1988): Molecular cloning and complete amino-acid sequence of form-I phosphoinositide-specific phospholipase C. *Nature*, 324:268–270.

75. Martin, J. L., Martin, B. M., Butler, L. E., Pumford, N. R., Thomassen, D., Gonzaga, H., Beaven, M. A., and Pohl, L. R. (1990): Trifluoroacetylated phosphoinositide specific phospholipase-C (PI-PLC) is a halothane induced neoantigen. *FASEB J.*, 4:2101, AB# 2363.

76. Martin, J. L., Kenna, J. G., Martin, B., and Pohl, L. R. (1989): Trifluoroacetylated protein disulfide isomerase is a halothane induced neoantigen. *Toxicologist*, 9:5.

77. Yamauchi, K., Yamamoto, T., Hayuashi, H., Koya, S., Taikawa, H., Toyoshima, K., and Horiuchi, R. (1987): Sequence of membrane associated thyroid hormone binding protein from bovine liver: Its identity with protein disulfide isomerase. *BBRC*, 146:1485–1492.

78. Edman, J. C., Ellis, L., Blancher, R. W., Roth, R. A., and Rutter, W. J. (1985): Sequence of protein disulfide isomerase and its implications of its relationship to thioredoxin. *Nature*, 317:269–272.

79. Freedman, R. B., Hawkins, H. C., Murant, S. J., and Reid, L. (1988): Protein disulfide isomerase: A homologue of thioredoxin implicated in the biosynthesis of secretory proteins. *Biochem. Soc. Trans.*, 16:96–99.

80. Koivu, J., Myllyla, R., Helaakoski, T., Pihlajaniemi, T., Tassanen, K., and Kivirikko, K. I. (1987): A single polypeptide acts both as the B subunit of prolyl 4-hydroxylase and as a protein disulfide-isomerase. *J. Biol. Chem.*, 262:6447–6449.

81. Pihlajaniema, T., Helaakoski, T., Tasanen, K., Myllyla, R., Huhtala, M. L., Koivu, J., and Kivirikko, K. I. (1987): Molecular cloning of the B-subunit of human prolyl 4-hydroxylase. This subunit and protein disulfide isomerase are products of the same gene. *EMBO J.*, 6:643–649.

82. Boado, R. J., Campbell, D. A., and Chopra, I. J. (1988): Nucleotide sequence of rat liver iodothyroxine 5'-monodeiodinase (5'MD): Its identity with the protein disulfide isomerase. *BBRC*, 155:1297–1304.

83. Gettha-Habib, G., Novia, R., Kaplan, H. A., and Lennarz, W. J. (1988): Glycosylation site binding protein, a component of oligosaccharyl transferase, is highly similar to three of the 57 kd luminal proteins of the ER. *Cell*, 54:1053–1060.

84. Wetterau, J. R., Combs, K. A., Spinner, S. N., and Joiner, B. J. (1990): Protein disulfide isomerase is a component of the microsomal triglyceride transfer protein complex. *J. Biol. Chem.*, 265:9800–9807.

85. Muno, S., and Pelham, H. R. B. (1986): An HSP 70 like-protein in the ER: Identity with the 78 kd glucose regulated protein and immunoglobin light chain binding protein. *Cell*, 46:291–300.

86. Bole, D. G., Hendershot, L. M., and Kemey, J. R. (1986): Post-transnational association of immunoglobin heavy chain binding protein with nascent heavy chains in non-secretory hybridomas. *J. Cell Biol.*, 102:1558–1566.

87. Booth, C., and Koch, G. L. E. (1989): Perturbation of cellular calcium induces secretion of luminal ER proteins. *Cell*, 59:729–732.

88. Waxman, D. J., Lapenson, D. P., Krishman, M., Bernard, O., Kreibich, G., and Alverez, F. (1988): Antibodies to liver/kidney microsome in chronic active hepatitis recognize cytochrome P-450. *Gastroenterology*, 95:1326–1331.

89. Kenna, J. G., Neuberger, J., and Williams, R. (1984): An enzyme-linked immunosorbent assay for detection of antibodies against halothane-altered hepatocyte antigens. *J. Immunol. Methods*, 75:3–14.

90. Kenna, J. G., Neuberger, J., and Williams, R. (1987): Specific antibodies to halothane-induced liver antigens in halothane-associated hepatitis. *Br. J. Anaesth.*, 59:1286–1290.

91. Satoh, H., Gillette, J. R., Takemura, T., Ferrans, V. J., Jelenich, S. E., Kenna, J. G., Neuberger, J., and Pohl, L. R. (1988): Investigation of the immunological basis of halothane-induced hepatotoxicity. In Biological Reactive Intermediates III, edited by J. J. Kocsis, D. J. Jollow, C. M. Witmer, J. O. Nelson, and R. Snyder, pp. 657–673. Plenum, New York.

92. Hubbard, A. K., Roth, T. P., Gandolfi, A. J., Brown, B. R., Webster, N. R., and Nunn, J. F.

(1988): Halothane hepatitis patients generate an antibody response toward a covalently bound metabolite of halothane. *Anesthesiology*, 68:791–796.

93. Martin, J. L., Kenna, J. G., and Pohl, L. R. (1990): Antibody for the detection of patients sensitized to halothane. *Anesth. Analg.*, 70:154–159.

94. Lewis, J. H., Zimmerman, H. J., Ishak, K. G., and Mullick, F. G. (1983): Enflurane hepatotoxicity. A clinicopathological study of 24 cases. *Ann. Intern. Med.*, 98:984–992.

95. van der Reis, L., Askin, S. J., Frecker, G. N., and Fitzgerald, W. J. (1974): Hepatic necrosis after enflurane anesthesia. *J.A.M.A.*, 227:76.

96. Ona, F. J., Patanella, H., and Ayub, A. (1980): Hepatitis associated with enflurane anesthesia. *Anesth. Analg.*, 59:146–149.

97. Chase, R. E., Holaday, D. A., Fiserova-Bergerova, V., Saidman, L. J., and Mack, F. E. (1971): The biotransformation of ethrane in man. *Anesthesiology*, 35:262–267.

98. Christ, D. D., Kenna, J. G., Kammerer, W., Satoh, H., and Pohl, L. R. (1988): Enflurane metabolism produces covalently-bound liver adducts recognized by antibodies from patients with halothane hepatitis. *Anesthesiology*, 69:833–838.

99. Holaday, D. A., Fiserova-Bergerova, V., Latto, I. P., and Zumbiel, M. A. (1975): Resistance of isoflurane to biotransformation in man. *Anesthesiology*, 43:325–332.

100. Gregorie, S., and Smiley, R. K. (1986): Acute hepatitis in a patient with mild factor IX deficiency after anesthesia with isoflurane. *Can. Med. Assoc. J.*, 135:645–646.

101. Carrigan, T. W., and Straughen, W. J. (1987): A report of hepatic necrosis and death following isoflurane anesthesia. *Anesthesiology*, 67:581–583.

102. Stoelting, R. K., Blitt, C. D., Cohen, P. J., and Merin, R. G. (1987): Hepatic dysfunction after isoflurane anesthesia. *Anesth. Analg.*, 66:147–153.

103. Christ, D. D., Satoh, H., Kenna, J. G., and Pohl, L. R. (1988): Potential metabolic basis for enflurane hepatitis and the apparent cross sensitization between enflurane and halothane. *Drug Metab. Dispos.*, 16:135–140.

104. Barton, J. D. M. (1980). Jaundice and halothane, *Lancet*, 1:1087.

105. Smith, R. M. (1980): Anesthesia for Infants and Children, 4th ed. C. V. Mosby, St. Louis.

106. Psacharopoulos, H. S., Mowat, A. P., Davies, M., Portmann, B., Silk, D. B. A., and Williams, R. (1980): Fulminant hepatic failure in childhood: An analysis of 31 cases. *Arch. Dis. Child.*, 55:252–258.

107. Crowe, G. R. (1977): Halothane hepatitis in children. *Med. J. Aust.*, 1:794.

108. Campbell, R. L., Small, E. W., Lesesne, H. R., Levin, K. J., and Moore, W. H. (1977): Fatal hepatic necrosis after halothane anesthesia in a boy with juvenile rheumatoid arthritis: A case report. *Anesth. Analg.*, 56:589–593.

109. Lewis, R. B., and Blair, M. (1982): Halothane hepatitis in a young child. *Br. J. Anaesth.*, 54:349–354.

110. Kenna, J. G., Nuuberger, J., Meili-Vergani, G., Mowat, A. P., and Williams, R. (1987): Halothane hepatitis in children. *Br. Med. J.*, 294:1209–2111.

111. Resurreccion, M. A., Casthely, P., Pimentel, C., Cottrel, J. E., and Veleck, F. (1981): Serum bromide post-halothane in infants and young children. *Anesthesiology*, 55:A 327.

112. Baren, F., Goudeau, A., Denis, F., Yonnet, B., Chiron, J. P., Coursaget, P., and Diop Mar, I. (1982): Immune response in neonates to hepatitis B vaccine. *Lancet*, 1:252–253.

113. Molina, D. M., and Rowland, F. S. (1974): Stratospheric sink for chlorofluoromethanes: chlorine atomic-catalyzed destruction of ozone. *Nature*, 249:810–812.

114. U.S. Environmental Protection Agency Federal Register (1988): 53:30566–30619.

115. Harris, J. W., Pohl, L. R., Martin, J. L., and Anders, M. W. (1991): Tissue acylation by the chlorofluorocarbon substitute 2,2-dichloro-1,1,1-trichloroethane (HCFC-123) Proceedings of the National Academy of Sciences, 88:1407–1410, 1991.

116. Sipes, I. G., and Brown, B. B. (1976): An animal model of hepatotoxicity associated with halothane anesthesia. *Anesthesiology*, 45:622–628.

117. Wood, M., Berman, M. L., Harbison, R. D., Hoyle, P., Phythyon, J. M., and Wood, J. J. (1980): Halothane-induced hepatic necrosis in triiodothyronine-pretreated rats. *Anesthesiology*, 52:470–476.

118. Uetrecht, J., Wood, A. J., Phythyon, J. M., and Wood, M. (1983): Contrasting effects on halothane hepatotoxicity in phenobarbital-hypoxia and triiodothyronine model; mechanistic implications. *Anesthesiology*, 59:196–201.

119. McClain, G. E., Sipes, I. G., and Brown, B. R. (1979): An animal model of halothane hepatotoxicity. *Anesthesiology*, 51:321–326.

120. Lunam, C. A., Cousins, M. J., and Hall, P. M. (1985): Guinea-pig model of halothane associated hepatotoxicity in the absence of enzyme induction and hypoxia. *J. Pharmacol. Exp. Ther.*, 232:802–809.
121. Lind, R. C., Gandolfi, A. J., Brown, B. R., and Hall, P. M. (1987): Halothane hepatotoxicity in guinea pigs. *Anesth. Analg.*, 66:222–228.
122. Lunam, C. A., Hall, P. M., and Cousins, M. J. (1989): The pathology of halothane hepatitis in a guinea-pig model: A comparison with human halothane hepatitis. *Br. J. Exp. Pathol.*, 70:533–541.
123. Biermann, J. S., Rice, S. A., Fish, K. J., and Serra, M. T. (1989): Metabolism of halothane in obese Fischer 344 rats. *Anesthesiology*, 71:431–437.
124. Bentley, J. B., Vaughan, R. W., Gandolfi, A. J., and Cork, R. C. (1982): Halothane biotransformation in obese and non-obese patients. *Anesthesiology*, 57:94–97.
125. Rice, S. A., and Fish, K. J. (1986): Anesthetic metabolism and renal function in obese and non-obese Fischer 344 rats following enflurane of isoflurane anesthesia. *Anesthesiology*, 65:28–34.
126. Young, S. R., Stoelting, R. K., Peterson, C., and Mandura, J. (1975): Anesthetic biotransformation and renal function in obese patients during and after methoxyflurane or halothane anesthesia. *Anesthesiology*, 42:451–457.
127. Miller, M. S., Gandolfi, A. J., Vaughan, R. W., and Bentley, J. B. (1980): Disposition of enflurane in obese patients. *J. Pharmacol. Exp. Ther.*, 215:292–296.
128. Bentley, J. B., Gandolfi, A. J., and Cork, R. C. (1982): Halothane biotransformation in obese and non-obese patients. *Anesthesiology*, 57:94–97.
129. Neuberger, J. M., Kenna, J. G., and Williams, R. (1987): Halothane hepatitis: Attempt to develop an animal model. *Int. J. Immunopharmacol.*, 9:123–131.
130. Callis, A. H., Brooks, S. D., Roth, T. P., Gandolfi, A. J., and Brown, B. B.: Characterization of a halothane-induced humoral response in rabbits. *Clin. Exp. Immunol.*, 67:343–351.
131. Roth, P. T., Hubbard, A. K., Gandolfi, A. J., and Brown, B. B. (1988): Chronology of halothane-induced antigen expression in halothane exposed rabbits. *Clin. Exp. Immunol.*, 72:330–336.
132. Van Dyke, R. A., (1982): Hepatic centrilobular necrosis after exposure to halothane, enflurane or isoflurane. *Anesth. Analg.*, 61:812–819.
133. Strunin, L., Harrison, L. J., and Davies, J. M. (1983): Etiology of halothane hepatotoxicity. *Anesthesiology*, 58:391.
134. Gelman, S. (1986): Halothane hepatotoxicity—again? *Anesth. Analg.*, 65:831–834.
135. Pohl, L. R., Satoh, H., Christ, D. D., and Kenna, J. G. (1988): The immunologic and metabolic basis of drug hypersensitivities. *Annu. Rev. Pharmacol.*, 28:367–387.
136. Farrell, G. C. (1989): Mechanisms of halothane-induced liver injury: Is it immune or metabolic idiosyncracy? *J. Gastroenterol. Hepatol.*, 3:465–482.

Clinical Immunotoxicology, edited by
D. S. Newcombe, N. R. Rose, and J. C. Bloom.
Raven Press, Ltd., New York © 1992.

12

Selective Interactions of Cancer Chemotherapeutic Agents with the Host Immune System

Wafik S. El-Deiry

The Johns Hopkins Oncology Center, Baltimore, Maryland

The immune system is being found to play an ever more complex and integral role in host defense, i.e., surveillance and elimination of tumor cells. Immune deficiencies, whether inherited, acquired, or drug-induced, are all associated with an increased incidence of various malignancies (14,22,25,62). In the case of drug-induced immunosuppression (e.g., postorgan transplantation), removal of the immunosuppressive drug is often associated with secondary tumor regression.

Conversely, posttransplantation graft-versus-host disease provides another component to host defense through its antitumor effects. Classic cytotoxic chemotherapeutic drugs interact with the immune system by various mechanisms: (a) through direct cytotoxicity toward tumor cells, they inhibit release of substances that interact with host immunity or directly inhibit tumor-induced activation of suppressor T cells; (b) through direct (nonspecific) toxicity toward the cells of the bone marrow or peripheral blood, necessary for normal immune function; (c) through selective effects on subsets of effector cells, resulting in imbalances in the immune system, which may be either deleterious or beneficial to the host; and (d) through effects on lymphokine expression or function.

Biomodulators are under basic science and clinical investigation with the hope that immunomodulation by these agents will supplement and enhance the host antitumor response, alter the behavior of the tumor, or decrease the toxicity of concurrently used cytotoxic agents.

Several excellent reviews discuss the immunological effects/immunomodulation by chemotherapeutic agents (15,16,19). This review focuses on specific mechanisms of interaction between selected chemotherapeutic agents, immunosuppressive agents, or biological response modifiers and the immune host defense system, with emphasis on their mechanisms of immunotoxicity.

Before embarking on a discussion of specific agents and their specific targets within the immune system, a brief summary of general effects of anticancer drugs on host defense is presented. Cancer chemotherapeutic drugs are most effective when a majority of the cells within a tumor are in the cell cycle. The drugs target dividing cells by various mechanisms, including inhibition of DNA, RNA, or protein synthesis, mitotic arrest, cross-linking, damage through DNA strand breaks or chain termination, and competition for metabolites important for replication and cell division. Unfortunately, their effects are not limited to the dividing cells within a particular tumor but rather involve all dividing cells within the body. The consequences are, in general, predictable and encountered frequently in clinical practice. These include common side effects such as hair loss, nausea, mucositis, or diarrhea related to sloughing of the dividing cells within the gastrointestinal mucosa; bone marrow suppression resulting in anemia that frequently requires blood transfusions; thrombocytopenia that may cause bruising or serious bleeding if not corrected with platelet transfusions; and neutropenia, which may be associated with serious or life-threatening infections. Breakdown in the mucosal barriers increases the risk of bacterial seeding of the bloodstream, with increased risk of septic complications. Bone marrow suppression is also frequently associated with the development of systemic fungal infections or occasionally opportunistic infections. In general, the dose intensity of a chemotherapeutic drug or regimen correlates with the duration of aplasia, and the risk of infectious complications also correlates with the depth and duration of neutropenia. One of the major advances in the field of oncology has been the development of therapeutic regimens that combine different mechanisms of anti-tumor action to decrease specific side effects of particular agents. Efforts are also in progress to use biological agents that stimulate the patient's bone marrow to regenerate, thus shortening the period during which host defenses are most compromised. In addition to the previously described general effects of cancer chemotherapeutic drugs, a variety of drugs have been found to have additional effects on host defenses through their particular interaction with elements of the immune system.

The thiopurine drugs, 6-mercaptopurine (6-MP) and azathioprine (AZA), provided some of the first data on the interactions between the immune system and chemotherapeutic drugs. A variety of investigations determined that 6-MP interfered with cell metabolism by several mechanisms (4–6,26,30,43,48,52,53,60). Metabolites of 6-MP are known to cause the following changes: (a) inhibition of purine phosphoribosyltransferase, (b) incorporation of 6-MP metabolites into cellular RNA and DNA, and (c) inhibition of *de novo* purine ribonucleotide synthesis, e.g., pseudofeedback inhibition of phosphoribosylpyrophosphate aminotransferase. These different mechanisms of 6-MP action may vary in their significance, depending on the type of cell attacked by this chemotherapeutic agent. Further, there are differences between the mechanisms of cytotoxic and proliferative activity of 6-MP and AZA. Inhibition of purine nucleotide synthesis by either the parent molecule, 6-MP, or its metabolites does not account for the delayed cytotoxic effects of this drug (54–56). For example, 6-methylthioinosine treatment markedly reduces purine nucleotide pools and cellular proliferation but has little effect on cell viability (63,64). In contrast, thioguanine exposure causes cytotoxicity but has little effect on purine ribonucleotide pools in 6-MP-treated cells (15,16). Thioguanine nucleotides appear to be selectively incorporated into DNA as compared with RNA (54,55), and inhibitors of DNA synthesis protect cells from thioguanine-induced cytotoxicity, whereas RNA synthesis inhibitors do not (54,55). The role of thioguanine nucleotides in cytotoxic responses has recently been verified for humans in whom the enzyme, thiopurine methyltransferase, shows low activity (38,39). In such genetically altered individuals, the inability to catabolize 6-MP to nontoxic metabolites increases the tissue levels of 6-thioguanine nucleotides, which are correlated with bone marrow depression and neutropenia (38,39). Thus, the incorporation of thiopurine nucleotides into cellular DNA is probably the primary mechanism of 6-MP and AZA cytotoxicity. Since the metabolism of azathioprine is slightly different from that of 6-MP, some have postulated that the imidazolyl component of azathioprine may account for some of its immunosuppressive activity (29,60).

Since bone marrow suppression leads to a decrease of immune cells, such an alteration undoubtedly contributes to some of the immunosuppressive effects of these drugs, but whether such mechanisms account for all of the immunosuppressive effects from these drugs remains to be seen.

Perhaps the best known, longest studied, and most understood classic chemotherapeutic agent with respect to its interaction with the immune system is the drug cyclophosphamide (Cytoxan) (8,49). Cyclophosphamide is an alkylating agent, first described in 1958 (2) as a chemotherapeutic agent and subsequently found to have effects on the immune system. In the early 1960's, the ability of various chemotherapeutic agents to inhibit the immune response was investigated, and dose-response relationships were generated (13). Cyclophosphamide, 6-thioguanine, and 6-MP were found to be much more effective in suppressing antibody production in mice as compared with vincaleukoblastine, triethylenemelamine, and 5-fluorouracil. Optimal inhibition of antibody production occurred with exposure of mice to chemotherapy 2 days prior to antigen exposure.

In the middle to late 1960's, a paradoxical effect of exaggerated and prolonged delayed hypersensitivity was observed in the skin of guinea pigs sensitized by dinitrochlorobenzene if they were first exposed to cyclophosphamide for 5 days (41). In the early 1970's, the effects of cyclophosphamide on the structure and function of lymphoid tissue were investigated (58,59). Treatment of mice or guinea pigs with high (sublethal or lethal) doses of cyclophosphamide resulted in the selective depletion of lymphocytes from lymph follicles from the corticomedullary junction in lymph nodes and nonthymus areas in the spleen. These geographical areas are associated with lymphocyte proliferation in the development of a cell-mediated immune response and are similar to the effects of irradiation of lymphoid tissues. It subsequently became clear that low doses of cyclophosphamide, which do not inhibit antibody production, are effective in the augmentation of delayed type hypersensitivity (3), possibly through effects on suppressor T cells. Further studies demonstrated that cyclophosphamide treatment of mice before immunization resulted in a strong augmentation of their capacity to generate *in vivo* antigen-specific cytotoxic T lymphocytes (47). The differential sensitivity of suppressor cell-mediated immune mechanisms, over the effector arm of the immune response, forms the basis for immune augmentation by cyclophosphamide. BALB/c mice given 3-methylcholanthrene, a tumor-inducing agent, and injected with cyclophosphamide every 10 days had a striking delay in the appearance of primary sarcomas (28).

In the early 1980's, it was observed that a variety of cancer chemotherapeutic agents (both cell cycle–specific and cell cycle–nonspecific), including mitomycin C, doxorubicin, 5-fluorouracil, vincristine, cyclocytidine, and methotrexate, all significantly enhance delayed hypersensitivity reactions in mice after intermittent high dosing, as in clinical practice (23). It was speculated that differential (delayed or insufficient) recovery of lymphocyte subsets after chemotherapy (interruption of normal suppressor cell function) may explain this apparently general phenomenon of potentiation of delayed hypersensitivity with anticancer drugs.

Recent studies with low doses of cyclophosphamide have attempted to exploit its ability to augment the immune response in order to achieve tumor regression (7,11, 12,17,23,28,31–33,65). Berd and coworkers (11) demonstrated augmentation of cell-mediated immunity (increase in the magnitude of delayed type hypersensitivity skin reactions) in advanced metastatic cancer patients following low-dose cyclophosphamide administration. In a group of patients with metastatic melanoma, Berd and Mastrangelo (12) found that treatment with cyclophosphamide plus melanoma vaccine resulted in a progressive depletion of the CD4 + , 2H4 + suppressor-inducer T-cell subset of peripheral blood lymphocytes (not CD8 + suppressor or the suppressor subpopulations as defined by expression of leu-15). They further found no evidence that activated suppressor or inducer cells, as defined by expression of the interleukin-2 receptor (Tac) or the activation antigen, Ta1, were reduced by cyclophosphamide plus vaccine treatment.

Wise and colleagues (65) studied the immunomodulatory activity of low-dose cyclophosphamide in mice bearing large MOPC-315 plasmacytomas. Although these tumors are sensitive to the chemotherapeutic effects of cyclophosphamide, there is also a contribution of antitumor immunity to control the tumor mass after the drug and its metabolites have cleared. Prior to cyclophosphamide therapy, spleen cells from these mice are depressed in their ability to generate an *in vitro* cytotoxic response to the plasmacytoma. However, following cyclophosphamide, the spleen cells generate a specific and sustained antiplasmacytoma response (65).

Using a cyclophosphamide-resistant murine lymphoma as a model, Awwad and North (7) demonstrated a sustained and augmented level of immunity following cyclophosphamide treatment associated with immunologically mediated tumor regression. Because the therapeutic effect of cyclophosphamide could be inhibited by passive transfer of L3T4 + T cells from normal donor mice, it was felt that this therapeutic effect is likely attributable to the preferential destruction of these precursor suppressor T cells.

Two recent studies have demonstrated improved therapeutic effects with the combination of adoptive immunotherapy with interleukin-2, lymphokine-activated killer cells, and cyclophosphamide (17,33). Hosokawa and associates (33) showed that the 3 LL lung carcinoma in C57BL/6 mice was inhibited in terms of local recurrence as well as pulmonary metastases when cyclophosphamide was combined with interleukin-2. Furthermore, there was a markedly increased accumulation and concentration of lymphokine-activated killer cells in the tumor treated with cyclophosphamide. These cyclophosphamide-treated tumors regressed completely in most cases, so that the number of tumor cells that had to be eliminated by the killer cells was much smaller in the cyclophosphamide-treated group. Using another murine tumor model, the 3-methylcholanthrene-induced sarcoma mentioned above, Eggermont and Sugarbaker (17) showed that combinations of cyclophosphamide with interleukin-2 or interleukin-2 plus lymphokine-activated killer cells had superior antitumor activity when compared with the effects of single agent treatment. Several hypotheses were put forth to explain the enhanced antitumor effects: (a) reduction in tumor bulk by cyclophosphamide, allowing a greater tumor reducing effect by interleukin-2, (b) damage of tumor cells by cyclophosphamide to a degree that makes them more susceptible to lysis by lymphokine-activated killer cells, or possibly effects of immunotherapy on tumor cells to make them more susceptible to chemotherapy, (c) potentiation of immunotherapy by cyclophosphamide by removal of suppressor cell function, (d) cyclophosphamide removal of a cytotoxic T-lymphocyte population competing for exogenous interleukin-2, and (e) effects of interleukin-2 on liver and kidney function to alter cyclophosphamide metabolism and elimination, thus enhancing its antitumor effect.

Recent studies on the mechanisms of immunosuppression by cyclophosphamide have focused on its metabolites (36), phosphoramide mustard and acrolein. Phosphoramide mustard is thought to mediate the immunosuppressive and antitumor effects of cyclophosphamide by binding to DNA and inhibiting cell proliferation. Acrolein is thought to inhibit the immune response through its interaction with sulfhydryl groups of important cellular macromolecules.

In summary, the effects of cyclophosphamide are numerous and complex, ranging from high-dose suppression of antibody production to low-dose stimulation of delayed type hypersensitivity and depletion of suppressor T lymphocytes. The drug has proven effects in augmenting the host antitumor response and provides added benefits when combined with biological response modifiers. Its metabolites have both activity and toxicity. The molecular mechanisms underlying its interactions with the immune system, however, remain unknown.

Another commonly used chemotherapeutic agent whose interaction with the immune system has been under investigation for many years is doxorubicin (1,10,15, 18–20,40,42,45,57,61,66). The contribution of host defense mechanisms to the antitumor effects of doxorubicin has been known since the early 1970's, offering this drug a selective advantage in terms of efficacy compared with its closely related analogue, daunorubicin. Vecchi and coworkers (61) found that both doxorubicin and daunomycin inhibited DNA synthesis and reduced bone marrow stem cells to a similar extent. However, doxorubicin induced a greater reduction in the number of antibody-producing cells after primary stimulation with sheep erythrocytes, whereas daunorubicin was more suppressive on the secondary response to the same antigen. Mantovani and colleagues (42) provided evidence for the role of host defense mechanisms in the antitumor activity of doxorubicin. They demonstrated that doxorubicin had greater therapeutic efficacy than daunorubicin in treating the more immunogenic tumors in mice. Further, prior treatment with immunosuppressant DTIC (5-(3,3-dimethyl-1-triazenyl)-1H-imidazole-4-carboxamide) markedly impaired the efficacy of doxorubicin in immunogenic tumor models.

Orsini and associates (45) demonstrated augmentation of cell-mediated immunity of spleen cells in culture with allogeneic tumor cells after treatment with doxorubicin or daunorubicin versus no treatment or treatment with cyclophosphamide. It is felt that augmented cell-mediated immunity by doxorubicin is somehow related to modulation of cytotoxic T-cell progenitors, with a relative sparing of macrophages (18). Doxorubicin did not selectively interact with T-helper or T-suppressor cells. Suppression of natural killer cell activity by doxorubicin is felt to be related to prostaglandin E_2 levels, resulting in decreased recognition and lysis of tumor cells. Prostaglandin E_2 is a product of macrophages; studies with indomethacin in culture resulted in augmentation of natural killer cell activity of spleen cells and slight decreases in phagocytic activity (18). Studies by Wood and Lotzova (66) recently demonstrated that doxorubicin exposure of colon cancer cells in culture resulted in a resistance to natural killer cell–mediated lysis. It was found that interleukin-2 stimulated natural killer cell effectors were able to overcome the doxorubicin-induced resistance to lysis. The mechanism of resistance to natural killer cell–mediated lysis is not well understood but is not apparently related to alteration in the binding of the effector to the doxorubicin-treated targets.

Foa and coworkers (20) investigated the augmentation of cytotoxic T-cell and lymphokine–activated killer cell response by doxorubicin and mitomycin C. They used electron micrographs to study the membrane interactions between the effectors and their targets. Although changes in target size and changes in membrane characteristics were induced by the drugs, they did not observe any change in either the size or the folding of the interacting areas between killers and targets. They speculated on the possible consequences of drug-membrane interactions, e.g., effects of physicochemical properties, receptor levels, or adhesion molecules.

Further, studies of the effects on interleukin-2 release by chemotherapeutic drugs by Abdul-Hamied and Turk (1) exposed a key difference among bleomycin, doxorubicin, and cyclophosphamide. Both bleomycin and doxorubicin significantly increased the amount of interleukin-2 activity produced by spleen cells stimulated by concanavalin A, whereas cyclophosphamide inhibited interleukin-2 production under the same conditions. Again, neither bleomycin nor doxorubicin enhancement of interleukin-2 release could be linked with either enrichment of T-helper cells or depletion of suppressor cells in the spleen. Additionally, there was only slight enhancement of interleukin-1 production from peritoneal exudate cells in comparison to the profound elevation of interleukin-2 levels by spleen cells with either bleomycin or doxorubicin, suggesting that the role of macrophages and the mechanisms of enhanced interleukin-2 production need further investigation. Of note, either 4-hydroperoxycyclophosphamide or mafosfamide (cyclophosphamide derivatives) addition to rat splenocytes resulted in a significant inhibition of interleukin-2 release.

Recently, Maccubbin and associates (40) provided further direct evidence for the role of prostaglandin E_2 in the immunomodulatory effects of doxorubicin. Doxorubicin-treated spleen cells produced increased amounts of prostaglandin E_2 and manifested reduced natural killer cell and lymphokine-activated killer cell activities and elevated Fc-dependent phagocytosis. Exogenous prostaglandin E_2 inhibited natural killer cell activity in a dose-dependent fashion, and the addition of indomethacin reversed effects of doxorubicin on both the natural killer cell and phagocytic activities observed with cultured spleen cells. A role for indomethacin in palliation or therapy of cancer is mentioned, with attention to studies showing higher levels of target killing by cytotoxic T lymphocytes after the addition of indomethacin to either normal or doxorubicin-treated spleen cells.

An association between increased sialic acid content of K562 cells and doxorubicin-induced resistance to natural killer cell–mediated lysis has been investigated (10). Neuraminidase treatment resulted in an obvious enhancement of susceptibility to natural killer cell–mediated lysis, probably caused by increased target-effector binding.

A general phenomenon of lymphokine-activated killer cell induction following combination chemotherapy has recently been described (37). MVAC (methotrexate, vinblastine, doxorubicin [adriamycin], and cisplatin) therapy for patients with bladder cancer, PEB (cisplatin, etoposide, and bleomycin) therapy for testicular cancer, and MA (methotrexate, doxorubicin [adriamycin]) therapy for testicular cancer were all found to induce a strong lymphokine-activated killer cell–like activity in the peripheral blood of patients approximately 1 month following combined chemotherapy. The recognition specificity of these effector cells was broad and included not only natural killer cell–resistant Raji cells and natural killer cell–sensitive K562 human myelogenous leukemia cells but also human bladder tumor T24 cells, human prostatic cancer PC-3 cells, and murine fibrosarcoma UV female cells. The target specificities were very similar regardless of the chemotherapeutic regimen used. The contribution of this induction phenomenon to the mechanism of antitumor drugs is still under investigation.

The antihelminthic drug, suramin, a potent inhibitor of cell growth, with the ability to prevent lymphoid and nonlymphoid tumor progression *in vivo*, is also an immunosuppressive agent. Mills and coworkers (44) demonstrated that suramin induces a concentration-dependent decrease in binding of interleukin-2 to its receptor complex and murine T lymphocytes (44). The growth inhibitory properties of suramin were found to be reversed by interleukin-2 in a murine system and partially reversed with human cells. The mechanism whereby interleukin-2 receptor activation results in cell proliferation is felt to be related to interleukin-2-induced tyrosine phosphorylation, which is also inhibited by suramin and not via phosphatidylinositol hydrolysis, with its associated changes in intracellular calcium or protein kinase C activation.

A variety of drugs with immunosuppressive properties are currently being used in the treatment of cancer patients, including steroids, cyclosporine, thalidomide, and AZA. Steroids have widespread uses, including the treatment of Hodgkin's and non-Hodgkin's lymphomas, leukemias, chemotherapy-associated nausea and vomiting, edema related to brain metastases or spinal cord compression, and graft-versus-host disease. The other immunosuppressive agents mentioned and used in the treatment of graft-versus-host disease also induce a graft-versus-tumor effect associated with the disease. Behrens and Goodwin reviewed the known effects of steroids on the immune system (9) and referenced several excellent reviews. The glucocorticoids have numerous complex interactions with the host immune system resulting in powerful immunosuppression. Their effects include (a) a lymphocytopenia with particular depletion of T-helper cells within hours; (b) variable effects on immunoglobulin production, including decreased IgG, IgA, and IgM levels within weeks of steroid treatment or increased immunoglobulin levels under certain conditions that may be related to effects on suppressor cells; (c) interference with early B-cell activation events that may be related to inhibition of RNA and DNA synthesis with a block in G_0 to G_1 transition; (d) inhibition of cell-mediated immunity and anergy thought to be related to impaired macrophage recruitment and inhibition of T-lymphocyte function; (e) inhibition of early T-cell activation and proliferative responses that is characterized by suppression of T-lymphocyte blast formation, suppression of T-lymphocyte responses to antigen stimulation, inhibition of mixed lymphocyte reaction, inhibition of T-suppressor cells, and variable effects on natural killer cells; (f) inhibition of lymphokine production, i.e., inhibition of interleukin-1 production, inhibition of Ia antigen expression on macrophages, profound inhibition of interleukin-2 production, inhibition of interleukin-2 mRNA synthesis, partial inhibition of interleukin-2 receptor production, and blockage of interferon-gamma production by T cells at the transcription level; (g) decreased Fc receptor expression with decreased Fc receptor–mediated clearance by the reticuloendothelial system; and (h) antiinflammatory effects related to inhibition of arachidonic acid metabolism and release, which may be associated with increased "lipomodulin" production and consequent inhibition of natural killer cells and antibody-dependent cell-mediated cytotoxicity.

Insight into mechanisms of immunosuppression and a possible wider involvement of basic cellular processes of signal transduction are being gained from studies of cyclosporine and unrelated structures that appear to act through remarkably similar mechanisms (21,24,27,34,35,46,50,51). Cyclosporine, a cyclic peptide, has found widespread clinical use as an immunosuppressive agent after organ transplant and after bone marrow transplantation. The novel macrolide FK506, a newly discovered potent immunosuppressive agent, which is under investigation in the clinical arena, is a potent inhibitor of T-cell activation. Both cyclosporine and FK506 inhibit specific lymphokine production by activated T cells. Specifically, these agents have been found to inhibit production of interleukin-2, interleukin-3, interleukin-4, GMCSF, tumor necrosis factor-alpha, and interferon-gamma. They have not been found to affect bone marrow colony formation or lymphokine-dependent proliferation (i.e., inhibition of T-cell proliferation could be reversed by addition of recombinant interleukin-2). Cyclosporine has been found to directly inhibit interleukin-2 transcription through a mechanism that involves inhibition of DNA binding of lymphocyte-specific factors to promoter/enhancer regions critical for interleukin-2 gene expression.

The inhibition of T-cell proliferation and lymphokine production by cyclosporine and FK506 has been linked to the effects of these agents on signal transduction pathways that cause a measurable rise in intracellular calcium. For example, in the case of interleukin-2, inhibition of production occurs when human lymphocytes are activated via the CD3/T-cell receptor complex but not when the same cells are triggered via the CD28 pathway. Similarly, other lymphokine genes that are inhibited can be made resistant when an alternative activation pathway is utilized.

Specific and distinct binding proteins have been found in the cytoplasm that interacts with cyclosporine and FK506. Both cyclophilin, a highly conserved cytosolic protein with cyclosporine binding activity, and FKBP, the FK506 binding protein, catalyze the cis-trans isomerization of peptidyl-proline bonds. These isomerization activities are inhibited by binding of the immunosuppressive agents and correlate with immunosuppression. These observations have led to the hypothesis that these peptidyl-prolyl isomerases may play a critical role in lymphocyte signal transduction. However, it has not been proved that cyclophilin and FKBP are direct mediators of the immunosuppressive activities of cyclosporine and FK506. In fact, there are results that strongly imply that inhibition of the enzymatic activity of FKBP does not directly result in suppression of calcium-associated signal transduction pathways and interleukin-2 expression. Both FK506 and another immunosuppressive agent, rapamycin, compete for FKBP. However, rapamycin appears to lack the selectivity for suppression of calcium-associated signal transduction pathways in the lymphocyte and does not block accumulation of interleukin-2 mRNA induced by any mode of activation.

SUMMARY

Agents used in the treatment of human cancer interact with host defenses in a variety of ways. These include general effects such as toxicity to gastrointestinal mucosa resulting in perturbation of mucosal barriers, which increases the risk of bacterial invasion. Toxicity to the bone marrow results in neutropenia, which decreases the ability to fight infection and predisposes the host to systemic fungal infections (when prolonged). Other general effects include potentiation of delayed hypersensitivity, possibly via differential recovery of lymphocyte subsets following chemotherapy-induced bone marrow suppression, and a general phenomenon of lymphokine-activated killer cell induction following combination chemotherapy.

Specific interactions of drugs with host defense, and in particular the host immune system, include (a) inhibition of humoral immunity by high doses of cyclophosphamide and other drugs mentioned previously; (b) differential sensitivity of suppressor cell–mediated immune mechanisms by low doses of cyclophosphamide, resulting in immune augmentation; (c) suppression of natural killer cell activity by doxorubicin, possibly related to prostaglandin E_2 levels, (d) enhancement of interleukin-2 release by bleomycin and doxorubicin, under conditions resulting in decreased interleukin-2 levels by spleen cells treated with cyclophosphamide; (e) decreased interleukin-2 binding to its receptor complex by suramin, (f) multiple effects of steroids on all arms of the immune system detailed previously, and (g) interaction of the immunosuppressive drugs cyclosporine and FK506 with signal transduction pathways as well as inhibition of lymphokine production, which in the case of cyclosporine and interleukin-2, is probably mediated by inhibition of DNA binding of lymphocyte-specific factors to promoter/enhancer regions critical for interleukin-2 gene expression.

The interactions of agents used in the treatment of cancer with the immune system are being exploited in order to maximize the host-antitumor response. Lymphokines are being used clinically to increase sensitivity of tumors to killing (by increasing tumor growth fraction), to shorten the time period during which host defenses are perturbed, and to decrease toxicity.

REFERENCES

1. Abdul-Hamied, T. A., and Turk, J. L. (1987): Enhancement of interleukin-2 release in rats by treatment with bleomycin and Adriamycin in vivo. *Cancer Immunol. Immunother.*, 25:245–249.
2. Arnold, H., et al. (1958): Chemotherapeutic action of a cyclic nitrogen mustard phosphamide ester (B-518-ASTA) in experimental tumors of the rat. *Nature*, 181:931.
3. Askenase, P. W., et al. (1975): Augmentation of delayed-type hypersensitivity by doses of cyclophosphamide which do not affect antibody responses. *J. Exp. Med.*, 141:697–702.
4. Atkinson, M. R., and Murray, A. W. (1965): Inhibition of purine phosphoribosyltransferases of Ehrlich ascites-tumour cells by 6-mercaptopurine. *Biochem. J.*, 94:64–70.
5. Atkinson, M. R., Morton, R. K., and Murray, A. W. (1964): Inhibition of adenylosuccinate synthetase and adenylosuccinate lyase from Ehrlich ascites-tumor cells by 6-thioguanine 5′-phosphate. *Biochem. J.*, 92:398–404.
6. Atkinson, M. R., Morton, R. K., and Murray, A. W. (1963): Inhibition of inosine 5′-phosphate dehydrogenase from Ehrlich ascites-tumor cells by 6-thioguanine 5′-phosphate. *Biochem. J.*, 89:167–172.
7. Awwad, M., and North, R. J. (1989): Cyclophosphamide-induced immunologically mediated regression of a cyclophosphamide-resistant murine tumor: A consequence of eliminating precursor L3T4 + suppressor T-cells. *Cancer Res.* 49:1649–1654.
8. Bartlett, R. R. (1988): Cyclophosphamide. In The Pharmacology of Lymphocytes. Handbook of Experimental Pharmacology, vol. 85, edited by M. A. Bray and J. Morley, pp. 453–469. Springer-Verlag, New York.
9. Behrens, T. W., and Goodwin, J. S. (1988): Glucocorticoids. In The Pharmacology of Lymphocytes: Handbook of Experimental Pharmacology, vol. 85, edited by M. A. Bray and J. Morley, pp. 425–439. Springer-Verlag, New York.
10. Benoist, H., et al. (1988): Association of Adriamycin-induced resistance to NK-mediated lysis with sialic acid level and immunological reactivity of transferrin receptors and glycophorin A. *Int. J. Cancer*, 42:299–304.
11. Berd, D., et al. (1984): Potentiation of human cell-mediated and humoral immunity by low-dose cyclophosphamide. *Cancer Res.*, 44:5439–5443.
12. Berd, D., and Mastrangelo, M. J. (1988): Effect of low dose cyclophosphamide on the immune system of cancer patients: Depletion of CD4 + , 2H4 + suppressor-inducer T-cells. *Cancer Res.*, 48:1671–1675.
13. Berenbaum, M. C., and Brown, I. N. (1964): Dose response relationships for agents inhibiting the immune response. *Immunology*, 7:65–71.

14. Berlinger, N. T., and Good, R. A. (1980): Suppressor cells in healthy relatives of patients with hereditary colon cancer. *Cancer*, 45:1112–1116.
15. Braun, D. P., and Harris, J. E. (1981): Modulation of the immune response by chemotherapy. *Pharmacol. Ther.*, 14:89–122.
16. Bray, M. A., and Morley, J. (eds.) (1988): The pharmacology of lymphocytes. In Handbook of Experimental Pharmacology, vol. 85, edited by M. A. Bray and J. Morley. Springer-Verlag, New York.
17. Eggermont, A. M. M., and Sugarbaker, P. H. (1988): Efficacy of chemoimmunotherapy with cyclophosphamide, interleukin 2 and lymphokine activated killer cells in an intraperitoneal murine tumor model. *Br. J. Cancer*, 58:410–414.
18. Ehrke, M. J., et al. (1982): Selective effects of Adriamycin on murine host defense systems. *Immunol. Rev.*, 65:55–78.
19. Ehrke, M. J., and Mihich, E. (1984): Immunologic effects of anticancer drugs. In Clinical Chemotherapy, vol. 3, edited by M. P. Kuemmerle, pp. 475–499. Thieme, Stuttgart.
20. Foa, C., et al. (1987): Study of CTL and LAK contacts to target cells after treatment with mitomycin C and Adriamycin. *Immunol. Invest.*, 16:241–262.
21. Foxwell, B. M. J., Woerly, G., and Ryffel, B. (1990): Inhibition of interleukin 4 receptor expression on human lymphoid cells by cyclosporin. *Eur. J. Immunol.*, 20:1185–1188.
22. Gatti, R. A., and Good, R. A. (1971): Occurrence of malignancy in immunodeficiency diseases: A literature review. *Cancer*, 28:89–98.
23. Goto, M., et al. (1981): Enhancement of delayed hypersensitivity reaction with varieties of anticancer drugs: A common biological phenomenon. *J. Exp. Med.*, 154:204–209.
24. Granelli-Piperno, A. (1990): Lymphokine gene expression in vivo is inhibited by cyclosporin A. *J. Exp. Med.*, 171:533–544.
25. Guanti, G., et al. (1989): Depressed level of natural killer cells in cancer family syndrome. *Cancer Immunol. Immunother.*, 30:307–311.
26. Hakala, M. T., and Nichol, C. A. (1959): Studies on the mode of action of 6-mercaptopurine and its ribonucleoside on mammalian cells in culture. *J. Biol. Chem.*, 234:3224–3228.
27. Harding, M. W., Galat, A., Uehling, D. E., and Schreiber, S. L. (1989): A receptor for the immunosuppressant FK506 is a cis-trans peptidyl-prolyl isomerase. *Nature*, 341:758–760.
28. Hellstrom, I., and Hellstrom, K. E. (1978): Cyclophosphamide delays 3-methylchloranthrene sarcoma induction in mice. *Nature*, 275:129–130.
29. Hitchings, G. H. (1967): Immunosuppressive drugs. Summary and concluding remarks. *Fed. Proc.*, 26:958–960.
30. Hitchings, G. N., and Elion, G. B. (1967): Mechanisms of action of purine and pyrimidine analogs. In Cancer Chemotherapy, II, edited by I. Brodsky, S. Benham, Kahn, and J. H. Moyer, pp. 23–32. Grune & Stratton, New York.
31. Hoon, D. S. B., et al. (1990): Suppressor cell activity in a randomized trial of patients receiving active specific immunotherapy with melanoma cell vaccine and low dosages of cyclophosphamide. *Cancer Res.*, 50:5358–5364.
32. Hooner, S. K., et al. (1990): Cyclophosphamide and abrogation of tumor-induced suppressor T cell activity. *Cancer Immunol. Immunother.*, 31:121–127.
33. Hosokawa, M., et al. (1988): Improved therapeutic effects of interleukin-2 after the accumulation of lymphokine-activated killer cells in tumor tissue of mice previously treated with cyclophosphamide. *Cancer Immunol. Immunother.*, 26:250–256.
34. Kahan, B. D. (1989): Cyclosporin. *N. Engl. J. Med.*, 321:1725–1738.
35. Kasaian, M. T., and Biron, C. A. (1990): Cyclosporin A inhibition of interleukin 2 gene expression, but not natural killer cell proliferation, after interferon induction in vivo. *J. Exp. Med.*, 171:745–762.
36. Kawabata, T. T., et al. (1990): Mechanisms of in vitro immunosuppression by hepatocyte-generated cyclophosphamide metabolites and 4-hydroperoxycyclophosphamide. *Biochem. Pharmacol.*, 40:927–935.
37. Kiyohara, T., et al. (1988): Induction of lymphokine-activated killer-like cells by cancer chemotherapy. *J. Exp. Med.*, 168:2355–2360.
38. Lennard, L., Van Loon, J. A., Lilleyman, J. S., and Weinshilboum, R. M. (1987): Thiopurine pharmacogenetics in leukemia: Correlation of erythrocyte thiopurine methyltransferase activity and 6-thioguanine nucleotide concentrations. *Clin. Pharmacol. Ther.*, 41:18–25.

39. Lennard, L., Van Loon, J. A., and Weinshilboum, R. M. (1989): Pharmacogenetics of acute aza-thioprine toxicity: Relationship to thiopurine methyl-transferase genetic polymorphism. *Clin. Phar-macol. Res.*, 46:149–154.

40. Maccubbin, D. L., et al. (1990): Indomethacin modulation of Adriamycin induced effects on multi-ple cytolytic effector functions. *Cancer Immunol. Immunother.*, 31:373–380.

41. Maguire, H. C., Jr., and Ettore, V. L. (1967): Enhancement of dinitrochlorobenzene (DNCB) con-tact sensitization by cyclophosphamide in the guinea pig. *J. Invest. Dermatol.*, 48:39–43.

42. Mantovani, A., et al. (1979): Role of host defense mechanisms in antitumor activity of Adriamycin and daunomycin in mice. *J. Natl. Cancer Inst.*, 63:61–66.

43. McCollister, R. J., Gilbert, W. R., Ashton, D. M., and Wyngaarden, J. B. (1962): Pseudofeed-back inhibition of purine synthesis by 6-mercaptopurine and other purine analogues. *J. Clin. Invest.*, 41:1383.

44. Mills, G. B., et al. (1990): Suramin prevents binding of interleukin 2 to its cell surface receptor: A possible mechanism for immunosuppression. *Cancer Res.*, 50:3036–3042.

45. Orsini, F., et al. (1977): Increased primary cell-mediated immunity in culture subsequent to Adria-mycin or daunomycin treatment of spleen donor mice. *Cancer Res.*, 37:1719–1726.

46. Randak, C. (1990): Brabletz, T., Hergenrother, M., Sabotta, I., and Serfling, E. (1990): Cyclo-sporin A suppresses the expression of the interleukin 2 gene by inhibiting the binding of lymphocyte-specific factors to the IL-2 enhancer. *EMBO J.*, 9:2529–2536.

47. Rollinghoff, M., et al. (1977): Cyclophosphamide-sensitive T lymphocytes suppress the in vivo generation of antigen-specific cytotoxic T lymphocytes. *J. Exp. Med.*, 145:455–459.

48. Scannell, J. P., and Hitchings, G. H. (1966): Thioguanine in deoxyribonucleic acid from tumors of 6-mercaptopurine-treated mice. *Proc. Soc. Exp. Biol. Med.*, 122:627–629.

49. Shand, F. L. (1979): The immunopharmacology of cyclophosphamide. *Int. J. Immunopharmacol.*, 1:165–171.

50. Siekierka, J. J., Hung, S. H. Y., Poe, M., Lin, C. S., and Sigal, N. H. (1989): A cytosolic binding protein for the immunosuppressant FK506 has peptidyl-prolyl isomerase activity but is distinct from cyclophilin. *Nature*, 341:755–757.

51. Sigal, N. H., Siekierka, J. J., and Dumont, F. J. (1990): Observations on the mechanism of action of FK506: A pharmacologic probe of lymphocyte signal transduction. *Biochem. Pharmacol.*, 40: 2201–2208.

52. Silberman, H. R., and Wyngaarden, J. B. (1961): 6-mercaptopurine as substrate and inhibitor of xanthine oxidase. *Biochim. Biophys. Acta*, 47:178–180.

53. Simpson, L., Bennett, L. L., and Golden, J. (1962): Effects of 6-mercaptopurine (MP) on the synthesis of purines in ascites tumor cells. *Proc. Am. Assoc. Cancer Res.*, 3:361.

54. Tidd, D. M., and Paterson, A. R. P. (1974): A biochemical mechanism for the delayed cytotoxic reaction of 6-mercaptopurine. *Cancer Res.*, 34:738–746.

55. Tidd, D. M., and Paterson, A. R. P. (1974): Distinction between inhibition of purine nucleotide synthesis and the delayed cytotoxic reaction of 6-mercaptopurine. *Cancer Res.*, 34:733–737.

56. Tidd, D. M., Kim, S. C., Harakova, K., Mariwaki, A., and Paterson, A. R. P. (1972): A delayed cytotoxic reaction for 6-mercaptopurine. *Cancer Res.*, 32:317–322.

57. Tomazic, V., et al. (1980): Modulation of cytototoxic response against allogeneic tumor cells in culture by Adriamycin. *Cancer Res.*, 40:2748–2755.

58. Turk, J. L., et al. (1972): Functional aspects of the selective depletion of lymphoid tissue by cyclo-phosphamide. *Immunology*, 23:493–501.

59. Turk, J. L., and Poulter, L. W. (1972): Selective depletion of lymphoid tissue by cyclophos-phamide. *Clin. Exp. Immunol.*, 10:285–296.

60. Van Scoik, K. G., Johnson, C. A., and Porter, W. R. (1985): The pharmacology and metabolism of the thriopurine drugs 6-mercaptopurine and azathioprine. *Drug Metab. Rev.*, 16:157–174.

61. Vecchi, A., et al. (1976): A characterization of the immunosuppressive activity of Adriamycin and daunomycin on humoral antibody production and tumor allograft rejection. *Cancer Res.*, 36:1222–1227.

62. Waldmann, T. A., Strober, W., and Blaese, R. M. (1972): Immunodeficiency disease and malig-nancy: Various immunologic deficiencies of man and the role of immune processes in the control of malignant disease. *Ann. Intern. Med.*, 77:605–628.

63. Warnick, C. T., and Paterson, A. R. P. (1973): Effect of methylthioinosine on nucleotide concen-trations in L5178Y cells. *Cancer Res.*, 33:1711–1715, 1973.

64. Warnick, C. T., and Paterson, A. R. P. (1972): The effect of methylthioinosine on purine ribo-nucleotide levels in murine lymphoma cells. *Proc. Am. Assoc. Cancer Res.*, 13:51.
65. Wise, J. A., et al. (1988): Effect of low-dose cyclophosphamide therapy on specific and nonspecific T cell dependent immune responses of spleen cells from mice bearing large MOPC-315 plasma-cytomas. *Cancer Immunol. Immunother.*, 27:191–197.
66. Wood, W. J., and Lotzova, E. (1989): Adriamycin induced resistance to natural killer (NK) medi-ated cytotoxicity. *Cancer*, 64:396–403.

13

Pulmonary Hypersensitivity Disorders

I. Leonard Bernstein

*Division of Immunology, Department of Medicine,
University of Cincinnati Medical Center, Cincinnati, Ohio*

In contrast to the wider range of immunological responses that clinical immunotoxicology encompasses, the subspecialty of pulmonary immunotoxicology is chiefly concerned with the direct effects of systemic or inhaled exogenous agents on lung and bronchial tissues. At times, the pathological expression of respiratory immune disease is unique, but more often tissue injury patterns mimic those caused by toxins or infectious agents. For example, bronchiectasis is a complication of both allergic bronchopulmonary aspergillosis and inhaled toxic gases (e.g., ammonia) (11). In addition, autoimmune epiphenomena may appear during the course of fibrogenic lung diseases such as asbestosis and silicosis, despite the nonimmunological background of these diseases. Nevertheless, significant immunotoxicological mechanisms have been investigated and implicated in the pathogenesis of pulmonary hypersensitivity disorders induced by drugs, chemicals, and other occupational substances. The purpose of this discussion is a selective update of current progress in these specific clinical entities with an emphasis on the occupational aspects of immunologically induced pulmonary diseases.

Drug-induced pulmonary lesions have been recognized more frequently since the advent of modern chemotherapy. Apart from the life-threatening asthmatic and anaphylactic complications that can occur after exposure to many organic compounds, the chief categories of drug-related pulmonary immune diseases are listed in Table 1. Many drugs have been identified as causes of both acute and/or chronic pneumonia-like infiltrates. A partial compilation of such drugs is presented in Table 2 (19). Drug-associated pulmonary infiltrates are usually accompanied by eosinophilia, and open biopsies of such lesions also reveal chronic eosinophilic infiltrates. Sulfonamides and related analogues (e.g., nitrofurantoin) have often been associated with these pulmonic syndromes. Sulfonamide-induced lung lesions may or may not be associated with systemic reactions. Recently, lymphocytes derived from sulfonamide-sensitive patients have proved to be most susceptible to cytotoxic sulfonamide metabolites generated from a mouse hepatic microsomal preparation (20). Many of these patients also have the slow acetylator phenotype. This de-

TABLE 1. *Morphological classification of pulmonary drug reactions*

Pneumonitis: alveolar or interstitial
   Acute
   Chronic
   Lupus-related
   Fibrosis

creased ability to catabolize a reactive toxic metabolite, combined with a secondary immunological response to this metabolite, may result in the clinical manifestation of these lesions. Antigen-induced lymphocyte proliferation has also been demonstrated in a few patients after inhalation treatment with cromolyn sodium, a very rare adverse reaction to this drug (21). Pulmonary lesions and pleuropericardial effusions may be observed in patients with drug-related lupus erythematosus. Among the drugs that have been reported to induce these reactions, procainamide has the highest incidence of drug-induced lupus (7). Immunological mechanisms have been explored most actively in procainamide-treated patients, 100% and 30% of whom develop antinuclear autoimmune antibodies and clinical symptoms, respectively, if the drug is continued for a sufficient period of time. It has been proposed that oxidation of the primary aromatic amine of procainamide may lead to the formation of a reactive metabolite that ultimately induces immune abnormalities (24). There is also evidence that metabolism of the primary arylamine of procainamide may lead to production of procainamide hydroxylamine. This compound

TABLE 2. *Partial list of agents causing drug-induced pneumonitis*

Nitrofurantoin
Sulfonamides
Para-aminosalicylic acid
Sulfasalazine
Methotrexate
Phenytoin
Minocycline
Penicillin
Isoniazid
Procarbazine
Carbamazepine
Imipramine
Methylphenidate
Dantrolene
Chlorpropamide
Mecamylamine
Mephenytoin
Naproxen sodium
Cromolyn sodium

may undergo nonenzymatic oxidation to a nitroso metabolite, which may bond to proteins and histones. These multivalent conjugates could then induce classic auto-antibodies (23). Several drugs (cyclophosphamide, busulfan, and bleomycin) have fibrosis-stimulating properties and may be associated with either interstitial or pleural fibrosis (12,14). Whether immunological factors are involved in the genesis of these reactions is unknown. However, neither drug hypersensitivity nor toxic reactive metabolites have been demonstrated in the most common form of lung fibrosis, idiopathic pulmonary fibrosis.

Progress in elucidating immunotoxicological mechanisms of drug-induced respiratory disease is limited by two factors: (1) the low incidence of drug immunotoxicity involving only the lower airways and alveoli; and (2) the natural inclination of physicians to switch to alternative drugs having less immunotoxic potential. These limitations have precluded prospective mechanistic investigations in drug-sensitive patients. It is therefore not surprising that major research in the field of pulmonary immunotoxicology is currently focused on occupational environmental substances that affect relatively large numbers of exposed workers. Moreover, the pathogenesis of these work-related problems often can be studied in greater detail by prospective epidemiological and laboratory experiments. The remainder of this discussion is concerned with diagnosis, differential diagnosis, immunopathogenetic mechanisms, and relevant examples that illustrate the important contributions being made to pulmonary immunotoxicology by investigation of occupationally induced immunological lung diseases (18).

The immunopathology of lung diseases caused by occupational antigens includes the four main categories of human hypersensitivity shown in Table 3. Type I reactions are mediated by specific IgE antibodies that sensitize mast cells and basophils throughout the body by combining with high affinity IgE receptors in the membranes of these cells. Once sensitization has been established, subsequent contact with the specific allergen—usually by inhalation in the workplace situation—results in cross-linking of the allergen with two adjacent cell fixed antibody molecules, thereby leading to complex activation of signals within the membrane, which ultimately causes release of preformed mediators (histamine) and the generation of membrane phospholipid-derived sulfidopeptides and platelet-activating factor. Potent chemotactic mediators are also released. This complex cascade of events may cause systemic symptoms (anaphylaxis) or localized symptoms (asthma, rhinitis, gastrointestinal disorders), depending on the route of exposure, the dose of allergen,

TABLE 3. *Classification of human hypersensitivity*

Type	Antibody	Immunocyte
I	Reagin (IgE, IgG$_4$)	B
II	Cytotoxic (IgM, IgG)	B
III	Immune complex (IgM, IgG)	B
IV	Delayed (cell-mediated)	T

and the amount of antibody bound to tissues. Many industrial proteins and reactive chemicals readily induce this form of human hypersensitivity. Under these conditions the primary target organ is the lower airways, but both upper and lower airways may be involved. At first the allergic inflammatory response evokes only an immediate reaction after inhalation exposure to the allergen, but if exposure continues for a longer period of time, the allergic inflammatory response becomes progressively more severe and ultimately results in both immediate and late asthmatic responses—the so-called late phase or dual response.

Type II reactions are mediated by cytotoxic IgM or IgG antibodies and also cause activation of complement after interaction with corresponding specific antigens. The classic pulmonary lesion corresponding to this category of antibody response is Goodpasture's syndrome, in which cytotoxic antibodies are produced against lung and renal basement membrane antigens. In this disease, cytotoxic reactions in the lung ultimately result in extensive pulmonary hemorrhage and death. Although no direct correlate of this syndrome has yet been encountered in industrial medicine, multiple hemorrhagic lesions of the lung associated with a hemolytic anemia have been reported in four workers after exposure and sensitization to trimellitic anhydride (27). Both pulmonary lesions and the hemolytic anemias cleared completely after these workers were removed from further exposure to this chemical compound. Similar pulmonary hemorrhagic lesions have been produced in an animal rat model (26).

Type III diseases are mediated by toxic immune complexes that are formed in slight antigen excess and may activate either classic or alternate complement pathways and in some cases both. Although high levels of specific IgG and/or precipitating antibodies may be associated with immune complex–mediated diseases, these are by no means pathognomonic of tissue damage. Tissue damage mediated by soluble immune complexes can only be demonstrated by direct evidence of necrotizing vasculitis or by deposition of immunofluorescent antibodies in tissues. The chief pulmonary pathological entities in this category include Wegener's granulomatosis, hypersensitivity angiitis, and periarteritis nodosa. Since etiological factors can rarely be demonstrated in these conditions, little is known about the immunological genesis and persistence of these diseases. After exposure and sensitization to trimellitic anhydride, some workers developed a late respiratory system syndrome that is characterized by fever, myalgias, and chills occurring 6 or more hours after exposure (27). These workers also exhibited high levels of IgG antibodies. Based on the latter immune responses and the late occurrence of symptoms, it was postulated but not proved that this syndrome could have a type III immunopathogenetic background. Methylene diphenyldiisocyanate–induced hypersensitivity pneumonitis may be associated with the presence of specific precipitating antibodies, but it is unlikely that type III mechanisms alone account for the complex histopathological sequelae of hypersensitivity pneumonitis (25).

The prototype of cell-mediated reactivity (type IV) in the pulmonary system is the tuberculous histopathological response. Delayed hypersensitivity T lymphocytes account for the classic round cell (lymphocytes and macrophages) infiltrates associated with these diseases. T lymphocytes and macrophages produce a variety of substances that are important immunomodulators of the type IV immune response. Included among these are fibrosis-generating factors, macrophage inhibitory factor, leukocyte inhibitory factor, and several types of histamine releasing factors. Berylliosis is the classic example of how severe and progressive cell-mediated sensitization can be after inhalation of a simple chemical compound. Cell-mediated immune responses have also been observed after exposure to a variety of other occupational chemicals, but the immunopathogenetic significance of these associations remains to be determined. Some relevant examples are discussed later in this chapter.

The clinical diagnosis of pulmonary immunotoxicological problems requires special attention to detailed history taking with emphasis on prior drugs taken, the extent and duration of inhalation exposure, allergic susceptibility, coprecipitating factors (smoking, alpha$_1$-antitrypsin deficiency), and the nature of the immunogen. Physical examination is rarely helpful. Similarly, the chest x-ray study has limited diagnostic discrimination. Pulmonary function testing can be very helpful in cases of lower airways obstruction and diseases affecting the alveolar membranes. Many of the techniques mentioned in Chapter 2 have useful applications in the diagnosis of occupational immune-mediated lung disease. The direct skin test may be the most sensitive indicator of IgE-mediated sensitivity. Both IgE and IgG humoral antibodies may be detected by specific *in vitro* methods. Patch tests and/or tuberculin-like intradermal tests may be useful *in vivo* tests for confirming the presence of delayed hypersensitivity. Several *in vitro* correlates of cell-mediated immunity have been utilized as objective measurements of type IV hypersensitivity reactions. Under special circumstances, direct inhalation challenges performed under controlled laboratory conditions may be indicated to corroborate the presence of occupational asthma or hypersensitivity pneumonitis.

Occupational asthma is one of the most promising human models for future investigation of pulmonary immunotoxicological phenomena. If investigated properly, outbreaks of occupational asthma should be assessed as mini–air pollution epidemiological models, the components of which are sources of exposure, release, dispersion, impaction, and biomedical effects. The proper evaluation of these air pollution compartments requires expert assistance from aerosol scientists, chemists, industrial hygienists, toxicologists, immunologists, and physician specialists. The vast majority of pulmonary immunotoxicological contributions from our laboratory have occurred as a result of our interest in a variety of work-related asthma problems.

The initial approach to the assessment of occupational asthma is to differentiate asthma from other obstructive airways diseases (6). The reactive airways dysfunction syndrome may be confused with immune-mediated asthma. This syndrome is characterized by persistent bronchospasm appearing after a single massive exposure to a toxic gas such as ammonia, sulfur dioxide, or nitrous oxide. Initially, the symptoms of the reactive airways dysfunction syndrome cannot be distinguished from those of bronchitis, but when it becomes obvious that the bronchospasm is persisting for long periods of time, the disease resembles asthma more than bronchitis. Bronchiolitis obliterans is an end stage fibrosing process in the respiratory bronchiole after exposure to highly irritative gases and vapors. The respiratory epithelium is denuded after the acute inhalation injury, infection by respiratory tract flora occurs, and the inflammatory sequelae of organizing pneumonitis and/or peribronchial fibrosis ensue. Small airways obstruction may also be associated in the adult acute respiratory distress syndrome, fibrotic pulmonary diseases (silicosis, asbestosis), emphysema, and hypersensitivity pneumonitis. The recognition that obstructive dysfunction exists in this heterogeneous group of nonasthmatic clinical entities is an absolute prerequisite to proper differential diagnosis of occupational asthma.

Occupationally associated asthma may have several types of clinical presentations. Preexistent asthma may be aggravated by nonspecific stimuli or irritants at work. If the job involves cold exposure, for example, preexistent asthma is almost always aggravated. Exercise and subtoxic levels of sulfur dioxide are also common irritants. The classic case of occupationally induced asthma occurs after a variable period of exposure or "sensitization" to the offending agent, during which time the worker is asymptomatic. Thereafter, the worker may experience immediate symptoms of bronchospasm shortly after exposure is resumed. The immediate nature of symptoms is most apparent on Mondays after a weekend of nonexposure to the occupational agent. In other cases, symptoms may be minor on Monday mornings but may gradually become more severe during the rest of the week as exposure becomes more intense. Symptomatic responses become progressively worse as late phase asthmatic responses begin to appear. The late phase response may appear anywhere from 2 to 12 hours after subsidence of the acute asthmatic response. Therefore, it is not unusual for many workers with severe occupational asthma to complain of persistent asthma at night and in some cases even after 1 or 2 work-free days. There are also valid examples of patients without a significant immediate phase bronchospastic response but with a much more severe late clinical response pattern. The terminology for these varied responses recognizes three categories: (a) immediate responders, (b) late responders, and (c) dual responders. Recently, a new aspect of occupational asthma—persistence of asthma after removal from exposure—has been recognized with greater frequency (8,16). Long-term clinical and pulmonary function measurements of workers removed from the work environment as long as 4 years after the onset of occupational asthma have demonstrated that as many as 60% of the terminated work force may have persistent asthma. This is a very important problem for future research in pulmonary immunotoxicology because it suggests not only that immune-generated disease may persist for long periods of time without further exposure to the original immunogen but also that the original immunotoxicological process may elicit a long-term nonspecific host response.

Nonimmunological factors must be clearly distinguished from immunological ones as causes of occupational asthma (2). Nonspecific bronchial hyperresponsiveness commonly occurs in workers exposed to cotton, flax, or hemp dusts. Immunological factors cannot be demonstrated in the vast majority of workers who develop toluene diisocyanate–induced asthma, even though there is always a latent incubation period and symptoms develop at very low exposure levels (<20 ppb). Organophosphates cause asthma presumably as pharmacological antagonists by inhibiting cholinesterase activity at vagus nerve terminal branches. A variety of industrial dusts (e.g., aluminum, talc) may stimulate irritant nerve receptors in the tracheobronchial tree. Exercise, exposure to cold, and subirritant threshold levels of sulfur dioxide are well-known reflex-induced causes of asthma. Liberation of anaphylatoxins (C3a and C5a) may act as direct histamine-releasing agents on mast cells and basophils, thereby leading to smooth muscle spasm. Both organic grain dusts and plicatic acid, the chief organic acid in Western red cedar, possess this unique property.

The pulmonary immunotoxicologist is concerned primarily with industrial agents that function as immunogens. High molecular weight substances such as proteins and polysaccharides are both antigenic and immunogenic. They also have multiple epitopic domains that account for heterogeneous immune responses in the intact animal. Proteins are of special importance in this regard because much has been learned about peptide domains on these molecules and how important they are in eliciting immune responses. In contrast, low molecular weight materials such as drugs and chemicals are antigenic but lack immunogenic properties. According to the classic hypothesis of Landsteiner, low molecular weight molecules must first be conjugated to carrier proteins before acquiring the property of immunogenicity. Even low molecular weight molecules may have several epitopes or reactive sites that, after combination with proteins at various side groups (e.g., amino acid, carboxyl), may form new antigenic determinants within the protein molecule.

The list of high and low molecular weight immunogens and allergens is extensive and is covered in greater detail elsewhere (2). Exposure to high molecular weight material substances such as laboratory animal proteins, enzymes, and a variety of plant proteins is likely to induce classic IgE-mediated reactions in atopic, susceptible workers. These immune sequelae can be readily demonstrated by direct skin tests and several *in vitro* specific IgE diagnostic tests.

Among the industrial low molecular weight compounds that we have investigated extensively are various acid anhydride compounds, a variety of diisocyanates, platinum salts, and salts of several transition metals. Precise prevalence statistics about exposure and sensitization to these compounds are not available, but some estimates were provided by the National Institute of Occupational Safety and Health several years ago (6). It is estimated that 200,000 workers are exposed to acid anhydrides that are used extensively in the plastic and resin industries and are dispersed as dusts, aerosols, and vapors. The rate of sensitization in this group of workers may be as high as 20%. About 160,000 workers are now exposed to diisocyanates. The rate of sensitization or asthma in this group has been estimated to be within the range of 5 to 10%. Although a relatively small number of workers are exposed to platinum salts in platinum heavy refining operations, the rate of sensitization among this group of workers is estimated to be as high as 35%.

Basic immunochemical principles must be appreciated and applied before immunotoxicological investigations can be undertaken. Preparatory methods for respective immunological reagents vary, depending on the innate reactivity of the chemical compound itself, the number and reactivity of intermediate metabolites, and the types of chemical interactions with carrier proteins. Generally, an attempt is made to restrict the number of haptenic (chemical) combining sites on each molecule of protein, although this can be difficult to accomplish in a precise manner when highly reactive chemicals such as diisocyanates are involved. Nevertheless, oversubstitution of haptenic ligands can usually be prevented by limiting the time of incubation of hapten with protein (22). In some cases it is possible to obtain preferential binding with certain residues (e.g., lysine) by prior chemical blocking of other reactive moieties within the protein molecule. Techniques used for chemical characterization of ligand binding vary, depending upon the nature of specific chemical interactions. Most investigators have used human serum albumin as the carrier protein because it is a common transport protein and it also has a generous number of lysine residues to which many of these chemicals are readily attached. It is also important to realize that immunological specificity can be directed toward the hapten alone, carrier protein, or new antigenic determinants created by the ligand binding process. Such specificities must be tested by appropriate inhibition experiments using simple salts of the respective ligands or monoamino acid conjugates of the ligands. Such immunochemical characterizations have become a fertile field of research for industrial pulmonary immunotoxicologists. The remainder of this chapter discusses several relevant immune-mediated occupational asthma problems and how immunochemical technology may be applied to gain further insights into pathogenetic mechanisms.

Although the clinical features of diisocyanate-induced asthma are highly suggestive of a sensitization process, the current status of immunopathogenesis in this disease is highly controversial. Several groups of investigators have observed that specific IgE sensitization occurs in a minority (5 to 10%) of workers with toluene diisocyanate–induced asthma (1). On the other hand, our laboratory has reported that a majority of clinically symptomatic toluene diisocyanate workers develop delayed hypersensitivity to this compound, as indexed by positive leukocyte inhibitory factor tests (10). There is as yet no direct evidence that these immunological findings are related to clinical asthma in these workers. Cross-sectional surveys have also been conducted among workers exposed to methylene diphenyldiisocyanate (13). The use of this compound in foundry operations and polyurethane foam packaging kits has increased dramatically in recent years. It has a higher molecular weight than toluene diisocyanate and is available chiefly in the polymeric form as it is dispersed through the work environment. This unique property, as compared to toluene diisocyanate, may account for higher percentages of sensitized workers with clearly identifiable methylene diphenyldiisocyanate–specific skin and positive radioallergosorbent test (RAST). Moreover, both symptomatic and asymptomatic workers were found to have significant levels of methylene diphenyldiisocyanate–specific IgG antibodies. None of these exposed workers had precipitating antibodies, but there have been several individual case reports of methylene diphenyldiiso-cyanate–induced hypersensitivity pneumonitis associated with methylene diphenyl-diisocyanate precipitins (25). Similar to what occurs in toluene diisocyanate–sensitive workers, positive leukocyte inhibitory factor tests also occur in symptomatic methylene diphenyldiisocyanate workers. In fact, a positive leukocyte inhibitory factor test was the only immunological finding in one of our workers with severe asthma and a well-documented dual response after bronchial challenge with a sub-toxic dose (<20 ppb) of diisocyanate.

Occupational asthma induced by acid anhydride compounds is clearly associated with IgE-dependent mechanisms. This was first demonstrated in a phthalic an-hydride worker whose sensitivity was confirmed by direct bronchial tests, positive prick tests, and positive RASTs (15). Similar immunoreactivity was observed in other groups of workers exposed to trimellitic anhydride, hexahydrophthalic an-hydride, himic anhydride, and tetrachlorophthalic anhydride (3). Type I sensitiza-tion to these agents was confirmed by one or more objective tests of immediate hypersensitivity. This clinical experience suggested that acid anhydride–induced asthma might be a preferred human model in the clinical discipline of pulmonary immunotoxicology. Extensive immunochemical investigations were therefore un-dertaken to characterize various ligand specificities and cross-reactivities (4). Using chemically defined acid anhydride coupled human serum albumin conjugates and various sodium salts of the respective acid anhydride compounds, it was possible to compare relative inhibitory capacities (in molar equivalents) of homologous and heterologous antigens in various groups of proven acid anhydride–sensitive work-ers. These studies revealed heterogeneity of IgE antibody responses among individ-ual workers. For example, two types of phthalic anhydride–sensitive workers were identified. One phthalic anhydride–sensitive individual developed IgE hapten-spe-cific antibodies to the phthalic anhydride moiety alone as assessed by the equimolar inhibitory capacity of the corresponding sodium phthalate salt. In contrast, another phthalic anhydride worker's serum had no evidence of hapten-specific antibodies but reacted only to the complete conjugate, indicating that immunological specific-ity was directed to the new antigenic determinant formed by combination of phthalic anhydride with lysine residues on the human serum albumin molecule. The new antigenic determinant is most likely phthalimide which, by itself, also has inhibitory properties. Hexahydrophthalic anhydride–sensitive workers showed specificity only toward the new antigenic determinant moiety, but one himic anhydride–sensi-tive individual showed specificities directed both to the hapten and the new anti-genic determinant. The latter individual's serum also cross-reacted with hexa-hydrophthalic anhydride. The cross-reacting antibodies were directed against both the heterologous hapten and the new antigenic hexahydrophthalic anhydride deter-minant. These series of experiments revealed that both hapten and new antigenic determinant specificities exist in human IgE antibody systems, thereby confirming once again the elegant experiments originally described by Landsteiner for IgG antibody and cell-mediated host responses. The ease with which antibodies were induced against new antigenic determinants on homologous human proteins also suggests that autoantigens formed after various types of occupational exposures could serve as possible models of human autoimmune disease.

Hypersensitivity reactions to platinum and other precious metal salts constitute another important human model of pulmonary immunotoxicology. The incidence of immediate hypersensitivity reactions to chlorinated platinum salts is very high. The majority of sensitized workers first develop rhinoconjunctivitis, which is almost always followed by the appearance of clinical asthma. IgE sensitization is readily corroborated by simple prick skin test reactions to very dilute concentrations of platinum salts (5). One group of investigators also reported positive RAST reactions to platinum salt–human albumin conjugates (9). However, this serological assay could not be confirmed in our laboratory, and alternative immunological reagents were developed. It was determined that irreversible binding of platinum occurred after combination with its specific metallo-binding protein, maleic dehydrogenase. Using this stable reagent, positive RAST findings were demonstrated in the majority of sera from workers with platinum asthma (5). Moreover, the sensitivity of this assay was greatly enhanced by a technique designed to remove traces of free platinum from the sera of sensitive workers. It was postulated that traces of platinum in serum were leached from stored platinum fat depots and that this unbound serum platinum interfered with the RAST assay by acting as an inhibitory hapten. Removal of free platinum from the sera of sensitive workers with polyacrylamide gel significantly improved the sensitivity of the RAST assay. Several other intriguing observations about platinum-sensitive workers require further investigations. Platinum-sensitive workers who had been removed from the workplace for periods ranging from 6 months to 4 years still exhibited very high levels of total IgE and platinum-specific RAST reactions. In addition, most of them still exhibited markedly positive skin test responses to platinum salts. None of these workers had been exposed directly to platinum after their work experiences were terminated. The persistence of high degrees of specific platinum sensitivity in these workers is as yet unexplained. To some extent, it is possible that continuation of platinum exposure could be due to leaching of trace amounts of platinum from stored fat depots. However, it is unlikely that this process would continue as long as 4 years. It has also been suggested that platinum itself could act as an immunomodulatory adjuvant. Preliminary experimental data in a rat model suggest that this might be a viable alternative hypothesis (17).

This brief survey of human pulmonary immunotoxicology indicates that this newly emerging specialty is in the phenomenology stage of scientific inquiry. Nevertheless, current research trends are promising in several areas of drug and occupational chemical immunotoxicity. The scientific data concerning autoantigens formed by toxic drug metabolites and occupational reactive chemicals are now established to the point where molecular biological probes could lead to increased understanding of the pathological and physiological effects of these substances. Cell-mediated immunity is associated with many forms of occupationally associated pulmonary lesions—including asthma—and further research about the possible toxic effects of cell-derived lymphokines merits more detailed investigation. Finally, it is probable that the immunomodulatory roles of inhaled immunogens and nonimmunogens will also be a fertile area of active future research.

REFERENCES

1. Bernstein, I. L. (1982): Isocyanate-induced pulmonary diseases: A current perspective. In Symposium Proceedings on Occupational Immunologic Lung Disease, edited by R. Patterson and R. A. Goldstein. *J. Allergy Clin. Immunol.* 70:24–31.
2. Bernstein, I. L. (1985): Occupational asthma. In Allergy, edited by A. P. Kaplan. Churchill Livingstone, Inc., New York.
3. Bernstein, I. L., and Bernstein, D. I. (1984): Respiratory allergy to synthetic resins. *Clin. Immunol.*, 4:83–101.
4. Bernstein, D. I., Gallagher, J. S., D'Souza, L., et al. (1984): Heterogeneity of specific-IgE responses in workers sensitized to acid anhydride compounds. *J. Allergy Clin. Immunol.*, 74:794–801.
5. Biagini, R. E., Bernstein, I. L., Gallagher, J. S., et al. (1985): The diversity of reaginic immune responses to platinum and palladium metallic salts. *J. Allergy Clin. Immunol.*, 76:794–802.
6. Brooks, S. M., and Kalica, A. R. (1987): NHLBI Workshop Summary. Strategies for elucidating the relationship between occupational exposures and chronic air-flow obstruction. *Am. Rev. Respir. Dis.*, 135:268–273.
7. Budinsky, R. A., Roberts, S. M., Coats, E. A., et al. (1987): The formation of procainamide hydroxylamine by rat and human liver microsomes. *Drug Metab. Dispos.*, 15:37–43.
8. Chan-Yeung, M., MacLean, L., and Paggiaro, P. L. (1987): Follow-up study of 232 patients with occupational asthma caused by western red cedar (*Thuja plicata*). *J. Allergy Clin. Immunol.*, 79:792–796.
9. Cromwell, O., Pepys, J., Parish, W. E., et al. (1979): Specific IgE antibodies to platinum salts in sensitized workers. *Clin. Allergy*, 9:109–117.
10. Gallagher, J. S., Tse, C. S. T., Brooks, S. M., et al. (1981): Diverse profiles of immunoreactivity in toluene diisocyanate (TDI) asthma. *J. Occup. Med.*, 23:610–616.
11. Hoeffler, H. B., and Greenberg, S. D. (1982): Bronchiectasis following pulmonary ammonia burn. *Arch. Pathol. Lab.*, 106:686–687.
12. Karnofsky, D. A. (1967): Late effects of immunosuppressive anticancer drugs. *Fed. Proc.*, 26:925–933.
13. Liss, G. M., Bernstein, D. I., Moller, D. R., et al. (1988): Pulmonary and immunologic evaluation of foundry workers exposed to methylene diphenyldiisocyanate (MDI). *J. Allergy Clin. Immunol.*, 82:55–61.
14. Littler, W. A., Ogilvie, C. (1970): Lung function in patients receiving busulphan. *Br. Med. J.*, 4:530–532.
15. Maccia, C. A., Bernstein, I. L., Emmett, E. A., et al. (1976): *In vitro* demonstration of specific IgE in phthalic anhydride hypersensitivity. *Am. Rev. Respir. Dis.*, 113:701–704.
16. Moller, D. R., Brooks, S. M., McKay, R. T., et al. (1986): Chronic asthma due to toluene diisocyanate. *Chest*, 90:494–499.
17. Murdoch, R. D., and Pepys, J. (1986): Enhancement of antibody production by mercury and platinum group metal halide salts. Kinetics of total and ovalbumin-specific IgE synthesis. *Int. Arch. Allergy Appl. Immunol.*, 80:405–411.
18. Patterson, R. and Goldstein, R. A. (eds.) (1982): Symposium Proceedings on Occupational Immunologic Lung Disease. *J. Allergy Clin. Immunol.*, 70:1–72.
19. Rossing, T. H. (1986): Pulmonary infiltrates with eosinophilia (PIE) syndrome and asthma. *Med. Grand Rounds*, 4:84–93.
20. Shear, N. H., Spielberg, S. P., Grant, D. M., et al. (1986): Differences in metabolism of sulfonamides predisposing to idiosyncratic toxicity. *Ann. Intern. Med.*, 105:179–184.
21. Sheffer, A. L., Rocklin, R. E., and Goetzl, E. J. (1975): Immunologic components of hypersensitivity reactions to cromolyn sodium. *N. Engl. J. Med.*, 293:1220–1224.
22. Tse, C. S. T., and Pesce, A. J. (1979): Chemical characterization of isocyanate-protein conjugates. *Toxicol. Appl. Pharmacol.*, 51:39–46.

23. Uetrecht, J. P. (1985): Reactivity and possible significance of hydroxylamine and nitroso metabolites of procainamide. *J. Pharmacol. Exp. Ther.*, 232:420–425.
24. Uetrecht, J. P., Sweetman, B. J., Woosley, R. L., et al. (1984): Metabolism of procainamide to a hydroxylamine by rat and human hepatic microsomes. *Drug Metab. Dispos.*, 12:77–81.
25. Zeiss, C. R., Kanellakes, T. M., Bellone, T. D., et al. (1980): Immunoglobulin E-mediated asthma and hypersensitivity pneumonitis with precipitating antihapten antibodies due to diphenylmethane diisocyanate (MDI) exposure. *J. Allergy Clin. Immunol.*, 65:346–352.
26. Zeiss, C. R., Levitz, D., Leach, C. L., et al. (1987): A model of immunologic lung injury induced by trimellitic anhydride inhalation: Antibody response. *J. Allergy Clin. Immunol.*, 79:59–63.
27. Zeiss, C. R., Patterson, R., Pruzansky, J. J., et al. (1977): Trimellitic anhydride-induced airway syndromes: Clinical and immunologic studies. *J. Allergy Clin. Immunol.*, 60:96–103.

Clinical Immunotoxicology, edited by
D. S. Newcombe, N. R. Rose, and J. C. Bloom.
Raven Press, Ltd., New York © 1992.

14

The Immunopathogenesis of Pulmonary Responses to Environmental and Chemical Pollutants

David S. Newcombe

*Department of Environmental Health Sciences, Johns Hopkins University,
School of Hygiene and Public Health, Baltimore, MD*

In humans, the immune system consists of primary lymphoid tissues (thymus, bone marrow, and fetal liver) and secondary lymphoid tissues (spleen, lymph nodes, gut-associated lymphoid tissues, and bronchial-associated lymphoid tissues) in addition to the cells derived from these organs and tissues. Except for bone marrow, primary and secondary lymphoid organs are usually not available for immunopathological analyses in the living host. However, cells derived from these organs for the regulation of innate and adaptive immunity are accessible, and immunological analyses of these cells are useful both in evaluating immune-mediated tissue responses and in characterizing immunotoxic mechanisms.

Peripheral blood cells and bronchoalveolar lavage (BAL) specimens have been used to assess inflammatory and immune responses and to identify and characterize disorders of the respiratory tract and lung. The latter organ systems also represent a primary portal of entry for toxic substances and have direct links to vascular compartments that distribute toxicants to their sites of toxic action, storage, detoxification, or elimination. Thus, immunotoxicological changes could be reflected in the cells and soluble constituents recovered from peripheral blood and BAL after exposure to toxic substances.

This chapter reviews the pathogenesis of immune-mediated injuries of the animal and human lung associated with environmental and occupational exposures. Its purpose is to characterize both the specific and nonspecific immunological responses of the lung to a variety of substances that implicate the immune system of the lung in the pathogenesis of the diseases resulting from environmental and/or occupational exposures. In some cases, the immunological responses fall into well-defined types of immunopathological processes, such as the IgE-mediated hypersensitivity responses observed with occupational asthma, whereas other cases, such as silicosis, defy distinct classification into specific types of immunopathological processes but do alter components of the host's immune system.

The clinical expression of the environmental and occupational disorders to be dealt with here has been described in detail in a variety of other publications and is not discussed in this chapter.

IMMUNE SYSTEM OF THE LUNG

The conducting airways of the lung have two separate immune defense systems: (a) mononuclear phagocytic cells and mast cells localized to the surface of the large and small conducting airways (100,236,300,350), and (b) bronchus-associated lymphatic tissue (BALT) consisting of lymphatic follicles with germinal centers in the submucosal lamina propria (36,206,367). Although most of the luminal macrophages probably represent cells laden with debris being transported by the mucociliary escalator, some bronchial macrophages are tightly adherent to epithelial cells, and their functions as tissue macrophages are incompletely characterized. The lymphoid aggregates of the BALT system appear to be comparable to Peyer's patches in the small bowel, since they can repopulate the lung with IgA-synthesizing cells. Specialized epithelial cells (M cells) form the surface area over the BALT and these M cells have the unique capacity to ingest and transport antigens across the bronchial mucosa to the BALT system, where such antigens may be presented to helper lymphocytes (36,412). Other investigations have suggested that alveolar macrophages may process antigens and then migrate through the bronchial epithelium and present processed antigen to the BALT (350).

Distal airways also have several immune systems, including alveolar macrophages and small numbers of lymphocytes residing in the alveolar space, lymphoid aggregates without germinal centers, and lymphatic channels arising from submucosal lymphoid aggregates with connections to the BALT. The primary precursor of the alveolar macrophage is the bone marrow–derived monocyte, but additional sources also exist for these macrophages (527). Less than 10% of alveolar macrophages can be renewed by self-replication, and there is a suggestion that lung tissue macrophages may migrate from the interstitial spaces to the alveolus (39). The longevity of the alveolar macrophage in humans is unknown but is probably longer than 30 days. Macrophages migrate from the alveolar space and respiratory mucosa during the transport of foreign body–laden cells up the mucociliary escalator to the pharnyx, and such cells are then either swallowed or expectorated. Some alveolar macrophages migrate to the BALT system via specialized bronchial epithelium, and others may cross the epithelial layers and gain access to the peribronchial lymphatics, where they may be transported to the tracheobronchial lymph nodes.

In the nonsmoker, lymphocytes represent about 10% of the cell population recovered by BAL, and such lymphocytes are functionally competent (Table 1). Of these lymphocytes, 85% are small (<8 μm in diameter) and 10% are large (>9 μm). T lymphocytes account for 60% to 80%, B lymphocytes for 5% to 10%, and null cells

TABLE 1. *Bronchoalveolar lavage lymphocyte profiles in nonsmoker healthy humans*

Total lymphocyte cell numbers	$1.05 - 1.80 \times 10^6$/lavage
Lymphocytes (% of total)	
T-lymphocytes	70
Helper/inducer	50
Suppressor/cytotoxic	30
Killer T-lymphocytes	7
B-lymphocytes	5–10
Untypeable lymphocytes	5

Modified from Reynolds, H. Y. (1986): *J. Allergy Clin. Immunol*, 78:833, with permission.

without lymphocyte markers account for the remainder of the cells (206,341,570). Some of these null cells represent nonfunctional, large, granular lymphocytes (natural killer cells). The ratio of helper to suppressor lymphocytes in BAL specimens is similar to that in the peripheral blood (1.6:1). Since the ratio of helper to suppressor cells is comparable to that in the peripheral blood, the suggestion has been made that lung lymphocytes originate in blood. The ultimate fate of these cells has not been determined.

In the extraalveolar spaces, lymphatic channels may exist, and these spaces also contain mononuclear cells, including macrophages, lymphocytes, and plasma cells. Such perivascular accumulations of cells provide ready access to regional lymph nodes. Thus, the cellular constituents of the lung clearly indicate that this organ has the capacity to generate immune responses and that such responses may contribute to lung pathology.

TYPE I HYPERSENSITIVITY

In the human, airborne dusts, gases, vapors, and fumes make initial contact with the skin and/or respiratory tract, and the latter organ systems utilize cells of the immune system to detect, localize, and dispose of those substances foreign to the host. The immune responses generated are usually sufficient to protect the host from tissue invasion and damage by these foreign substances but adequately regulated to avoid pathological changes during the detoxification and disposal processes. However, pathological responses may occur in the setting of diminished or absent immune responsivity, altered immunoregulation leading to an exaggerated or inappropriate adaptive immune response, or an overwhelmed immune system. Coombs and Gel classified such immunopathological responses as types I, II, III, and IV hypersensitivity reactions (101). The first three responses are antibody-dependent and represent humoral immune responses. Type IV reactions are cell-mediated responses and are dependent on the presence of T cells and macrophages.

In the lung, type I hypersensitivity reactions are exemplified by the induction of IgE-mediated asthma after exposure to a variety of inorganic or organic substances (Table 2). The pathogenesis of these asthmatic attacks requires the production of

TABLE 2. *Occupational asthma*

Vectors	Industries	Skin tests
High Molecular Weight Substances		
Animal products (vertebrates)	Laboratory workers	
	Veterinarians	+
	Animal handlers	
Animal products (birds)	Pigeon breeders	+
	Poultry workers	+
	Bird fanciers	
Insect products		
Mite (grain)	Grain workers	+
Locust	Laboratory workers	
Fly (river)	River occupations/sites	
Fly (screw worm)	Flight crews	
Cockroach	Laboratory workers	+
Cricket	Field workers	+
Moth (bee)	Fish bait breeders	+
Butterfly	Entomologists	
Plants		
Buckwheat	Bakers	
Castor bean	Oil extractors	+
Coffee bean	Food processor	+
Grain dust	Grain handlers	+
Hops (*Humulus lupulus*)	Brewery workers	
Tea	Tea workers	+
Tobacco leaf	Tobacco manufacturer	+
Wheat/rye flour	Bakers/millers	+
Biologic enzymes		
B. Subtilis	Detergent workers	+
Bromelin	Pharmaceutical industry	+
Flaviastase	Pharmaceutical industry	
Fungal amylase	Manufacturing, bakers	
Pancreatin	Pharmaceutical industry	
Paparin	Laboratory/packing	+
Pepsin	Pharmaceutical industry	+
Trypsin	Plastics/pharmaceutical industry	+
Vegetables		
Gum acacia	Printers	+
Gum tragacanth	Gum manufacturing	
Other		
Crab	Crab processing	+
Hoya	Oyster farming	
Prawn	Prawn processing	+
Silkworm larva	Sericulture	+
Low Molecular Weight Substances		
Anhydrides		
Phthalic anhydride	Plastics/resins	+
Tetrachlorophthalic anhydride	Plastics/resins	+
Trimetallic anhydride	Plastics/resins	+
Diisocyanates		
Diphenylmethane diisocyanate	Foundries	+
Hexamethylene diisocyanate	Spray painting	+
Toluene diisocyanate	Plastics/varnish	+
Drugs		
Amprolium hydrochloride	Poultry feed mixer	+
Cephalosporins	Pharmaceutical	+

TABLE 2. *Continued*

Vectors	Industries	Skin Tests
Methyldopa	Pharmaceutical	+
Penicillins	Pharmaceutical	+
Phenylglycine acid chloride	Pharmaceutical	+
Piperazine hydrochloride	Chemists	+
Psyllium	Laxative manufacturing	+
Salbutamol intermediate	Pharmaceutical	+
Spiramycin	Pharmaceutical	+
Sulfone chloramides	Manufacturer, brewer	+
Tetracycline	Pharmaceutical	+
Metals		
Chromium	Tanning	+
Cobalt	Hard metal industry	+
Nickel	Metal plating	+
Platinum	Platinum refinery	+
Tungsten carbide	Hard metal industry	
Vanadium	Hard metal industry	
Other chemicals		
Azodicarbonamide	Plastics/rubber	
Dimethyl ethanolamine	Spray painting	+
Dioazonium salt	Photocopying/dye	+
Ethylene diamine	Photography	+
Formalin	Hospital staff	+
Freon	Refrigeration	+
Furfuryl alcohol	Foundry mold making	+
Hexachlorophene	Hospital staff	+
Paraphenylene diamine	Fur dying	+
Persulfate salts and henna	Hairdressing	+
Urea formaldehyde	Insulation/resin	+

Modified from Chan-Yeung and Lam, ref. 87, with permission.

cytotropic IgE antibodies in response to antigen exposure; these antibodies bind through their Fc receptors to tissue mast cells, causing their sensitization (282). On occasion, cytotoxic IgG antibodies may be generated that bind to mast cells or basophils (184). On reexposure to antigen, multivalent antigens seek IgE or rarely IgG tissue–fixed antibodies, and one antigen molecule reacts with two Fc receptor–anchored IgE antibodies, resulting in a cross-linkage between the antibody molecules. This bridging of IgE antibodies triggers an enzymatically regulated cascade of reactions that causes the degranulation of the mast cell (283,372,373). Subsequent dissolution of these granules releases preformed allergic mediators such as histamine, heparin, neutrophil chemotactic factor, tryptase, kininogenase, and eosinophilic chemotactic factor of anaphylaxis. The cross-linkage of IgE antibodies also initiates the synthesis of potent lipid mediators derived from arachidonic acid such as prostaglandin D_2 (PGD_2), leukotrienes B_4, C_4, and D_4, and platelet-activating factor.

All these mediators and perhaps others to be better defined contribute to the induction of asthmatic bronchitis (2,118,365,382). Histamine release results in vasodilation, increased capillary permeability, chemokinesis, and bronchoconstriction. The leukotrienes also have vasoactive properties, cause bronchoconstriction, and are chemokinetic and chemotactic. In addition, these latter agents, together with PGD_2, cause mucosal edema and mucus secretion. The kinins generated from kininogenase activity also cause vasodilation and edema. Complement fragments (C3a), lymphokines, antigen-specific T-cell factors, and diesel exhaust particles may amplify mast cell degranulation and mediator release. The complement fragment, C3a, is generated from complement by the activity of tryptase released from mast cells, and lymphokines secreted by lymphocytes induce the release of histamine from basophils. This histamine-releasing activity is independent of the IgE-mediated histamine release. Diesel exhaust particles may also act as adjuvants in the production of IgE antibodies (522). Thus, these small (1 μm) diesel particles, together with a sensitizing antigen, may significantly increase the levels of IgE antibodies. Other environmental pollutants, such as sulfur dioxide, nitrogen oxides, diesel fumes, and fly ash, also have the capacity to increase mucosal permeability and may increase the quantity of antigen available for reaction with IgE-sensitized cells (121,231,288,314,360–362). In addition to antigen, anti-IgE receptor antibodies, antiidiotype antibodies, anti-Fc receptor antibodies, and lectins can trigger the release of mediators from IgE-sensitized cells. IgG_4, like IgE, can also sensitize mast cells, but the frequency of IgG-mediated hypersensitivity reactions is low (75, 243,257,413,419,420,491).

Several risk factors may contribute to the expression of type I hypersensitivity reactions. Abnormal states of hypersensitivity (atopy) recognized by a family history of allergic disorders, elevated serum IgE levels, and in some cases histocompatibility locus antigen (HLA) associations with such allergic diatheses may signal an increased susceptibility to type I hypersensitivity responses (58,87). Cigarette smoking, through its capacity to increase epithelial permeability, may also contribute to the enhanced penetration of antigens known to cause hypersensitivity responses, but the actual role of cigarette smoke in the induction of such responses is controversial (64–66,85,105,278,289,344,547,560,576). Evidence to support both an increased and decreased risk to smokers is described in the literature (87). Most patients with occupational asthma express nonspecific bronchial hyperreactivity to methacholine. Since this hyperreactivity may decrease when occupational exposures are removed, environmental exposure appears to be the primary vector rather than some undefined predisposition to bronchial hyperreactivity (68,331). Genetic studies of monozygotic and dizygotic twins have not characterized any genetic factors as the cause of airway responsivity to methacholine (572). Thus, despite the increased frequency of bronchial reactivity in patients with occupational asthma, this condition appears to be associated with the occupational exposure rather than with a genetic or ill-defined state of bronchial reactivity present in the host prior to environmental exposure.

Immune-mediated hypersensitivity reactions must be differentiated from other types of bronchoconstriction. Reflex bronchoconstriction occurs when patients with bronchial asthma are exposed to cold air, inert particles, or noxious gases that react with irritant receptors to cause bronchoconstriction (56,180,274,563). Since such irritants may aggravate preexisting asthma, they are not considered primary vectors of occupational asthma. Inflammatory bronchoconstriction results from exposure to irritants such as hydrogen sulfide, diethylene diamine fumes, smoke, or fumes from many chemicals used in a variety of industrial processes (194). In such cases, pathological examination shows extensive infiltration of the airways with inflammatory cells, mucosal damage, and tissue sloughing as well as hypertrophy of the bronchial submucosal glands (55,57,89,141). Changes associated with bronchial asthma are not always present in these irritant-mediated bronchial responses. Finally, pharmacological bronchoconstriction is a term derived from the observation that some work environments are contaminated by substances that behave like pharmacological agonists (70,83,148,427,466). Such substances are not considered vectors of occupational asthma because they do not manifest certain classic findings (e.g., eosinophilia, nonspecific hyperactivity) associated with asthma. Cotton dust, organophosphorus chemicals, isocyanates, and plicatic acid have been considered by some workers to represent environmental agents causing so-called pharmacological bronchoconstriction (33,68,86,119,148,403,559). Nonetheless, the mediators of such diseases remain incompletely defined in some cases and do not always support existing theories (60).

The absence of skin reactivity to a specific antigen and IgE antibodies and pathological changes in the airways that are more consistent with inflammation than asthma *may* help differentiate inflammation-induced bronchoconstriction from classic occupational asthma. Nonetheless, asthma caused by low molecular weight substances may be especially difficult to characterize, since these molecules may not be immunogenic by themselves. They often bind to tissue or serum proteins to facilitate their immunogenicity, and the formation of IgE antibodies against such a hapten-protein conjugate makes it exceedingly difficult both to characterize the antigen involved and to identify the IgE responses to such antigens. Plicatic acid, the compound responsible for Western red cedar asthma, and isocyanates such as toluene diisocyanate may represent low molecular weight substances of the sort in which the role of IgE antibodies may be controversial (11,28,69,71–73,85,114,192,297,410, 524,530), but the frequency of the asthma suggests a more selective mechanism than the simple induction of airways inflammation (88,537). As can be seen by comparing high and low molecular weight substances (see Table 2), high molecular weight compounds account for a much higher prevalence of specific IgE antibodies than do low molecular weight compounds (87). Thus, high molecular weight substances such as biological enzymes used in detergents and the pharmaceutical industry, dusts from insects, grain dusts, and animal products in most cases cause immediate skin reactivity to the appropriate antigen and usually induce specific IgE antibodies (15,18,34,41,45,46,61,94,120,139,173,181,204,235,249,250,262, 263,272,356,381,404,446,504,516,553).

Mast cells and alveolar macrophages are the key cellular operatives from which the chemical mediators of occupational asthma are released, and these cell types do not represent a homogeneous population of cells (25,58,140,244,273,342,440, 474,493,494,503). Mast cells have been shown to vary both in their morphology and their staining properties. Connective tissue mast cells found near blood vessels demonstrate different morphology, granule number, and size as well as pharmacological properties, depending on their tissue site (58). Mucosal mast cells, residents of the gastrointestinal tract and lung, increase in number in response to various pathological processes and appear to be regulated by T-cell factors. High affinity Fc_E receptors are present on mast cells and basophils, whereas low affinity receptors are present on T and B cells, monocytes, alveolar macrophages, and eosinophils (58,185,298,372,511). When cross-linked by their reaction with antigen, these receptors cause the release of lysosomal enzymes and the synthesis of leukotrienes that participate in asthmatic reactions (25,157). Mucosal mast cells produce primarily leukotriene C_4 (58), whereas corrective tissue mast cells generate 40 times more PGD_2 than leukotriene C_4. Recent investigations have focused on defining mast cell subsets by differences in their mediator production, response to secretagogues, and drug-induced alterations in mediator release. Improved characterizations of mast cell subsets recovered by BAL may also lead to a better understanding of the clinical subsets of occupational asthma.

Alveolar macrophages are also a heterogeneous population of cells derived, for the most part, from peripheral blood monocytes that produce a variety of mediators, including monokines (such as interleukin-1), arachidonic acid derivatives, and other substances with physiological activity. Human monocytes, precursors of alveolar macrophages, also clearly express heterogeneity in their physical properties, immunological responses, and mediator production (140,244,273,342,444,474, 493,494). On the basis of these findings alone, one might also expect alveolar macrophages, also clearly express heterogeneity in their physical properties, immunological responses, and mediator production (140,244,273,342,444,474,493, 494). On the basis of these findings alone, one might also expect alveolar macrophages to express heterogeneity, since they could arise from different monocyte precursors. A number of studies have now documented alveolar macrophage heterogeneity (140,244,273,342,444,474,493,494). Such heterogeneity may play a role in the variation of host responses to antigens. Macrophages are also a source of the mediators involved in the biphasic responses (immediate and late reactions) observed in occupational asthma. The synthesis and release of leukotrienes are not immediate responses but are triggered by antigen challenge and can be contrasted with the direct release of preformed mediators such as histamine (171,228,565). It fluid only during late phase responses (87). Leukotriene B_4, a neutrophil chemotaxin, in association with neutrophil chemotactic factor and eosinophil chemotactic factor of anaphylaxis, factors preformed and released from mast cell granules, cause the recruitment of inflammatory cells to the airways, and such recruitment contributes to the late phase asthmatic reaction.

In summary, type I hypersensitivity reactions in the lung are initiated by low and high molecular weight substances that cause the generation of cytotropic IgE, which sensitizes the host's mast cell by binding to its Fc receptor. Subsequent antigen challenge results in a cross-linking of the mast cell–bound IgE and causes the release of pharmacoactive substances that mediate bronchoconstriction, mucus release, and inflammatory cell chemotaxis. Such immediate and late phase mediators contribute to the initiation and persistence of the asthmatic bronchitis observed after occupational exposure to specific antigens.

TYPE II HYPERSENSITIVITY

Hypersensitivity type II, like type I, requires the presence of antibodies directed, in this case, against specific cell and tissue basement membranes. The mechanism for the induction of such antibody synthesis remains incompletely understood, but exposure to hydrocarbon fumes has been associated with the development of Goodpasture's syndrome, a disorder usually observed in young males with pulmonary hemorrhage, glomerulonephritis, and the linear deposit of immunoglobulins and complement on pulmonary alveolar and glomerular basement membranes (31,54, 229,269). Other age groups and females may also be affected by this disorder (415, 550). Hydrocarbon exposure appears to alter nonimmunogenic basement membrane such that an antigen not recognized as self is exposed, which triggers the synthesis of antibodies (29,79,178,305,310,312,330,396,447,485,577). The chemical determinants of these "neoantigens" that are not recognized as self have been characterized as carbohydrates associated with type IV collagen (301). In fact, evidence suggests that the glomerular basement membrane antigen responsible for initiating antibody synthesis is most probably a collagenase-resistant glycoprotein (398,564). These antitissue antibodies are usually of the IgG class, but rarely IgA antibodies have been detected (47,193,320,368,369). Such antibodies bind directly to alveolar and glomerular basement membranes, usually in association with complement.

There are two primary mechanisms by which damage to target cells and tissues may occur in type II hypersensitivity: (a) complement activation by antibody and the deposition of the C5b67-9 membrane attack complex on target cells (102, 107,111,387,557), and (b) interaction between C3b complement fragments and Fc immunoglobulin components, which act as recognition factors for inflammatory and immune cells recruited to the target tissue site that have C3b, C4b, and Fc receptors (166,538,539,568). The generation of C5a complement fragment results in neutrophil and monocyte chemotaxis, causes granulocyte aggregation, releases proteolytic enzymes from inflammatory cells, and stimulates oxidant production and the synthesis of leukotrienes (90,165,170,215,225–227,358,364,400,556). These C5a-mediated processes contribute to tissue damage (365). C3b and C4b complement fragments facilitate the binding of bacteria, viruses, and immune complexes to professional phagocytes and trigger IgG-mediated phagocytosis by neutrophils, monocytes, and macrophages through activation of their CR1 (complement) receptor, which in turn triggers a respiratory burst as a result of CR receptor activation and endocytosis (551). Complement fragments also concentrate immune complexes on antigen-presenting cells, and C3 may increase immune complex solubility by disrupting immunoglobulin lattices. In cases in which the targets of phagocytes are large, i.e., indigestible molecules such as basement membranes, a process known as frustrated phagocytosis occurs. The phagocyte, frustrated in its attempt to completely endocytose its target substance, releases its lysosomal enzymes to the extracellular milieu in an attempt to digest the target and causes damage to tissues and cells in the vicinity. Further, in the process of the phagocytosis of opsonized tissue components or other particles, phagocytes such as eosinophils, neutrophils, monocytes, macrophages, and killer cells demonstrate increased lysosomal enzyme activity and produce reactive oxygen intermediates. Such components not only mediate the destruction of pathogens and assist in the remodeling of damaged tissues but also may be vectors of immunopathologically mediated tissue and cell damage in type II hypersensitivity reactions. The role of killer cells remains to be elucidated in such hypersensitivity reactions, but these cells, like cytotoxic T cells, have the capacity to destroy other cells.

The membrane attack complex is formed by the selective binding of C5 to the C5 convertase enzyme (179). The subsequent nonenzymatic formation of the membrane attack complex is accomplished by the sequential binding of C5b, C6, and C7, which results in a hydrophobic complex capable of inserting itself into cell membrane lipid layers. Then, C8 and C9 bind to this membrane component and C9 polymerizes to form pores, permitting the leakage of intracellular components. Such cell leakage eventually results in cell death.

Animal models of Goodpasture's syndrome have clearly shown that the circulating anti–basement membranes are pathogenic because these antibodies can transfer glomerular damage to normal, healthy animals (145,213). In fact, the recipients of renal transplants who have circulating antiglomerular basement membrane antibodies develop glomerulonephritis in the transplanted kidney. Antiglomerular basement membrane antibodies are usually cross-reactive with alveolar basement membranes, but lung damage has been difficult to induce in experimental models (32,145). The latter findings may indicate that lung injury may be essential to the fixation of these antitissue antibodies that subsequently cause lung damage. These anti–basement membrane antibodies appear to be selective, since they do not react with glomerular basement membranes isolated from kidneys manifesting abnormal basement membrane components such as occurs in patients with some forms of hereditary nephritis (145).

Mercuric chloride in nontoxic amounts has been shown to cause the transient formation of antiglomerular basement membrane antibodies in Brown Norway (BN) rats (475). This disease appears to be a two-stage process with the production of anti–basement membrane antibodies initially and subsequently the formation of immune complexes with organ deposition (32). These mercury-treated rats develop lymphadenopathy, immunoglobulinemia (IgE and IgG), and antinuclear antibodies (30,143,268,421). The immunoglobulin elevations observed in these rats are striking, especially the IgE elevations. In some ways they resemble the responses observed in type I hypersensitivity reactions. In association with proteinuria and the nephrotic syndrome, these BN rats generate antiglomerular basement membrane antibodies that are deposited on kidney basement in a linear fashion (145). Further studies have shown that these antibodies react with type IV collagen, laminin, proteoglycan, and entactin (30,190). Despite the cross-reactivity of these antibodies with alveolar basement membrane in other settings, the alveolar basement membrane is not involved in the immunopathological reactions observed in the mercury-treated BN rat (32,145). This may indicate that alveolar damage is necessary for the deposition of alveolar basement membrane antibodies. Interestingly, the disease in BN rats can be transferred to normal BN rats by T cells from mercuric chloride–treated rats (422). In the human, chronic mercury poisoning may be associated with pulmonary and renal symptoms, including the nephrotic syndrome, but few studies have examined immunopathogenetic factors in such patients. Certainly, transfer of the lesion by T cells speaks to a cell-mediated process rather than a humoral one.

In summary, the association of type II hypersensitivity reactions with environmental toxins is tentative. Hydrocarbon fume exposure has been reported in patients with Goodpasture's syndrome, but no one has a large enough series of cases to confirm this association. Further, lung damage is difficult to induce in experimental models, so that toxic exposures in animal models have not been intensively investigated. Mercury causes the appearance of antiglomerular basement membrane antibodies in mice and rats, but human toxicity to this chemical has not been fully evaluated from this perspective. Type II hypersensitivity does not appear to be a major effector of immunotoxic responses in the lung.

TYPE III HYPERSENSITIVITY REACTIONS

Like type II hypersensitivity reactions, type III reactions also require antibodies, but they react with antigens to form immune complexes that trigger inflammatory processes. The antigens necessary for the formation of immune complexes may arise from endogenous or exogenous sources. Extrinsic antigens are the only known cause of environmental/occupational diseases resulting from type III hypersensitivity, and the pathogenesis of these disorders may be the result of type IV hypersensitivity reactions, since the formation of immune complexes may be a secondary phenomenon (251,371).

Extrinsic allergic alveolitis represents a family of hypersensitivity disorders that arise from the inhalation of extrinsic antigens, which then react with circulating antibodies to form immune complexes (451,470,489,490). The antibodies induced by these extrinsic antigens are, for the most part, IgG antibodies. Reexposure to the inhaled antigen may lead to immune complex formation if antibody levels are sufficient to react with antigens.

Precipitating antibodies are found in many patients with pigeon breeder's lung and farmer's lung, well-characterized forms of extrinsic allergic alveolitis, but they are also present in entirely asymptomatic healthy farm workers (75,103,104). Therefore, the role of immune complexes formed from the interaction of antigen with precipitating antibodies in the pathogenesis of this disorder remains in question. In fact, such data have led to the conclusion that type IV hypersensitivity reactions (see discussion to follow) are more significant contributors to the pathogenesis of these disorders than are type III reactions (451,470).

Immune complexes cause tissue damage by the following mechanisms: the generation of complement products, the reaction with Fc receptors, and the release of lysosomal enzymes (113). The generation of complement products such as C3a and C5a, as discussed previously, results in the chemotaxis of inflammatory cells and the release of vasoactive mediators that complement the inflammatory cell recruitment process by increasing vascular permeability. In addition to the interaction of the Fc portions of immune complexes with Fc receptors on neutrophils and monocytes during endocytosis, platelet Fc receptors interact with immune complexes to cause platelet aggregation and the production of microthrombi. Frustrated phagocytosis, protected from lysosomal neutralizing proteins, may occur when phagocytic cells attack tissue-fixed immune complexes. All these processes contribute to the tissue damage associated with immune complex tissue injury.

A key factor in the generation of immune complex–mediated disease is the balance between the clearance of immune complexes by the reticuloendothelial system and the tissue deposition of these complexes. Immune complex clearance is usually rapid, and removal is by the macrophages of the liver (Kupffer's cells) or tissue macrophages (256). The CR1 receptor on erythrocytes rapidly binds immune complexes and transports them to reticuloendothelial cells for endocytosis and removal from the circulation. Immune complex clearance is significantly decreased when C3b and Fc cell receptors are deficient or defective and immune complexes are unable to bind to these receptors. Large complexes are cleared more rapidly than smaller complexes, since they fix more complement and are bound more readily by erythrocytes and phagocytic cells (256).

Both systemic and local factors affect the tissue deposition of immune complexes. Vasoactive substances that increase vascular permeability enhance the tissue deposition of immune complexes. In antibody excess, large complexes are formed, whereas antigen excess produces small complexes. The most likely complexes to deposit in tissues are complexes formed at the zone of equivalence where antigen and antibody levels are nearly equal. Thus, the size of immune complexes depends on antigen valence, antibody titer, and antibody affinity. Positively charged immune complexes are more apt to interact with negatively charged basement membranes, and different immunoglobulin classes vary in their avidity for tissue binding. Certain antigens also have greater affinity for tissue substances than others and may, therefore, play a central role in the tissue localization and deposition of immune complexes. Finally, the cell receptors essential for immune complex clearance may be deficient or defective, leading to an overloading of the phagocytic system essential for immune complex disposal. There is no systematic way to predict the degree of immune complex–mediated tissue damage, and for this reason, prevention is a sentinel issue in the management of immune complex–mediated disorders. Removal of the host from chronic antigen exposure either by changing the environment or by treating a persistent infection should be undertaken to prevent immune complex formation.

Precipitating antibodies are sometimes identified by the appearance of the characteristic Arthus reaction in the skin, and such a reaction has been used as evidence both for the formation of soluble immune complexes and for their possible role in disease pathogenesis (175). In hosts that have been repeatedly immunized, significant levels of precipitating antibody (IgG) may develop. Subsequent delivery of antigen by subcutaneous or intradermal injection results in edema and hemorrhage at the injection site within 8 hours (256). A biopsy sample reveals the deposition of immune complexes and complement in the walls of skin capillaries. This acute response is accompanied by neutrophil infiltration and platelet clumping. Later, the neutrophils are replaced by mononuclear cells. This pathological response has all the earmarks of an immunologically mediated vasculitis.

As noted previously, hypersensitivity pneumonitis has been considered an immune complex disorder, but recent evidence has shifted in support of a type IV cell-mediated hypersensitivity response as the cause for this disorder (451,470). Caution must be used when implicating immune complex pathogenesis because predisposing antibodies are often present in asymptomatic patients, complement levels frequently do not decrease when patients are challenged with antigen, and measurable levels of circulating immune complexes often do not correlate with disease activity (175,469). Further, no tissue-specific antigens have been identified in suspected immune complex–mediated lung diseases, and tissue deposition of immune complexes infrequently correlates with the development of changes in tissue pathology.

In conclusion, no single immunopathogenetic mechanism appears to be operative in hypersensitivity pneumonitis. Despite normal serum IgE levels and a low incidence of eosinophilia, some patients with pigeon breeder's disease acquire asthma-like symptoms after inhalation challenge with pigeon antigens (382). Further, these same antigens cause an immediate skin wheal and flare reaction. Such immediate type reactions have led some workers to speculate that sensitizing antibodies may mediate certain responses in some cases of extrinsic allergic alveolitis (40). Lung biopsy specimens showing *Micropolyspora faeni* antigen, immunoglobulin, and complement in bronchial walls lead others to suggest that type II hypersensitivity may play a role in farmer's lung (252,450). The presence of circulating precipitating antibodies against specific antigens; the demonstration of immunoglobulins, complement, and antigen in lung biopsy specimens; and the occurrence of an Arthus-type reaction in skin biopsies after antigen rechallenge have been used as evidence that hypersensitivity pneumonitis is an immune complex disorder (type III hypersensitivity) (425,479,562). The absence of serum complement changes after inhalation challenge with specific antigen, the relation of precipitating antibodies to exposure and not disease, and the absence of the vasculitic lesions of immune complex–mediated disease do not support a type III hypersensitivity reaction (382,469). At present, most of the experimental findings support a cell-mediated immunopathological mechanism. The histopathological appearance of macrophages, lymphocytes, and noncaseating granulomas in lung specimens is indicative of a cell-mediated response (175,469). Further, both peripheral blood and bronchoalveolar lymphocytes proliferate and produce lymphokines in response to pigeon antigens in pigeon breeder's disease (246,482). The presence of an excess of T-suppressor lymphocytes in BAL from symptomatic patients and activated macrophages and lymphocytes provides further evidence of a type IV hypersensitivity reaction in this disorder. Further, peripheral blood lymphocytes express more suppressor activity in samples obtained from asymptomatic pigeon breeders than in those from symptomatic breeders (303,382). The clinical and laboratory expression of hypersensitivity pneumonitis clearly suggests that a cell-mediated process is involved, and such data may assist in differentiating this disorder from sarcoidosis, which may mimic its clinical presentation. Hypersensitivity pneumonitis is a disorder characterized by the exposure to organic dusts or occupational antigens, often related to decaying material containing thermophilic actinomycetes and the subsequent development of peripheral airways disease in the absence of hilar adenopathy (sarcoidosis) or systemic organ involvement (sarcoidosis). The pathology of such lung lesions is characterized by a mononuclear cell infiltrate with a predominance of macrophages and T lymphocytes that may evolve into a granulomatous process. Peripheral blood leukocytosis without eosinophilia and elevated serum and bronchoalveolar levels of IgA, IgG, and IgM are often detected in association with precipitating antibodies to appropriate antigens. IgE levels are not elevated. Bronchoalveolar lavage evaluations show a predominance of alveolar macrophages and lymphocytes that are activated and of suppressor-cytotoxic T lymphocytes in contrast to the helper-inducer predominance observed in sarcoidosis.

TYPE IV HYPERSENSITIVITY REACTIONS

The hallmark of type IV hypersensitivity reactions is their mediation by cells rather than antibodies and their transfer to nonsensitized individuals by T lymphocytes. If the recipient of the transferred cells is subsequently challenged by the same antigen that produced the sensitized lymphocytes, the recipient's sensitized T cells undergo transformation and proliferation, as measured by radiolabeled thymidine uptake. The recognition of antigen by T-cell receptors causes T-cell activation by stimulating membrane-localized phospholipase C to hydrolyze phosphatidylinositol 4,5-biphosphate, resulting in the generation of the second messengers, diacylglycerol and inositol 1,4,5-triphosphate (518). Diacylglycerol activates protein kinase C, leading to the phosphorylation of Na^+-H^+ exchange protein and a resultant increase in intracellular pH. The latter process causes phosphorylation of proteins and the activation of genes responsible for the synthesis of lymphokines. Inositol 1,4,5-triphosphate increases calcium release from intracellular stores, which binds to the cytoplasmic protein, calmodulin. This calcium-calmodulin complex then binds to cytoplasmic kinases and induces protein phosphorylation, leading to the activation of nuclear genes responsible for the new protein synthesis necessary for lymphokine generation. The biological roles of these lymphokines are responsible for the pathogenetic responses seen with type IV hypersensitivity reactions.

Four types of delayed hypersensitivity reactions (type IV or cell-mediated hypersensitivity) are observed in individuals who have been sensitized by antigen: the Jones-Mote reaction (cutaneous basophil hypersensitivity), contact hypersensitivity, tuberculin-type hypersensitivity, and granulomatous hypersensitivity (146,159, 160,199,200,292,299,445,453,531). Clinically, the Jones-Mote reaction occurs within 12 hours of contact with a nontuberculin antigen and reaches a peak at 24 hours (22,532). The lesion itself is edematous and red but lacks the induration seen with tuberculin sensitivity on skin biopsy. Histopathological examination of the Jones-Mote reaction reveals skin infiltration with lymphocytes and basophils but without the fibrin deposits seen in delayed hypersensitivity of the tuberculin type. Such reactions are characteristic of some types of human contact dermatitis and skin allograft rejections. Since T lymphocytes produce a lymphokine with basophil chemotactic properties and since the hypersensitivity can be transferred by T lymphocytes to unsensitized recipients, cutaneous basophil hypersensitivity appears to be a T-cell–dependent reaction. Further, animal experiments have shown that cyclophosphamide alters the pathology of the Jones-Mote reaction such that basophil infiltration is diminished and replaced by a mononuclear cell (532,575). This observation provides indirect evidence that T-suppressor cells are significant components of this response, since cyclophosphamide acts primarily to alter T-suppressor cells.

Tuberculin-type hypersensitivity represents the classic delayed reaction usually seen when sensitive patients are injected intradermally with soluble microbial antigens. The response to these antigens is the prototype of delayed type hypersensitivity, since its outset is delayed and mediated by T lymphocytes without the need for humoral immune factors such as antibodies. The histopathological appearance of such reactions is characterized by T-lymphocyte infiltration of the skin in a perivascular distribution (436,440). Small numbers of monocytes accompany the lymphocytes. Helper T lymphocytes exceed suppressor T cells by a ratio of 2:1, whereas blood lymphocyte ratios do not reflect this increase in skin T-helper cells. The T-lymphocyte response reaches a peak in 48 to 72 hours. Langerhans'-type cells are observed in the dermis between 24 and 48 hours after their migration from the epidermis. Macrophages and lymphocytes have been determined to be activated by staining with antibodies with specificity for HLA-DR antigens, interleukin-2 receptors, and activated lymphocytes. Epidermal keratinocytes express HLA-DR antigens at 48 to 96 hours, and lymphocyte infiltration of the epidermis also occurs in this same time frame. Occasional large granular lymphocytes (natural killer cells) are also observed in the epidermis. There is no blister formation in the intraepithelial areas of the epidermis, and pathological changes are primarily confined to the dermis without basophil infiltration. Thus, skin biopsy distinguishes this delayed type hypersensitivity reaction from Jones-Mote and contact hypersensitivity reactions.

Contact hypersensitivity is a major cause of occupational dermatitis, and it may be either allergic or irritant in nature (22,359). The contact antigen usually enters the skin at its site of exposure and may initiate T-cell sensitivity by itself or combine with normal skin proteins to form a hapten-protein conjugate that sensitizes lymphocytes. The pathological changes observed after rechallenge with such sensitizing antigens usually begin 3 to 4 hours after antigen contact. Mononuclear cell infiltrates are seen in the dermis in a perivascular distribution, and these cells begin to migrate to the epithelium by 8 hours. In this lesion, the dendritic Langerhans' cells are the primary antigen-presenting cells, even though macrophages are observed in the dermis and epidermis. Langerhans' cells are also observed in efferent lymph nodes shortly after antigen challenge occurs in sensitized hosts. By 24 to 48 hours, there is a marked increase in macrophages, Langerhans' cells, and lymphocytes in both the dermis and epidermis. Both helper and suppressor lymphocytes have been identified, with an excess of helper cells. Some basophils have been observed but not in the numbers seen in the Jones-Mote reaction. By 48 hours, the epidermis shows spongiosis with an eczematous reaction. Keratinocytes and infiltrating macrophages are also activated and by 48 to 72 hours express class II HLA molecules. Thus, in contrast to tuberculin-type hypersensitivity, contact hypersensitivity is primarily an epidermal reaction with Langerhans' cell proliferation and subsequent mediation of antigen presentation by these same cells. The skin response peaks at a time identical to that of the tuberculin-type hypersensitivity response but primarily involves the epidermis.

Together with contact hypersensitivity, granulomatous reactions represent the most prevalent disorders induced by environmental agents, and these reactions are more serious than those of contact hypersensitivity. Granulomatous hypersensitivity reactions can be divided into nonimmunological, foreign body granulomas, and immunological hypersensitivity reactions (48) (Table 3). The foreign body granuloma has little relevance to environmental exposures except where it must be differentiated from an immunological hypersensitivity response. Foreign bodies are usually nonantigenic and cause a nonspecific inflammatory response through their interaction with tissue and plasma components. The products of the reaction between such foreign bodies and tissue components define the characteristics of the cellular response, but usually macrophages with ingested foreign bodies predominate in the chronic lesion, and the relatively low chemical irritancy of a foreign body results in a low turnover time for the macrophages (4,48,416,462,463). Such a granuloma has been called a low turnover granuloma. Foreign bodies with greater chemical reactivity, such as silica, cause cell membrane damage, the release of hydrolytic enzymes, and cell death (48,159). Tissue repair of such cell damage results in fibrosis. This active foreign body granuloma has a higher macrophage turnover rate than the low turnover, inactive foreign body lesion. Rechallenge with the same foreign body does not change the size or kinetics of the tissue response.

Immune-type granulomas or hypersensitivity granulomas are caused by the persistence of either soluble or insoluble antigens that are slowly degraded, with continual antigen release resulting in chronic tissue irritation and delayed hypersensitivity. Histopathological examination shows that the development of these lesions is primarily dependent on blood monocytes that are recruited to the lesion by chemotaxins generated in the tissue and plasma (48,328). Monocytes at the site of the reaction mature into macrophages and become activated by the lymphokines secreted by effector lymphocytes involved in antigen presentation. Epithelioid cells are derived from activated macrophages and surround granulomas. Their exact role in granuloma pathogenesis is unknown. These polygonal cells with interdigitating

TABLE 3. *Granulomatous lesions*

Nonimmunological foreign body:
   Inactive
      Talc
      Bentonite
      Plastic beads
      Carrageenan
   Active
      Silica
   Experimental
      Bentonite particles
      Plastic beads (divinyl-benzene copolymers)
      Streptococcal cell wall fragments
      Trehalose-6,6^1-dimycolate (cord factor)
Immunological hypersensitivity:
   Infectious
      Bacteria
      Virus
      Fungi
      Worms
   Metal-induced
      Zirconium
      Beryllium
   Unknown etiology
      Sarcoid
   Experimental
      Bacillus Calmette-Guerin
      Antigen extracts (e.g., pigeon droppings)
      Schistosome egggranuloma
      Antigen-coated bentonite

cell membranes contain large quantities of granular endoplasmic reticulum and have a well-developed Golgi apparatus, but such cells do not express Fc receptors and are unable to phagocytose substituents found in the lesion. The structural components of epithelioid cells suggest a secretory role. Langhans'-type giant cells are classic components of granulomas and represent the fusion products of macrophages. This fusion process may initially occur during the phagocytosis of indigestible material, but subsequently these giant cells manifest a decrease in Fc and C3 receptors concomitant with a loss of phagocytic activity. Despite these changes, the cytoplasm of these cells is rich in lysosomal enzymes with the capacity to damage and digest extracellular constituents. Lymphocytes are the second most common cell type in granulomas, making up about 10% to 15% of the granuloma cell population. Using monoclonal antibodies with specificity for lymphocytes, both T and B lymphocytes and plasma cells have been identified in such lesions. Basophils, eosinophils, and mast cells represent a small percentage of the cells in granulomas, but neutrophils are found only during the initial stages of the granuloma development. Fibroblasts play a role in the early development of granulomas as a connective tissue matrix that maintains a scaffolding for the cellular components of the granuloma.

As might be expected, a variety of different substances have been shown to induce granulomatous responses, and the pathogenesis of granuloma formation has been investigated in detail in several clinical and experimental settings. The classic inducers of nonimmune granulomas are plastic beads composed of divinyl-benzene copolymers, bentonite particles, glycolipid, streptocccal cell wall fragments, and the toxic glycolipid, trehalose-6,6^1-dimycolate (cord factor) (48). The clinical expression of foreign body granulomas is best exemplified by the silicotic granuloma (48). Immune granuloma-inducers are represented by a variety of effector substances known to cause granulomas in humans and used as models in animals to characterize the features of such immune granulomas. In animal models, bacillus Calmette-Guerin, the antigens evoking extrinsic allergic alveolitis such as extracts of pigeon droppings and *Micropolyspora faeni* antigen, the schistosome egg granuloma, and bentonite antigen-coated particles induce immune granulomas (48). The human counterparts to these granulomas include silicosis, berylliosis, hard metal disease, hypersensitivity pneumonitis, and a variety of granulomatous reactions associated with bacterial infections (tuberculosis, leprosy, salmonellosis, brucellosis, listeriosis, syphilis, Q fever), viral infections (cat scratch fever), helminthic infections (schistosomiasis, trichinosis, filariasis, capillariasis), and fungal infections (histioplasmosis, blastomycosis, paracoccidioidomycosis, cryptococcosis, coccidioidomycosis), and chlamydial (lymphogranuloma venereum) infections (48). There are also a number of granulomas of unknown cause: sarcoidosis, primary biliary cirrhosis, granulomatous ileitis and colitis, and certain vasculitides. In fact, sarcoidosis has been a primary contributor to knowledge about immune granulomas. Chronic granulomatous reactions of the skin may also be observed with zirconium, nickel, or chromium exposure (160).

Understanding the pathogenesis of immune type IV hypersensitivity granulomas requires the differentiation of this lesion from a foreign body granuloma (5,328). No single pathological feature distinguishes these two lesions. Such differentiation requires a constellation of findings rather than a single component. Although nonimmune granulomas may contain fewer lymphocytes than immune granulomas, the complete absence of lymphocytes is not an absolute characteristic of the foreign body granuloma. The absence of epithelioid cells has been the most consistent feature of foreign body granulomas, but muramyl dipeptide and plastics, which are foreign body agents, cause the generation of epithelioid cells. Although the absence of these macrophage-derived cells suggests a nonimmune granuloma, their presence in a lesion does not exclude a foreign body reaction. Further, foreign body granulomas may be associated with immunological features and lead to confusion over the type of granuloma. For example, patients with silicosis frequently have alterations in systemic immune function (291). Titers of antinuclear antibodies and rheumatoid factor are increased in silicosis, and these patients often manifest a polyclonal hypergammaglobulinemia without an associated increase in B lymphocytes. Cell-mediated immunity is often intact in silicosis, but decreased responses to T-cell mitogens have been observed (380). Such changes may depend on the dose of silica and the stage of the disease. Even though antibody formation does occur with foreign body granulomas, the absence of T cells sensitized by such antibodies and the inability to transfer hypersensitivity with lymphocytes documents the nonimmune character of these granulomatous reactions. It is also held that nonimmune granulomas do not produce lymphokines, but the production of these cytokines has not been investigated thoroughly in foreign body granulomas.

In summary, immune granulomas require a persistent or slowly digested antigen that is taken up by monocytes and macrophages and processed for presentation to T lymphocytes. Antigen presentation to specific T cells requires monocyte HLA-DR expression and the release of interleukin-1 during this process. T lymphocytes to which antigen has been presented express interleukin-2 receptors and release lymphokines, including interleukin-2. Interleukin-2 causes appropriately sensitized T cells to proliferate, and like interleukin-1, acts as a chemoattractant for T lymphocytes. Both macrophages and T lymphocytes are activated and release mediators that contribute to the pathogenesis of the disorder and may induce tissue damage. Among the lymphokines secreted by such T cells are monocyte chemotactic factors, migration inhibition factors, and macrophage activating factors. These and other immunoactive products are essential for the establishment of the presence of immune granulomas. The character and extent of the immune response in immune granulomatous disorders depend on the amount of antigen, the duration of antigen exposure, the genetic background of the host, and the modulation of the immune response by T-suppressor lymphocytes.

UNCLASSIFIABLE IMMUNOLOGICAL ABERRATIONS

Additional environmental and occupational disorders have immune dysfunctions that do not easily fit into the Coombs and Gel classification. The immunopathogenesis of these disorders is incompletely understood, and caution is necessary in the interpretation of published data because factors other than the disease must be considered as possible contributors to their immunopathology. For example, immunological changes have been described in certain pneumoconioses, but their role in the pathogenesis of these disorders remains incompletely understood. In addition, aging, cigarette smoking, and other parameters not associated with specific disease mechanisms may account for immunological changes alone or in concert with disease-related factors. Since no functional classification has been devised to segregate those immune dysfunctions that are not directly associated with specific diseases from those that are related directly to a documented clinical disorder, well-characterized immune abnormalities in environmental and occupational disorders are discussed under separate headings.

Age-Related Immune Dysfunction

Defects in both cell-mediated and humoral immunity have been described with increasing age (125,237). In aging populations, the total number of peripheral blood T lymphocytes is usually but not universally (24) reported to be decreased (84,241,394,458). No changes in the absolute number of T-helper lymphocytes have been observed with aging, but a variety of conflicting results in T-suppressor lymphocyte numbers have been described and probably represent the heterogeneity that would be seen in a population of older individuals (24,212,216,242,486). In addition to changes in lymphocyte subpopulations, functional changes in lymphocytes from aging populations have also been described. *In vitro* lymphocyte proliferation is decreased in the aged, and that defect appears not to be caused by an alteration in the receptor for the proliferative stimulus (561). The production of interleukin-2 as well as other lymphokines decreases with age, and this may be the mechanism by which proliferative responses are diminished (207,508). The data regarding lymphotoxic functions and delayed hypersensitivity testing in older populations are conflicting (62,98,126,147,169,313,395,424,476). Some workers have reported anergy to antigens administered intradermally, but others have not substantiated these findings (62,98,126,147,313). A decrease in delayed cutaneous hypersensitivity may be observed with aging, but the test procedures must be carefully monitored, and multiple antigens should be tested. As with delayed cutaneous hypersensitivity, some workers have shown that cytotoxic T lymphocytes and natural killer cell activities are reduced with age (169,313,424,476). These data have been well established in animals (149,164,558), but as noted previously, they are more controversial in humans. Thus, no uniform conclusions have been drawn as to the effects of aging on cytotoxic cell activity. From a functional standpoint, aging populations manifest an increased frequency of autoantibody production, although they show a decreased production of antibodies to foreign antigens (125). The mechanism for these disparate responses is not well understood but appears to be multifactorial. Aged B lymphocytes have a decreased response to polyclonal B-cell activators, and these changes are likely to contribute to the decrease in antibody responses to foreign antigens (309,569). Alterations in T-suppressor cell function may also contribute to the variations observed in autoantibody production. Nonetheless, the mechanistic explanations accounting for the differences between antibody production to self-antigens and foreign antigens as well as the increased incidence of benign monoclonal gammopathies in aging populations remain incompletely characterized. Variations in suppressor T-cell subsets may contribute to the opposing responses to self- and foreign antigens, but this may not be the complete answer. No consistent abnormalities in monocyte function have been described in association with aging, but lymphocytes from aging populations appear to be less responsive to mediators produced by monocytes. A well-described example of this phenomenon is the increased sensitivity of senescent lymphocytes to the immunosuppressive effects of prostaglandins as measured by *in vitro* lymphocyte proliferation and antibody synthesis (9,128,230). Such suppressive effects return to normal when prostaglandins are removed from the assay or their synthesis and release by monocytes is inhibited.

Cigarette Smoke

Cigarette smoke, a common environmental pollutant, also causes changes in the immune system. Cigarette smokers have increased numbers of leukocytes in both their peripheral blood and BAL fluid (17,37,106,258,276,402,407,452,552). Serum immunoglobulin levels are decreased in smokers (172,201,270,502) and in heavy smokers, a decreased ratio of helper to suppressor T lymphocytes has been observed (377). Some studies have shown decreased lymphocyte proliferation to mitogens and diminished natural killer cell activity as well as numbers of natural killer cells (131), but such findings have not been universal (428,431,455). Natural killer cell activity is reduced in the peripheral blood and BAL fluid of cigarette smokers (523). Smoking and asbestos exposure interact to reduce natural killer cell activity (134). These immune system alterations observed with aging and cigarette smoking emphasize the need for assessing these factors when evaluating changes in environmental and occupational disease. These and other confounding factors must be excluded before a disease-associated immune dysfunction can be determined.

Asbestosis

Asbestosis is the most common chronic environmental disorder causing interstitial lung disease and is a precursor of lung cancer in some patients. Elevated levels of immunoglobulins (IgG, IgM, and IgA) and an increased frequency of antinuclear antibodies and rheumatoid factors are well documented in asbestosis (333–336, 427,535). Antinuclear antibody positivity appears to correlate with the degree of lung fibrosis and with severe fibrosis. More than 80% of patients with asbestosis have positive antinuclear antibodies (333,337,534). Although antinuclear antibodies are usually in the IgM class, IgG class antinuclear antibodies also occur in a frequency higher than normal in asbestosis (333). Polyclonal immunoglobulinemia is also characteristic of asbestosis, and some patients have circulating immune complexes (335). Asbestosis also manifests defects in cellular immune function, as noted by the suppressed delayed cutaneous hypersensitivity observed in some patients (198,295). A decrease in T-cell subsets in the peripheral blood has also been identified in patients with asbestosis (135,198,247,346,378,529). Further, there is a decrease in peripheral blood T-cell proliferation to phytohemagglutin (PHA) in some but not all patients with asbestosis (77,254), and some evidence exists to suggest that differences in response to PHA are related to the type of asbestos fiber (52,294). Perhaps more relevant to the association between cancer and asbestos exposure is the finding that chrysotile asbestos fibers suppress *in vitro* human natural killer cell activity, and this cell activity is diminished in nonsmoking asbestos workers (209,326,571).

The role of these immune dysfunctions in asbestosis is incompletely understood (132). The changes in cellular immunity observed in this disease have suggested to some that patients with asbestosis are immunosuppressed, and the immunosuppressed state may be a precursor of the malignant disorders associated with asbestosis. Further, decreased natural killer cell numbers and function in cigarette smokers with asbestosis may also contribute to the expression of neoplastic disorders in such populations (209).

Silicosis

Silicosis has many immune features in common with asbestosis. As in asbestosis, serum antinuclear antibodies and rheumatoid factor titers are often increased (109,136). Antinuclear antibody titers are especially elevated in patients with silicosis who have progressive massive fibrosis. Circulating immune complexes are also present in 25% to 30% of patients with silicosis (137). Polyclonal hypergammaglobulinemia is also a component of silicosis, but no change in B-lymphocyte numbers has been observed in this disorder in contrast to asbestosis in which B cells may either be increased or decreased (116,133,135,198,483). Silica-exposed cultures of human peripheral blood mononuclear cells produce more immunoglobulins when stimulated with pokeweed mitogen or specific antigen than do cells not exposed to silica (408). Thus, silica behaves like an adjuvant, and humoral immunity is stimulated. The mechanism for such B-cell hyperactivity is not understood.

Cell-mediated immunity is also altered in silicosis, and such changes depend, in part, on the stage of the disease. The number of circulating T cells and their proliferative response to T-cell mitogens such as PHA are normal in patients with uncomplicated silicosis (116,483). However, in silicosis associated with progressive massive fibrosis, T-cell proliferation to both PHA and concanavalin A is depressed (116). Humans show no change in delayed cutaneous hypersensitivity regardless of the stage of the disease (483). In mononuclear cell cultures, T-lymphocyte responses to PHA are enhanced, probably as a result of the release of interleukin-1 from monocytes (408,480). In animals exposed to silica, alveolar macrophages examined for their functional capacities show variable results, depending on the dose and duration of exposure to silica. In general, macrophages from the lung demonstrate increased secretory activity, as measured by the release of lysosomal and cytoplasmic enzymes and chemotactic factors from inflammatory cells (131,376, 507). There also appears to be heterogeneity among the alveolar macrophage populations recovered by lung lavage, and such differences may account for the stages of disease observed with silicosis (385). The cytotoxic effects of silica may also alter the capacity of lung macrophages to become activated and may vary the immunopathogenic responses mediated by activated macrophages (115). Despite the presence of immunological factors in silicosis, their role in the pathogenesis of this disorder remains incompletely defined. Often the term silicotic granuloma is used to describe the pathological appearance of a silicotic nodule, but this terminology should not convey the idea that such nodules represent type IV hypersensitivity responses. In fact, such nodules do not exhibit the classic features of a granulomatous response except for the presence of giant cells and dust-laden macrophages and lymphocytes in the outer layer of the nodule.

In summary, silicosis is a fibrotic lung disease primarily associated with humoral immune dysfunction, and its progression is not clearly related to the immunopathological changes observed. It must be differentiated from conditions associated with silicate deposition in the lung. Unlike silicon dioxide, the mediator of silicosis, most silicates are nonfibrogenic. Silicatosis results from exposures to talc

(374,473,526,543), kaolin and china stone (239,287,338,383,492,549), slate (108,205), mica (117,434), Fuller's earth (76,468,528), zeolite (81), graphite, and aluminum silicate (214,390). The fibrotic scarring of silicatosis is quite different from the appearance of silicotic nodules. Occasionally, silicates cause a granulomatous response with an appearance similar to that of type IV hypersensitivity reactions containing giant and epithelioid cells. Since the macrophages of these lesions are loaded with birefringent silicate particles, such reactions can easily be differentiated from classic type IV responses.

Berylliosis

Beryllium and its salts are chemical irritants that can cause inflammatory responses of ocular tissues and the respiratory tract, but with the exception of the inflammatory cells involved in these tissue reactions, no immune mechanisms have been characterized to account for these responses (280a,525). Acute exposures associated with beryllium may result in a toxic pneumonitis (325). In addition to these irritant and toxic effects, the skin can become sensitized to beryllium, causing a chronic dermatitis (325). Acute disorders associated with beryllium exposure occur infrequently and are easily managed by removal of the host from exposure.

Chronic berylliosis is the more common disorder observed today in relation to beryllium exposures and may express itself after a long latent period. Chronic berylliosis is a systemic granulomatous disorder with a focus in the respiratory tract that causes tissue reactions suggestive of a delayed type hypersensitivity reaction (325). Interstitial beryllium granulomas are primarily found in the lung, but noncaseating granulomas have been observed in a wide array of tissue sites, including bone, muscle, liver, and salivary glands (182). In the lung, such granulomatous reactions may proceed to lung fibrosis. The immunopathogenesis of this chronic disorder is supported by several factors. Initial epidemiological studies demonstrated a high frequency of case findings outside the workplace, which suggested an immunological mechanism to the observers (155,515). Multiple beryllium exposures are necessary for the development of pulmonary disease (325), and noncaseating granulomas of skin occur in response to the intradermal injection of beryllium salts (357). T lymphocytes in the peripheral blood and alveolar lavage fluid from suspected cases proliferate in response to beryllium (19,110,130,158,245,441,456, 459,460,566). Such observations clearly suggested that beryllium or a beryllium-protein adduct was the antigen responsible for a T-cell–mediated lung disorder (290). On the other hand, beryllium increases the proliferation of B lymphocytes and spleen cells to mitogens as well as the replication of lymph node cells to recall antigens (240,401,442). Beryllium also increases the expression of macrophage markers of activation, such as Ia antigens. These findings suggest a nonspecific adjuvant-like effect of beryllium on the immune system.

In animal models of chronic berylliosis, genetic factors have been determined to play a role in the expression of this disease. Some guinea pig strains appear to be resistant to granuloma development, whereas other strains are susceptible (20,21). Thus, genetic factors may also contribute to the expression of the human disorder, and based on animal investigations, these susceptibility traits may be related to *h*istocompatibility *l*ocus *a*ntigens (438,540). Finally, beryllium salts are phagocytosed by alveolar macrophages, and such particulate forms may be partially cytotoxic to macrophages, resulting in the release of lysosomal enzymes that are likely to contribute to the chronic inflammatory response of this disease (325).

Hard Metal Lung Disease

Hard metal lung disease remains somewhat of an enigma, but increasing evidence suggests that an immunopathogenetic mechanism probably accounts for some clinical expressions of this disorder (16). Hard metal is defined as an alloy of tungsten carbide with other metals such as cobalt, titanium, nickel, chromium, tantalum, and niobium. Recent studies have focused on cobalt as the etiological vector of the asthmatic responses and fibrosing alveolitis seen after hard metal exposures. Animal studies have shown that tungsten alone is inert and does not induce bronchoconstriction when used as a provocative agent (127,248,296,375,478). Further, workers exposed to cobalt alone have developed occupational asthma in the absence of any tungsten carbide (129,203). Since hard metal disease occurs in exposed populations at a low frequency (1% to 5%), it appears that lung disease in such workers is related to a hypersensitivity-like disorder rather than an overt toxic reaction to the metal (93,329).

Recent investigations implicate an immunopathogenetic mechanism for this disorder, since cobalt is a known skin sensitizer (176,467) and can induce lymphocyte transformation (545). In a small population of cobalt-exposed workers with asthma, IgE antibodies specific for cobalt adducted to human serum albumin have been detected. Such studies have also demonstrated selective binding of radiolabeled cobalt to human serum, which is blocked by preabsorption with unlabeled cobalt (500). Patch testing of cobalt-sensitive workers shows only 25% to be positive, whereas no control subjects respond (500). Challenge with cobalt chloride results in immediate asthmatic reactions in 25% of cobalt-sensitive workers. In another 25% of cobalt-sensitive workers, both late and immediate asthmatic reactions develop, and 50% of these hypersensitive workers manifest only late asthmatic reactions. No control subjects have been found to have positive reactions to cobalt chloride challenge, and no abnormalities in serum complement or immunoglobulin levels have been observed in hard metal–sensitive workers. IgE levels are increased in only a small percentage of these cobalt-sensitive workers.

Although the pathogenesis of cobalt-induced asthma is not completely understood, the history of chest symptoms associated with cobalt exposure, the presence of IgE antibodies specific for cobalt conjugated to human serum albumin, and positive challenge tests to cobalt chloride are very suggestive of a type I hypersensitivity response. Other investigators suggest that the pathogenesis of such cobalt-related disorders may be from an increased susceptibility of alveolar macrophages to activation by cobalt or an increased responsiveness of target tissues to bronchoactive mediators in the presence of cobalt.

Clinical observations of diamond polishers with interstitial lung disease and fibrosis have led to some confusion about the immunopathogenesis of hard metal lung disease. The presence of multinucleated giant cells in lung biopsies and BAL specimens raises the suspicion of a granulomatous process (1,8,122,129). Further, no correlation between cobalt-induced dermatitis, a skin sensitization process, and cobalt-induced pulmonary disease has been observed. Cobalt-induced dermatitis is associated with an increase in lymphocyte proliferation of peripheral blood mononuclear cells exposed to cobalt chloride, but no such evaluations have been reported thus far in patients with cobalt-induced pulmonary disease. In fact, lymphocytosis is not a common characteristic of BAL specimens obtained from patients with cobalt-induced lung disease (8,122). Thus, there may be different responses of the human host to cobalt exposure, some of which may lead to a type I hypersensitivity response, whereas others may be caused by different immunopathological or nonimmunological mechanisms.

Cadmium and Other Heavy Metals

A variety of metals (e.g., cadmium, lead, mercury, selenium, zinc, arsenic, and nickel) alter the immune system in animals and humans (7,38,80,162,208,232,321, 429,505,512,513,554,555). Such effects, in some cases, are difficult to interpret because both stimulation and suppression of humoral and cell-mediated immunity have been demonstrated. Factors such as the dose, the duration of exposure, the animal species, the capacity to generate metallothionein, and the methods of study have often not been evaluated. Nonetheless, recent studies using state-of-the-art assays for immune functions and focusing on mechanisms have begun to document specific metal-induced effects on the immune system. Even though cadmium appears not to be a major cause of immunological lung dysfunction, it serves as a good example of metal-induced immune dysfunctions and is discussed in some detail as a model for the elucidation of such metal-related effects.

Cadmium is a common environmental pollutant with a half-life (20 to 30 years) and a vapor pressure higher than those of other metals. In its gaseous state, it combines with oxygen and condenses to form cadmium oxide. The latter is a particulate of respirable size (266,267). Cadmium is present as a soluble substance in water and food and in particulate form from the emissions of welding, smelting, electroplating, and automobile exhausts. Cigarette smoke, pigments, and metal alloys are also significant sources of cadmium. The primary toxic effects of this metal are those associated with renal, hepatic, and testicular damage and bone decalcification (183,355,430). Cadmium pneumonitis, an acute chemical pneumonitis, and emphysema associated with chronic exposure have also been observed in cadmium-exposed populations (23).

Few studies have evaluated the role of cadmium's immunotoxic effects on diseases associated with this heavy metal. This is especially true when one considers the chemical pneumonitis and pulmonary fibrosis associated with cadmium exposure. Some monocyte and macrophage membrane enzymes are sulfhydryl-dependent, and exposure to cadmium, a potent sulfhydryl reactant and inhibitor, has been incompletely evaluated in relation to the biological functions regulated by these sulfhydryl-dependent reactions (43). Thus, although few investigations have focused on the role of the immune system in cadmium toxicity, this might be a fertile area for future investigation.

Cadmium appears to affect all components of the animal immune system, including T and B lymphocytes, monocytes, and cytotoxic T cells. Cadmium concentrations in the range of 10^{-5}M to 10^{-4}M significantly reduce the capacity of mouse peritoneal macrophages to ingest IgG- and IgM-opsonized erythrocytes (245). Such effects are not mediated via Fc or complement receptors because binding to macrophages remains unaffected by cadmium. Further, receptor migration remains intact, leaving cell signaling and cellular responses to such signals as the most likely targets of cadmium. Other studies have shown that cadmium is directly toxic to macrophages and may activate macrophages under certain conditions (322,353,354). In contrast to the results of studies showing unimpaired mouse peritoneal macrophage Fc and complement receptors in the presence of cadmium, erythrocyte antibody rosette formation is impaired when alveolar macrophages exposed to cadmium are used as the erythrocyte antibody substrate (238). These studies suggest that alveolar macrophage Fc receptors are altered by cadmium. Further, alterations in macrophage mobility, response to macrophage inhibiting factor, and cytotoxic activity have been attributed to the presence of cadmium (162,308).

Functional abnormalities in pulmonary bacterial clearance in mice exposed to an aerosol of cadmium chloride delivering between 80 and 2000 $\mu g/m^3$ over a 2-hour period have been described (195,197). After exposure to cadmium, mice are given a bacterial aerosol of *Streptococcus pyogenes* either immediately after the cadmium treatment or 24 hours later. Mice exposed to cadmium chloride concentrations greater than 100 $\mu g/m^3$ and an immediate bacterial challenge show a significantly increased mortality and shortened length of survival when compared with control mice not exposed to cadmium. In mice with a delayed bacterial challenge (24 hours), increased mortality is observed with a dose of 550 $\mu g/m^3$ or 1,675 $\mu g/m^3$ cadmium chloride. At cadmium chloride concentrations of 325 $\mu g/m^3$, viable organisms increase up to 2 days after bacterial challenge, and the number of bacteria in the lung reaches a plateau at 10^5 viable *Streptococci* per lung. In contrast, control lungs contain less than 10 viable microbes per lung at 4 days. Thus, cadmium chloride treatment significantly decreases the pulmonary clearance of *Streptococci*. The mechanism by which this alteration in clearance occurs may relate, in part, to the significant decrease in the viability of alveolar macrophages observed after cadmium chloride treatment in rats. At doses of 1,500 $\mu g/m^3$ in this species, there is about an 11% decrease in macrophage viability in cells obtained from cadmium chloride-treated rats as compared with controls (197). There is also a significantly lower number of macrophages obtained by lavage in rats lavaged immediately after cessation of the aerosolization of 1,500 μg calcium chloride per cubic meter.

Thus, cadmium, at relatively high doses, clearly has a significant effect on pulmonary bacterial clearance in rats and mice. Nonetheless, the principal effects of cadmium on macrophage activity remain incompletely resolved. Improved assays for receptors and a better understanding of the mechanisms of motility, chemotaxis, and monokine production should resolve the conflicting concepts about cadmium's effects on bacterial clearance.

Recent studies of lymphocyte activation have delineated a mechanism that might explain the signaling defect observed in cadmium-exposed macrophages (92). At high concentrations (100 μM), cadmium interferes with PHA-induced lymphocyte activation and proliferation. This is a time- and dose-dependent process, and little or no effect is observed if T cells are treated with cadmium 3 or 4 hours after PHA stimulation. Focusing on the metabolic events in the early stages of cell division, cadmium chloride (50 μM) has been determined to decrease both interleukin-2 receptor expression and interleukin-2 production (92). Neither of these processes is completely obliterated by high cadmium levels, and more than one process may be involved in the inhibition of T-dependent and T-independent mitogen stimulation of lymphocytes. In mice exposed to 10 to 50 μg/ml of cadmium for 3 weeks, lymphocyte DNA synthesis is modestly increased as compared with unexposed animals. Such experimental results suggest that cadmium itself is a weak mitogen. Cadmium reduces the generation of inositol triphosphate by human lymphocytes in culture and increases its rate of disappearance (92). In addition, a more rapid production of inositol phosphate has been observed in cadmium-containing cells than in cells in which inositol triphosphate has been measured in the absence of cadmium. Thus, the production of inositol triphosphate is significantly reduced by cadmium. Since cadmium blocks both calcium channels and the calcium-mobilizing messenger, inositol triphosphate, the effects of this metal may be mediated by altering the influx of calcium and suppressing the calcium-requiring processes of the cell. In addition to blocking calcium channels, cadmium also inhibits the binding of phorbol dibutyrate to specific receptors on peripheral blood lymphocytes and blocks lymphocyte activation by phorbol myristate acetate (92). Such receptor inhibition provides additional evidence for a cadmium-induced alteration in signal transduction. Further, cadmium ($10^{-3} - 10^{-4}$M) inhibits protein kinase C activation by calcium (388). These data all support a cadmium-induced defect in signal transduction and intracellular processing of messages.

Another mechanism relevant to cadmium's effects on immunoactive cells is its capacity to cause a dose-dependent increase in prostaglandin E_2 (PGE_2), a substance with known immunosuppressive activity (521). At present, cadmium has only been shown to release PGE_2 from osteoblast-like cells, but it is reasonable to expect that similar effects might be observed with monocytes and macrophages.

As noted previously, cadmium induces dichotomous responses in humoral immunity. Mice drinking water containing 10 to 50 ppm cadmium chloride have a significant decrease in their *in vitro* T-lymphocyte–dependent antibody production to sheep red blood cells (44). Only nonadherent cells exposed to cadmium trigger the suppression of antibody production. In contrast to these findings, T-cell–independent *in vivo* and *in vitro* antibody production against dinitrophenyl-aminoethylcarbamylmethyl-Ficoll (DNP-Ficoll) and *Escherichia coli* is enhanced in mice provided with drinking water with 10 to 50 ppm of cadmium chloride. These experiments show that T–dependent antibody production is suppressed whereas T–independent antibody synthesis is increased under the same conditions of exposure. Since T–independent antibody responses are macrophage- or B-lymphocyte–dependent, immunosuppression does not appear to affect these cell functions. Further evidence of the absence of an immunosuppressive effect on macrophage-dependent antibody production has been derived from experiments in which cadmium-exposed macrophages and cadmium-unexposed lymphocytes are used to generate antibodies against sheep red blood cells (44). Such experiments demonstrate no suppression of antibody production.

Since antibody responses to the T lymphocyte and the macrophage-independent antigen, *E. coli* lipopolysaccharide, are enhanced in the presence of cadmium, such data have implicated cadmium as a B-lymphocyte stimulator (437,546). This concept receives further support from data demonstrating increased B-lymphocyte blastogenesis after cadmium exposure (42,323,386). Cadmium-treated mice also show either a direct or an indirect polyclonal activation of B lymphocytes with an associated induction of antinuclear antibodies (406). Long-term cadmium chloride exposure also causes glomerular amyloidosis in rabbits, a pathological process with immunological overtones (82). Further, cadmium can induce an immune complex nephritis in Sprague-Dawley rats treated with 100 to 200 ppm of cadmium chloride (293). Antinuclear antibody induction appears to be strain-specific like other metal-induced autoimmune manifestations (406). Strains of ICR mice are particularly susceptible to antinuclear antibody induction since 50 percent of low-dose (3 ppm) cadmium-treated animals acquire antinuclear antibodies, whereas BALB/c strains require 30 to 300 ppm of cadmium chloride to generate antinuclear antibodies. No immune-mediated nephritis has been observed in ICR or BALB/c mice treated for 10 weeks with high (300 ppm) and low (3 ppm) doses of cadmium chloride. Earlier investigations have shown that immature B cell (bone marrow plaque-forming cells) numbers are significantly decreased in the presence of cadmium (512). Thus, *in vivo* cadmium exposure may cause cell-specific bone marrow suppression. Spleen plaque-forming cells appear to be unaffected by cadmium treatment and may even show increased activity (proliferation) in the presence of cadmium.

Phorbol esters (TPA) induce phosphatidylinositol turnover in B lymphocytes by activating phospholipase C, and such increased phosphatidylinositol turnover leads to the release of both diacylglycerol and intracellular calcium stores from the endoplasmic reticulum. Both calcium and diacylglycerol acting together activate protein kinase C. As noted previously, components of this signal transducing mechanism are involved in lymphocyte activation, and such a process is inhibited by cadmium (280). In contrast, the proliferation of B lymphocytes from murine spleens does not appear to be inhibited by cadmium. Investigations have not yet determined whether

T and B lymphocyte activation occurs by different mechanisms or different roles for accessory cells account for this apparently dichotomous effect of cadmium.

Genetic susceptibility to cadmium-induced immunosuppression has been evaluated in DBA/2, BALB/c, and C3H/He mice (405). Such studies have shown that differences in cadmium susceptibility in these strains do not arise from intrinsic abnormalities in their lymphocytes but are more likely related to altered cadmium metabolism. These results correlate well with other studies demonstrating differences in mortality, metallothionein induction, and autoantibody production in inbred strains of mice.

Although cadmium has been shown to have significant effects on the immune system, few investigations have focused on the role of immune dysfunctions related to the lung. Emphysema has been reported as a complication of cadmium exposure, but such exposures have not been separated from the effects of cigarette smoke, a well-characterized vector of emphysema (123,183,332). Acute inflammatory responses to cadmium have been defined by BAL studies in animals (253,260, 261,266). Numbers of inflammatory cells in lavage fluids increase after short-term cadmium exposure, and neutrophil and macrophage aggregates are found in cadmium-exposed lungs. Lysosomal enzyme activities are also increased in these lung lavage fluids. Despite these studies, little is known about the capacity of lung macrophages to present antigen in the presence of cadmium or to produce monokines such as interleukin-1. Epidemiological data determining the frequency of lung infection and the duration of such infections have not been well documented.

A variety of other metals may cause lung disorders (Table 4), and some involve the immune system (7). Industrial metals such as platinum salts, chromates, cobalt, nickel sulfate, nickel carbonyl, and vanadium have all been documented to trigger attacks of occupational asthma (7,59,78,122,366). Typically, the asthmatic attacks associated with metal exposure begin several hours after exposure, but immediate reactions have been observed with platinum salts. In the case of nickel salts, IgE and IgG antibodies have been detected that react with nickel serum albumin conjugates (138). In the case of the others, these metals probably induce tissue protein denaturation with the creation of neoantigens to which antibodies are formed. The pathogenesis of such occupational asthmas has been discussed in detail under type I hypersensitivity reactions.

Other metal-induced lung diseases such as the interstitial pneumonia and fibrosis observed with hard metal disease have been discussed previously in association with cobalt exposure, and the granulomatous disorder seen with beryllium exposure has also been described as a type IV hypersensitivity disorder.

There has been some suggestion that metal fume fever induced by zinc, copper, magnesium, aluminum, nickel, iron, manganese, and antimony fumes may be an immunological reaction rather than an acute toxic chemical response (472). A little evidence is beginning to be generated in support of this hypothesis.

Finally, exposure to chromates and nickel compounds has been clearly documented to be associated with lung cancer (418). Whether such an association is related to immune dysfunction, cigarette smoking as a confounding factor, or some

TABLE 4. *Metal toxicity and lung disease*

Chemical Pneumonitis	Granulomatous Lung Disease
Cadmium fumes	Beryllium
Manganese fumes	Pneumoconiosis
Mercury fumes	Iron (benign)
Nickel carbonyl fumes	Cerium
Zinc chloride fumes	Antimony (benign)
Vanadium pentoxide fumes	Barium (benign)
Lithium hydride	Emphysema
Osmium	Cadmium
Selenium	Chronic Bronchitis and Cold
Titanium chloride	Aluminum
Uranium fluoride	Cadmium
Zirconium chloride	Cobalt
Gold salt therapy	Iron
Metal Fume Fever	Manganese
Beryllium	Titanium (?)
Cadmium	Lung Fibrosis
Cobalt	Aluminum (rare)
Manganese	Beryllium (granulomatous)
Mercury	Cobalt (fibrosing alveolitis)
Tin	Lanthanons
Zinc	Lung Cancer
Copper	Antimony (?)
Iron	Arsenic
Lead	Beryllium (?)
Magnesium	Cadmium (?)
Nickel	Cobalt (?)
Arsenic	Iron ore mining (? radon)
Hard Metal Lung Disease	Nickel
Cobalt	Uranium
Bronchial Asthma	
Complex platinum salts	
Nickel	
Chromium	
Aluminum	
Cobalt	

other mechanism has yet to be determined. Thus, metals are the vectors of lung diseases ranging from asthma to fibrosis and cancer. With the exception of occupational asthma, little is known about the mechanisms by which metals cause lung dysfunction. However, a number of studies have evaluated the effects of metals on pulmonary macrophage functions.

Until recently, investigations of metal-induced lung disease have been primarily concerned with the clinicopathological expression of the exposed workers. Pneumonitis and broncholitis attributable to manganese dioxide exposure have been described, but the mechanism of this chemically induced disorder has not been completely evaluated (352). Mononuclear cell infiltrations are observed in the lungs of exposed workers, and large macrophage-like cells appear to be the target of cytotoxic effects. Similar effects have been described in workers exposed to nickel carbonyl (519). Pathological examinations of the lungs of patients who succumbed to their disease show alveolar spaces filled with pigment-laden histiocytes, and hepatic Kupffer cells are also engorged with a similar pigment. Nickel carbonyl is extremely toxic, and a 30 ppm exposure for 30 minutes is usually fatal. Alterations in adenosine triphosphatase and RNA polymerase have been implicated in the toxic responses, but little else has been evaluated. Whether phagocytic cell activity is diminished has not been evaluated. Copper sulfate used to prevent mildew in grape vineyards has given rise to a granulomatous disorder of the lung aptly called vineyard sprayer's lung (433,548). The pathology of this disorder is characterized in its early stages by macrophage desquamation and the subsequent formation of histiocytic granulomas. Infections, fibrosis, and cavitation may all occur in this disorder, suggesting a pathogenic response similar to that observed in coal miner's pneumoconiosis. There is a high rate of tuberculin anergy in these copper sulfate-exposed workers, giving rise to the speculation that immune dysfunction plays a part in this disease. The increased frequency of cancer in vineyard sprayers relates to the use of arsenic in the spray rather than a copper sulfate–mediated condition.

In addition to these clinical studies after human exposure, animal studies of lavaged cells have been performed to assess the effects of metals on alveolar macrophage viability and function (38,99,555). Viability of macrophages has been shown to decrease to levels of less than 50% of control tissue cultures at concentrations of 0.1 mM for cadmium and vanadate and 4 to 5 mM for nickel, manganese, and chromium. Only *in vitro* cadmium exposures have been shown to maintain cell numbers identical to those of controls at concentrations that significantly lower their viability. Other metals cause a significant reduction in these cell numbers in association with a decrease in their *in vitro* viability. The latter cells also show a decrease in acid phosphatase activity, a marker of macrophage lysosomal enzymes, presumably as a result of enzyme release into the extracellular milieu. With the exception of nickel, there is a direct correlation between viability and a decrease in phagocytic capacity by macrophages. Nickel impairs phagocytosis at a concentration much lower than is needed to reduce cell viability. Such data are probably related to the capacity of nickel to bind adenosine triphosphatase and adenosine triphosphate, which blocks the adenosine triphosphate energy release and utilization necessary for phagocytosis.

Well-characterized defects in the generation of immune responses have been delineated for lead exposure, and ever-present pollutant commonly found in the environment and a frequent occupational hazard (324,399,542). Lead has been demonstrated to enhance and inhibit the expression of plaque-forming cells in mice, and cell-mediated immunity, as measured by challenges with *Listeria monocytogenes*, shows an increased mortality in lead-exposed animals as compared with controls. Further, delayed hypersensitivity is suppressed in mice exposed to lead. Recent investigations of cell-mediated immunity in mice have also demonstrated that autologous mixed lymphocyte reactions are stimulated by lead exposure, whereas antigen presentation is suppressed. No defect in phagocytosis or interleukin-1 has been found to account for such findings. Unfortunately, the mechanisms by which lead causes such defects in cell-mediated immunity remain unresolved.

These data suggest that metals may clearly alter lung macrophage-dependent processes, including those related to immune reactions. Despite these documented changes in macrophage biology, relatively little evidence is available in the medical literature in support of metal-induced immune dysfunctions. Even though few reports of immune-mediated lung diseases after metal exposure have been described, the models represented by berylliosis and metal-induced occupational asthma indicate the need for careful evaluations of lung functions and pulmonary immune responses in individuals exposed to metals.

Ozone

Oxidants such as ozone, nitrogen oxides, and sulfur oxides are common contaminants of ambient air (91,211,349,384,514,574). These gases arise from a number of different sources and their generation, in some instances, is interdependent. Ozone arises, in part, from exchanges between stratospheric ozone and tropospheric air (349). Ozone is also generated by complex photochemical reactions between organic vapors (olefinic hydrocarbons, formaldehyde, *m*-xylene), nitrogen oxides, and ultraviolet radiation. Methane gas from biogenic decay as well as isoprene and terpenes from trees also contribute to ozone formation. Industrial processes and vehicular traffic also result in the formation of ozone.

Ozone is the most potent airborne oxidant. It has two free electrons and can form free radicals that have the propensity to oxidize tissue components. For this reason, ozone is more reactive than nitrogen and sulfur oxides, but it is less water-soluble than the latter two compounds. The current ambient air quality standard for ozone is 120 ppb or 235 $\mu g/m^3$ body surface area for a maximum exposure time of 1 hour (349). More than half the United States population resides in areas where this standard is exceeded, and such data emphasize the need to understand the short- and long-term health effects of this compound. Exposure to oxidants in doses that exceed the usual and acceptable standards may result in changes in pulmonary function, may account for an increased incidence of asthma and other respiratory disorders, and may increase the susceptibility of exposed hosts to infections as a result of altered lung defense mechanisms. There is also evidence that ozone increases the risk for lung cancer.

The focus of this discussion is concerned with the immunopathogenic effects of oxidants that may result from changes in mechanical systems regulating host lung defenses (mucociliary escalator), nonspecific alterations in inflammatory and immune cells essential for host defenses, or specific defects in lung immune responses used for protection against and prevention from invasive infectious agents. In reviewing these processes, it must be recognized that animal responses to ozone may not reflect the human reaction to ozone, and extrapolations from animals to humans may be inappropriate. This is best illustrated by the delay in mucociliary clearance observed in animals exposed to ozone, whereas human exposures lead to accelerated mucociliary clearances (177,302,304). Other variables also play a role in determining the health effects of ozone. These include the dose, the duration of exposure, the mixture of pollutants contaminating the ozone, and the physical activity of the exposed host. For these reasons, oxidant studies usually characterize physiological changes occurring after acute, short-term exposures or after chronic, longer term exposures. Since exercise increases the dose delivered to the respiratory tract, airborne measurements are not comparable to tissue doses. All these factors must be considered in order to derive a true representation of how airborne pollutants affect human health.

More than adequate evidence exists to show that airborne pollutants, including ozone, increase the susceptibility to infection in animals (96,97,222,223, 426,487,498,544). These studies have been structured to evaluate the morbidity and mortality of ozone exposure in animals who have subsequently been challenged with bacteria. Such experiments are not a true reflection of an increased susceptibility to infectious agents because microbes, in the natural state, are not always delivered to the human host in the same doses used in animal experiments. Nonetheless, these animal investigations clearly indicate that ozone does induce defects in lung host defense functions, even though the microbial dose necessary to exploit such deficiencies has not been precisely defined for humans.

In terms of ozone-related immunosuppression of lung defense functions, two central mechanisms are likely to contribute to this dysfunction: alterations in the function of lung defense cells and specific changes in the immune responses essential for the integrity of host defenses. Studies in rabbits exposed to ozone at 1 to 3 ppm for 3 hours have demonstrated that changes in both the functions and numbers of pulmonary cells occur after such exposures (97). Alveolar macrophage numbers decrease, whereas the number of neutrophils increases in lung lavage samples. The peak increment in neutrophils occurs about 10 hours after ozone exposure and declines gradually over 24 hours (97). A significant decrease in alveolar macrophage phagocytic capacity has also been measured by *in vitro* assays of phagocytosis. Further, there is also a decrease in the number of macrophages engaged in phagocytosis (97). These responses have been observed at ozone concentrations as low as 0.33 ppm, with a maximum response at 4 ppm. Similar results have been observed using radiolabeled bacteria to assess *in vivo* antibacterial defenses. Since nasal lavage is a useful marker of inflammatory cell response after ozone exposure, investigations have been performed in rats to determine whether such nasal responses reflected pulmonary inflammatory responses (275). For these studies, rats have been exposed to various concentrations of ozone (0, 0.12, 0.8, and 1.5 ppm) for 6 hours and then sacrificed either immediately after exposure or at 3, 18, 42, or 66 hours after exposure. No significant change in nasal lavage neutrophil content has been observed with 0.12 ppm ozone until 18 hours after exposure, and no concurrent change in BAL neutrophil numbers has been observed at this and later time points. In rats exposed to 0.8 ppm of ozone, neutrophils in the nasal lavage fluid are increased in the immediate postexposure samples, but no concomitant change in BAL neutrophil content is observed at that time point. However, as the numbers of neutrophils in the BAL fluid increase to reach a maximum at 42 hours after exposure, there is an accompanying decrease in the numbers of nasal lavage neutrophils. Interestingly, rats exposed to 1.5 ppm of ozone show significant increases in neutrophil numbers in BAL samples obtained at 3, 18, and 42 hours after ozone exposure, but such changes are not accompanied by any significant alterations in nasal lavage neutrophil numbers. The results of these studies suggest that at low ozone concentrations (0.12 to 0.8 ppm), nasal lavage samples may represent a reflection of pulmonary changes in neutrophil numbers, but at higher doses, nasal lavage samples probably underestimate the neutrophil changes occurring in the lung.

Since ozone exposure in animals decreases lung antibacterial defense mechanisms and cells with antibacterial activity infiltrate the lung and nasal passages of ozone-exposed mammals, a key question is why infections are increased after ozone exposure in animals and whether similar conditions exist in humans. As will be seen in the subsequent descriptions, a variety of different mechanisms have been proposed, but no one factor appears to have been implicated as a cause of increased infection in ozone-exposed animals. Such studies have clearly documented an increased incidence of infections with pathogenic streptococci, *Klebsiella pneumoniae*, *Staphylococcus aureus* as well as *Listeria monocytogenes* and influenza A virus (95,379,443,487,544). These studies have concluded, for the most part, that defective antibacterial macrophage defenses are primarily responsible for this increased susceptibility to infection, but the actual mechanisms remain elusive. In recent studies of ozone-exposed rats, T-cell–mediated immunity to *L. monocytogenes* also appears to be impaired by ozone. Such changes are particularly evident if ozone exposure occurs during an infection with this organism. Both delayed type hypersensitivity after ear challenge with formalin-killed bacteria and antigen-specific lymphoproliferative responses are significantly depressed in animals exposed to ozone in the presence of *L. monocytogenes* infection (544).

Since asthmatics show nonspecific airways hyperactivity similar to the findings observed in ozone-exposed animals and humans and the increasing frequency of asthma in humans has been postulated to be associated, to some degree, with ozone (air pollutant) exposure (26,218,389,514), animal studies have been performed to examine the responses of allergic animals to antigens known to provoke allergic airways responses. Both immediate and late phase asthmatic responses are altered by short-term ozone exposures (1 ppm for 5 minutes), but the mechanisms by which these alterations occur have not been completely characterized (311,533). The alteration of antigen-induced bronchoconstriction after ozone exposure in dogs sensitive to *Ascaris* serum antigen does not appear to be related to the tissue invasion with polymorphonuclear leukocytes. The late phase bronchoconstrictor response is completely blocked when ozone is administered in conjunction with the antigen. This effect occurs in the setting of increased mast cell numbers in the airways.

Other investigations have demonstrated a significant increase in IgE in the airways of mice exposed to ozone and then given a standard dose of aerosolized antigen (ovalbumin) (202). Total numbers of IgE cells have been shown to be increased in mice that received aerosolized antigen as compared with mice that did not receive antigen. On the other hand, ozone-exposed mice have a much more marked increase in IgE cells when compared with controls and mice receiving only aerosolized antigen. Precipitating antibodies have not been detected in the sera of animals challenged with aerosolized antigen. The effects of ozone on IgE antibody production after delivery of aerosolized antigen have also been examined. Relatively high doses of ozone were used in these short-term experiments (0.8 ppm ozone for 1, 2, or 4 weeks), and the timing of the antigen administration is critical to eliciting an ozone-induced effect. Primary IgE antibody production is unaffected by ozone when antigen is administered by the intraperitoneal route, whereas the administration of aerosolized antigen after ozone exposure and the subsequent intraperitoneal immunization with antigen cause a significant suppression of IgE antibody production (414). On the basis of these results, it has been postulated that the suppression of IgE is caused either by altered helper T-cell function or by the activity of a radiation-resistant suppressor T cell. Mice exposed to ozone (0.8 ppm for varying times up to 2 weeks) also show a significant suppression of the primary antibody response to a T-dependent antigen, sheep red blood cells (188). On the other hand, no significant change in antibody response has been observed at this ozone dose with the T-independent antigen, DNP-Ficoll. These effects correlate with a decrease in thymus weights.

In addition to these ozone-induced effects on antibody production, recent investigations have demonstrated that ozone exposure at 1 ppm for varying periods of time up to 7 days caused a suppression of pulmonary natural killer cell activity (63). Adaptation to ozone exposure occurs, since the observed suppression in natural killer cell activity is not seen if ozone exposure continues beyond 7 days. The mechanism for this repair of natural killer cell activity remains unknown, and in fact, the mechanism by which suppression of natural killer cell activity is induced is not understood. The direct effect of an adherent suppressor cell as a cause for these findings has not been excluded. Prostaglandin E_2, a known inhibitor of natural killer cell cytotoxicity, could account for this ozone-induced suppression of pulmonary natural killer cell activity, and studies show that ozone increases PGE_2 levels in BAL fluids (see Chapter 15). Since natural killer cell activity plays a significant role in host defenses against tumors and viral infections, examination of these parameters is appropriate. Despite the role of these cells in viral infection, little direct support for alterations in the morbidity and mortality from viral infections in ozone-exposed mammals can be documented. In fact, there is evidence that ozone reduces the severity of influenza virus infection in mice. Thus, the effects of ozone exposure on viral infection in animals remains incompletely understood. Natural killer cell activity also participates in tumor surveillance, but its part in that function has not been apportioned in relation to other immunosurveillance mechanisms. Initial studies using a mouse adenoma assay show that ozone delivered at concentrations of 0.31 ppm for 103 hours per week every other week for 6 months or 0.50 ppm for 102 continuous hours during the first week of each month for 6 months causes an increased number of lung tumors as compared with what occurs in mice exposed to room air alone (255). Under these conditions, ozone has been determined to behave like a tumor promoter when combined with urethane (2 mg per mouse intraperitoneally) given prior to exposure to 0.31 ppm ozone as described above or the same urethane dose given at the end of the 0.5 ppm ozone administered at monthly intervals. When ozone is given after urethane, no tumor-promoting capacity has been observed. Animals given both ozone and urethane have a significant increase in lung tumor formation. It has been suggested that ozone causes more cells to become susceptible to the carcinogenic properties of urethane. Using different mouse strains, ozone decreases the number of tumors when administered in association with urethane, and it has been postulated that ozone may either increase or decrease the susceptibility of cells to carcinogens (340). The latter effect could be mediated by a cytotoxic mechanism. Further, the difference in genetic makeup of animals may clearly play a role in the ultimate outcome. Whether natural killer cells could significantly alter such tumor expression is unknown, and obviously exposure conditions also have a major influence on the resultant effects. The effects of ozone on mouse fibrosarcoma NR-FS metastases also emphasize the multifactorial nature of the process (315). In these studies, ozone exposure (0.1, 0.2, 0.4, or 0.8 ppm) for 1, 3, 5, 7, or 14 days causes an increase in the number of fibrosarcoma metastases compared to that observed in mice not exposed to ozone. Both the duration of exposure and the dose influence the rate of metastases; higher doses and longer times of exposure increase the number of metastases. The corollary of this is also true. Modulation of cytotoxic natural killer cells and perhaps cytotoxic macrophages may play a role in regulating metastatic disease.

In summary, macrophages and natural killer cells may play a significant role in host defenses against bacterial and viral infections as well as in tumor expression, but the detailed mechanisms of their effect and the degree of contribution to tumorigenesis or infection remain almost completely unknown. Thus, the effects of airborne pollutants on these processes remain only partially understood.

Despite the body of evidence implicating ozone as a mediator of lung disease and immune dysfunction, the underlying mechanisms accounting for ozone toxicity remain incompletely characterized. The earliest observations describe an ozone-induced decrease in the phagocytic properties of pulmonary alveolar macrophages (97). Further investigations attempting to evaluate the decrease in both phagocytic capacity and antibacterial defenses have assessed the levels of lysosomal enzymes in alveolar macrophages (279). Acid phosphatase, beta-glucuronidase, and lysozyme levels have all been determined to be low in rabbits exposed to 0.25 ppm ozone for 3 hours, with a maximal depression after 3 ppm for the same time period. Further, the depression of lysosomal enzyme levels in macrophages is no longer apparent within 24 hours. Other workers have shown that rabbit alveolar macrophages have increased osmotic fragility after ozone exposure at relatively high doses (10 ppm for 3 hours) (141). Ozone or an ozone metabolite may alter macrophage plasma membranes or macrophage lysosomal membranes. Additional evidence of altered membrane integrity comes from studies of concanavalin A agglutinability of ozone-exposed alveolar macrophages (0.5 ppm for 60 minutes *in vitro*) (220). Both a significant reduction in agglutination by concanavalin A after ozone exposure and no change in the number of concanavalin A binding sites have been observed. Since the number of concanavalin A receptors is not reduced by ozone,

ozone may alter the transduction of the concanavalin A receptor message via a change in alveolar macrophage membrane fluidity. Nitrogen dioxide (2.4 ppm for 60 minutes), another airborne pollutant and oxidant, causes an increased agglutination with concanavalin A treatment (220). These studies clearly demonstrate differences between the effects of these two oxidants on alveolar macrophages. Cigarette smokers' macrophages also show greater agglutination by concanavalin A than macrophages recovered from nonsmokers. Such results suggest that nitrogen oxides may cause these effects in cigarette smokers and emphasize the potential differences in the effects of ozone and nitrogen oxides in cigarette smoke.

Defective macrophage migration could suppress the capacity of the host to respond to bacterial challenges, and a significant decrease in the *in vitro* mobility of alveolar macrophages obtained by lavage from rhesus monkeys exposed to 0.8 ppm ozone for 7 days has been shown compared with mobility of macrophages not exposed to ozone (484). A change in macrophage kinetics with a diminished migratory capacity and a decrease in the removal of macrophages over time has been suggested from such ozone data. Ozone-exposed macrophages do respond to chemotaxins contained in lung lining material. Subsequent investigations confirm a decrease in rat alveolar macrophage mobility after *in vivo* ozone exposure and demonstrate its reversibility with time (142,363). Despite these changes in macrophage mobility, rabbit alveolar macrophages retain the capacity to release chemotactic and/or chemokinetic factors for neutrophils and monocytes after ozone exposure (0.1 to 1.2 ppm for 2 hours) (142). The threshold level for the release of the chemoattractant for peripheral blood neutrophils occurs at ozone exposure doses of 0.1 to 0.3 ppm for 2 hours. After 1.2 ppm ozone, macrophages also appear to release a factor that stimulates monocyte migration. These findings are perfectly consistent with the pathological findings in humans exposed to ozone, but the mechanism by which this pollutant enhances the release of such chemoattractants remains unknown. Ozone has also been determined to cause a decrease in interferon production by rabbit alveolar macrophages, but studies in humans after ozone exposure do not show any change in interferon production (259,499). Thus, it can be concluded that many macrophage functions are altered by ozone, but the mechanisms for these alterations remain unknown.

Recent studies have evaluated the capacity of ozone exposure in rats to generate oxygen-derived oxidants, including superoxide radical, hydroxyl radical, and hydrogen peroxide (161). The rationale for such experiments was to determine whether changes in either bactericidal activity or cytotoxic responses could be correlated with the presence or absence of oxidant formation. Rats exposed to 2 ppm ozone for 4 hours show a significant decrease in superoxide generation by lung cell populations lavaged immediately after ozone exposure. Such effects last for nearly 3 days after ozone exposure. These changes could reflect the direct effects of ozone on resident alveolar macrophages, altered inflammatory cell populations, or both processes. Using luminol-amplified chemiluminescence, which is a measure of oxidants primarily derived from peroxidase-mediated reactions, a significant increase in TPA-stimulated and opsonized zymosan-stimulated chemiluminescence has been observed in ozone-exposed lavaged samples as compared with samples of controls (161). The correlation of this increment with the degree of neutrophil migration to the lung provides strongly suggestive evidence that polymorphonuclear leukocytes account for these changes in chemoluminescence. The inhibitors of chemoluminescence, superoxide dismutase and sodium azide, have been used to further characterize the cells responsible for this increment in chemoluminescence. Sodium azide inhibits the myeloperoxidase-dependent chemoluminescence generated by neutrophils, whereas superoxide dismutase inhibits primarily macrophage-generated superoxide. As might be expected, azide significantly inhibits the enhanced chemoluminescence observed 24 hours after ozone exposure when the percentage of neutrophils in lavages has peaked. Further, taurine chloramine generation has only been observed in cells obtained 24 hours after ozone exposure and not in cells from control animals. Since myeloperoxidase-dependent hypochlorous acid generation is essential for the reaction with taurine to form chloramines, taurine chloramine generation observed in this time sequence suggests that its formation results from the presence of neutrophil myeloperoxidase in the lavage fluid. Interestingly, macrophages in the presence of exogenous myeloperoxidase can also generate taurine chloramine, and BAL fluid obtained from ozone-exposed rats contains free myeloperoxidase, whereas this enzyme is absent from air-exposed control lavages. These data make a strong case for the contribution of oxidants to the ozone-induced alterations in immune and inflammatory cells, but no evidence has been presented as to the mechanism by which such oxidants damage various immune cell functions.

In summary, ozone induces multiple defects in animal immune systems, with an increased frequency of infection being the most significant clinical expression of these ozone-induced abnormalities. In the human, the picture is less clear, since little or no evidence exists that an increased incidence of lung infection occurs in relation to ozone exposure. Some evidence exists to implicate ozone as a carcinogen, and there are immune system dysfunctions observed in animals that could be related to an increased incidence of cancer. Epidemiological studies have demonstrated that asthma is on the increase in humans, and the focus of oxidant-induced injury should probably be related to this observation. What is strikingly obvious from the reported studies in both humans and animals is the absence of a clear mechanism by which ozone alters immune cells and their function. Many studies suggest that free radicals play a major role in ozone-induced tissue and cell alterations, but the way in which this occurs has yet to be defined. It is entirely possible that such ozone-induced changes are multifactorial, but the identification of a specific mechanism for ozone-induced immune dysfunction would permit a more precise evaluation of the role of this oxidant in the immunopathogenesis of human lung diseases.

Nitrogen Oxides

Nitrogen oxides arise from decaying organic matter, forest fires, atmospheric lightning, and volcanic debris, and such sources represent the primary environmental origins of these oxidants. Over 300,000 tons of such oxidants are also produced annually in the United States from a wide variety of industrial processes, and more than 10 million tons are generated from fuel combustion (397). Industrial production of nitrogen oxides includes such diverse processes as welding, exposure to the products of internal combustion engines, agricultural silos, textile and food bleaching, and the manufacture of nitric acid and jewelry (306,445a). For nitrogen dioxide, the current ambient air quality standard for 24-hour concentrations must not exceed, on the average, 100 μg/m^3 on an annual basis (124). The World Health Organization recommends that hourly exposures to nitrogen dioxide not exceed 190 to 320 μg/m^3 for 1 hour (124).

Nitrogen oxides are the other major class of airborne oxidants that increase susceptibility to respiratory infections in animals (151–153,221,281,284,285,417,423), but little evidence for this effect can be found in the literature concerned with human exposure to nitrogen dioxide (217,471,510). However, epidemiological evidence of increased respiratory infections in children exposed to nitrogen dioxide has been published (510). There is also a sufficient body of evidence to demonstrate an increase in airway obstruction after nitrogen oxide exposure in humans, despite the fact that nitrogen dioxide is less soluble than ozone and may be less capable of reaching small airways (27,74,411). For these reasons, it is important to seek nitrogen dioxide (NO$_2$)–induced changes in immune cell numbers and their functions. Further, although most investigations center on NO$_2$, there are other oxides of nitrogen to which humans are exposed and that may cause more significant effects on the immune system of the lung than NO$_2$.

A variety of studies have been performed in animals to address lung defense mechanisms from three different perspectives: alterations in lung cell populations and their lung defense functions, susceptibility to infectious agents, and immune responses of the lung.

Alterations in Lung Cell Populations and Functions

Investigations document a significant increase in the percentage of polymorphonuclear leukocytes obtained by lavage from rabbits exposed to 8, 16, 20, 36, and 60 ppm NO$_2$ for 3 hours (196). This increment is first observed at doses of 8 ppm NO$_2$ and at 20 ppm NO$_2$; more than 10% of the BAL cells are neutrophils. Comparisons between ozone and nitrogen dioxide have found that 2 ppm ozone (9.08 mmol/m^3) causes an increase in neutrophils comparable to the numbers observed with 25 ppm NO$_2$ (0.98 mmol/m^3) (196). Thus, ozone is a more potent inducer of neutrophil aggregation than NO$_2$. After a single dose of 40 ppm NO$_2$ for 3 hours, the peak increase in neutrophil numbers recovered by lavage (20 × 10^6 neutrophils) has been observed 6 to 9 hours after exposure, and elevated neutrophil numbers persist for 72 hours after exposure. A significant decrease in macrophage phagocytic capacity is also observed after such *in vivo* exposures (196). *In vitro* exposure of macrophages to NO$_2$ also impairs their capacity for phagocytosis (392). Subsequent studies have demonstrated an increased capacity for phagocytosis in alveolar macrophages obtained from rats exposed to 40 ppm NO$_2$ for 4 hours/day for 1 day (509). In these experiments phagocytosis is measured by the uptake of opsonized sheep red blood cells in contrast to the use of bacteria in those experiments showing depressed macrophage phagocytosis. In the experiments using opsonized red blood cells, a single-day exposure caused a greater increment in phagocytic capacity compared with a 7-day exposure to NO_2. Nonetheless, increased phagocytosis is also observed after a 7-day exposure, but exposures for 2 weeks produce no change in the ability of macrophages to phagocytose erythrocytes.

After a 2-hour *in vitro* exposure of macrophages to either 10 or 20 ppm NO_2, increased cytotoxic activity has been observed against syngeneic mammary adenocarcinoma cells (509). Exposure to nitrogen dioxide at 40 ppm for 2 hours does not increase the cytotoxic activity of macrophages, but after low-dose NO_2 (10 ppm) a time-related increase in cytotoxic activity is seen. No cytotoxic activity is observed when normal syngeneic cells are the target of NO_2-exposed macrophages (509). Similar experiments to assess macrophage activation have been performed with macrophages obtained by lavage after NO_2 exposure in an intact animal. *In vitro* activation induced by lipopolysaccharide, muramyl dipeptide, or macrophage activating factor after low-dose, short-term NO_2 exposure (4 hours) results in an increase in rat macrophage cytotoxic activity when compared with cells obtained from unexposed rats (509). Cells recovered from animals exposed to NO_2 and then incubated for 24 hours before assaying their cytotoxic activity show no enhancement of this function. Such experiments clearly demonstrate that multiple NO_2 exposures are less effective in their capacity to activate macrophages than single NO_2 exposures. In addition, the effect of NO_2 on the cytotoxic capacity of these cells is a time-dependent process; such effects are no longer observed when cells are incubated for more than 24 hours after exposure (509). On the basis of these experiments, acute NO_2 exposures appear to enhance immunological reactivity, whereas chronic NO_2 exposures result in tolerance.

Rats exposed continuously to 30 ppm NO_2 for 3 to 6 weeks have been used to quantitate the changes in the cellular content of lung lavages (210). An immediate and significant increase in neutrophils has been observed under these conditions, which peaks on day 2 of NO_2 exposure and then rapidly decreases to levels of two- to sixfold above controls for the entire 20 weeks of NO_2 exposure. Macrophage numbers in the lavage from these same experiments actually decrease on day 2 of NO_2 exposure, but after 7 days of exposure, macrophage numbers increase to twice those observed in air-exposed controls. Macrophage numbers subsequently decrease to normal after 14 days of exposure. Lymphocytes in the lavage from NO_2-exposed animals increase abruptly after the onset of NO_2 exposure and reach a peak around day 7 (210). By 2 weeks, lymphocyte numbers have fallen below normal levels and remain at their usual low levels in lavage fluid for the remainder of the exposure period. Although these studies clearly delineate the changes in the lung cell populations associated with continuous NO_2 exposure in rats, no functional analyses were performed on the cells recovered by lavage.

From these and other data, it is clear that neutrophils accumulate in the lung in response to NO_2 exposures and that macrophage function is altered. In some experiments, macrophages show decreased phagocytic capacity, whereas in others, NO_2 exposure enhances macrophage phagocytic and tumoricidal activities (509,520). Whether these opposing functional changes relate to differences in the way macrophages respond from different animal species or some other factors, such as NO_2 dose, experimental conditions, or sample handling, remains to be defined. As might be expected, the capacity of alveolar macrophages to generate superoxide anion has also been evaluated using a nonphagocytic stimulus (phorbol myristate acetate) in animals exposed to NO_2 (6). In NO_2-exposed rats (24 ppm-hours), a significant decrease in superoxide production has been observed when such data are compared with the superoxide generated by air-exposed rats and NO_2-exposed rats receiving NO_2 doses less than 24 ppm-hours. NO_2 doses between 35 and 50 ppm-hours decrease superoxide production to levels of less than 50% of controls. Such changes may contribute to the increased susceptibility of animals to infection. Confirmatory studies linking decreased phagocytosis and superoxide production after low doses of NO_2 (4 to 8 ppm for 5 to 7 days) have also been published (520). In addition to these changes in superoxide anion production, a decrease in hexose monophosphate shunt activity after NO_2 exposure has been observed that is consistent with the decrements in phagocytic activity observed by others (3).

To determine the effects of NO_2 on the inflammatory process in the lung, the generation of neutrophil chemotactic factor by human alveolar macrophages and the release of interleukin-1, an activator of many immune cell activities, has been examined (435). After exposure to 5, 10, and 15 ppm of NO_2 for 3 hours, it has been determined that no differences between the capacities of air-exposed controls and NO_2-exposed human macrophages to release interleukin-1 exist. Further, no NO_2-induced alteration in the quantity of neutrophil chemotactic factor released by these NO_2 exposed and unexposed macrophages has been found. Another cellular component that contributes significantly to localized inflammatory processes is the lymphokine, migration inhibitory factor, which has the ability to maintain macrophages at the site of an inflammatory reaction. Baboon alveolar macrophages obtained by lavage from animals exposed to 2 ppm NO_2 for 8 hours per day for 5 days a week for 6 months do not respond to migration inhibitory factor derived from antigen-stimulated autologous lymphocytes (233). Thus, NO_2 exposure in animals appears to alter the responsiveness of macrophages to lymphokines that assist in the repair of localized inflammatory reactions.

Susceptibility to Infectious Agents

Central to the NO_2 exposure issue in animals is the reported increased susceptibility to infection in such animals. Further, the influx of polymorphonuclear leukocytes induced by NO_2 exposure should enhance the biocidal and virucidal capacities of the lung. However, in animals exposed to NO_2, these antibacterial and antiviral defense mechanisms appear to be diminished by NO_2. Early workers studying the effects of NO_2 on virus infections have demonstrated that alveolar macrophages from rabbits exposed to 25 ppm of NO_2 for 3 hours are unable to develop resistance to rabbit pox virus infection when an infective dose of parainfluenza 3 virus is administered within 24 hours after NO_2 exposure (541). These NO_2-exposed macrophages are also unable to produce interferon, a substance known to have antiviral activity. The mechanisms accounting for such alterations in these host defense functions have not been delineated. Monkeys exposed chronically to NO_2 (1 ppm continuously for 393 days) show no alteration in their capacity to produce serum neutralizing antibody against a monkey-adapted influenza strain when compared with air-exposed and virus-challenged controls (167,168).

A more realistic approach to the effects of NO_2 on viral infections has been taken by investigators using murine cytomegalovirus infection as a model (457). In these studies, mice were exposed for 2 consecutive days to 5 ppm NO_2 for 6 hours prior to the delivery of murine cytomegalovirus by intratracheal inoculation. After viral inoculation, NO_2 exposure is continued for 4 days at the same dose to CD-1 mice. The results of these studies show that more than 70% of NO_2-exposed mice develop viral bronchopneumonia associated with murine cytomegalovirus proliferation in contrast to air-exposed control mice, which are free of any pneumonia and show no evidence of viral replication. A dose-response curve based on the NO_2 exposure dose was derived from these experiments. About 4 ppm NO_2 results in a 50% infection rate in mice given an identical viral inoculum, and the viral dose necessary to infect NO_2-exposed mice was 100-fold lower than the dose required to infect air-exposed control mice. In addition to these findings, *in vivo* phagocytosis by macrophages has been evaluated by comparing radiolabeled gold ingestion in NO_2-exposed and air-exposed mice (457). Macrophage phagocytosis is also significantly decreased in animals exposed to 5 ppm NO_2 using the same exposure conditions cited previously. These same NO_2-exposed animals are also less efficient in their capacity to destroy murine cytomegalovirus as compared with their air-exposed controls. Thus, NO_2 exposure alters certain macrophage-dependent antiviral activities. The possibility that natural killer cells may contribute to these defective antiviral activities has not been excluded. These animal data provide a reasonable body of evidence that implicates NO_2 as an agent capable of altering antiviral defenses in animals.

Lung Defense Mechanisms

A number of investigations have clearly demonstrated that NO_2 impairs lung antibacterial defenses (150–153,221,281,417). Such studies have addressed the mechanisms by which antibacterial lung defenses are altered as well as attempted to characterize the effects of NO_2 on different classes of bacteria. The general conclusion from all these studies is that NO_2 affects different lung defense mechanisms, depending on the pollutant dose, the time of exposure, and the bacterial strain under study. It is reasonably well established that animal lungs challenged with *Staphylococcus aureus* do not mount an inflammatory response (351), and bacterial disposal is primarily dependent on alveolar macrophage phagocytosis and intracellular killing (221,409) whereas organisms like *Proteus mirabilis* cause the recruitment of neutrophils to the lungs and are likely to be dependent on ingestion and killing by both neutrophils and macrophages (432,448,449). Experiments with *Proteus pneumotropica* have been used to examine the response of lung defense mechanisms to an organism endogenous to mice (53,286), and studies with this organism and NO_2 exposure suggest that yet another lung defense mechanism, antibody generation against *P. pneumotropica*, may play a role in the antibacterial defenses against this organism (284,285). Mice exposed to 4 ppm of NO_2 for 4 hours have defective antibacterial defenses against an aerosol inhalation of a constant number of *S. aureus*, and this defective host defense system is dose-dependent (284,285). With *P. mirabilis* aerosol inhalation, no difference in bacterial killing is observed between control and experimental mice at a dose of 5 ppm NO_2 for 4 hours. At NO_2 doses of 10 and 15 ppm for 4 hours, there is an enhancement in intrapulmonary killing of *P. mirabilis*, and this increment in bacterial killing is associated with an increase in neutrophils in the lavage obtained from mice exposed to these NO_2 doses. Nonetheless, at a dose of 20 ppm of NO_2, there is a suppression of intrapulmonary killing of *P. mirabilis*. Finally, 5 ppm NO_2 exposure for 4 hours produces no differences in bacterial killing between control and pollutant-exposed animals, whereas exposure to 10 ppm NO_2 for the same time period results in a significant suppression of *P. pneumotropica* killing (284,285). At 15 and 20 ppm of NO_2, no significant change in bacterial killing is observed between control and experimental mice, but at 25 and 30 ppm NO_2, there is a reappearance of suppressed bacterial killing. A neutrophil influx into the lungs occurs when mice are challenged with *P. pneumotropica* and exposed to either air or NO_2 (10 ppm), and relatively little difference in the numbers of neutrophils is observed when control (air-exposed) and experimental mice are compared.

Several additional parameters have been evaluated with respect to NO_2 exposures and antibacterial defense mechanisms. These include data relating investigations of pathogen-free animals, genetic strains with resistance and susceptibility to organisms, and animals exposed to mixtures of pollutants. Studies of mice strains exposed to NO_2 and infectious aerosols of murine *Mycoplasma pulmonis* provide solid experimental evidence that NO_2 enhances pulmonary infections with this organism in pathogen-free mice (417). Such effects have been documented both by an increase in the numbers of *Mycoplasma* organisms and the severity of the pneumonic infiltrate but not by an increase in susceptibility to the organism. Since strains both susceptible and resistant to *M. pulmonis* show abnormalities resulting from NO_2 exposure, no specific genotype appears to be responsible for the pathology associated with NO_2 exposure. However, there are differences in the mortality rates between C3H/HeN-susceptible mice and C57BL/6N-resistant mice that may indicate interactions between the NO_2 dose, the concentration of organisms, and the genetic makeup of the host.

Mixed pollutant exposures obviously may reflect what occurs with air pollution and may provide a more realistic view of the pathogenesis of those dysfunctions associated with exposures to pollutants. Studies using ozone and NO_2 show that *S. aureus* bactericidal dysfunction is observed only when one pollutant exceeds its threshold value (221). In another study, using a single exposure of ozone and NO_2 for 5 hours, mice exposed to an infectious challenge with *Staphylococcus pyogenes* by aerosol have increased mortality, and the effects of these pollutants are additive (152). Data from mixtures of these two pollutants given as multiple doses (20 daily 3-hour exposures) appear to have a synergistic effect on mortality. Subsequent studies by these same investigators have demonstrated that mixed exposure of 0.5 ppm NO_2 and 0.1 ppm ozone in animals both before and after the aerosol bacterial challenge significantly increased susceptibility to pneumonia when compared with animals given postaerosol delivery of pollutants (153). Other investigations have supported the concept that exercise increases the quantity of pollutant delivered to the lung, which could alter host resistance to infection (281). The occurrence of an increased mortality rate when ozone or NO_2 is administered to exercising mice compared with mice that were not exercised appears to support this conclusion.

Thus, it appears that genetic factors may affect lung responses to airborne pollutants, but evidence for this is far from conclusive. Mixed exposures of NO_2 and ozone seem to be additive, and therefore airborne pollutant mixtures may be more deleterious than an identical dose of a single agent. Continuous exposure to a pollutant during an infection seems to be more harmful than when pollutant exposures end with the introduction of aerosolized bacteria. Thus, the advice to remain in a pollutant-free environment during the course of a respiratory tract infection seems unwarranted.

Immune Responses of the Lung

Defective cellular and humoral immunity may also play a role in the increased expression of infections associated with exposures of animals to NO_2. Investigations have demonstrated circulating substances in guinea pigs exposed to NO_2 that cause latex agglutination when such substances are used to coat latex particles and are then reacted with lung proteins (14). The titers of these serum antibodies are higher in guinea pigs exposed to 5 ppm NO_2 for 4 hours daily for 2 months than in air-exposed control animals. Exposure to 15 ppm NO_2, under similar conditions, gives agglutination titers that far exceed those of control animals. The character of these serum substances induced by NO_2 exposure has not been delineated. Subsequent investigations have evaluated the effect of NO_2 exposure on the generation of serum neutralization and hemagglutination-inhibition antibodies after vaccination with influenza virus (154). Under conditions in which Swiss albino mice have been exposed to 0.5 ppm NO_2 for 5 days per week with daily peak exposures of 2 ppm NO_2 over a 12-week period, there is a significant depression of serum neutralization antibody in NO_2-exposed mice compared with air-exposed controls. No difference has been detected in the capacity of NO_2 to depress antibody formation between mice preexposed to the pollutant prior to immunization or mice exposed after immunization. Serum immunoglobulin levels measured after NO_2 exposures show a marked suppression in serum IgM, IgA, and IgG_2 levels, whereas IgG_1 levels are significantly elevated in response to NO_2 (154). These responses are dependent on the exposure of mice to NO_2 after vaccination, since these changes are not observed if mice are exposed to room air after vaccination. Serum IgM, IgA, IgG, and IgG_2 levels are elevated in nonvaccinated mice exposed to NO_2 when compared with levels in air-exposed controls. Chronic NO_2 exposures (10 ppm NO_2 for 2 hours for 5 days over 30 weeks) suppress serum antibody responses to T-dependent antigen but do not alter responses to T-independent antigens (271). Chronic NO_2 exposures (15 weeks) also suppress spleen cell responses to PHA as compared with air-exposed controls. In addition, graft-versus-host responses of spleen cells are suppressed in NO_2-exposed mice as compared with unexposed controls (271). No significant differences between NO and NO_2 exposures have been characterized in these mice (271). The effects of NO_2 exposures on the generation of antibody-forming cells have been examined by varying the time of immunization in relation to the time of NO_2 exposure. Acute NO_2 exposure (26 ppm for 24 hours) either preceded by or followed by intratracheal immunization with sheep red blood cells results in an increase in IgM antibody-forming cells in lung-associated lymph nodes (481). In rats immunized 1 day after NO_2 exposure, there is a striking increase in IgG antibody-forming cells, whereas rats immunized 3 days after NO_2 exposure show a slight depression in IgG antibody-forming cells. Epithelial repair has been suggested as the modulator of the response to antigen. Antibody-forming cells are limited to lung-associated lymph nodes, and no such cells are observed in cervical lymph nodes or spleen. Intraperitoneal administration of antigen does not cause any differences in the number of IgM and IgG antibody-forming cells between NO_2-exposed and air-exposed rats (481). More refined examinations of the kinetics of antibody production and primary antibody responses have been undertaken to evaluate the effects of acute NO_2 exposure on humoral immunity. Using BALB/c mice, a significant suppression of primary antibody responses to intravenous sheep red blood cells has been observed after exposures of 20 or 40 ppm NO_2 for 12 hours (189). Presumably, NO_2 directly or indirectly alters spleen functions in exposed animals, since NO_2 suppresses the number of plaque-forming spleen cells. A decreased number of thymus cells has also been detected, and the decreases in thymus cells are greater than those observed for spleen plaque-forming cells.

In vitro studies have also been performed to examine the sensitivity of T and B lymphocytes to NO_2 exposure and to measure the effects of such exposure on cell-mediated immune processes. *In vitro* studies have used spleen cells from rats exposed to 20 ppm NO_2 for 12 hours (187). Both primary and secondary antibody responses are suppressed compared with responses of spleen cells obtained from air-exposed control rats. In primary antibody responses, B-lymphocyte function is reduced rather than T-lymphocyte function. On the other hand, with secondary antibody responses, NO_2 causes a suppression of primed T-cell functions. Such findings have been compared to the differential sensitivity of T and B cells to irradiation.

Evaluations of cellular immunity have also been performed using rats exposed to varying doses of NO_2 for 24 hours before intratracheal immunization with sheep red blood cells (265). Antigen-specific lymphoproliferation has then been measured with lymphoid cell suspensions from either thoracic lymph nodes or spleens. Enhanced cellular immunity is observed in rats exposed to 26 ppm NO_2 using either lymph node or spleen preparations. Such enhancement is comparable to that observed after immunization with bacillus Calmette-Guerin and sheep red blood cells. Rat alveolar macrophages show a dose (NO_2)-response increase in random migratory activity which, at some NO_2 doses, is greater than macrophages obtained from bacillus Calmette-Guerin–immunized animals. Thus, NO_2-exposed animals may be more susceptible to hypersensitivity disorders or autoimmune diseases.

More recent animal studies have examined T-lymphocyte subsets after chronic NO_2 exposures (0.25 ppm for 7 weeks or 0.35 ppm for 12 weeks) (454). These studies show that NO_2 dose results in lower percentages of total splenic T lymphocytes, T-helper/inducer, and T-cytotoxic/suppressor subsets as well as natural killer cells. Acute NO_2 exposures (4 ppm for 8 hours) have been used to detect the most susceptible population of cells (112). Large cytotoxic-suppressor T lymphocytes appear to be the most susceptible lymphocyte subset. Such cells are also the ones that are noted to have abnormal functions or changes in their numbers in organ-specific or generalized autoimmune disorders.

Several studies have also addressed the roles of stress and diet as contributors to the changes in immune function induced by NO_2 (12,13,50,51). Studies in adrenalectomized mice have clearly demonstrated that the effects of NO_2 on humoral immunity are independent of stress-induced endogenous steroids (13). Subsequent investigations have confirmed these observations in the same strain of mice ($C57B\frac{1}{6}$) and extended the studies to show that diminished food intake during NO_2 exposure contributes to the decrease in humoral immunity observed with NO_2 exposures (13).

Mixed exposures of ozone and NO_2 show suppression of antibody production to sheep red blood cells but not to the T-independent antigen, DNP-Ficoll (186). NO_2 exposure (4 ppm for 3, 7, 14, and 56 days) has no effect on T-dependent antibody production and with mixed exposures, suppression of antibody production after 56 days of exposure has not been observed. Such studies provide evidence that mixed pollutant exposures alter immune function in a variable fashion, depending on exposure conditions and the pollutants used.

In summary, NO_2 clearly suppresses humoral immunity, and exposures to this pollutant significantly reduce both primary and secondary antibody synthesis against T-dependent antigens. T-independent antibody synthesis is unaltered by NO_2 exposures. Cellular immune responses, as measured by lymphoproliferation, appear to be enhanced by NO_2 exposure, and such responses may make the host more susceptible to hypersensitivity disorders and autoimmune diseases. Poor nutrition leading to starvation may aggravate the effects of NO_2 exposures on the immune system, but stress, as assessed by corticosteroid production, appears to have no effect on NO_2-induced changes in humoral immunity.

Sulfur Dioxide

Sulfur dioxide is a common airborne pollutant with a suffocating odor; it is a byproduct of industrial processes consuming fossil fuels as well as more specific manufacturing processes in which it is used as a bleaching, fumigating, or preserving agent. It is also generated in the manufacture of sodium sulfite and sulfuric acid (307,536). Sulfur oxides also arise from the combustion of fossil fuels (89,307). This irrigating gas forms sulfurous acid when mixed with water, which dissociates into bisulfite, sulfite, and hydrogen ions (174). It can also be oxidized to sulfur trioxide. Such sulfur derivatives are the major contributors to acid rains.

Most respired sulfur dioxide (SO_2) is converted to sulfurous acid on contact with the moist mucous membranes in the upper respiratory tract; the acid then dissociates into sulfite and hydrogen ions (174). Little SO_2 reaches the lower respiratory tract (370). Further, ammonia produced by the respiratory tract can neutralize SO_2 through the formation of ammonium sulfate (339). For SO_2 exposures, the Occupational and Safety Health Administration (OSHA) has set the limit at 5 ppm as a time-weighted average for an 8-hour work period (156). Levels of 2 ppm have been recommended to ensure a greater margin of safety.

In the human exposed to SO_2, several pathogenic responses have been identified that may be related to immune-mediated responses (191). These include the initiation of bronchoconstriction and the increased sensitivity of asthmatics to SO_2 exposures (180,393,495–497). Such findings are most pertinent to the suggestion that airborne pollutants may contribute to the increasing frequency of asthma in the general population. There are also a few studies to suggest that individuals exposed to SO_2 and other airborne pollutants are more susceptible to respiratory tract infections (219,264,277,439).

The relationship between SO_2 exposure and influenza infections has been evaluated in animals. Such studies have shown that viral infections are more virulent when infected animals are exposed to relatively high doses of SO_2 (10 to 20 ppm daily for 7 days) after inoculation with an influenza virus adapted to mice (163). Sulfur dioxide dose-response experiments demonstrate an excess morbidity from SO_2 beginning at total doses in the range of 7 to 10 ppm $\times$ 7 days. If the SO_2 exposure (25 ppm for 7 days) occurs prior to inoculation with virus, influenza pneumonia is also observed more frequently in SO_2-exposed animals when compared with air-exposed controls (163). No mechanism for the morbidity associated with SO_2 exposure and influenza infection has been characterized to explain these data, but the SO_2 dose used in these studies was 100 times greater than the SO_2 concentration observed in New York. Other pollutants interacting with SO_2 may be more pertinent to exposures in humans.

Mixed pollutant exposures in guinea pigs using SO_2 in conjunction with carbon particles have been performed to evaluate the capacity of lungs to kill and clear bacteria (464,465). Animals exposed to coal dust and SO_2 show a decrease in bactericidal activity. Such changes occur both in animals exposed to coal dust alone and to mixtures of coal dust and SO_2. Immune processes are also suppressed by the latter mixture, and enormous doses of SO_2 (500 ppm) decrease the production of antibodies in guinea pigs and rabbits (234).

More detailed studies using BALB/c mice and *Escherichia coli* aerosolization after exposure to SO_2 alone, carbon particles alone, and mixtures of carbon and SO_2 have been used to characterize the effects of these pollutants on the immune system (573). Animals were exposed to 2 ppm SO_2 alone, 558 ± 154 µg carbon/m^3 alone, or SO_2 2 ppm and 554 ± 142 µg carbon/m^3. After 135 days of exposure, SO_2 alone causes a significant increase in the numbers of antibody-forming cells in the spleen along with increased agglutination titers in the serum as compared to exposures to carbon alone or mixtures of carbon and SO_2 (573). All animals show an increase in plaque-forming cells in their mediastinal lymph nodes, and this change is most significant in animals exposed to the combination of SO_2 and carbon particles. After 192 days, significant immunosuppression is observed in all animals compared with animals exposed for shorter time periods. The expression of enhanced antibody-forming cells in association with SO_2 exposure suggests that this pollutant has adjuvant properties perhaps related to tissue damage and an enhanced access of the antigen to antibody-synthesizing cells. Other published data show an increased sensitization of guinea pigs to anaphylaxis after exposure to high SO_2 concentrations and an increased amount of serum antialbumin antibody in association with the administration of albumin as an antigen (360,361). More recently, this adjuvant-like response has been confirmed in studies exposing mice for 5 hours/day for 5 days/week for 103 days to either 0.2 mg ozone/m^3 or to a mixture of ozone at the same concentration along with 13.2 mg SO_2/m^3 and ammonium sulfate aerosol of 1.04 ± 0.14 mg/m^3 (10). No difference in animal mortality is observed after aerosolization of streptococcus group C organisms between ozone-exposed and mixed-exposure animals. Nonetheless, the mortality rate exceeds that observed in air-exposed animals in both the mixed exposure and ozone-exposed groups. Lung bactericidal activity is significantly greater in the mixture exposed group compared with controls and with the ozone-exposed mice (10). Such results are postulated to be the result of macrophage activation.

Significant increments in the blastogenic responses to PHA and alloantigens have also been observed in animals after mixed exposures compared with air-exposed animals, and these mice also show an enhanced response to the T-cell mitogens, PHA and concanavalin A, compared with ozone-treated animals (10). The response to alloantigens is also greater in this group than the levels observed in ozone-exposed mice. Splenic B-cell function and antigen processing are not altered by exposures to ozone and the mixture of ozone, SO_2, and ammonium sulfate. No further evaluations of the effects of SO_2 on immune responses in humans or animals have been reported in the last decade, but work has continued to focus on the capacity of SO_2 to induce bronchoconstriction in both animals and humans (35,67,316–319,327,347,348,391,461,477,488,495,501,506,514,517,567). Of relevance to these investigations is the possible role that immune cells might play in the mediation of SO_2-induced bronchoconstriction as well as the sulfite ion responsible for such changes. Observations relating to the capacity of SO_2 to induce bronchoconstriction were made in the early 1960's and have been confirmed in numerous studies of human volunteers and animals since that time.

In summary, airborne pollutants clearly alter both the lung immune system and respiratory function in animals, whereas in humans there is less direct evidence that such airborne pollutants express immunotoxicity toward the immune system of the lung. The major premise on which such pollutants have been investigated is the assumption that they play a role in the increased frequency of asthma observed in the general population and possibly an increased frequency of respiratory tract infections related to airborne pollutant exposure. No absolute answers have emerged from investigations of these pollutants, but they do represent models for the evaluation of environmental pollutants as mediators of immunotoxic lung responses.

CONCLUSIONS

As has been characterized by this and other chapters in this book, the respiratory tract and lung carry out specific immune functions to protect the exposed host from damage to these and other organs. Studies of the immunopathogenesis of environmental and chemical pollutants have kept pace with the evolution of immunology as a scientific discipline, but there is more to be understood as immunology progresses to the stage of unraveling immune responses at the molecular level. Of even greater significance is the imminent potential for the use of human gene products to alter immunopathological responses to chemical and environmental pollutants.

Although most emphasis has been placed on the identification and characterization of mechanisms of toxicity, there remains the real possibility that such defined mechanisms may be used to design ways to avoid pathological responses, and in the case of chemical pollutants, to synthesize similar industrial agents with less toxicity. Further, the need to identify individuals with increased susceptibility to environmental exposures and the factors that govern such increased responsiveness offer the possibility of preventing immunotoxic damage by regulating host exposures.

A better understanding of immunopathogenesis as related to chemical pollutants also offers a unique opportunity to identify immunoactive pathways incompletely characterized at this time, and such chemically targeted reactions may also define biomarkers of immunotoxicity. Further, identification of specific defects in these immune pathways mediated by chemicals could provide additional insight into the biochemical basis of immune responses and the pathogenesis of incompletely understood immune dysfunctions such as autoimmunity.

The Bhopal, India disaster serves to emphasize the need for a continuing evaluation of immune reactions even as they may relate to chemicals used in commerce in an attempt to understand the possible immunotoxic potential of these agents. This is especially true with respect to carcinogenesis, in the study of which the focus has been on chemical carcinogens acting directly on host structures to cause abnormal cell growth and proliferation. However, the association of drug-induced immunosuppression and/or immune dysregulation in those with congenital immune defects that are known precursors of cancer has been incompletely evaluated in relation to environmental exposure and induced altered immunity. Similarly, chemical-chemical interactions have been overlooked to a large extent, and such interactions are especially relevant to the lung because cigarette smoke contains a wide array of toxic chemicals readily available for reaction with other chemicals in the environment.

REFERENCES

1. Abraham, J. L. (1986): Lung pathology in 22 cases of giant cell interstitial pneumonia (GIP) suggests GIP is pathognomonic of cobalt (hard metal) disease. 3rd International Conference on Environmental Lung Disease, Montreal.
2. Ackerman, S. J., Kephart, G. M., Habermann, T. M., Greipp, P. R., and Gleich, G. J. (1983): Localization of eosinophil granule major basic protein in human basophils. *J. Exp. Med.*, 158:946–961.
3. Acton, J. D., and Myrvick, Q. N. (1972): Nitrogen dioxide effects on alveolar macrophages. *Arch. Environ. Health*, 24:48–52.
4. Adams, D. O. (1976): The granulomatous inflammatory response. *Am. J. Pathol.*, 84:164–191.
5. Adams D. O., and Hamilton, T. A. (1989): The activated macrophage and granulomatous inflammation. *Curr. Top. Pathol.*, 79:151–167.
6. Amoruso, M. A., Witz, G., and Goldstein, B. D. (1981): Decreased superoxide radical production by rat alveolar macrophages following inhalation of ozone or nitrogen dioxide. *Life Sci.*, 28:2215–2221.
7. Anonymous (1984): Metals and the lung. *Lancet*, 1:903–904.
8. Antilla, S., Sutinen, S., Paananen, M., Kreus, K. E., Sivonen, S. J., and Grekula, A. (1986): Hard metal lung disease: A clinical, histological, ultrastructural and x-ray micro-analytical study. *Eur. J. Respir. Dis.*, 69:83–94.
9. Antonaci, S., Jirillo, E., and Lucivero, G. (1980): Humoral immune response in aged humans: Suppressor effect of monocytes on spontaneous plaque forming cell generation. *Clin. Exp. Immunol. Immunopathol.*, 17:203–211.
10. Aranyi, C., Vana, S. C., Thomas, P. T., Bradof, J. N., Fenters, J. D., Graham, J. A., and Miller, F. J. (1983): Effects of subchronic exposure to a mixture of O_3, SO_2, and $(NH_4)_2 SO_4$ on host defenses of mice. *J. Toxicol. Environ. Health*, 12:55–71.
11. Avery, S. B., Stetson, D. M., Pan, P. M., and Matthews, K. P. (1969): Immunological investigation of individuals with toluene diisocyanate asthma. *Clin. Exp. Immunol.*, 4:585–596.
12. Azoulay-Dupuis, E., Bouley, G., Moreau, J., Muffat-Joly, M., and Pocidalo, J. J. (1987): Evidence for humoral immunodepression in NO_2-exposed mice: Influence of food restriction and stress. *Environ. Res.*, 42:446–454.
13. Azoulay-Dupuis, E., Lavacher, M., Muffat-Joly, M., and Pocidalo, J. J. (1985): Humoral immunodepression following acute NO_2 exposure in normal and adrenalectomized mice. *J. Toxicol. Environ. Health*, 15:149–162.
14. Balchum, O. J., Buckley, R. D., Sherwin, R., and Gardner, M. (1963): Nitrogen dioxide inhalation and lung antibodies. *Arch. Environ. Health*, 10:274–277.
15. Baldo, B. A., Krilis, S., and Wrigley, C. W. (1980): Hypersensitivity to inhaled flour antigens. *Allergy*, 35:45–56.
16. Balmes, J. R. (1987): Respiratory effects of hard-metal dust exposure. *Occup. Med. State of the Art Rev.*, 2:327–344.
17. Banks, D. C. (1971): Smoking and leukocyte counts. *Lancet*, 2:815.
18. Bar-Sela, S., Teichtahl, H., and Lutsky, I. (1984): Occupational asthma in poultry workers. *J. Allergy Clin. Immunol.*, 73:271–275.
19. Bargon, J., Kronenberger, H., Bergman, L., Buhl, R., Meier-Sydow, J., and Mitrou, P. (1986): Lymphocyte transformation test in a group of foundry workers exposed to beryllium and non-exposed controls. *Eur. J. Respir. Dis.*, 146:211–215.

20. Barna, B. P., Chang, T., Pillarisetti, S. G., and Deodhar, S. D. (1981): Immunologic studies of experimental beryllium lung disease in the guinea pig. *Clin. Immunol. Immunopathol.*, 20:402–411.
21. Barna, B. P., Deodhar, S. D., Chiang, T., Gautam, S., Edinger, M., Chang, T., and McMahon, J. T. (1984): Experimental beryllium-induced lung disease. II. *Int. Arch. Allergy Appl. Immunol.*, 73:49–55.
22. Barnetson, R. St. C., and Gawkrodger, D. (1989): Hypersensitivity-type IV. In Immunology, edited by I. Roitt, J. Brostoff, D. Mate, pp. 22.1–22.10. Gower Medical Publishing, London.
23. Barnhart, S., and Rosenstock, L. (1984): Cadmium chemical pneumonitis. *Chest*, 86:789–791.
24. Barrett, D. J., Stenmark, S., Wara, D. W., and Ammann, A. J. (1980): Immunoregulation in aged humans. *Clin. Immunol. Immunopathol.*, 17:203–211.
25. Barrett, K. E., and Metcalfe, D. D. (1987): Heterogeneity of mast cells in the tissues of the respiratory tract and other organ systems. *Am. Rev. Respir. Dis.*, 135:1190–1195.
26. Bates, D. V. (1989): Ozone—myth and reality. *Environ. Res.*, 50:230–237.
27. Bauer, M. A., Utell, M. J., Morrow, P. E., Speers, D. M., and Gibb, F. R. (1986): Inhalation of 0.30 ppm nitrogen dioxide potentiates exercise-induced bronchospasm in asthmatics. *Am. Rev. Respir. Dis.*, 134:1203–1208.
28. Baur, X., and Fruhmann, G. (1981): Specific IgE antibodies in patients with isocyanate asthma. *Chest*, 80(Suppl.):73–76.
29. Beirne, G. J., and Brennan, J. T. (1972): Glomerulonephritis associated with hydrocarbon solvents. *Arch. Environ. Health*, 25:365–369.
30. Bellon, B., Capron, M., Druet, E., Verroust, P., Vial, M. C., Sapin, C., Girard, J. F., Foidart, J. M., Mahieu, P., and Druet, P. (1982): Mercuric chloride induced auto-immune disease in Brown-Norway rats: Sequential search for anti-basement membrane antibodies and circulating immune complexes. *Eur. J. Clin. Invest.*, 12:127–133.
31. Benoit, F. L., Rulon, D. B., Theil, G. B., Doolan, P. D., and Watten, D. H. (1964): Goodpasture's syndrome. *Am. J. Med*, 37:424–444.
32. Bernaudin, J. F., Druet, E., Belair, M. F., Pinchon, M. C., Sapin, C., and Druet, P. (1979): Extrarenal immune complex type deposits induced by mercuric chloride in the Brown Norway rat. *Clin. Exp. Immunol.*, 38:265–273.
33. Bernstein, I. L. (1982): Isocyanate-induced pulmonary disease: A current perspective *J. Allergy Clin. Immunol.*, 70(Suppl.):24–31.
34. Bernton, H. S., McMahon, T. F., and Brown, H. (1972): Cockroach asthma. *Br. J. Dis. Chest*, 66:61–66.
35. Bethel, R. A., Epstein, J., Sheppard, D., Nadel, J. A., and Boushey, H. A. (1983): Sulfur dioxide-induced bronchoconstriction in freely breathing, exercising, asthmatic subjects. *Am. Rev. Respir. Dis.*, 128:987–990.
36. Bienenstock, J. (1980): Bronchus-associated lymphoid tissue. In Cellular Biology of the Lung, edited by G. Cumming and G. Bonsiguone. Plenum Press, New York.
37. Billimoria, J. D., Pozner, H., Metselaar, B., Best, F. W., and James, D. C. O. (1975): Effects of cigarette smoking on lipids, lipoproteins, blood coagulation, fibrinolysis and cellular components of human blood. *Atherosclerosis*, 21:61–76.
38. Bingham, E., Barkley, W., Zerwas, M., Stemmer, K., and Taylor, P. (1972): Responses of alveolar macrophages to metals. I. Inhalation of lead and nickel. *Arch. Environ. Health*, 25:406–414.
39. Bitterman, P. B., Saltzman, L. E., Adelberg, S., Ferrans, V. J., and Crystal, R. G. (1984): Alveolar macrophage replication: One mechanism for the expansion of the mononuclear phagocyte population in the chronically inflamed lung. *J. Clin. Invest.*, 74:460–469.
40. Bjermer, L., Engstrom-Laurent, A., Lundgren, R., Rosenhall, L., and Hallgren, R. (1987): Hyaluronate and type III procollagen peptide concentrations in bronchoalveolar lavage fluid as markers of disease activity in farmer's lung. *Br. Med. J.*, 295:803–806.
41. Bjorksten, F., Backman, A., Jarvinen, K., Lehti, H., Savilohte, E., Syvanen, P., and Karkkarnen, F. (1977): IgE specific to wheat and rye flour protein. *Clin. Allergy*, 7:473–483.
42. Blakely, B. R. (1985): The effect of cadmium chloride on the immune response in mice. *Can. J. Comp. Med.*, 49:104–108.
43. Blakely, B. R., and Archer, D. L. (1981): The effects of lead acetate on the immune response of mice. *Toxicol. Appl. Pharmacol.*, 61:18–26.
44. Blakely, B. R., and Tomar, R. S. (1986): The effect of cadmium on antibody responses to antigens with different cellular requirements. *Int. J. Immunopharmacol.*, 8:1009–1015.

45. Blands, J., Diamant, B., Kallos, P., Kallos-Deffner, L., and Lowenstein, H. (1976): Flour allergy in bakers. *Int. Arch. Allergy Appl. Immunol.*, 52:392–409.
46. Block, G., Tse, K. S., Kijek, K., Chan, H., and Chan-Yeung, M. (1983): Baker's asthma: Clinical and immunological studies. *Clin. Allergy*, 13:359–370.
47. Border, W. A., Baehler, R. W., Bhathena, D., and Glassock, R. J. (1979): IgA antibasement membrane nephritis with pulmonary hemorrhage. *Ann. Intern. Med.*, 91:21–25.
48. Boros, D. L. (1978): Granulomatous inflammation. *Prog. Allergy*, 24:183–267.
49. Botham, P. A. Davis, G. E., and Teasdale, E. L. (1987): Allergy to laboratory animals: A prospective study of its incidence and of the influence of atopy in its development. *Br. J. Ind. Med.*, 44:627–632.
50. Bouley, G., Azoulay-Dupuis, E., and Gaudebout, C. (1986): Impaired acquired resistance of mice to *Klebsiella pneumoniae* infection induced by acute NO_2 exposure. *Environ. Res.*, 41:497–504.
51. Bouley, G., Azoulay-Dupuis, E., Moreau, J., Muffat-Joly, M., and Pocidalo, J. J. (1987): Evidence for humoral immunodepression in NO_2-exposed mice. Influence of food restriction and stress. *Environ. Res.*, 42:446–454.
52. Bozelka, B. E., Gaumer, H. R., Nordberg, J. E., and Salvaggio, J. E. (1983): Asbestos-induced alterations of human lymphoid cell mitogenic response. *Environ. Res.*, 30:281–290.
53. Brennan, P. C., Fritz, T. E., and Flynn, R. J. (1969): Murine pneumonia. A review of the etiologic agents. *Lab. Anim. Care*, 19:360–371.
54. Briggs, W. A., Johnson, J. P., Teichman, S., Yaeger, H. C., and Wilson, C. B. (1979): Antiglomerular basement membrane antibody mediated glomerulonephritis and Goodpasture's syndrome. *Medicine*, 58:348–361.
55. Brooks, S. M., and Lockey, J. (1981): Reactive airways disease syndrome (RADS). A newly defined occupational disease. *Am. Rev. Respir. Dis.*, 123:A133.
56. Brooks, S. M., Mintz, S., and Weiss, E. (1972): Changes occurring after freon inhalation. *Am. Rev. Respir. Dis.*, 105:640–643.
57. Brooks, S. M., Weiss, M. A., and Bernstein, I. L. (1985): Reactive airways dysfunction syndrome (RADS). Persistent airways hyperreactivity after high level irritant exposure. *Chest*, 88:376–384.
58. Brostof, J., and Hall, T. (1989): Hypersensitivity-type I. In Immunology, edited by I. M. Roitt, J. Brostoff, and D. K. Male, pp. 19.1–19.19. Gower Medical Publishing, London.
59. Browne, R. C. (1955): Vanadium poisoning from gas turbines. *Br. J. Indust. Med.*, 12:57–59.
60. Buck, M. G., Schachter, E. N., and Wall, J. H. (1982): Partial composition of a low molecular weight cotton bract extract which induces acute airway constriction in humans. In Proceedings of the Sixth Cotton Dust Research Conference, edited by P. J. Wakekyn, pp. 19–23. National Cotton Council, Memphis.
61. Burge, P. S., Edge, G., O'Brien, M., Harries, M. G., Hawkins, R., and Pepys, J. (1980): Occupational asthma in a research centre breeding locusts. *Clin. Allergy*, 10:355–363.
62. Burke, B. L., Steele, R. W., Beard, O. W., Wood, J. S., Cain, T., and Marmer, D. J. (1982): Immune response to varicella-zoster in the aged. *Arch. Intern. Med.*, 142:291–293.
63. Burleson, G. R., Keyes, L. L., and Stutzman, J. D. (1989): Immunosuppression of pulmonary natural killer activity by exposure to ozone. *Immunopharmacol. Immunotoxicol.*, 11:715–735.
64. Burrows, B., Bloom, J. W., Traver, G. A., and Cline, M. G. (1987): The course and prognosis of different forms of chronic airways obstruction in a sample from the general population. *N. Engl. J. Med.*, 317:1309–1314.
65. Burrows, B., Halonen, M., Barbee, R. A., and Lebowitz, M. D. (1981): The relationship of serum immunoglobulin E to cigarette smoking. *Am. Rev. Respir. Dis.*, 124:523–525.
66. Burrows, B., Martinez, F. D., Halonen, M., Barbee, R. A., and Cline, M. G. (1989): Association of asthma with serum IgE levels and skin-test reactivity to allergens. *N. Engl. J. Med.*, 320:271–277.
67. Burton, G. G., Corn, M., Gee, B. L., Vasallo, C., and Thomas, A. P. (1969): Response of healthy men to inhaled low concentrations of gas-aerosol mixtures. *Arch. Environ. Health*, 18:681–692.
68. Butcher, B. T., Jones, R. N., O'Neill, C. E., Glindmeyer, H. W., Diem, J. E, Venkatram, D., Weill, H., and Salvaggio, J. E. (1977): Longitudinal study of workers employed in the manufacture of toluene diisocyanate. *Am. Rev. Respir. Dis.*, 116:411–421.
69. Butcher, B. T., Mapp, C., Reed, M. A., O'Neil, C. E., and Salvaggio, J. E. (1982): Evidence for carrier specificity of IgE antibodies detected in sera of isocyanate exposed workers. *J. Allergy Clin. Immunol.*, 69(Suppl.):123.

70. Butcher, B. T., O'Neil, C. E., and Jones, R. N. (1983): The respiratory effects of cotton dust. *Clin. Chest Med.*, 4:63–70.

71. Butcher, B. T., O'Neil, C. E., Reed, M. A., and Salvaggio, J. E. (1980): Radioallergosorbent testing of toluene diisocyanate-reactive individuals using p-tolyl isocyanate antigen. *J. Allergy Clin. Immunol.*, 66:213–216.

72. Butcher, B. T., Salvaggio, J. E., O'Neil, C. E., Weill, H. and Gang, O. (1976): Toluene diisocyanate pulmonary disease. Immunopharmacologic and mecholyl challenge studies. *J. Allergy Clin. Immunol.*, 59:223–227.

73. Butcher, B. T., Salvaggio, J. E., Weill, H., and Ziskind, M. M. (1976): Toluene diisocyanate (TDI) pulmonary disease: Immunologic and inhalation challenge studies. *J. Allergy Clin. Immunol.*, 58:89–100.

74. Bylin, G., Lindvall, T., Rehn, T., and Sundin, B. (1985): Effects of short-term exposure to ambient nitrogen dioxide concentrations on human bronchial reactivity and lung function. *Eur. J. Respir. Dis.*, 66:205–217.

75. Calvanico, N. J., Ambegaonkar, S. P., Schlueter, D. P., and Fink, J. M. (1980): Immunoglobulin levels in bronchoalveolar lavage fluid from pigeon breeders. *J. Lab. Clin. Med.*, 96:129–140.

76. Campbell, A. H., and Gloyne, S. R. (1942): A case of pneumoconiosis due to inhalation of Fuller's earth. *J. Pathol.*, 54:75–79.

77. Campbell, M. J., Wagner, M. M. F., Scott, M. P., and Brown, D. G. (1980): Sequential immunological studies in an asbestos-exposed population. II. Factors affecting lymphocyte function. *Clin. Exp. Immunol.*, 39:176–182.

78. Card, W. I. (1935): A case of asthma sensitivity to chromates. *Lancet*, 2:1348–1349.

79. Carlier, B., Schroeder, E., and Mahieu, P. (1980): A rapidly and spontaneously reversible Goodpasture's syndrome after carbon tetrachloride inhalation. *Acta Clin. Belg.*, 35:193–198.

80. Casarett, L. J., Casarett, M. G., and Whalen, S. A. (1971): Pulmonary cell responses to metallic oxides. *Arch. Intern. Med.*, 127:1090–1098.

81. Casey, K. R., Shigeoka, J. W., Rom, W. N., and Moatamed, E. (1985): Zeolite exposure and associated pneumoconiosis. *Chest*, 6:837–840.

82. Castano, P. (1971): Chronic intoxication by cadmium experimentally induced in rabbits. A study of kidney ultrastructure. *Pathol. Microbiol.*, 37:280, 1971.

83. Castellan, R. M., Millner, P. D., Cocke, J. B., Bragg, L., Perkins, H., Jacobs, R. R., Olenchock, S. A., and Hankinson, J. L. (1984): Acute bronchoconstriction induced by cotton dust: Dose-related response to endotoxin and other dust factors. *Ann. Intern. Med.*, 101:157–163.

84. Ceuppens, J. L., and Goodwin, J. S. (1982): Regulation of immunoglobulin production in pokeweed mitogen-stimulated cultures of lymphocytes from young and old adults. *J. Immunol.*, 128:2429–2434.

85. Chan-Yeung, M. (1982): Immunologic and non-immunologic mechanisms in asthma due to western red cedar (*Thuja plicata*). *J. Allergy Clin. Immunol.*, 70:32–37.

86. Chan-Yeung, M., Giclas, P., and Henson, P. (1980): Activation of the complement by plicatic acid: The chemical compound responsible for asthma due to western red cedar (*Thuja plicata*). *J. Allergy Clin. Immunol.*, 65:333–337.

87. Chan-Yeung, M., and Lam, S. (1986): Occupational asthma. *Am. Rev. Respir. Dis.*, 133:686–703.

88. Chan-Yeung, M., Vedal, S., Kus, J., MacLean, L., Enarson, D., and Tse, K. (1984): Symptoms, pulmonary function and bronchial hyperreactivity in western red cedar compared with those in office workers. *Am. Rev. Respir. Dis.*, 130:1038–1041.

89. Charan, N. B., Myers, C. G., Lakshminarayan, S., and Spencer, T. M. (1979): Pulmonary injuries associated with acute sulfur dioxide inhalation. *Am. Rev. Respir. Dis.*, 119:555–560.

90. Chenoweth, D. E., and Hugli, T. E. (1978): Demonstration of specific C5a-related synthetic peptides on intact human polymorphonuclear leukocytes. *Proc. Natl. Acad. Sci. U.S.A.*, 75:3943–3947.

91. Chiaramonte, L. T., Bongiorno, J. R., Brown, R., and Laano, M. E. (1970): Air pollution and obstructive respiratory disease in children. *N.Y. State J. Med.*, 70:394–398.

92. Cifone, M. G., Alesse, E., Procopio, A., Paolini, R., Morrone, S., Di Eugenio, R., Santoni, G., Santoni, A. (1989): Effects of cadmium on lymphocyte activation. *Biochem. Biophys. Acta*, 1011:25–32.

93. Coates, E. O., Sawyer, H. J., Rebuck, J. W., Kvale, P. A., and Sweet, L. W. (1973): Hypersensitivity bronchitis in tungsten carbide workers. *Chest*, 64:390.

94. Cockcroft, A., Edwards, J., McCarthy, P., and Anderson, N. (1981): Allergy in laboratory animal workers. *Lancet*, 1:827–830.

95. Coffin, D. L., and Blommer, E. J. (1965): *J. Air Pollut. Control Assoc.*, 15:523.

96. Coffin, D. L., and Gardner, D. E. (1972): Interaction of biological agents and chemical air pollutants. *Ann. Occup. Hyg.*, 15:219–234.

97. Coffin, D. L., Gardner, D. E., Holzman, R. S., and Wolock, J. (1968): Influence of ozone on pulmonary cells. *Arch. Environ. Health*, 16:633–636.

98. Cohn, J. R., Buckley, C. E., Hohl, C. A., Tyson, G., and Neish, D. D. (1983): Persistent cutaneous cellular immune responsiveness in a nursing home population. *J. Am. Geriatr. Soc.*, 31:261–265.

99. Coin, P. G., and Stevens, J. B. (1986): Toxicity of cadmium chloride in vitro: Indices of cytotoxicity with the pulmonary alveolar macrophage. *Toxicol. Appl. Pharmacol.*, 82:140–150.

100. Connell, J. T. (1971): Asthmatic deaths. Role of the mast cell. *J.A.M.A.*, 215:769–776.

101. Coombs, R. R. A., and Gel, P. G. H. (1968): Classification of allergic reactions responsible for clinical hypersensitivity and disease. In Clinical Aspects of Immunology, edited by P. G. H. Gel and R. R. A. Coombs, vol. 2, pp. 575–596. Blackwell Scientific, Oxford.

102. Cooper, N. R. (1985): The classical complement pathway. Activation and regulation of the first complement component. *Adv. Immunol.*, 37:151–216.

103. Cormier, Y., Belanger, J., Beaudoin, J., Laviolette, M., Beaudoin, R., and Hebert, J. (1984): Abnormal bronchoalveolar lavage in asymptomatic dairy farmers. Study of lymphocytes. *Am. Rev. Respir. Dis.*, 103:1046–1049.

104. Cormier, Y., Belanger, J., Leblanc, P., and Laviolette, M. (1986): Bronchoalveolar lavage in farmer's lung disease: Diagnostic and physiological significance. *Br. J. Ind. Med.*, 43:401–405.

105. Cormier, Y., Gagnon, L., Berube-Genest, F., and Fournier, M. (1988): Sequential bronchoalveolar lavage in experimental extrinsic alveolitis. The influence of cigarette smoking. *Am. Rev. Respir. Dis.*, 137:1104–1109.

106. Corre, F., Lellouch, J. and Schwartz, D. (1971): Smoking and leukocyte-counts. *Lancet*, 2:632–634.

107. Couser, W. G., Baker, P. J., and Adler, S. (1985): Complement and the direct mediation of immune glomerular injury: A new perspective. *Kidney Int.*, 28:879–890.

108. Craighead, J. E., and Emerson, R. J. (1986): Slateworker's pneumoconiosis: Lung disease due to a mixture of slate and silicate dust. In Silica, Silicosis and Cancer: Controversy in Occupational Medicine. Cancer Research Monographs, edited by D. F. Goldsmith, D. M. Winn, and G. M. Shy, p. 533. Praeger Publishers, New York.

109. Craighead, J. E., Kleinerman, J., Abraham, J. L., Gibbs, A. R., Green, F. H. Y., and Juliano, E. B. (1988): Diseases associated with exposure to silica and nonfibrous silicate minerals. Silicosis and silicate disease committee. *Arch. Pathol. Lab. Med.*, 112:673–720.

110. Cullen, M. R., Kominsky, J. R., Rossman, M. D., Cherniak, M. G., Rankin, J. A., Balmes, J. R., Kern, J. A., Daniel, R. P., Palmer, L., Naegel, G. P., McManus, K., and Cruz, R. (1987): Chronic beryllium disease in a precious metal refinery. Clinical epidemiologic and immunologic evidence for continuing risk from exposure to low level beryllium fumes. *Am. Rev. Respir. Dis.*, 135:201–208.

111. Cybulsky, A. V., Rennke, H. G., Feintzeig, I. D., and Salant, D. J. (1986): Complement-induced glomerular epithelial cell injury: Role of the membrane attack complex in rat membraneous nephropathy. *J. Clin. Invest.*, 77:1096–1107.

112. Damji, K. S., and Richters, A. (1989): Reduction in T lymphocyte subpopulations following acute exposure to 4 ppm nitrogen dioxide. *Environ. Res.*, 49:217–224.

113. Daniele, R. P., Henson, P. M., Fantone, J. C., Ward, P. A., and Dreisin, R. B. (1981): Symposium on immune complex injury of the lung: State of the art. *Am. Rev. Respir. Dis.*, 124:738–755.

114. Danks, J. M., Cromwell, O., Buckingham, J. A., Newman-Taylor, A. J., and Davies, R. J. (1981): Toluene diisocyanate-induced asthma: Evaluation of antibodies in the serum of affected workers against a tolyl mono-isocyanate protein conjugate. *Clin. Allergy*, 11:161–168.

115. Dauber, J. H. (1988): Immunologic diseases caused by inorganic dusts. In Immunology and Immunologic Diseases of the Lung, edited by R. P. Daniele, pp. 451–480. Blackwell Scientific Publications, Boston.

116. Dauber, J. H., Finn, D. R., and Daniele, R. P. (1976): Immunologic abnormalities in anthrasilicosis. *Am. Rev. Respir. Dis.*, 113(Suppl.): No. 2, Pt. 2:94.

117. Davies, D., and Cotton, R. (1983): Mica pneumoconiosis. *Br. J. Ind. Med.*, 40:22–27.

118. Davies, G. E., Thompson, A. V., Niewola, Z., Burrows, G. E., Teasdale, E. L., Bird, D. J., and Phillips, D. A. (1983): Allergy to laboratory animals: A retrospective and a prospective study. *Br. J. Ind. Med.*, 40:442–449.

119. Davies, R. J., Butcher, B. T., O'Neil, C. E., and Salvaggio, J. E. (1977): The in vitro effect of toluene diisocyanate on lymphocyte cyclic adenosine monophosphate production by isoproterenol, prostaglandin and histamine. A possible mode of action. *J. Allergy Clin. Immunol.*, 60:223–229.

120. Davies, R. J., Green, M., and McSchofield, N. M. (1976): Recurrent nocturnal asthma after exposure to grain dust. *Am. Rev. Respir. Dis.*, 114:1011–1019.

121. Davis, D. J., Gallo, J., Hu, E., Boucher, R. C., and Bromberg, P. A. (1980): The effects of ozone on respiratory epithelial permeability. *Am. Rev. Respir. Dis.* 121(Suppl.):231.

122. Davison, A. G., Haslam, P. L., Corrin, B., Coutts, H., Dewar, A., Riding, W. D., Studdy, P. R., and Newman-Taylor, A. J. (1983): Interstitial lung disease and asthma in hard-metal workers: Bronchoalveolar lavage, ultrastructural, and analytical findings and the results of bronchial provocation tests. *Thorax*, 38:119–128.

123. Davison, A. G., Taylor, A. J. N., Darbyshire, J., Chettle, D., Guthrie, C. J. G., O'Malley, D., Mason, H. J., Fayers, P. M., Venables, K. M., Pickering C. A. C., Franklin, D., Scott, M. C., Holden, H., Wright, A. L., and Gonepertz, D. (1988): Cadmium fume inhalation and emphysema. *Lancet*, 1:663–667.

124. Dawson, S. V., and Schenker, M. B. (1979): Health effects of inhalation of ambient concentrations of nitrogen dioxide. *Am. Rev. Respir. Dis.*, 120:281–292.

125. Delafuente, J. C. (1985): Immunosenescence: Clinical and pharmacologic considerations. *Med. Clin. North Am.*, 69:475–486.

126. Delafuente, J. C., Eisenberg, J. D., and Hoelzer, D. R. (1983): Tetanus toxoid as an antigen for delayed cutaneous hypersensitivity. *J.A.M.A.*, 249:3209–3211.

127. Delahant, A. (1955): An experimental study of the effects of rare metals in animal lungs. *A.M.A. Arch. Ind. Health*, 12:116.

128. Delfraissy, J. F., Galanaud, P., Wallon, C., Balavoine, J. F., and Dormont, J. (1982): Abolished in vitro antibody response in elderly: Exclusive involvement of prostaglandin-induced T suppressor cells. *Clin. Immunol. Immunopathol.*, 24:377–385.

129. Demedts, M., Gheysens, B., Nagel, J., Verbeken, E., Lauweryns, J., van den Eeckhout, A., Lahaye, D., Gyselen, A. (1984): Cobalt lung in diamond polishers. *Am. Rev. Respir. Dis.*, 130:130–135.

130. Deodhar, S. D., Barna, B., and Van Orstrand, H. S. (1973): A study of the immunologic aspects of chronic berylliosis. *Chest*, 63:309–313.

131. deShazo, R. D. (1982): Current concepts about the pathogenesis of silicosis and asbestosis. *J. Allergy Clin. Immunol.*, 70:41–49.

132. deShazo, R. D., Daul, C. B., Morgan, J. E., Diem, J. E., Hendrick, D. J., Bozelka, B. E., Stankus, R. P., Jones, R., Salvaggio, J. E., and Weill, H. (1986): Immunologic investigations in asbestos-exposed workers. *Chest*, 89:162S–165S.

133. deShazo, R. D., Hendrick, J. H., Diem, J. E., Nordberg, J. A., Baser, Y., Bevier, D., Jones, R. N., Barkman, H. W., Salvaggio, J. E., and Weill, H. (1983): Immunological aberrations in asbestos cement workers: Dissociation from asbestosis. *J. Allerg. Clin. Immunol.*, 72:454–461.

134. deShazo, R. D., Morgan, J., Bozelka, B., and Chapman, Y. (1988): Natural killer cell activity in asbestos workers. Interactive effects of smoking and asbestos exposure. *Chest*, 94:482–485.

135. deShazo, R. D., Nordberg, J., Baser, Y., Bozelka, B., Weill, H., and Salvaggio, J. (1983): Analysis of depressed cell-mediated immunity in asbestos workers. *J. Allergy Clin. Immunol.*, 71:418–424.

136. Doll, N. J., Stankus, R. P., and Barkman, H. W. (1983): Immunopathogenesis of asbestosis, silicosis, and coal workers' pneumoconiosis. *Clin. Chest Med.*, 4:3–14.

137. Doll, N. J., Stankus, R. P., Hughes, J., Weill, H., Gupta, R. C., Rodriguez, M., Jones, R. N., Alspaugh, M. A., and Salvaggio, J. E. (1981): Immune complexes and autoantibodies in silicosis. *J. Allergy Clin. Immunol.*, 68:281–285.

138. Dolovich, J., Evans, S. L, and Nieboer, E. (1984): Occupational asthma from nickel sensitivity. I. Human serum albumin in the antigenic determinant. *Br. J. Indust. Med.*, 41:51–55.

139. doPico, G. A., Jacobs, S., Flaherty, D., and Rankin, J. (1982): Pulmonary reactions to durum wheat: A constituent of grain dust. *Chest*, 81:55–61.

140. Dougherty, G. J., and McBride, W. H. (1984): Macrophage heterogeneity. *J. Clin. Lab. Immunol.*, 14:1–11.

141. Dowell, A. R., Lohrbauer, L. A., Hurst, D., and Lee, S. D. (1970): Rabbit alveolar macrophage damage caused by in vivo ozone inhalation. *Arch. Environ. Health*, 21:121–127.

142. Driscoll, K. E., and Schlesinger, R. B. (1988): Alveolar macrophage-stimulated neutrophil and monocyte migration: Effects of in vitro ozone exposure. *Toxicol. Appl. Pharmacol.*, 93:312–318.

143. Druet, P. (1989): Contribution of immunological reactions to nephrotoxicity. *Toxicol. Lett.*, 46:55–64.

144. Druet, P., Druet, E., Potdevin, F., and Sapin, C. (1978): Immune type glomerulonephritis induced by HgCl$_2$ in the Brown Norway rat. *Ann. Immunol.* (Inst. Pasteur), 129c:777–792.

145. Druet, P., Jacquot, C., Baran, D., Kleinknecht, D., Fillastre, J. P., and Mery, J. P. (1987): Immunologically mediated nephritis induced by toxins and drugs. In Nephrotoxicity in the Experimental and Clinical Situation, edited by P. H. Bach and E. A. Lock, pp. 727–770. MTP Press, Lancaster.

146. Dvorak, H. F., Dvorak, A. M., Simpson, B. A., Richerson, H. B., Leskowitz, S., and Karnovsky, M. J. (1970): Cutaneous basophil hypersensitivity. II. Light and electron microscopic description. *J. Exp. Med.*, 132:558–582.

147. Dworsky, R., Paganini-Hill, A., and Arthur, M. (1983): Immune responses of healthy humans 83–104 years of age. *J. Natl. Cancer Inst.*, 71:265–268.

148. Edwards, J. (1981): Mechanisms of disease induction. *Chest*, 79(Suppl.):38–43.

149. Effros, R. B., and Walford, R. L. (1983): Diminished T-cell response to influenza virus in aged mice. *Immunology*, 49:387–392.

150. Ehrlich, R. (1966): Effect of nitrogen dioxide on resistance to respiratory infections. *Bacteriol. Rev.*, 30:604–614.

151. Ehrlich, R. (1980): Interaction between environmental pollutants and respiratory infections. *Environ. Health Perspect.*, 6:89–100.

152. Ehrlich, R., Findlay, J. C., Fenters, J. D., and Gardner, D. E. (1977): Health effects of short-term inhalation of nitrogen dioxide and ozone mixtures. *Environ. Res.*, 14:223–231.

153. Ehrlich, R., Findlay, J. C., and Gardner, D. E. (1979): Effects of repeated exposures to peak concentrations of nitrogen dioxide and ozone on resistance to streptococcal pneumonia. *J. Toxicol. Environ. Health*, 5:631–642.

154. Ehrlich, R., Silverstein, E., Maigetter, R., and Fenters, J. D. (1975): Immunologic response in vaccinated mice during long-term exposure to nitrogen dioxide. *Environ. Res.*, 10:217–223.

155. Eisenbud, M., and Lisson, J. (1983): Epidemiological aspects of beryllium-induced nonmalignant lung disease: A 30-year update. *J. Occup. Med.*, 25:196–202.

156. Ellenhorn, M. J., and Barceloux, D. G. (1988): Medical Toxicology. Diagnosis and Treatment of Human Poisoning. Elsevier, Amsterdam.

157. Enerback, L. (1981): The gut mucosal mast cell. *Monogr. Allergy*, 17:222–232.

158. Epstein, P. E., Dauber, J. H. Rossman, M. D., and Daniele, R. P. (1982): Bronchoalveolar lavage in a patient with chronic berylliosis: Evidence for hypersensitivity pneumonitis. *Ann. Intern. Med.*, 97:213–216.

159. Epstein, W. L. (1967): Granulomatous hypersensitivity. *Prog. Allergy*, 11:36–88.

160. Epstein, W. L. (1971): Metal-induced granulomatous hypersensitivity in man. *Adv. Biol. Skin*, 11:313–335.

161. Esterline, R. L., Bassett, D. J. P., and Trush, M. A. (1989): Characterization of the oxidant generation by inflammatory cells lavaged from rat lungs following acute exposure to ozone. *Toxicol. Appl. Pharmacol.*, 99:229–239.

162. Exon, J. H. (1984): The immunotoxicity of selected environmental chemicals, pesticides and heavy metals. In Chemical Regulation of Immunity in Veterinary Medicine, pp. 355–368. Alan R. Liss, New York.

163. Fairchild, G. A., Roan, J., and McCarroll, J. (1972): Atmospheric pollutants and the pathogenesis of viral respiratory infection. Sulfur dioxide and influenza infection in mice. *Arch. Environ. Health*, 25:174–182.

164. Falchetti, R., Cafiero, C., and Caprino, L. (1982): Impaired T-cell functions in aged guinea pigs restored by thymostimulin (TS). *Int. J. Immunopharmacol.*, 4:181–186.

165. Falk, W., and Leonard, E. J. (1981): Specificity and reversibility of chemotactic deactivation of human monocytes. *Infect. Immun.*, 32:464–468.

166. Fearon, D. T. (1980): Identification of the membrane glycoprotein that is the C3b receptor of the human erythrocyte, polymorphonuclear leukocyte, B lymphocyte and monocyte. *J. Exp. Med.*, 152:20–30.

167. Fenters, J. D., Ehrlich, R., Findlay, J., Spangler, J., and Tolkacz, V. (1971): Serologic response

in squirrel monkeys exposed to nitrogen dioxide and influenza virus. *Am. Rev. Respir. Dis.*, 104:448–451.

168. Fenters, J. D., Findlay, J. C., Port, C. D., Ehrlich, R., and Coffin, D. L. (1973): Chronic exposure to nitrogen dioxide. Immunologic, physiologic, and pathologic effects on virus-challenged squirrel monkeys. *Arch. Environ. Health*, 27:85–89.

169. Fernandes, S., and Gupta, S. (1981): Natural killing and antibody-dependent cytotoxicity by lymphocyte subpopulations in young and aging humans. *J. Clin. Immunol.*, 1:141–148.

170. Fernandez, H. N., Henson, P. M., Otani, A., and Hugli, T. E. (1978): Chemotactic response to C3a and C5a anaphylatoxins. I. Evaluation of C3a and C5a leukotaxis in vitro and under simulated in vivo conditions. *J. Immunol.*, 120:109–115.

171. Ferreri, N. R., Zeiger, R. S., and Spiegelberg, H. L. (1988): IgG-, IgA- and IgE-induced release from leukotriene C_4 by monocytes isolated from patients with atopic dermatitis. *J. Allergy Clin. Immunol.*, 82:556–567.

172. Ferson, M., Edwards, A., Lind, A., Milton, G. W., and Hersey, P. (1979): Low natural killer-cell activity and immunoglobulin levels associated with smoking in human subjects. *Int. J. Cancer*, 23:603–609.

173. Figley, K. D. (1940): Mayfly (*Ephemerida*) hypersensitivity. *J. Allergy*, 11:376–387.

174. Fine, J. M., Gordon, T., and Sheppard, D. (1987): The roles of pH and ionic species in sulfur dioxide- and sulfite-induced bronchoconstriction. *Am. Rev. Respir. Dis.*, 136:1122–1126.

175. Fink, J. N. (1984): Hypersensitivity pneumonitis. *J. Allergy Clin. Immunol.*, 74:1–9.

176. Fisher, T., and Rystedt, I. (1983): Cobalt allergy in hard metal workers. *Contact Dermatitis*, 9:115–121.

177. Frager, N. B., Phalen, R. F., and Kenoyer, J. L. (1979): Adaptations to ozone in reference to mucociliary clearance. *Arch. Environ. Health*, 34:51–57.

178. Franchini, I., Cavatorta, A., Falzoi, M., Lucertini, S., and Mutti, A. (1983): Early indicators of renal damage in workers exposed to organic solvents. *Int. Arch. Occup. Environ. Health*, 52: 1–9.

179. Frank M. M., and Fries, L. F. (1989): Complement. In Fundamental Immunology, edited by W. E. Paul, pp.688–692. Raven Press, New York.

180. Frank, N. R., Amdur, M. O., Worcester, J., and Whittenberger, J. L. (1962): Effects of acute controlled exposure to SO_2 on respiratory mechanics in healthy male adults. *J. Appl. Physiol*, 17:252–258.

181. Franz, T., McMurrain, K. D., Brooks, S., and Bernstein, I. L. (1971): Clinical immunologic and physiologic observations in factory workers exposed to *B. subtilis* enzyme dust. *J. Allergy*, 47:170–180.

182. Freiman, D. G., and Hardy, H. L. (1970): Beryllium disease: The relation of pulmonary pathology to clinical course and prognosis based on a study of 130 cases from the U.S. Beryllium Case Registry. *Hum. Pathol.*, 1:25–44.

183. Friberg, L., Piscator, M., Nordberg, G. F., and Kjellstrom, T. (1974): Cadmium in the Environment, 2nd ed., pp. 93–204. CRC Press, Cleveland.

184. Frick, O. L. (1987): Immediate hypersensitivity. In Basic and Clinical Immunology, edited by D. P. Stites, J. D. Stobo, and J. V. Wells, pp. 197–227. Appleton and Lange, Norwalk, Conn.

185. Froese, A. (1984): Receptors for IgE on mast cells and basophils. *Prog. Allergy*, 34:142–187.

186. Fujimaki, H. (1989): Impairment of humoral immune responses in mice exposed to nitrogen dioxide and ozone mixtures. *Environ. Res.*, 48:211–217.

187. Fujimaki, H., and Fujio, S. (1981): Effects of acute exposure to nitrogen dioxide on primary antibody response. *Arch. Environ. Health*, 36:114–119.

188. Fujimaki, H., Ozawa, M., Imai, T., and Shimizu, F. (1984): Effect of short-term exposure to O_3 on antibody response in mice. *Environ. Res.*, 35:490–496.

189. Fujimaki, H., Shimizu, F., and Kubota, K. (1981): Suppression of antibody response in mice by acute exposure to nitrogen dioxide: *In vitro* study. *Environ. Res.*, 26:490–496.

190. Fukatsu, A., Brentjens, J., Killen, P., Kleinman, H., Martin, G., and Andres, G. (1987): Glomerular immune deposits in rats injected with mercuric chloride ($HgCl_2$). *Kidney Int.*, 31:320.

191. Galea, M. (1964): Fatal sulfur dioxide inhalation. *Can. Med. Assoc. J.*, 91:345–347.

192. Gallagher, J. S., Tse, C. S. T., Brooks, S. M., and Bernstein, I. L. (1981): Diverse profiles of immunoreactivity in toluene diisocyanate (TDI) asthma. *J. Occup. Med.*, 23:610–616.

193. Gallo, G. (1971): Electron studies in kidneys with linear deposition of immunoglobulin in glomeruli. *Am. J. Pathol.*, 61:377–385.

194. Gandevia, B. (1970): Occupational asthma I. *Med. J. Aust.*, 2:332–335.

195. Gardner, D. E., and Graham, J. A. (1976): Increased pulmonary disease mediated through altered bacterial defenses. In Pulmonary Macrophage and Epithelial Cells. Proceedings Sixteenth Annual Hanford Biology Symposium, edited by C. L. Saunders, R. P. Schneider, G. E. Doyle, and H. A. Ragan, pp. 1–21. ERDA Symposium Series, Richland, Washington.

196. Gardner, D. E., Holzman, R. S., and Coffin, D. L. (1969): Effects of nitrogen dioxide on pulmonary cell populations. *J. Bacteriol.*, 98:1041–1043.

197. Gardner, D. E., Miller, F. J., Illing, J. W., and Kirtz, J. M. (1977): Alterations in bacterial defense mechanisms of the lung induced by inhalation of cadmium. *Bull. Eur. Physiopathol. Resp.*, 13:157–174.

198. Gaumer, H. R., Doll, N. J., Kaimal, J., Schuyler, M., and Salvaggio, J. E. (1981): Diminished suppressor cell function in patients with asbestosis. *Clin. Exp. Immunol.*, 44:108–116.

199. Gawkrodger, D. J., Carr, M. M., McVittie, E., Guy, K., and Hunter, J. A. A. (1987): Keratinocyte expression of MHC class II antigens in allergic sensitization and challenge reactions and in irritant contact dermatitis. *J. Invest. Dermatol.*, 88:11–16.

200. Gawkrodger, D. J., McVittie, E., Carr, M. M., Ross, J. A., and Hunter, J. A. A. (1986): Phenotypic characterization of the early cellular responses in allergic and irritant contact dermatitis. *Clin. Exp. Immunol.*, 66:590–598.

201. Gerrard, J. W., Heiner, P. C., Ko, C. J., Mink, J., Meyers, A., Dosman, J. A. (1980): Immunoglobulin levels in smokers and nonsmokers. *Ann. Allergy*, 44:261–262.

202. Gershwin, L. J., Osebold, J. W., and Zee, Y. C. (1981): Immunoglobulin E-containing cells in mouse lung following allergen inhalation and ozone exposure. *Int. Arch. Allergy Appl. Immunol.*, 65:266–277.

203. Gheysens, B., Auwerx, J., van den Eeckhout, A., and Demedts, M. (1985): Cobalt-induced bronchial asthma in diamond polishers. *Chest*, 88:740–744.

204. Gibbons, H. L., Dille, J. R., and Cowley, R. G. (1965): Inhalant allergy to the screwworm fly. *Arch. Environ. Health*, 10:424–430.

205. Gibbs, A., Craighead, J. E., and Pooley, F. (1988): The pathology of slateworkers pneumoconiosis in Wales and Vermont. In Inhaled particles, pp. 273–276. Pergamon Press, London.

206. Gil, J., and Daniele, R. P. (1988): Morphology of the lung's immune system. In Immunology and Immunologic Diseases of the Lung, edited by R. P. Daniele, pp. 21–54. Blackwell Scientific Publications, Boston.

207. Gillis, S., Kozak, R., Durante, M., and Weksler, M. E. (1981): Immunological studies of aging: Decreased production of and response to cell growth factor by lymphocytes from aged humans. *J. Clin. Invest.*, 67:937–942.

208. Gilmour, M. I., Taylor, F. G. R., and Wathes, C. M. (1989): Pulmonary clearance of *Pasteurella haemolytica* and immune responses in mice following exposure to titanium dioxide. *Environ. Res.*, 50:184–194.

209. Ginns, L. C., Ryu, J. H., Rogol, P. R., Sprince, N. L., Oliver, L. C., and Larsson, C. J. (1985): Natural killer cell activity in cigarette smokers and asbestos workers. *Am. Rev. Respir. Dis.*, 131:831–834.

210. Glasgow, J. E., Pietra, G. G., Abrams, W. R., Blank, J., Oppenheim, D. M., and Weinbaum, G. (1987): Neutrophil recruitment and degranulation during induction of emphysema in the rat by nitrogen dioxide. *Am. Rev. Respir. Dis.*, 135:1129–1136.

211. Glasser, M., Greenberg, L., and Field, F. (1967): Mortality and morbidity during a period of high level air pollution, New York, November 23 to 25, 1966. *Arch. Environ. Health*, 15:684–694.

212. Globerson, A., Abel, L., and Barzilay, M. (1982): Immmunoregulatory cells in aging mice. I. Concanavalin A-induced and naturally occurring suppressor cells. *Mich. Aging Dev.*, 19:293–306.

213. Glotz, D., Hirsch, F., Druet, E. and Druet, F. (1984): Activate anti-membrane basales (MB) d'antiserums anti-idiotype d'anticorps anti-MB. *Nephrologie*, 5:92.

214. Gloyne, S. R., Marshall, G., and Hoyle, C. (1949): Pneumoconiosis due to graphite dust. *Thorax*, 4:31–38.

215. Goetzl, E. J., and Austen, K. F. (1974): Stimulation of human neutrophil leukocyte aerobic glucose metabolism by purified chemotactic factors. *J. Clin. Invest.*, 53:591–599.

216. Goidl, E. A., Innes, J. B., and Weksler, M. E. (1976): Immunological studies of aging. II. Loss of IgG and high avidity plaque-forming cells and increased suppressor cell activity in aging mice. *J. Exp. Med.*, 144:1037–1048.

217. Goings, S. A. J., Kulle, T. J., Bascom, R., Sauder, L. R., Green, D. J., Hebel, J. R., and Clem-

ents, M. L. (1989): Effect of nitrogen dioxide exposure on susceptibility to influenza A virus infection in healthy adults. *Am. Rev. Respir. Dis.*, 139:1075–1081.

218. Golden, J. A., Nadel, J. A., and Boushey, H. A. (1978): Bronchial hyperirritability in healthy subjects after exposure to ozone. *Am. Rev. Respir. Dis.*, 118:287–294.

219. Goldsmith, J. R. (1968): Effects of air pollution on human health. In Air Pollution, edited by A. C. Stern, pp. 547–615. Academic Press, New York.

220. Goldstein, B. D., Hamburger, S. J., Falk, G. W., and Amoruso, M. A. (1977): Effect of ozone and nitrogen dioxide on the agglutination of rat alveolar macrophages by concanavalin A. *Life Sci.*, 21:1637–1644.

221. Goldstein, E., Lippert, W., and Warshauer, D. (1974): Defender against bacterial infection of the lung. *J. Clin. Invest.*, 54:519–528.

222. Goldstein, E., Tyler, W. S., Hoeprich, P. D., and Davis, C. E. (1971): Ozone and the antibacterial defense mechanisms of the murine lung. *Arch. Intern. Med.*, 127:1099–1102.

223. Goldstein, E., Tyler, W. S., Hoeprich, P. D., and Eagle, C. (1971): Adverse influence of ozone on pulmonary bactericidal activity of murine lung. *Nature*, 229:262–263.

224. Goldstein, E., Warshauer, D., Lippert, W., and Tarkington, B. (1974): Ozone and nitrogen dioxide exposure. Murine pulmonary defense mechanisms. *Arch. Environ. Health*, 28:85–90.

225. Goldstein, I. M. (1988): Complement: Biologically active products. In Inflammation. Basic Principles and Clinical Correlates, edited by J. I. Gallin, I. M. Goldstein, and R. Snyderman, pp. 55–74. Raven Press, New York.

226. Goldstein, I. M., Feit, F., and Weissman, G. (1975): Enhancement of nitroblue tetrazolium dye reduction by leukocytes exposed to a component of complement in the absence of phagocytosis. *J. Immunol.*, 114:516–518.

227. Goldstein, I. M., Roos, D., Weissman, G., and Kaplan, H. (1975): Complement and immunoglobulins stimulate superoxide production by human leukocytes independently of phagocytosis. *J. Clin. Invest.*, 56:1155–1163.

228. Goldyne, M. E., Burrish, G. F., Poubelle, P., and Borgeat, P. (1984): Arachidonic acid metabolism among human mononuclear leukocytes: Lipoxygenase-related pathways. *J. Biol. Chem.*, 259:8815–8819.

229. Goodpasture, E. W. (1919): The significance of certain pulmonary lesions in relation to the etiology of influenza. *Am. J. Med. Sci.*, 158:863–870.

230. Goodwin, J. S. (1982): Changes in lymphocyte sensitivity to prostaglandin E, histamine, hydrocortisone, X-irradiation with age. Studies in healthy elderly population. *Clin. Immunol. Immunopathol.*, 25:243–251.

231. Gordon, R. E., Case, B. W., and Kleinerman, J. (1983): Acute NO_2 effects on penetration and transport on horseradish peroxidase in hamster respiratory epithelium. *Am. Rev. Respir. Dis.*, 128:528–533.

232. Graham, J. A., Gardner, D. E., Waters, M. D., and Coffin, D. L. (1975): Effect of trace metals on phagocytosis by alveolar macrophages. *Infect. Immunity*, 11:1278–1283.

233. Greene, N. D., and Schneider, S. L. (1978): Effects of NO_2 on the response of baboon alveolar macrophages to migration inhibitory factor. *J. Toxicol. Environ. Health*, 4:869–880.

234. Greenwald, I. (1954): Effects of inhalation of low concentrations of sulfur dioxide upon man and other mammals. *Arch. Industr. Hyg.*, 10:455–475.

235. Gross, N. J. (1980): Allergy to laboratory animals: Epidemiologic, clinical and physiologic aspects, and a trial of cromolyn in its management. *J. Allergy Clin. Immunol.*, 66:158–165.

236. Guerzon, G. M., Pare, P. D., Michoud, M. C., and Hogg, J. C. (1979): The number and distribution of mast cells in monkey lungs. *Am. Rev. Respir. Dis.*, 119:59–66.

237. Gutowski, J. K., Innes, J. B., Weksler, M. E., and Cohen, S. (1986): Impaired nuclear responsiveness to cytoplasmic signals in lymphocytes from elderly humans with depressed proliferative responses. *J. Clin. Invest.*, 78:40–43.

238. Hadley, J. G., Gardner, D. E., Coffin, D. L., and Menzel, D. B. (1977): Inhibition of antibody-mediated rosette formation by alveolar macrophages: A sensitive assay for metal toxicity. *J. Reticuloendothel. Soc.*, 22:417–425.

239. Hale, L. W., Gough, J., King, E. J., and Nagelschmidt, G. (1956): Pneumoniosis of kaolin workers. *Br. J. Ind. Med.*, 13:251–259.

240. Hall, J. G. (1984): Studies on the adjuvant action of beryllium. I. Effects on individual lymph nodes. *Immunology*, 53:105–113.

241. Hallgren, H. M., Jackola, D. R., and O'Leary, J. J. (1983): Unusual pattern of surface marker

expression on peripheral lymphocytes from aged humans suggestive of a population of less differentiated cells. *J. Immunol.*, 131:191–194.

242. Hallgren, H. M., and Yunis, E. J. (1977): Suppressor lymphocytes in young and aged humans. *J. Immunol.*, 118:2004–2008.

243. Halpern, G. M. (1984): Serological markers of human allergic disease. II. Immunoglobulin G_4. *Immunol. Allergy Prac.*, 6:246–257.

244. Hance, A. J., Douches, S., Winchester, R. J., Ferrans, V. J., and Crystal, R. G. (1985): Characterization of mononuclear phagocyte subpopulations in the human lung by using monoclonal antibodies: Changes in alveolar macrophage phenotype associated with pulmonary sarcoidosis. *J. Immunol.*, 134:284–292.

245. Hanifin, J. M., Epstein, W. L., and Cline, M. J. (1970): In vitro studies of granulomatous hypersensitivity to beryllium. *J. Invest. Dermatol.*, 55:284–288.

246. Hansen, P. J., and Penny, R. (1974): Pigeon breeders disease: Study of cell-mediated response to pigeon antigens by the lymphocyte culture technique. *Int. Arch. Allergy Appl. Immunol.*, 47:498–507.

247. Hanton-Culver, H., Culver, B. D., and Kurosaki, T. (1988): Immune response in shipyard workers with x-ray abnormalities consistent with asbestos exposure. *Br. J. Ind. Med.*, 45:464–468.

248. Harding, H. E. (1950): Notes on the toxicology of cobalt metal. *Br. J. Ind. Med.*, 7:76–78.

249. Harfi, H. A. (1980): Immediate hypersensitivity to cricket. *Ann. Allergy*, 44:162–163.

250. Hargreave, F. E., and Pepys, J. (1972): Allergic respiratory reactions in bird fanciers, provoked by allergen inhalation provocation tests. *J. Allergy Clin. Immunol.*, 50:157–173.

251. Harmon, E. M. (1985): Immunologic lung disease. *Med. Clin. North Am.*, 69:705–714.

252. Harris, J. O., Bice, D., and Salvaggio, J. E. (1976): Cellular and humoral bronchopulmonary immune responses of rabbits immunized with thermophilic actinomycete antigen. *Am. Rev. Respir. Dis.*, 114:29–43.

253. Hart, B. A. (1986): Cellular and biochemical response of the rat lung to repeated inhalation of cadmium. *Toxicol. Appl. Pharmacol.*, 82:281–291.

254. Haslam, P. L., Turoszek, A. Merchant, J. A., and Turner-Warwick, M. (1978): Lymphocyte responses to phytohemagglutinin in patients with asbestosis and pleural mesothelioma. *Clin. Exp. Immunol.*, 31:178–188.

255. Hassett, C., Mustafa, M. G., Coulson, W. F., and Elashoff, R. M. (1985): Murine lung carcinogenesis following exposure to ambient ozone concentrations. *J. Natl. Cancer Inst.*, 75:771–777.

256. Hay, F. (1989): Hypersensitivity—type III. In Immunology, edited by I. Roitt, J. Brostoff, and D. Male, pp. 21.1–21.9. Gower Medical Publishing, London.

257. Heiner, D. C. (1984): Significance of immunoglobulin G subclasses. *Am. J. Med.*, 76(3A):1–6.

258. Helman, N., and Rubenstein, L. S. (1975): The effects of age, sex and smoking on erythrocytes and leukocytes. *Am. J. Clin. Pathol.*, 63:35–44.

259. Henderson, F. W., Dubovi, E. J., Harder, S., Seal, E., Jr., and Graham, D. (1988): Experimental rhinovirus infection in human volunteers exposed to ozone. *Am. Rev. Respir. Dis.*, 137:1124–1128.

260. Henderson, R. F., Rebar, A. H., and Denicola, D. B. (1979): Early damage indicators in the lungs. IV. Biochemical and cytologic response of the lung to lavage with metal salts. *Toxicol. Appl. Pharmacol.*, 51:129–135.

261. Henderson, R. F., Rebar, A. H., Pickrell, J. A., and Newton, G. J. (1979): Early damage indicators in the lung. III. Biochemical and cytological responses of the lung to inhaled metal salts. *Toxicol. Appl. Pharmacol.*, 50:123–136.

262. Hendrick, D. J., Daires, R. J., and Pepys, J. (1976): Baker's asthma. *Clin. Allergy*, 6:241–250.

263. Herxheimer, H. (1973): The skin sensitivity to flour of baker's apprentices. *Acta Allergol.*, 28:42–49.

264. Higgins, I. T. T. (1971): Effects of sulfur oxides and particulates on health. *Arch. Environ. Health*, 22:584–590.

265. Hillam, R. P., Bice, D. E., Hahn, F. F., and Schnizlein, C. T. (1983): Effects of acute nitrogen dioxide exposure on cellular immunity after lung immunization. *Environ. Res.*, 31:201–211.

266. Hirano, S., Tsukamoto, N., Higo, S., and Suzuki, K. T. (1989): Toxicity of cadmium oxide instilled into the rat lung. II. Inflammatory response in bronchoalveolar lavage fluid. *Toxicology*, 55:25–35.

267. Hirano, S., Tsukamoto, N., Kobayashi, E., and Suzuki, K. T. (1989): Toxicity of cadmium oxide

instilled into the rat lung. I. Metabolism of cadmium oxide in the lung and its effects on essential elements. *Toxicology*, 55:15–24.

268. Hirsch, F., Conderc, J., Sapin, C., Fournie, G., and Druet, P. (1982): Polyclonal effect of $HgCl_2$ in the rat, its possible role in an experimental auto-immune disease. *Eur. J. Immunol.*, 12:620–625.

269. Holdsworth, S., Boyce, N., and Thompson, N. M. (1985): The clinical spectrum of acute glomerulonephritis and lung hemorrage (Goodpasture's syndrome). *Q. J. Med.*, 55:75–86.

270. Holt, P. G. (1987): Immune and inflammatory function in cigarette smokers. *Thorax*, 42:241–249.

271. Holt, P. G., Finlay-Jones, L. M., Keast, D., and Papadimitrou, J. M. (1979): Immunologic function in mice chronically exposed to nitrogen oxides (NOx). *Environ. Res.*, 19:154–162.

272. Hook, W. A., Powers, K., and Siraganian, R. P. (1984): Skin tests, and blood leukocyte, histamine release of patients with allergies to laboratory animals. *J. Allergy Clin. Immunol.*, 73:457–465.

273. Hopper, K. E., Wood, P. R., and Nelson, D. S. (1979): Macrophage heterogeneity. *Vox. Sang.*, 36:257–274.

274. Horton, D. J., and Chen, W. Y. (1979): Effects of breathing warm humidified air on bronchoconstriction induced by body cooling and by inhalation of methacholine. *Chest*, 75:24–28.

275. Hotchkiss, J. A., Harkema, J. R., Sun, J. D., and Henderson, R. F. (1989): Comparison of acute ozone-induced nasal and pulmonary inflammatory responses in rats. *Toxicol. Appl. Pharmacol.*, 98:289–302.

276. Howell, R. W. (1970): Smoking habits and laboratory tests. *Lancet*, 2:152.

277. Huhti, E., Ryhanen, P., Vuopala, U., and Torkkanen, J. (1970): Chronic respiratory disease among pulp mill workers in an arctic area in northern Finland. *Acta Med. Scand.*, 187:433–444.

278. Hulbert, W. C., Walker, D. C., Jackson, A., and Hogg, J. C. (1981): Airway permeability to horseradish peroxidase in guinea pigs: The repair phase after injury by cigarette smoke. *Am. Rev. Respir. Dis.*, 123:320–326.

279. Hurst, D. J., Gardner, D. E., and Coffin, D. L. (1970): Effect of ozone on acid hydrolases of the pulmonary alveolar macrophage. *J. Reticulendothel Soc.*, 8:288–300.

280. Hurtenbach, U., Oberbarnscheidt, J., and Gleichman, E. (1988): Modulation of murine T and B cell reactivity after short-term cadmium exposure in vivo. *Arch. Toxicol.*, 62:22–28.

280a. Hygienic Guide Series (1964): Beryllium and its compounds. *Am. Ind. Hyg. Assoc. J.*, 25:614–617.

281. Illing, J. W., Miller, F. J., and Gardner, D. E. (1980): Decreased resistance to infection in exercised mice exposed to NO_2 and O_3. *J. Toxicol. Environ. Health*, 6:843–851.

282. Ishizaka, T., and Ishizaka, K. (1975): Biology of immunoglobulin E: Molecular basis of reaginic hypersensitivity. *Prog. Allergy*, 19:60–121.

283. Ishizaka, K., and Ishizaka, T. (1989): Allergy. In Fundamental Immunology, edited by W. E. Paul, pp. 867–888. Raven Press, New York.

284. Jakab, G. J. (1987): Modulation of pulmonary defense mechanisms by acute exposures to nitrogen dioxide. Proceedings of Third International Conference on Aerobiology, edited by G. Boehm and R. M. Leuschner. Birkhauser Verlag, Basel.

285. Jakab, G. J. (1987): Modulation of pulmonary defense mechanisms by acute exposures to nitrogen dioxide. *Environ. Res.*, 42:215–228.

286. Jakab, G. J., and Dick, E. C. (1973): Synergistic effect in viral-bacterial infection: Combined infection of the murine respiratory tract with Sendai virus and *Pasteurella pneumotropica*. *Infect. Immun.*, 8:762–768.

287. Jepson, W. B., Comyus, R. A., and Stewart, J. H. (1985): Pulmonary implications of the inhalation of china clay (kaolin) dust. Sixth International Symposium on Inhaled Particles. *Br. Occup. Hyg. Soc.*, pp. 108–109.

288. Jones, J. G., Minty, B. D., Lawler, P., Hulands, G., Crawley, J. C. W., and Veall, N. (1980): Increased alveolar epithelial permeability in cigarette smokers. *Lancet*, 1:66–67.

289. Jones, J. G., Minty, B. D., Royston, D., and Royston, J. P. (1983): Carboxyhaemoglobin and pulmonary epithelial permeability in man. *Thorax*, 38:129–133.

290. Jones, J. M., and Amos, H. E. (1975): Antigen formation in metal contact sensitivity. *Nature*, 256:499–500.

291. Jones, R. N., Turner-Warwick, M., Ziskind, M., and Weill, H. (1976): High prevalence of antinuclear antibodies in sandblaster's silicosis. *Am. Rev. Respir. Dis.*, 113:393–395.

292. Jones, T. D., and Mote, J. R. (1934): The phases of foreign sensitization in human beings. *N. Engl. J. Med.*, 210:120–123.
293. Joshi, B. G., Dwivedi, C., Powell, A., and Holscher, M. (1981): Immune complex nephritis in rats induced by long-term oral exposure to cadmium. *J. Comp. Pathol.*, 91:11–15.
294. Kagamimori, S., Scott, M. P., Brown, P. G., Edwards, R. D., and Wagner, M. M. F. (1980): Effects of chrysotile asbestos on mononuclear cells *in vitro. Br. J. Exp. Pathol.*, 61:55–60.
295. Kagan, E., Solomon, A., Cochrane, J. C., Beissner, E. I., Gluckman, J., and Rocks, P. H. (1977): Immunological studies of patients with asbestosis. I. Studies of cell-mediated immunity. *Clin. Exp. Immunol.*, 28:261–267.
296. Kaplun, Z. S., and Mezentseva, N. V. (1960): Experimental study on the toxic effects of dust in products of sintered metals. *J. Hyg. Epidemiol. Microbiol. Immunol.*, 4:390.
297. Karol, M. H., Ioset, H. H., Yves, C. A., and Alarie, Y. C. (1978): Tolyl-specific IgE antibodies in workers with hypersensitivity to toluene diisocyanate. *Am. Ind. Hyg. Assoc.*, 39:454–458.
298. Kay, A. B. (1985): Eosinophils as effector cells in immunity and hypersensitivity disorders. *Clin. Exp. Immunol.*, 62:1–12.
299. Katz, S. I., Heather, C. J., Parker, D., and Turk, J. L. (1974): Basophilic leukocytes in delayed hypersensitivity reactions. *J. Immunol.*, 113:1073–1078.
300. Kazmierowski, J. A., Fauci, A. S., and Reynolds, H. Y. (1976): Characterization of lymphocytes in bronchial lavage fluid from monkeys. *J. Immunol.*, 116:615–618.
301. Kefalides, N. A., Alper, R., and Clark, C. C. (1979): Biochemistry and metabolism of basement membranes. *Int. Rev. Cytol.*, 61:167–228.
302. Kehrl, H. R., Vincent, L. M., Kowalsky, R. J., Hortsman, D. H., O'Neill, J. J., McCartney, W. H., and Bromberg, P. A. (1987): Ozone exposure increases respiratory epithelial permeability in humans. *Am. Rev. Respir. Dis.*, 135:1124–1128.
303. Keller, R. H., Fink, J. N., Lyman, S., and Pedersen, G. (1982): Immunoregulation in hypersensitivity pneumonitis. I. Differences in T-cell and macrophage suppressor activity in symptomatic and asymptomatic pigeon breeders. *J. Clin. Immunol.*, 2:46–54.
304. Kenoyer, J. L., Phalen, R. F., and Davis, J. R. (1981): Particle clearance from the respiratory tract as a test of toxicity: Effect of ozone on short and long term clearance. *Exp. Lung Res.*, 2:111–120.
305. Keogh, A. M., Ibels, L. S., Allen, D. H., and Isbister, J. P. (1984): Exacerbation of Goodpasture's syndrome after inadvertent exposure to hydrocarbon fumes. *Br. Med. J.*, 288:188.
306. Key, M. M., Henschel, A. F., Butler, J., Ligo, R. N., Tabershaw, I. R., and Ede, L. (1977): Occupational Diseases. A Guide to Their Recognition, pp. 436–438. U.S. Department of Health, Education, and Welfare, Public Health Service, Centers for Disease Control, and National Institute for Occupational Safety and Health. U.S. Government Printing Office, Washington, D.C.
307. Key, M. M., Henschel, A. F., Butler, J., Ligo, R. N., Tabershaw, I. R., and Ede, L. (1977): Occupational Diseases. A Guide to Their Recognition, pp. 425–426. U.S. Department of Health, Education, and Welfare, Public Health Service, Centers for Disease Control, and National Institute for Occupational Safety and Health. U.S. Government Printing Office, Washington, D.C.
308. Kiremidjian-Schumacher, L. Stotzky, G., Dickstein, R. A., and Schwartz, J. (1981): Influence of cadmium, lead, and zinc on the ability of guinea pig macrophages to interact with macrophage inhibitory factor. *Environ. Res.*, 24:106–116.
309. Kishimoto, S., Tomino, S., and Mitsuya, H. (1980): Age-related decline in the in vitro and in vivo synthesis of anti-tetanus toxoid antibody in humans. *J. Immunol.*, 125:2347–2352.
310. Klavis, G., and Drommer, W. (1970): Goodpasture-syndrome and benzineinwirkung. *Arch. Toxicol.*, 26:40–50.
311. Kleeberger, S. R., Kolbe, J., Turner, C., and Spannhake, E. W. (1989): Exposure to 1 ppm ozone attenuates the immediate antigenic response of canine peripheral airways. *J. Toxicol. Environ. Health*, 28:349–362.
312. Kleinknecht, D., Morel-Maroger, L., Callard, P., Adhemar, J-P, and Mahieu, P. (1980): Anti-glomerular basement membrane nephritis after solvent exposure. *Arch. Intern. Med.*, 140:230–232.
313. Knicker, W. T., Anderson, C. T., McBryde, J. L., Roumiantzeff, M., and Lesourd, B. (1984): Multitest CMI for standardized measurement of delayed cutaneous hypersensitivity and cell-mediated immunity: Normal values and proposed scoring system for healthy adults in the U.S.A. *Ann. Allergy*, 52:75–82.

314. Knowles, M., Murray, G., Shallal, J., Askin, F., Ranga, V., Gatzy, J., and Boucher, R. (1984): Bioelectric properties and ion flow across excised human bronchi. *J. Appl. Physiol.*, 56:868–877.
315. Kobayashi, T., Todoroki, T., and Sato, H. (1987): Enhancement of pulmonary metastasis of murine fibrosarcoma NR-FS by ozone exposure. *J. Toxicol. Environ. Health*, 20:135–145.
316. Koenig, J. Q., Covert, D. S., Hanley, Q. S., Van Belle, G., and Pierson, W. E. (1990): Prior exposure to ozone potentiates subsequent response to sulfur dioxide in adolescent asthmatic subjects. *Am. Rev. Respir. Dis.*, 141:377–380.
317. Koenig, J. Q., Morgan, M. S., Horike, M., and Pierson, W. E. (1985): The effects of sulfur oxides on nasal and lung function in adolescents with extrinsic asthma. *J. Allergy Clin. Immunol.*, 76:813–818.
318. Koenig, J. Q., Pierson, W. E., Horike, M., and Frank, R. (1981): Effects of SO_2 plus NaCl aerosol combined with moderate exercise on pulmonary function in asthmatic adolescents. *Environ. Res.*, 25:340–348.
319. Koenig, J. Q., Pierson, W. E., Horike, M., and Frank, R. (1982): Effects of inhaled sulfur dioxide (SO_2) on pulmonary function in healthy adolescents: Exposure to SO_2 alone or SO_2 + sodium chloride droplet aerosol during rest and exercise. *Arch. Environ. Health*, 37:5–9.
320. Koffler, D., Sandson, J., Carr, R., and Kunkel, H. G. (1969): Immunologic studies concerning the pulmonary lesions in Goodpasture's syndrome. *Am. J. Pathol.*, 54:293–305.
321. Koller, L. D. (1980): Immunotoxicology of heavy metals. *Int. J. Immunopharmacol.*, 2:269–279.
322. Koller, L. D., and Roan, J. G. (1977): Effects of lead and cadmium on mouse peritoneal macrophages. *J. Reticuloendothel. Soc.*, 21:7–12.
323. Koller, L. D., Roan, J. G., and Isaacson-Kerkvliet, N. (1979): Mitogen stimulation of lymphocytes in CBA mice exposed to lead and cadmium. *Environ. Res.*, 19:177–188.
324. Kowolenko, M. Tracy, L., Mudzinski, S., and Lawrence, D. A. (1988): Effect of lead on macrophage function. *J. Leuk. Biol.*, 43:357–364.
325. Kriebel, D., Brain, J. D., Sprince, N. L., and Kazemi, H. (1988): The pulmonary toxicity of beryllium. *Am. Rev. Respir. Dis.*, 137:464–473.
326. Kubota, M., Kagamimori, S., Yokoyama, K., and Okada, A. (1985): Reduced killer cell activity of lymphocytes from patients with asbestosis. *Br. J. Ind. Med.*, 42:276–280.
327. Kulle, T. J., Sander, L. R., Shanty, F., Kerr, H. D., Farrell, B. P., Muller, W. R., and Milman, J. H. (1984): Sulfur dioxide and ammonium sulfate effects on pulmonary function and bronchial reactivity in human subjects. *Am. Ind. Hyg. Assoc. J.*, 45:156–161.
328. Kunkel, S. L., Chensue, S. W., Strelter, R. M., Lynch, J. P., and Remick, D. G. (1989): Cellular and molecular aspects of granulomatous inflammation. *Am. J. Respir. Cell. Mol. Biol.*, 1:439–447.
329. Kusaka, Y., Yokoyama, K., Sera, Y., Yamamoto, S., Sone, S., Kyono, H., Shirakawa, T., and Goto, S. (1986): Respiratory diseases in hard metal workers: An occupational hygienic study in a factory. *Br. J. Ind. Med.*, 43:474–485.
330. Lagrue, G., Kamalodine, T., Hirbec, G., Bernaudin, J-F, Guerrero, J., and Zaepova, F. (1977): Role de l'inhalation de substances toxiques dans la genese des glomerulonephrites. *Nouv. Presse Med.*, 6:3609–3613.
331. Lam, S., Wong, R., and Yeung, M. (1979): Nonspecific bronchial reactivity in occupational asthma. *J. Allergy Clin. Immunol.*, 63:28–34.
332. Lane, R., and Campbell, A. C. P. (1954): Fatal emphysema in two men making a copper cadmium alloy. *Br. J. Ind. Med.*, 11:118–122.
333. Lange, A. (1980): An epidemiological survey of immunological abnormalities in asbestos workers. I. Non-organ and organ-specific autoantibodies. *Environ. Res.*, 22:162–175.
334. Lange, A. (1980): An epidemiological survey of immunological abnormalities. II. Serum immunoglobulin levels. *Environ. Res.*, 22:176–183.
335. Lange, A., Nineham, L. J., Garncarek, D., and Smolik, R. (1983): Circulating immune complexes and antiglobulins (IgG and IgM) in asbestos-induced lung fibrosis. *Environ. Res.*, 31:287–295.
336. Lange, A., Skibinski, G., and Garncarek, D. (1980): The follow-up study of skin reactivity to recall antigens and E and EAC-RFC profiles in blood in asbestos workers. *Immunobiology*, 157:1–11.
337. Lange, A., Smolick, R., Zatonski, W., and Szymanska, J. (1974): Autoantibodies and serum immunoglobulin levels in asbestos workers *Int. Arch. Arbeitsmed.*, 32:313–325.

338. Lapenas, D., Gale, P., and Kennedy, T. (1983): Kaolin pneumoconiosis: Radiologic, pathologic and mineralogic findings. *Am. Rev. Respir. Dis.*, 4:282–288.

339. Larson, T. V., Covert, D. S., and Frank, N. R. (1977): Ammonia in the human airways: Neutralization of inspired acid sulfate aerosols. *Science*, 197:161–163.

340. Last, J. A., Warren, D. L., Pecquet-Goat, E., and Witschi, H. (1987): Modification by ozone of lung tumor development in mice. *J. Natl. Cancer Inst.*, 78:149–154.

341. Lawrence, E. C. (1988): Cellular immune responses of the lung. In Immunology and Immunologic Diseases of the Lung, edited by R. P. Daniele, pp. 97–114. Blackwell Scientific Publications, Boston.

342. Lehnert, B. E., and Morrow, P. E. (1984): Size, adherence, and phagocytic characteristics of alveolar macrophages harvested "early" and "later" during bronchoalveolar lavage. *J. Immunol. Methods*, 73:329–335.

343. Lerner, R. A., Glassock, R. J., and Dixon, F. J. (1967): The role of antiglomerular basement membrane antibody in the pathogenesis of human glomerulonephritis. *J. Exp. Med.*, 126:989–1004.

344. Leskowitz, S., Salvaggio, J. E., and Schwartz, H. J. (1972): An hypotheses for the development of atopic allergy in man. *Clin. Allergy*, 2:237–246.

345. Levy, L., Vredove, D. L., and Cook, G. (1986): In vitro reversibility of cadmium-induced inhibition of phagocytosis. *Environ. Res.*, 41:361–371.

346. Lew, F., Tsang, P., Holland, J. F., Warner, N., Selikoff, I. J., and Bekesi, J. G. (1986): High frequency of immune dysfunctions in asbestosis workers and in patients with malignant mesothelioma. *J. Clin. Immunol.*, 6:225–233.

347. Linn, W. S., Avol, E. L., Peng, R-C., Shamoo, D. A., and Hackney, J. D. (1987): Replicated dose-response study of sulfur dioxide effects in normal, atopic, and asthmatic subjects. *Am. Rev. Respir. Dis.*, 136:1127–1134.

348. Linn, W. S., Shamoo, D. A., Spier, C. E., Valencia, L. M., Anzar, V. T., Venet, T. G., and Hackney, J. D. (1983): Respiratory effects of 0.75 ppm sulfur dioxide in exercising asthmatics: Influence of upper-respiratory defenses. *Environ. Res.*, 30:340–348.

349. Lippmann, M. (1989): Health effects of ozone. A critical review. *JAPCA*, 39:672–695.

350. Lipscomb, M. F. (1988): The alveolar macrophage: Role in antigen presentation and accessory cell function. In Immunology and Immunologic Diseases of the Lung, edited by R. P. Daniele, pp. 79–96. Blackwell Scientific Publications, Boston.

351. Lipscomb, M. F., Onofrio, J. M., Nash, E. J., Pierce, A. K., and Toews, G. B. (1983): A morphologic study of the role of phagocytes in the clearance of *Staphylococcus aureus* from the lung. *J. Reticuloendothel. Soc.*, 33:429–442.

352. Lloyd-Davies, T. A., and Harding, H. E. (1949): Manganese pneumonitis. Further clinical and experimental observations. *Br. J. Indust. Med.*, 6:82–90.

353. Loose, L. D., Silkworth, J. B., and Simpson, D. W. (1978): Influence of cadmium on the phagocytic and microbial activity of murine peritoneal macrophages, pulmonary alveolar macrophages and polymorphonuclear neutrophils. *Infect. Immun.*, 22:378–381.

354. Loose, L. D., Silkworth, J. B., and Warrington, D. (1978): Cadmium-induced phagocyte cytotoxicity. *Bull. Environ. Contam. Toxicol.*, 20:582–588.

355. Luckey, T. D., and Venugopal, B. (1978): Metal Toxicity in Mammals, pp. 76–86. Plenum Press, New York.

356. Lutsky, I., Teichtahl, H., and Bar-Sela, S. (1984): Occupational asthma due to poultry mites. *J. Allergy Clin. Immunol.*, 73:56–60.

357. Maceira, J. M., Fukuyama, K., and Epstein, W. L. (1984): Appearance of T-cell subpopulations during the time course of beryllium-induced granuloma. *J. Invest. Dermatol.*, 83:314–316.

358. Marder, S. R., Chenoweth, D. E., Goldstein, I. M., and Perez, H. D. (1985): Chemotactic responses of human peripheral blood monocytes to the complement-derived peptides C5a and C5a des Arg. *J. Immunol.*, 134:3325–3331.

359. Mathias, C. G. T. (1987): Clinical and experimental aspects of cutaneous irritation. In Dermatotoxicology, edited by F. N. Marzulli and H. I. Maibach, pp. 173–189. Taylor and Francis, New York.

360. Matsumura, Y. (1970): The effects of ozone, nitrogen dioxide, and sulfur dioxide on the experimentally induced allergic respiratory disorder in guinea pigs. I. The effect on sensitization with albumin through the airway. *Am. Rev. Respir. Dis.*, 102:430–437.

361. Matsumura, Y. (1970): The effects of ozone, nitrogen dioxide, and sulfur dioxide on the experi-

mentally induced allergic respiratory disorder in guinea pigs. II. The effects of ozone on the absorption and the retention of antigen in the lung. *Am. Rev. Respir. Dis.*, 102:438–443.

362. Matsumura. Y. (1970): The effects of ozone, nitrogen dioxide, and sulfur dioxide on the experimentally induced allergic respiratory disorder in guinea pigs. III. The effect on the occurrence of dyspneic attacks. *Am. Rev. Respir. Dis.*, 102:444–447.

363. McAllen, S. J., Chiu, S. P., Phalen, R. F., and Rasmussen, R. E. (1981): Effect of in vivo ozone exposure on in vitro pulmonary alveolar macrophage mobility. *J. Toxicol. Environ. Health*, 7:373–381.

364. McCarthy, K., and Henson, P. M. (1979): Induction of lysosomal enzyme secretion by alveolar macrophages in response to the purified complement fragments C5a and C5a des Arg. *J. Immunol.*, 123:2511–2517.

365. McCombs, C. C., Michalski, J. P. Westerfield, B. T., and Light, R. W. (1982): Human alveolar macrophages suppress the proliferative response of peripheral blood lymphocytes. *Chest*, 82:266–271.

366. McConnell, L. H., Fink, J. N., Schleuter, D. P., and Schmidt, M. G. (1973): Asthma caused by nickel sensitivity. *Ann. Intern. Med.*, 78:888–890.

367. McDermott, M. R., Befus, A. D., and Bienenstock, J. (1982): A structural basis for immunity in the respiratory tract. *Int. Rev. Exp. Pathol.*, 23:47–111.

368. McPhaul, J. J., Jr., and Dixon, F. J. (1970): Characterization of human anti-glomerular basement membrane antibodies elicited from glomerulonephritis kidneys. *J. Clin. Invest.*, 49:308–317.

369. McPhaul, J. J., Jr., and Dixon, F. J. (1971): Characterization of immunoglobulin G anti-glomerular basement membrane antibodies eluted from kidneys of patients with glomerulonephritis. II. IgG subtypes and in vitro complement fixation. *J. Immunol.*, 107:678–684.

370. Mehlman, M. A., Norwell, M., and Dwyer, N. (1980): Toxic gases and fumes. In Public Health and Preventive Medicine, edited by J. M. Last, pp. 755–760. Appleton-Century-Crofts, New York.

371. Merrill, W. W., and Reynolds, H. Y. (1983): Bronchial lavage in inflammatory lung disease. *Clin. Chest Med.*, 4:71–84.

372. Metzger, H. (1988): Molecular aspects of receptors and binding factors for IgE. *Adv. Immunol.*, 43:277–312.

373. Metzger, H., Alcaraz, G., Hokman, R., Kinelt, J. P., Pribluda, V., and Quarto, R. (1986): The receptor with high affinity for immunoglobulin E. *Ann. Rev. Immunol.*, 4:419–470.

374. Miller, A., Teirstein, A. S., Bader, M. E., Bader, R. A., and Selikoff, I. J. (1971): Talc pneumoconiosis: Significance of sublight microscopic mineral particles. *Am. J. Med.*, 50:395–402.

375. Miller, C. W., Davis, M. W., and Goldman, A. (1953): Pneumoconiosis in the tungsten carbide tool industry. *A.M.A. Arch. Ind. Hyg. Occup. Med.*, 8:453–465.

376. Miller, K., Calverley, A., and Kagan, E. (1980): Evidence of a quartz-induced chemotactic factor for guinea pig alveolar macrophages. *Environ. Res.*, 22:31–39.

377. Miller, L. G., Goldstein, G., Murphy, M., and Ginns, L. C. (1982): Reverse alterations in immunoregulatory T-cells in smoking: Analysis by monoclonal antibodies and flow cytometry. *Chest*, 82:526–529.

378. Miller, L. G., Sparrow, D., and Ginns, L. C. (1983): Asbestos exposure correlates with alterations in circulating T cell subsets. *Clin. Exp. Immunol.*, 51:110–116.

379. Miller, S., and Ehrlich, R. (1958): Susceptibility to respiratory infections of animals exposed to ozone. I. Susceptibility to *Klebsiella pneumoniae. J. Infect. Dis.*, 103:145–149.

380. Miller, S. D., and Zarkower, A. (1974): Alterations of murine immunologic responses after silica dust inhalation. *J. Immunol.*, 113:1533–1543.

381. Mitchell, C. A., and Gandevia, B. (1971): Respiratory symptoms and skin reactivity in workers exposed to proteolytic enzyme in detergent industry. *Am. Rev. Respir. Dis.*, 104:1–12.

382. Moore, V. L., Fink, J. N., Barboriak, J. J., Ruff, L. L., and Schlueter, D. P. (1974): Immunologic events in pigeon breeder's disease. *J. Allergy Clin. Immunol.*, 53:319–328.

383. Morgan, W. K. C. (1983): Kaolin and the lung. *Am. Rev. Respir. Dis.*, 127:141–142.

384. Morrow, P. E. (1984): Toxicological data on NO_x: An overview. *J. Toxicol. Environ. Health*, 13:205–227.

385. Muller, K., and Kagan, E. (1977): The in vivo effects of quartz on alveolar macrophage membrane topography and on the characteristics of the intrapulmonary cell population. *J. Reticuloendothel. Soc.*, 21:307–316.

386. Muller, S., Gillert, K. E., Krause, C., Jautzke, G., Gross, V., and Diamanststein, T. (1979): Effects of cadmium on the immune system of mice. *Experientia*, 35:909–910.

387. Muller-Eberhard, H. J. (1984): The membrane attack complex. *Springer Semin. Immunopathol.*, 7:93–141.
388. Murakami, K., Whiteley, M. K., and Routtenberg, A. (1987): Regulation of protein kinase C activity by cooperative interaction of Zn2+ and Ca2+. *J. Biol. Chem.*, 262:13902-13906.
389. Murlas, C. G., and Roum, J. H. (1985): Sequence of pathologic changes in the airway mucosa of guinea pigs during ozone-induced bronchial hyperreactivity. *Am. Rev. Respir. Dis.*, 131:314–320.
390. Musk, A. W., Greville, H. W., and Tribe, A. E. (1980): Pulmonary disease from occupational exposure to an artifactual aluminum silicate used for cat litter. *Br. J. Ind. Med.*, 37:367–372.
391. Myers, D. J., Bigby, B. G., and Boushey, H. A. (1986): The inhibition of sulfur dioxide-induced bronchoconstriction in asthmatic subjects by cromolyn is dose-dependent. *Am. Rev. Respir. Dis.*, 133:1150–1153.
392. Myrvik, Q. N., and Evans, D. G. (1967): Metabolic and immunologic activities of alveolar macrophages. *Arch. Environ. Health*, 14:92–96.
393. Nadel, J. A., Salem, H., Tamplin, B., and Tokiwa, Y. (1965): Mechanism of bronchoconstriction during inhalation of sulfur dioxide. *J. Appl. Physiol.*, 20:164–167.
394. Nagel, J. E., Chrest, F. J., and Pyle, R. S. (1983): Monoclonal antibody analysis of T-lymphocyte subsets in young and aged adults. *Immunol. Commun.*, 12:223–237.
395. Nagel, J. E., Collins, G. D., and Adler, W. H. (1981): Spontaneous or natural killer cytotoxicity of K562 erythroleukemic cells in normal patients. *Cancer Res.*, 41:2284–2288.
396. Nathan, A. W., and Toseland, P. A. (1979): Goodpasture's syndrome and trichloroethane intoxication. *Br. J. Clin. Pharmacol.*, 8:284–286.
397. National Air Pollution Control Administration (1971): Air Quality Criteria for Nitrogen Oxides. Publication AP-84, National Air Pollution Control Administration, Washington, D.C.
398. Neale, T. J., and Wilson, C. B. (1982): Glomerular antigens in glomerulonephritis. *Springer Semin. Immunopathol.*, 5:221–249.
399. Needleman, H. L. (1989): The persistent threat of lead: A singular opportunity. *Am. J. Pub. Health*, 79:643–645.
400. Newcombe, D. S. (1988): Leukotrienes: Regulation of biosynthesis, metabolism, and bioactivity. *J. Clin. Pharmacol.*, 28:530–549.
401. Newman, L. S., and Campbell, P. A. (1987): Mitogenic effect of beryllium sulfate on mouse B lymphocytes but not T lymphocytes in vitro. *Int. Arch. Allergy Appl. Immunol.*, 84:223–227.
402. Noble, R. C., and Penny, B. B. (1975): Comparison of leukocyte count and function in smoking and nonsmoking young men. *Infect. Immun.*, 12:550–555.
403. Noweir, M. H. (1979): Highlights of broad-spectrum industrial-hygiene research activities in a developing country—Egypt. *Am. Ind. Hyg. Assoc. J.*, 40:839–859.
404. Ohman, J. L., Jr., Lowell, F. C., and Bloch, K. J. (1975): Allergens of mammalian origin. II. Characterization of allergens extracted from rats, mouse, guinea pig, rabbit pelts. *J. Allergy Clin. Immunol.*, 55:16–24.
405. Ohsawa, M., Masuko-Sato, K., Takahashi, K., and Otsuka, F. (1986): Strain differences in cadmium-mediated suppression of lymphocyte proliferation in mice. *Toxicol. Appl. Pharmacol.*, 84:379–388.
406. Ohsawa, M., Takahaski, K., and Otsuka, F. (1988): Induction of anti-nuclear antibodies in mice orally exposed to cadmium at low concentrations. *Clin. Exp. Immunol.*, 73:98–102.
407. Okuno, T. (1973): Smoking and blood changes. *J.A.M.A.*, 225:1387–1388.
408. Onofrio, J. M., Brady, M., and Hunninghake, G. W. (1983): Augmentation of immune responses in the lung by silica. *Am. Rev. Respir. Dis.*, 127:163.
409. Onofrio, J. M., Toews, G. B., Lipscomb, M. F., and Pierce, A. K. (1983): Granulocyte-alveolar macrophage interaction in the pulmonary clearance of *Staphylococcus aureus*. *Am. Rev. Respir. Dis.*, 127:335–341.
410. Oostdam, J. V., Moreno, R., Chan, H., Pare, P. D., Schellenberg, R. R., and Yeung, M. (1985): Animal models of western red cedar asthma. *Am. Rev. Respir. Dis.*, 131:Suppl. A9.
411. Orehek, J., Massari, J. P., Gayrard, G. C., Grimand, C., and Charpin, J. (1976): Effect of short-term, low level nitrogen dioxide exposure on bronchial sensitivity of asthmatic patients. *J. Clin. Invest.*, 57:301–307.
412. Owen, R. L. (1977): Sequential uptake of horseradish peroxidase by lymphoid follicle epithelium of Peyer's patches in normal unobstructed mouse intestine: An ultrastructural study. *Gastroen terology*, 72:440–451.
413. Oxelius, V-A. (1984): Immunoglobulin G subclasses and human disease. *Am. J. Med.*, 76(3A): 7–18.

414. Ozawa, M., Fujimaki, H., Imai, T., Honda, Y., and Watanabe, N. (1985): Suppression of IgE antibody production after exposure to ozone in mice. *Int. Arch. Allergy Appl. Immunol.*, 76:16–19.
415. Ozsoylu, S., Hicsonmez, G., Berkel, I., Say, B., and Tinaztepe, B. (1976): Goodpasture's syndrome: (Pulmonary haemosiderosis with nephritis). *Clin. Pediatr.*, 15:358–360.
416. Papadimitriou, J. M., and Spector, W. G. (1972): The ultrastructure of high and low turnover inflammatory granulomata. *J. Pathol.*, 106:37–43.
417. Parker, R. F., Davis, J. K., Cassell, G. H., White, H., Dziedzic, D., Blalock, D. K., Thorp, R. B., and Simecka, J. W. (1989): Short-term exposure to nitrogen dioxide enhances susceptibility to murine respiratory mycoplasmosis and decreases intrapulmonary killing of *Mycoplasma pulmonis*. *Am. Rev. Respir. Dis.*, 140:502–512.
418. Parkes, W. R. (1982): Lung cancer and occupation. In Occupational Lung Disorders, edited by W. R. Parkes, pp. 499–507. Butterworths, London.
419. Patterson, R., Addington, W., Banner, A. S., Byron, G. E., Franco, M., Herbert, F. A., Nicotra, M. B., Pruzansky, J. J., Rivera, M., Roberts, M., Yawn, D., and Zeiss, C. R. (1979): Antihapten antibodies in workers exposed to trimellitic anhydride fumes: A potential immunopathogenetic mechanism for the trimellitic anhydride pulmonary disease-anemia syndrome. *Am. Rev. Respir. Dis.*, 120:1259–1267.
420. Patterson, R., Suszko, I. M., Zeiss, C. R., and Pruzansky, J. J. (1981): Characterization of hapten-human serum albumins and their complexes with specific human antisera. *J. Clin. Immunol.* 1:181–185.
421. Pelletier, L., Pasquier, R., Guettier, C., Vial, M. C., Mandet, C., Nochy, D., Bazin, H., and Druet, P. (1988): HgCl₂ induces T and B cells to proliferate and differentiate in BN rats. *Clin. Exp. Immunol.*, 71:336–342.
422. Pelletier, L., Pasquier, R., Rossert, J., Vial, M-C, Mandet, C., and Druet, P. (1988): Autoreactive T cells in mercury-induced autoimmunity. Ability to induce the autoimmune disease. *J. Immunol.*, 140:750–754.
423. Parker, R. F., Davis, J. K., Cassell, G. H., White, H., Dziedzik, D., Blalock, D. K., Thorp, R. B., and Simecka, J. W. (1989): Short-term exposure to nitrogen dioxide enhances susceptibility to murine respiratory mycoplasmosis and decreases intrapulmonary killing of *Mycoplasma pulmonis*. *Am. Rev. Respir. Dis.*, 140:502–512.
424. Penschow, J., and Mackay, I. R. (1980): NK and K cell activity of human blood. Differences according to sex, age, and disease. *Ann. Rheum. Dis.*, 39:82–86.
425. Pepys, J. (1969): Hypersensitivity diseases of the lungs due to fungi and organic dusts. In Monographs in Allergy, vol. 4, pp. 1–147.
426. Pernis, B., Vigliani, E. C., Cavagna, C., and Finulli, M. (1961): The role of bacterial endotoxins in occupational diseases caused by inhaling vegetable dusts. *Br. J. Ind. Med.*, 18:120–129.
427. Pernis, B., Vigliani, E. C., and Selikoff, I. J. (1965): Rheumatoid factor in serum of individuals exposed to asbestos. *Ann. N.Y. Acad. Sci.*, 132:112–120.
428. Petersen, B. H., Steimel, L. F., and Callaghan, J. T. (1983): Suppression of mitogen-induced lymphocyte transformation in cigarette smokers. *Clin. Immunol. Immunopathol.*, 76:31–37.
429. Petrie, H. T., Klassen, L. W., Klassen, P. S., O'Dell, J. R., and Kay, H. D. (1989): Selenium and the immune response: 2. Enhancement of murine cytotoxic T-lymphocyte and natural killer cell cytotoxicity in vivo. *J. Leuk. Biol.*, 45:215–220.
430. Phillip, R. (1985): Cadmium-risk assessment of an exposed residential population. *J. R. Soc. Med.*, 78:328–333.
431. Phillips, B., Marshall, M. E., Brown, S., and Thompson, J. S. (1986): Effect of smoking on human natural killer cell activity. *Cancer*, 56:2789–2792.
432. Pierce, A. K., Reynolds, R. C., and Harris, G. D. (1977): Leukocytic response to inhaled bacteria. *Am. Rev. Respir. Dis.* 116:679–684.
433. Pimentel, J. C., and Marques, F. (1969): Vineyard sprayer's lung. A new occupational disease. *Thorax*, 24:678–688.
434. Pimentel, J. C., and Menezes, A. P. (1978): Pulmonary and hepatic granulomatous disorders due to inhalation of mica dusts. *Thorax*, 33:219–227.
435. Pinkston, P., Smeglin, A., Roberts, N. J., Jr., Gibb, F. R., Morrow, P. E., and Utell, M. J. (1988): Effects of in vitro exposure to nitrogen dioxide on human alveolar macrophage release of neutrophil chemotactic factor and interleukin-1. *Environ. Res.*, 47:48–58.
436. Platt, J. L., Grant, B. W., Eddy, A. A., and Michael, A. F. (1983): Immune cell populations in cutaneous delayed hypersensitivity. *J. Exp. Med.*, 158:1227–1242.

437. Poe, W. J., and Michael, J. G. (1974): The lack of cellular cooperation in the immune response to *E. coli* 0127. *J. Immunol.*, 113:1033–1038.
438. Polak, L., Barnes, J. M., and Turk, J. L. (1968): The genetic control of contact sensitivity to inorganic metal compounds in guinea pigs. *Immunology*, 14:707–711.
439. Poukkula, A., Huhti, E., and Makarainen, M. (1982): Chronic respiratory disease among workers in pulp mill. A ten-year follow up. *Chest*, 81:285–289.
440. Poulter, L. W., Seymour, G. J., Duke, O., Janossy, G., and Panayi, G. (1982): Immunohistological analysis of delayed-type hypersensitivity in man. *Cell. Immunol.*, 74:358–369.
441. Price, C. D., Pugh, A., Pioli, E. M., and Williams, W. J. (1976): Beryllium macrophage migration test. *Ann. N.Y. Acad. Sci.*, 278:204–211.
442. Price, R. J., and Skilleter, D. N. (1986): Mitogenic effects of beryllium and zirconium salts on mouse splenocytes in vitro. *Toxicol. Lett.*, 30:89–95.
443. Purvis, M. R., Miller, S., and Ehrlich, R. (1961): Effect of atmospheric pollutants on susceptibility to respiratory infection. I. Effect of ozone. *J. Infect. Dis.*, 109:238–242.
444. Raff, H. V., Picker, L. J., and Stobo, J. D. (1980): Macrophage heterogeneity in man. A subpopulation of HLA-DR-bearing macrophages required for antigen-induced T cell activation also contains stimulators for autologous-reactive T cells. *J. Exp. Med.*, 152:581–593.
445. Raffel, S., and Newel, J. M. (1958): The "delayed hypersensitivity" induced by antigen-antibody complexes. *J. Exp. Med.*, 108:823–841.
445a. Raffle, P. A. B., Lee, W. R., McCallum, R. I., and Murray, R. (1987): Hunter's Diseases of Occupations, 7th ed. pp. 384–388. Little, Brown and Company, Boston.
446. Randolph, H. (1934): Allergy responses to dust of insect origin. *J.A.M.A.*, 103:560–562.
447. Ravnskov, U. (1978): Exposure to organic solvents: A missing link in post-streptococcal glomerulonephritis? *Acta Med. Scand.*, 203:351–356.
448. Rehm, S. R., Gross, G. N., Hart, D. A., and Pierce, A. K. (1979): Animal model of neutropenia suitable for the study of dual phagocyte systems. *Infect. Immun.*, 25:199–303.
449. Rehm, S. R., Gross, G. N., and Pierce, A. K. (1980): Early bacterial clearance from murine lungs: Species-dependent phagocytic responses. *J. Clin. Invest.*, 66:194–199.
450. Reyes, C. N., Wenzel, F. J., Lawton, B. R., and Emanuel, D. A. (1982): The pulmonary pathology of farmer's lung disease. *Chest*, 81:142–146.
451. Reynolds, H. Y. (1986): Concepts of pathogenesis and lung reactivity in hypersensitivity pneumonitis. *Ann. N.Y. Acad. Sci.*, 465:287–303.
452. Reynolds, H. Y., and Newball, H. H. (1974): Analysis of proteins and respiratory cells obtained from human lungs by bronchial lavage. *J. Lab. Clin. Med.*, 84:559–573.
453. Richerson, H. B., Dvorak, H. F., and Leskowitz, S. (1970): Cutaneous basophil hypersensitivity. I. A new look at the Jones-Mote reaction. General characteristics. *J. Exp. Med.*, 132:546–557.
454. Richters, A., and Damji, K. S. (1988): Changes in T-lymphocyte subpopulations and natural killer cells following exposure to ambient levels of nitrogen dioxide. *J. Toxicol. Environ. Health*, 25:247–256.
455. Roder, J. C., and Pross, H. F. (1982): Biology of the human natural killer cell. *J. Clin. Immunol.*, 2:249–263.
456. Rom, W. M., Lockey, J. E., Bang, K. M., Dewitt, C., and Johns, R. E., Jr. (1983): Reversible beryllium sensitization in a prospective study of beryllium workers. *Arch. Environ. Health*, 38:302–307.
457. Rose, R. M., Fuglestad, J. M., Skornik, W. A., Hammer, S. M., Wolfthal, S. F., Beck, B. D., and Brain, J. D. (1988): The pathophysiology of enhanced susceptibility to murine cytomegalovirus respiratory infection during short-term exposure to 5 ppm nitrogen dioxide. *Am. Rev. Respir. Dis.*, 137:912–917.
458. Rosenkoetter, M., Antel, J. P., and Oger, J. J. F. (1983): Modulation of T lymphocyte differentiation antigens: Influence of aging. *Cell. Immunol.*, 77:395–401.
459. Rossman, M. D. (1988): Chronic beryllium disease. In Immunology and Immunologic Diseases of the Lung, edited by R. P. Daniele, pp. 351–359. Blackwell Scientific Publications, Boston.
460. Rossman, M. D., Kern, J. A., Elias, J. A., Cullen, M. R., Epstein, P. E., Preuss, O. P., Markham, T. N., and Daniele, R. P. (1988): Proliferative response of bronchoalveolar lymphocytes to beryllium. A test for chronic beryllium disease. *Ann. Intern. Med.*, 108:687–693.
461. Rubenstein, I., Bigby, B. G., Reiss, T. F., and Boushey, H. A., Jr. (1990): Short-term exposure to 0.3 ppm nitrogen dioxide does not potentiate airway responsiveness to sulfur dioxide in asthmatic subjects. *Am. Rev. Respir. Dis.*, 141:381–385.

462. Ryan, G. B., and Spector, W. G. (1969): Natural selection of long-lived macrophages in experimental granulomata. *J. Pathol.*, 99:139–151.
463. Rya, G. B., and Spector, W. G. (1970): Macrophage turnover in inflamed connective tissue. *Proc. R. Soc. Lond. [Biol.]*, 175:269–292.
464. Rylander, R. (1969): Alterations of lung defense mechanisms against airborne bacteria. *Arch. Environ. Health*, 18:551–555.
465. Rylander, R. (1970): Studies of lung defense to infections in inhalation toxicology. *Arch. Intern. Med.*, 126:496–499.
466. Rylander, R. K., Imbus, H. R., and Suh, M. W. (1979): Bacterial contamination of cotton as an indicator of respiratory effects among cardroom workers. *Br. J. Ind. Med.*, 36:299–304.
467. Rystedt, I., and Fisher, T. (1983): Relationship between nickel and cobalt in hard metal workers. *Contact Dermatitis*, 9:195–200.
468. Sakula, A. (1961): Pneumoconiosis due to Fuller's earth. *Thorax*, 16:176–179.
469. Salvaggio, J. E. (1987): Hypersensitivity pneumonitis. *J. Allergy Clin. Immunol.*, 79:558–571.
470. Salvaggio, J. E., and Reynolds, M. K. (1979): Hypersensitivity pneumonitis: State of the art. *Chest*, 75:270–274.
471. Samet, J. M. (1989): Nitrogen dioxide and respiratory infection. *Am. Rev. Respir. Dis.*, 139:1073–1074.
472. Sanderson, J. T. (1968): Hazards of the arc air gonging process. *Am. Occup. Hyg.*, 11:123–133.
473. Sandius, N., Bygden, A., and Bruce, T. (1967): Der staubinhalt einer silikotischen lunge eines steingutarbeiters. *Ber. Dtsck. Keran. Ges.*, 17:73–90.
474. Sandron, D., Reynolds, H. Y., Venet, A., Laval, A. M., Israel-Biet, D., and Chretien, J. (1986): Human alveolar macrophage subpopulations isolated on discontinuous albumin gradients: Functional data in normals and sarcoid patients. *Eur. J. Respir. Dis.*, 69:226–234.
475. Sapin, C., Druet, E., and Druet, P. (1977): Induction of anti-glomerular basement membrane antibodies in the Brown-Norway rat by mercuric chloride. *Clin. Exp. Immunol.*, 28:173–179.
476. Sato, T., Fuse, A., and Kuwata, T. (1979): Enhancement by interferon of natural cytotoxic activities of lymphocytes from human cord blood and peripheral blood of aged persons. *Cell. Immunol.*, 45:458–463.
477. Scanlon, P. D., Seltzer, J., Ingram, R. H., Jr., Reid, L., and Drazen, J. M. (1987): Chronic exposure to sulfur dioxide. Physiologic and histologic evaluation of dogs exposed to 50 or 15 ppm. *Am. Rev. Respir. Dis.*, 135:831–839.
478. Schepers, G. W. H. (1955): The biological action of tantalum oxide, cobaltic oxide, particulate cobalt metal, particulate tungsten metal, tungsten carbide and carbon and tungsten carbide and cobalt. *A.M.A. Arch. Ind. Health*, 12:121–146.
479. Schlueter, D. P., Fink, F. N., and Sosman, A. J. (1969): Pulmonary function in pigeon breeder's disease. A hypersensitivity pneumonitis. *Ann. Intern. Med.*, 70:457–470.
480. Schmidt, J. A., Oliver, C. N., Green, J., and Gery, I. (1982): Silica stimulated macrophages release a fibroblast proliferation factor identical to interleukin 1. *Fed. Proc.*, 41:438.
481. Schnizlein, C. T., Bice, D. E., Rebar, A. H., Wolfe, R. K., and Beethe, R. L. (1980): Effect of lung damage by acute exposure to nitrogen dioxide on lung immunity in the rat. *Environ. Res.*, 23:362–370.
482. Schuyler, M., Thigpen, T., and Salvaggio, J. E. (1978): Local pulmonary immunity in pigeon breeder's disease. *Ann. Intern. Med.*, 88:355–358.
483. Schuyler, M., Ziskind, M., and Salvaggio, J. (1977): Cell-mediated immunity in silicosis. *Am. Rev. Respir. Dis.*, 116:147–151.
484. Schwartz, L. W., and Christman, C. A. (1979): Alveolar macrophage migration. Influence of lung lining material and acute lung insult. *Am. Rev. Respir. Dis.*, 120:429–439.
485. Seeliger, K., and Huland, H. (1973): Kasuistischer beitrag zur atiologie des Goodpasture-Syndrome, *Med. Klin.*, 68:437–440.
486. Segre, D., and Segre, M. (1976): Humoral immunity in aged mice. II. Increased suppressor T cell activity in immunological deficient old mice. *J. Immunol.*, 116:735–738.
487. Selgrade, M. K., Illing, J. W., Starnes, D. M, Stead, A. G., Menache, M. G., and Stevens, M. A. (1988): Evaluation of effects of ozone exposure on influenza infection in mice using several indicators of susceptibility. *Fund. Appl. Toxicol.*, 11:169–180.
488. Seltzer, J., Scanlon, P. D., Drazen, J. M., Ingram, R. H., Jr., and Reid, L. (1984): Morphologic correlation of physiologic changes caused by SO_2-induced bronchitis in dogs. The role of inflammation. *Am. Rev. Respir. Dis.*, 129:790–797.

489. Semenzato, G. (1988): Current concepts on bronchoalveolar lavage cells in extrinsic allergic alveolitis. *Respiration*, 54(Suppl. 1):59–65.

490. Semenzato, G., Trentin, L, Zambello, R., Agostini, C., Cipriani, A., and Marcer, G. (1988): Different types of cytotoxic lymphocytes are involved in the cytolytic mechanisms taking place in the lung of patients with hypersensitivity pneumonitis. *Am. Rev. Respir. Dis.*, 137:70–74.

491. Shatz, M. Patterson, R., and Fink, J. (1979): Immunologic lung disease. *N. Engl. J. Med.*, 300:1310–1320.

492. Sheers, G. (1964): Prevalence of pneumoconiosis in Cornish kaolin workers. *Br. J. Ind. Med.*, 21:218–225.

493. Shellito, J., and Kaltreider, H. B. (1984): Heterogeneity of immunologic function among subfractions of normal rat alveolar macrophages. *Am. Rev. Respir. Dis.*, 129:747–753.

494. Shellito, J., and Kaltreider, H. B. (1985): Heterogeneity of immunologic function among subfractions of normal rat alveolar macrophages. II. Activation as a determinant of functional activity. *Am. Rev. Respir. Dis.*, 131:678–683.

495. Sheppard, D., Nadel, J. A., and Boushey, H. A. (1981): Inhibition of sulfur dioxide-induced bronchoconstriction by disodium cromoglycate in asthmatic subjects. *Am. Rev. Respir. Dis.*, 124:257–259.

496. Sheppard, D., Saisho, A., Nadel, J. A., and Boushey, J. A. (1981): Exercise increases sulfur dioxide-induced bronchoconstriction in asthmatic subjects. *Am. Rev. Respir. Dis.*, 123:486–491.

497. Sheppard, D., Wong, W. S., Uehara, C. F., Nadel, J. A., and Boushey, H. A. (1980): Lower threshold and greater bronchomotor responsiveness of asthmatic subjects to sulfur dioxide. *Am. Rev. Respir. Dis.*, 122:873–878.

498. Sherwood, R. L., Lippert, W. E., and Goldstein, E. (1986): Effect of 0.64 ppm ozone on alveolar macrophage lysozyme levels in rats with chronic pulmonary bacterial infection. *Environ. Res.*, 41:378–387.

499. Shingu, H., Sugiyama, M., Watanabe, M., and Nakajima, T. (1980): Effects of ozone and photochemical oxidants on interferon production by rabbit alveolar macrophages. *Bull. Environ. Contam. Toxicol.*, 24:433–438.

500. Shirakawa, T., Kusaka, Y., Fujimura, N., Goto, S., Kato, M., Heki, S., and Morimoto, K. (1989): Occupational asthma from cobalt sensitivity in workers exposed to hard metal dust. *Chest*, 95:29–37.

501. Shore, S. A., Kariya, S. T., Anderson, K., Skornik, W., Feldman, H. A., Pennington, J., Godleski, J., and Drazen, J. M. (1987): Sulfur dioxide-induced bronchitis in dogs. Effects on airway responsiveness to inhaled and intravenously administered methacholine. *Am. Rev. Respir. Dis.*, 135:840–847.

502. Silverman, N. A., Potvin, C., Alexander, J. C., and Chretien, P. B. (1975): *In vitro* lymphocyte reactivity and T-cell levels in chronic cigarette smokers. *Clin. Exp. Immunol.*, 22:285–292.

503. Siraganian, R. P. (1988): Mast cells and basophils. In Inflammation: Basic Principles and Clinical Correlates, edited by J. I. Gallin, I. M. Goldstein, and R. Snyderman, pp. 513–542. Raven Press, New York.

504. Slovak, A. J. M., and Hill, R. N. (1981): Laboratory animal allergy: A clinical survey of an exposed population. *Br. J. Ind. Med.*, 38:38–41.

505. Smialowicz, R. J., Rogers, R. R., Riddle, M. M., Garner, R. J., Rowe, D. G., and Luebke, R. W. (1985): Immunologic effects of nickel. II. Suppression of natural killer cell activity. *Environ. Res.*, 36:56–66.

506. Snell, R. E., and Luchsinger, P. C. (1969): Effects of sulfur dioxide on expiratory flow rates and total respiratory resistance in normal human subjects. *Arch. Environ. Health*, 18:693–698.

507. Snyderman, R., Shin, H. S., and Dannenberg, A. M. (1972): Macrophage proteinase and inflammation: The production of chemotactic activity from the fifth component of complement by macrophage proteinase. *J. Immunol.*, 109:896–898.

508. Sohnle, P. G., Collins-Lech, C., and Hukta, K. E. (1983): Kinetics of lymphokine production by lymphocytes from elderly humans. *Gerontology*, 29:169–175.

509. Sone, S., Brennan, L. M., and Cresia, D. A. (1983): In vivo and in vitro NO_2 exposures enhance phagocytic and tumoricidal activities of rat alveolar macrophages. *J. Toxicol. Environ. Health*, 11:151–163.

510. Speizer, F. E., Ferris, B., Jr., Bishop. Y. M. M., and Spengler, J. (1980): Respiratory disease rate and pulmonary functin in children associated with NO;d22 exposure. *Am. Rev. Respir. Dis.*, 121:3–10.

511. Spiegelberg, H. L. (1984): Structure and function of Fc receptors for IgE on lymphocytes, monocytes, and macrophages. *Adv. Immunol.*, 35:61–88.
512. Stelzer, K. J., and Pazdernik, T. L. (1983): Cadmium-induced immunotoxicity. *Int. J. Immunopharmacol.*, 5:541–548.
513. Stephenson, R. A., Luft, B. J., Pedrotti, P. W., and Remington, J. S. (1985): Inhibition of mouse natural killer cell activity by zinc. *J. Natl. Cancer Inst.*, 74:1067–1070.
514. Stern, B., Jones, L., Raizeene, M., Burnett, R., Meranger, J. C., and Franklin, C. A. (1989): Respiratory health effects associated with ambient sulfates and ozone in two rural Canadian communities. *Environ. Health*, 49:20–39.
515. Sterner, J. H., and Eisenbud, M. (1951): Epidemiology of beryllium intoxication. *Arch. Ind. Hyg. Occup. Med.*, 3:123–151.
516. Stevenson, D. D., and Matthews, K. P. (1967): Occupational asthma following inhalation of moth particles. *J. Allergy*, 39:274–283.
517. Stjernberg, N., Eklund, A., Nystrom, L., Rosenhall, L., Emmelin, A., and Stromavist, L.-H. (1985): Prevalence of bronchial asthma and chronic bronchitis in a commuity in northern Sweden; relation to environmental and occupational exposure to sulfur dioxide. *Eur. J. Respir. Dis.*, 67:41–49.
518. Stobo, J. D. (1988): Lymphocytes: Development and function. In Inflammation: Basic Principles and Clinical Correlates, edited by J. I. Gallin, I. M. Goldstein, and R. Snyderman, pp. 599–612. Raven Press, New York.
519. Sunderman, F. W., and Kincaid, J. F. (1954): Nickel poisoning. II. Studies on patients suffering from acute exposure to vapors of nickel carbonyl. *J.A.M.A.*, 155:889–894.
520. Suzuki, T., Ikeda, S., Kanoh, T., and Mizoguchi, I. (1986): Decreased phagocytosis and superoxide anion production in alveolar macrophages of rats exposed to nitrogen dioxide. *Arch. Environ. Contam.*, 15:733–739.
521. Suzuki, Y., Morita, I., Yamane, Y., and Murota, S. (1989): Cadmium stimulates prostaglandin E;d22 production and bone resorption in cultrued fetal mouse calvaria. *Biochem. Biophys. Res. Commun.*, 158:508–513.
522. Takafuji, S., Suzuki, S., Koizumi, K., Tadokoro, K., Miyamoto, T., Ikemori, R., and Muranaka, M. (1987): Diesel-exhaust particulates inoculated by the intranasal route have adjuvant activity for IgE production in mice. *J. Allergy Clin. Immunol.*, 79:639–645.
523. Takeuchi, M., Nagai, S., and Izumi, T. (1988): Effect of smoking on natural killer cell activity in the lung. *Chest*, 94:688–693.
524. Taylor, G. (1970): Immune responses to toluene diisocyanate (TDI) exposure in man. *Proc. R. Soc. Med.*, 63:379–380.
525. Tepper, L. B., Hardy, H. L., and Chamberlin, R. I. (1961): Toxicity of beryllium compounds. In Elsevier Monographs on Toxic Agents, edited by E. Browning, pp. 1–169. Elsevier, Amsterdam.
526. Terzakis, J. A., Shustak, S. R., and Stock, E. G. (1978): Talc granuloma identified by x-ray microanalysis. *J.A.M.A.*, 239:2371–2372.
527. Thomas, E. D., Ramberg, R. E., Sale, G. E., and Golde, D. W. (1976): Direct evidence for a bone marrow origin of alveolar macrophages in man. *Science*, 192:1016–1018.
528. Tonning, H. O. (1949): Pneumoconiosis from Fuller's earth. *J. Ind. Hyg. Toxicol.*, 31:41–45.
529. Tsang, P. H., Chu, F. N., Fischbein, A., and Bekesi, J. G. (1988): Impairments in functional subsets of T-suppressor (CD8) lymphocytes, monocytes, and natural killer cells among asbestos-exposed workers. *Clin. Immunol. Immunopathol.*, 47:323–332.
530. Tse, K. S., Chan, H., and Chan-Yeung, M. (1982): Specific IgE antibodies in workers with occupational asthma due to western red cedar. *Clin. Allergy*, 12:249–258.
531. Turk, J. L. (1980): Delayed Hypersensitivity, 3rd ed. Elsevier, Amsterdam.
532. Turk, J. L., and Parker, D. (1987): Immunological aspects of immediate and delayed skin hypersensitivity. In Dermatology, edited by F. N. Marzulli and H. I. Maibach, pp. 191–215. Taylor and Francis, New York.
533. Turner, C. R., Kleeberger, S. R., and Spannhake, E. W. (1989): Preexposure to ozone blocks the antigen-induced late asthmatic response of the canine peripheral airways. *J. Toxicol. Environ. Health*, 28:363–371.
534. Turner-Warwick, M. (1973): Immunological methods in occupational disorders. *Proc. R. Soc. Med.*, 66:927–930.
535. Turner-Warwick, M., and Parkes, W. R. (1970): Circulating rheumatoid and antinuclear factors in asbestos workers. *Br. Med. J.*, 3:492–495.

536. U.S. Department of Health, Education and Welfare, Public Health Service Center for Disease Control, National Institute for Occupational Safety and Health (1974): Criteria for a recommended standard: Occupational exposure to sulfur dioxide. U.S. Government Printing Office, Washington, D.C.

537. U.S. Department of Health, Education and Welfare (1978): NIOSH criteria for recommended standard occupational exposure to diisocyanate. National Institute for Occupational Safety and Health Publication No. 78–215, Washington, D.C.

538. Unkeless, J. C., Scigliano, E., and Freedman, V. H. (1988): Structure and function of human and murine receptors for IgG. *Ann. Rev. Immunol.*, 6:251–281.

539. Unkeless, J. C., and Wright, S. D. (1988): Phagocytic cells: Fc$_\gamma$ and complement receptors. In Inflammation. Basic Principles and Clinical Correlates, edited by J. I. Gallin, I. M. Goldstein, and R. Snyderman, pp. 343–362. Raven Press, New York.

540. Vacher, J. (1972): Immunological responses of guinea pigs to beryllium salts. *J. Med. Microbiol.*, 5:91–108.

541. Valand, S. B., Acton, J. D., and Myrvik, Q. N. (1970): Nitrogen dioxide inhibition of viral-induced resistance in alveolar monocytes. *Arch. Environ. Health*, 20:303–309.

542. Valway, S. E., Martyny, J. W., Muller, J. R., Cook, M., and Mangione, E. J. (1989): Lead absorption in indoor firing range users. *Am. J. Pub. Health*, 79:1029–1032.

543. Vallyathan, N. V., and Craighead, J. E. (1981): Pulmonary pathology in workers exposed to nonasbestiform talc. *Hum. Pathol.*, 12:28–35.

544. Van Loveren, H., Rombout, P. J. A., Wagenaar, S. S., Walvoort, H. C., and Vos, J. G. (1988): Effects of ozone on the defense to a respiratory *Listeria monocytogenes* infection in the rat. *Toxicol. Appl. Pharmacol.*, 94:374–393.

545. Veien, N. K., and Svejiaard, E. (1978): Lymphocyte transformation in patients with cobalt dermatitis. *Br. J. Dermatol.*, 99:191–196.

546. Veit, B. C., and Michael, J. G. (1983): The lack of thymic influence in regulating the immune response to *Escherichia coli* 0127 endotoxin. *J. Immunol.*, 109:547–553.

547. Venables, K. M., Topping, M. D., Howe, W., Luczynska, C. M., Hawkins, R., and Newman Taylor, A. J. (1975): Interaction of smoking and atopy in the production of specific IgE antibodies against a hapten protein conjugate. *Br. Med. J.*, 290:201–204.

548. Villar, T. G. (1974): Vineyard sprayer's lung. *Am. Rev. Respir. Dis.*, 110:545–555.

549. Wagner, P. C., Pooley, F. D., and Gibbs, A. R. (1986): Inhalation of china stove and china clay dusts: Relationship between the minerology of dust retained in the lungs and pathological changes. *Thorax*, 41:190–196.

550. Walker, R. G., Scheinkestel, L., Becher, G. J., Owen, J. E., Dowlding, J. P., and Kincaid-Smith, P. (1985): Clinical and morphological aspects of the management of crescentic anti-glomerular basement membrane antibody (anti-GMB) nephritis/Goodpasture's syndrome. *Clin. J. Med.*, 54:75–89.

551. Walport, M. (1989): Complement. In Immunology, edited by I. Roitt, J. Brostoff, and D. Male, pp. 13.1–13.16. Gower Medical Publishing, London.

552. Warr, G. A., Martin, R. R., and Holleman, C. L. (1976): Classification of bronchial lymphocytes from nonsmokers and smokers. *Am. Rev. Respir. Dis.*, 113:96–100.

553. Warren, P., Cherniack, R. M., and Tse, K. S. (1974): Hypersensitivity reactions to grain dust. *J. Allergy Clin. Immunol.*, 53:139–149.

554. Waters, M. D., Gardner, D. E., Aranyi, C., and Coffin, D. L. (1975): Metal toxicity for rabbit alveolar macrophages in vitro. *Environ. Res.*, 9:32–47.

555. Waters, M. D., Gardner, D. E., and Coffin, D. L. (1974): Cytotoxic effects of vanadium on rabbit alveolar macrophages in vitro. *Toxicol. Appl. Pharmacol.*, 28:253–263.

556. Webster, R. O., Hong, S. R., Johnston, R. B., Jr., and Henson, P. M. (1980): Biological effects of the human complement fragments C5a and C5a des Arg on neutrophil function. *Immunopharmacology*, 2:201–219.

557. Weigle, W. O., Goodman, M. G., Morgan, E. L., and Hugli, F. E. (1983): Regulation of immune response by components of the complement cascade and their activated fragments. *Springer Semin. Immunopathol.*, 6:173–194.

558. Weindruch, R., Devens, B. H., Raff, H. V., and Walford, R. L. (1983): Influence of dietary restriction and aging on natural killer cell activity in mice. *J. Immunol.*, 130:993–996.

559. Weiner, A. (1961): Bronchial asthma due to organic phosphate insecticide. *Ann. Allergy*, 19:397–401.

560. Weiss, S. T. (1987): Atopy and airways responsiveness in chronic obstructive pulmonary disease. *N. Engl. J. Med.*, 317:1345–1347.
561. Weksler, M. E., and Hausman, P. B. (1982): ffects of aging in the immune response. In Immunology, edited by D. P. Sites, J. D. Stobo, and H. H. Fudenberg, pp. 306–313. Lange Medical Publications, Los Altos.
562. Wenzel, F. J., Emanuel, D. A., and Gray, R. L. (1971): Immunofluorescent studies in patients with farmer's lung. *J. Allergy Clin. Immunol.*, 48:224–229.
563. Widdicombe, J. T., Kent, D. C., and Nadel, J. A. (1962): Mechanisms of bronchoconstriction during inhalation of dust. *J. Appl. Physiol.*, 17:613–616.
564. Wieslander, J., and Heinegard, D. (1985): The involvement of type IV collagen in Goodpasture's syndrome. *Ann. N.Y. Acad. Sci.*, 460:363–374.
565. Williams, J. D., Czop, J. K., and Austen, K. F. (1984): Release of leukotrienes by human monocytes on stimulation of their phagocytic receptor for particulate activators. *J. Immunol.*, 132:3034–3040.
566. Williams, W. R., and Williams, W. J. (1982): Development of beryllium lymphocyte transformation tests in chronic beryllium disease. *Int. Arch, Allergy Appl. Immunol.*, 67:175–180.
567. Witek, T. J., Jr., and Schachter, E. N. (1985): Airway responses to sulfur dioxide and methacholine in asthmatics. *J. Occup. Med.*, 27:265–268.
568. Wong, W. W., and Fearon, D. T. (1987): Human receptor for C3b/C4b: Complement receptor type I. *Methods Enzymol.*, 150:579–585.
569. Wrabetz, L. G., Antel, J. P., and Oger, J. J. F. (1982): Age-related changes in in vitro immunoglobulin secretion: Comparison of responses to T-dependent and T-independent polyclonal activators. *Cell. Immunol.*, 74:398–403.
570. Yamada, M., Tamura, N., Shirai, T., and Kira, S. (1986): Flow cytometric analysis of lymphocyte subsets in the bronchoalveolar lavage fluid and peripheral blood of healthy volunteers. *Scand. J. Immunol.*, 24:559–565.
571. Yoneda, T., Kitamura, H., Narita, N., Mikami, R., and Yokoyama, K. (1986): NK cell activity in asbestosis. *Eur. J. Respir. Dis.*, 68:64–67.
572. Zamel, N., Leroux, M., and Vanderdoelen, J. L. (1984): Airway response to inhaled methacholine in healthy nonsmoking twins. *J. Appl. Physiol.*, 56:936–939.
573. Zarkower, A. (1972): Alterations in antibody response induced by chronic inhalation of SO;d22 and carbon. *Arch. Environ. Health*, 25:45–50.
574. Zeidberg, L. D., Prindle, R. A., and Landau, E. (1961): The Nashville air pollution study. I. Sulfur dioxide and bronchial asthma. *Am. Rev. Respir. Dis.*, 84:489–503.
575. Zembala, M., and Asherson, G. L. (1973): Depression of the T cell phenomenon of contact sensitivity by T cells from unresponsive mice. *Nature*, 244:277–278.
576. Zetterstrom, O., Osterman, K., Machado, L., and Johanson, S. G. O. (1981): Another smoking hazard: Revised serum IgE concentration and increased risk of occupational asthma. *Br. Med. J.*, 283:1215–1217.
577. Zimmerman, S. W., Groehler, K., and Beirne, G. J. (1975): Hydrocarbon exposure and chronic glomerulonephritis. *Lancet*, 2:199–201.

Clinical Immunotoxicology, edited by
D. S. Newcombe, N. R. Rose, and J. C. Bloom.
Raven Press, Ltd., New York © 1992.

15

Bronchoalveolar Lavage and Bronchial Reactivity in Humans Associated with Environmental and Chemical Exposures

David S. Newcombe* and Peter B. Terry†

**Department of Environmental Health Sciences, Johns Hopkins University,
School of Hygiene and Public Health, Baltimore, MD; †Asthma and Allergy Center,
Francis Scott Key Medical Center, Baltimore, MD*

Bronchoalveolar lavage (BAL) has been a useful technique for determining the diagnosis, prognosis, and response to therapy in some pulmonary disorders (25,75, 81,84,127,160,163,172,229,266,268,276,312,321,328,341). Analyses of cell types, their distribution, and their response to stimuli as well as the measurement of biological and chemical markers in cell-free lavage fluid have also been used extensively as research tools for investigations of the pathogenesis of disorders of the lower respiratory tract and the oronasal passages (17,74,262,265,268,284,353). Such clinical and research studies have also had a significant impact on the understanding of environmental and occupational lung disease, but much more is yet to be learned from such procedures, since only a few occupational disorders have been studied intensively by this technique.

This chapter reviews the cellular and soluble components of BAL specimens recovered from both the healthy human host and from patients with disorders mediated by environmental and chemical substances. The purpose is to describe the most up-to-date procedures for performing lavage in humans and to document the findings from such procedures in humans who have had exposure to environmental pollutants and industrial chemicals. Although there is a large body of literature related to BAL findings in animals, the focus of this discussion is on humans.

The procedure for lung lavage and the methods for the analysis of cells and extracellular molecules are the most significant variables that affect the interpretation of conclusions derived from lung lavage studies. Bronchoalveolar lavage procedures are only partially standardized, and techniques continue to evolve; therefore it is useful to emphasize certain aspects of the procedure. A minimal amount of topical anesthesia should be used in order to avoid pharyngeal spasm and to ensure patient comfort during the procedure. Excess anesthesia may alter the assessment of phospholipase-dependent cellular responses. Administration of large volumes of saline may cause an impairment in pulmonary function, and for this reason, total volumes of 150 ml or less are generally used (158,192). Since correlations with other published data arc generally essential, the lavage site is usually restricted to the right middle lobe or lingula, from which most data in the literature have been derived. As might be imagined, the initial aliquot of lavage is representative either of material recovered from the bronchial airways or of a mixture of material from this site and the alveolar spaces. When the initial lavage fluid volume is low ($<$ 20 ml), its contribution to the total sample is unlikely to significantly alter the average content of the whole sample (75). Recently, fractional collections of bronchial lavage fluid have been used to separate bronchial and alveolar samples (265). Further, with the use of bronchoscopes with inflated balloon catheters, it has been possible to isolate the bronchial and alveolar spaces and the lavage material recovered from such spaces (265). The generalization that BAL samples from a single site are representative is, of course, not always true. In many diseases such as sarcoidosis, idiopathic pulmonary fibrosis, and systemic autoimmune disorders, several sites must be sampled to ensure that lavage samples are representative (75).

An accurate analysis of the cell populations recovered by lavage is essential for separating diffuse pulmonary disorders into specific diagnostic categories (Table 1). In general, inflammatory and immune lung disorders are separated on the basis of whether neutrophils or lymphocytes are the predominant cell type observed in association with alveolar macrophages. Cytocentrifuge preparations usually underestimate lymphocyte numbers when differential cell counts are determined by this method. Nearly 20% to 50% of the total number of recovered lymphocytes may disappear as a result of centrifugation (75,284). Such an error can lead to false conclusions regarding the nature of the underlying process. Collecting lavage cells on a Millipore filter and staining them with hematoxylin-eosin is a more precise method for determining differential cell counts and avoiding the errors inherent in the cytocentrifuge procedure. Mast cells stain poorly with Diff-Quik, whereas they are easily detected with the Wright-Giemsa stain. Flow cytometry has also been useful in the determination of cell subsets and receptors, but such technology has serious limitations because it requires large numbers of cells and cells from cigarette smokers are autofluorescent, which abrogates the accurate measurement of membrane antigens using fluorescent markers (75).

Measurements of the extracellular components of BALs have been difficult to quantitate because no universal denominator for such measurements has been found to be appropriate for all clinical settings. Lavage extracellular markers have been expressed as a fraction of the total lavage volume recovered, as the total quantity of the marker recovered, or as the fraction of the lavage marker related to the concentration of a low molecular weight compound such as albumin. None of these methods is entirely satisfactory, but most investigators now report such data as a function of the lavage albumin concentration. Obviously, in conditions in which an alveolitis exists or plasma protein leakage occurs, such a ratio is imprecise. Another acceptable way to measure extracellular substances is to express them as the total amount in the lavage without concentrating the specimen. Concentrating specimens

TABLE 1. *Bronchoalveolar lavage analyses: comparisons between various disease states*

	Normal	Asbestos	Silicosis	IPF	CTD	HP
Alveolar Macrophage (%)	88.0 ± 1.0	86.0 ± 1.9	88.0 ± 1.0	75.0 ± 2.9	69.0 ± 5.1	29.0*
Lymphocytes	9.5 ± 0.6	9.4 ± 1.7	9.6 ± 0.9	11.4 ± 2.0	10.5 ± 2.4	62.0
Neutrophils	1.8 ± 0.3	2.8 ± 0.5	1.5 ± 0.3	9.1 ± 1.0	18.3 ± 5.3	8.5
Eosinophils	0.4 ± 0.1	1.9 ± 0.6	0.5 ± 0.1	3.9 ± 0.9	2.3 ± 0.9	0.5
Total cells/mL $\times 10^4$	23 ± 2	34.4 ± 5	27.1 ± 2.4	43.7 ± 13	35.8 ± 8.5	
Total protein µg/mL	89.7 ± 3.0	124.2 ± 9.9	116.9 ± 7.6	173.8 ± 18.1	189.2 ± 48.1	
IgG	8.2 ± 0.4	15.9 ± 1.6	14.9 ± 1.7	30.3 ± 3.5	27.4 ± 5.5	
IgA	6.5 ± 0.4	10.1 ± 1.2	10.6 ± 1.3	16.6 ± 2.2	23.0 ± 5.8	
IgM	0.2 ± 0.0	0.5 ± 0.1	0.3 ± 0.0	0.8 ± 0.1	1.2 ± 0.4	
Albumin	40.8 ± 1.6	51.9 ± 4.6	55.1 ± 4.8	56.6 ± 9.2	50.5 ± 6.5	

IPF = Idiopathic Pulmonary Fibrosis; CTD = Connective tissue disease; HP = Hypersensitivity pneumonitis.
Data from Supplement to *Am. Rev. Respir. Dis.*, ref. 269.
*Reynolds H. Y., Fulmer J. D., et al., ref. 269.

can lead to a loss of up to 20% of the protein in the sample (75). In order to express concentrations on a molar basis, the volume of bronchial or alveolar lining fluid in which these components are dissolved must be known. Small molecules, such as urea or methylene blue, have been used to estimate this volume, since they rapidly equilibrate with lining fluid (17,264). In the case of methylene blue, the dilution of this marker by lining fluid can be calculated when it is added to the saline used for lavage. The methylene blue method has not been received favorably because this dye has a tendency to bind to cell membranes and resists free partitioning (266). Urea measurements appear to provide a more accurate reflection of lining fluid volumes and have been used with some success to express extracellular molecule concentrations in molar quantities (266).

In normal, healthy, nonsmoking adults, the total cell count in BAL specimens is between 1 and 1.5×10^6 cells per milliliter of lavage fluid, and alveolar macrophages represent 80% to 90% of the total cell number, with lymphocytes accounting for an additional 10% and neutrophils, basophils, and eosinophils making up the remainder of the cells (Table 2). Since the majority of macrophages are derived from peripheral blood monocytes, a spectrum of cells exists in the lung, from immature to mature alveolar macrophages. Immature macrophages are smaller in size than mature macrophages and contain only a few lysosomal structures, whereas mature macrophages are larger in size and contain multilamellar structures within large vacuoles. Double staining with fluorescent antibodies and FACS analyses shows that immature lung macrophages recovered by BAL are $CD14^+RFD9^-$, whereas mature macrophages are $CD14^- RFD9^+$ (169). Thus, CD14 is down-regulated during macrophage maturation, and its measurement could be used to characterize differences in macrophage maturation in various lung disorders.

Of the total number of lymphocytes, T lymphocytes represent about 65% to 70%, B lymphocytes are about 5% to 10%, and the remainder are null cells. T-helper cells are the predominant subset of T lymphocytes, and the ratio of T-helper to T-suppressor cells is approximately 1.6 (266). This ratio mirrors what is observed in the peripheral blood. In classifying lung diseases into inflammatory and immune disorders, the percentages of neutrophils and lymphocytes are the primary factors on which division into these categories is made (172,266,267). Neutrophils are rarely, if ever, found in percentages greater than 1% of the total cells recovered by lavage in normal healthy adults. When neutrophils represent more than 1% of the total

TABLE 2. *Bronchoalveolar lavage cellular counts: smokers and nonsmokers*

	Total cell count	Differential cell counts (%)		
		MO	PMN	LYMPH
Nonsmokers	$19.8 \pm 2.3 \times 10^6$	87.4 ± 1.3	1.5 ± 0.2	9.3 ± 0.8
Light Smokers (> 10 pk-yrs)	$58.2 \pm 5.8 \times 10^6$	93.0 ± 0.9	3.3 ± 0.9	4.0 ± 0.5
Heavy Smokers (> 20 pk-yrs)	$102.0 \pm 12.1 \times 10^6$	92.0 ± 0.5	3.5 ± 0.6	3.7 ± 0.5

From Reynolds and Chretien, ref. 268.

TABLE 3. *Acellular components of bronchoalveolar lavage fluid in normal subjects*

Component	Quantity	Primary source/function
Albumin	32%	Serum
Transferrin	0.1%	Serum
Immunoglobulins		
IgA (11S component and monomer)	5%	Serum
IgG_1	6.5%	Serum
IgG_2	2.8%	Serum
IgG_3	0.4%	Serum
IgG_4	0.5%	Serum
IgG	10%	Serum
IgM	trace	Serum
IgE	0.0001%	Serum
Complement components		
Properdin factor B	P	Serum
C3 through C6	P	Serum
Lactoferrin	P	Serum
Free secretory component	1%	Bronchial epithelium
Carcinoembryonic antigen	42 ng/mg protein	Bronchial epithelium
Keratin	P	Bronchial epithelium
Mucus glycoproteins	P	Bronchial epithelium
Laminin	P	Structural protein
Fibronectin	7 μg/mg albumin	Structural protein
N-acetyl-B-D-glucosaminidase	P	Enzyme
Collagenase	13 ng/mg protein	Enzyme
Elastase (neutrophil)	P	Enzyme
Prekallikrein activator (lung)	P	Enzyme
Hageman factor activator	P	Enzyme
Angiotensin convertase	4.5 units/10^7 cells	Enzyme
Alpha-1-proteinase inhibitor	51 μg/mg albumin	Enzyme inhibitor
Low M.W. trypsin inactivator	P	Enzyme inhibitor
Neutrophil elastase inhibitor	P	Enzyme inhibitor
Prostaglandins	P	Cellular products
Thromboxane B_2	P	Cellular products
Leukotrienes	P	Cellular products
Lysozyme	10.1 units/10^7 macrophages	
Carbohydrates	8.83 ± 4.5 μg/ml lavage fluid	
Polar lipids	44.1 ± 41.5 μg/ml lavage fluid	
Nonpolar lipids	77.8 ± 76.8 μg/ml lavage fluid	
Lipid phosphorus	1.1 ± 0.33 μg/ml lavage fluid	
Phosphatidylcholine	83.8 ± 7.5*	
Phosphatidylglycerol	12.3 ± 4.6	
Phosphatidylinositol	1.2 ± 1.9	
Phosphatidylethanolamine	0.3 ± 0.5	
Phosphatidylserine	0.7 ± 0.8	
Phosphatidic acid	0.4 ± 0.5	

*Percent of total phospholipid detected
P = present

cells, a variety of causes must be considered, including bleeding into bronchi from trauma during bronchoscopy, cigarette smoking, inflammatory interstitial lung disease, or inflammatory airway disease.

Lymphocytes rarely represent more than 10% of the total numbers recovered by lavage, and when such percentages are exceeded, an immunological process must be excluded as a cause of such changes. The classic environmental and occupational disorders in which lymphocytes predominate are hypersensitivity pneumonitis, silicosis, and berylliosis, whereas those with a predominance of neutrophils include cigarette smoking and asbestosis.

In addition to the cell content of lavage fluid, consideration must be given to its acellular components (Table 3). Protein concentrations are usually determined in unconcentrated lavage by sensitive methods for protein measurement. Molecules greater in size than 160 kDa are usually not detectable because of the limits of permeability of the endothelium and alveolar epithelium. Albumin has been used extensively as the denominator for the measurement of other molecules present in the acellular lavage.

More recent studies have also utilized assays of cell-mediated immunity to characterize the immune responses that might contribute to the changes in the BAL and the pathological alterations in lung tissues. Of particular importance to environmental and occupational lung diseases are new techniques that permit a more precise analysis of particulate recovered by BAL. The scanning electron microscope can identify and quantitate particulate in alveolar macrophages recovered by lavage, and x-ray spectral analyses and electron probes provide a more precise chemical characterization of particulates (8,33,349).

AGING

Although the lung and immune system both undergo changes with the increasing age of the host (95,145), no systematic evaluations of BAL specimens or bronchial reactivity have been undertaken to determine whether such changes are reflected in the cellular or acellular content of lavages or airways reactivity as a function of the host's age. Since the immune system may express specific impairments with increasing age, such studies might be useful.

CIGARETTE SMOKING

There are distinct changes in the cellular and acellular compositions of BAL fluid in cigarette smokers. The absolute number of macrophages is significantly increased when compared with those cell numbers in nonsmokers (see Table 1). In cigarette smokers, the total cell count is increased by four- to sixfold, with alveolar macrophages representing more than 90% of the total and neutrophils making up between 1% and 4% of the total cell number (see Table 1). Lymphocytes also account for between 1% and 5% of the total, which is significantly less than the numbers found in lavage fluids of nonsmokers. Thus, the total number of macrophages and neutrophils increases with cigarette smoking. Macrophage morphologic appearance is distinctly different in smokers. The plasma membrane of the cigarette smoker's macrophage loses its fine ruffled appearance, and its cytoplasm is filled with pigmented inclusion bodies from the particulate present in cigarette smoke. Macrophages from smokers also contain increased numbers of lysosomes and phagolysosomes. As a result of these cigarette smoke–induced changes in the macrophage plasma membrane, these cells do not spread well on glass surfaces and may or may not respond efficiently to macrophage chemotaxins (97,344). Such changes may be related to the dose and/or character of the smoke. Further, antigen presentation to lymphocytes may be significantly reduced (195,213).

In contrast to the changes in macrophages, the percentage of lymphocytes in the BAL fluid of smokers is reduced (80,171,270,345), but the total number of lymphocytes recovered by lavage does not differ from the numbers observed in nonsmokers (345). Despite the absence of differences in total numbers of lymphocytes between smokers and nonsmokers, there is a significant decrease in the percentage of T-helper/T-inducer cells that is associated with little or no change in the percentage of suppressor/cytotoxic T cells (67,198). Thus, the ratio of T-helper to T-suppressor cells is reduced below the normal level of 1.6:1. In addition to these changes in lymphocyte subsets, the responses to the T-cells mitogens, phytohemagglutinin and concanavalin A, are significantly reduced when compared with the proliferative responses observed in nonsmokers (198).

The key change in the BAL cellular components from cigarette smokers is an increase in the percentage of neutrophils, which is almost always greater than 1% of the total cell population recovered by lavage. A number of other abnormalities have also been noted in lavage fluid from cigarette smokers that become important in differentiating changes owing to environmental and occupational diseases from those induced by cigarette smoke. Macrophage C3 receptors are decreased in cigarette smokers, and the response of these cells to macrophage inhibition factor is diminished (343,345). The secretion of superoxide anion and elastase by macrophages is increased (167,174). Neutrophil elastase presumably ingested by alveolar macrophages is believed to be a key contributor to the pathogenesis of emphysema. The production of neutrophil chemotactic factor is decreased, and the synthesis and release of the arachidonic acid metabolites, prostaglandin E_2 and leukotriene B_4, are decreased (196,197). The lysosomal enzyme content of smoker's macrophages is increased, as is the quantity of alpha-1-antiproteinase (268). The free secretory component of IgA is decreased in the acellular fluid (217). The level of IgG is increased, particularly the IgG_4 fraction (219). Further, alpha-1-protease activity is inhibited (129,268). There are a number of additional abnormalities in the BAL specimens from smokers that must also be considered when such fluids are used as markers of exposure (1,44,115,218,334). Thus, the diversity and number of lavage abnormalities observed in cigarette smokers emphasize the caution that must be exercised in the interpretation of observed BAL changes used to detect an environmental or occupational disorder in cigarette smokers.

TYPE I HYPERSENSITIVITY DISORDERS

In the past decade, occupational asthma has become an increasingly recognized cause of obstructive pulmonary disease, and the performance of BAL in asthmatics has become a less serious concern. Thus, more clinical data on the response of airways to occupational or environmental chemicals have become available.

In settings in which high molecular weight allergens are common, IgE-mediated asthma is the rule, whereas after exposure to low molecular weight components, clear-cut immunopathological mechanisms remain to be characterized (112) (Table 4). With respect to the IgE-mediated disorders, it is important to recognize the timing of the pulmonary response. Initially, there may be a significant delay in the onset of symptoms, making it difficult to relate exposure to symptoms. Thus, exposure may have occurred for time periods up to 3 years or more before symptoms appear, as exemplified by allergic asthma induced by exposure to laboratory animals (82,144,170,314,314a). Such symptoms may frequently be associated with rhinitis, conjunctivitis, or urticaria, suggesting a nonoccupational etiology (60,82). Either an early or a late bronchial response may be observed after exposure, and in some instances, both early and late reactions may occur. If obstructive symptoms and signs occur within 8 hours after exposure, it is easy to relate exposure to such reactions. On the other hand, later responses are likely to be completely disassociated from the true allergen exposure. Since symptoms may persist for long periods of time after removal of the individual from the allergen, early recognition of occupational and environmental chemicals that cause asthma is essential if recovery is to occur over time.

To characterize the changes in BAL fluids associated with occupational asthma, studies have utilized bronchoprovocation with allergens to delineate changes in such lavage fluid from that of asymptomatic asthmatics, allergen-challenged asthmatics, and normal subjects (92,101,110,137,220). When compared with normal subjects, asthmatics with mild disease have a slight increase in the number of eosinophils in the recovered BAL fluid (110). The remainder of the cell differential findings of the lavages are comparable to what has been described in normal, healthy volunteers. Since severe asthmatics have not been extensively examined by BAL analyses, the changes in the lavages from such patients cannot be evaluated. In asthmatic patients challenged by aerosol with the allergen to which they are sensitive, there are significant differences in the BAL composition compared with the BAL of normal control subjects. Both eosinophil and neutrophil numbers are increased in the lavage fluid after aerosol challenge of asthmatic patients (111). Such changes are observed within 2 to 4 hours after aerosol administration. The increase in neutrophil count is also associated with increased airway reactivity, which returns to normal as the neutrophil count falls to the normal range. If the changes in BAL composition after local deposition of the allergen are observed, similar increases in neutrophils and eosinophils occur, but such changes are not immediate. Forty-eight hours after allergen deposition both neutrophil and eosinophil numbers are increased, but at 96 hours, neutrophil counts have returned to normal, whereas eosinophil counts are still increased (111).

Since neutrophil and eosinophil chemotactic activity has been measured in the peripheral blood after allergic responses, these mediators are likely to be the mediators for the increase in these cell types (178,357). Studies have, indeed, identified

TABLE 4. *Occupational asthma*

Vectors	Industries	Skin tests
High Molecular Weight Substances		
Animal products (vertebrates)	Laboratory workers	
	Veterinarians	+
	Animal handlers	
Animal products (birds)	Pigeon breeders	+
	Poultry workers	+
	Bird fanciers	
Insect products		
Mite (grain)	Grain workers	+
Locust	Laboratory workers	
Fly (river)	River occupations/sites	
Fly (screw worm)	Flight crews	
Cockroach	Laboratory workers	+
Cricket	Field workers	+
Moth (bee)	Fish bait breeders	+
Butterfly	Entomologists	
Plants		
Buckwheat	Bakers	
Castor bean	Oil extractors	+
Coffee bean	Food processor	+
Grain dust	Grain handlers	+
Hops (*Humulus lupulus*)	Brewery workers	
Tea	Tea workers	+
Tobacco leaf	Tobacco manufacturer	+
Wheat/rye flour	Bakers/millers	+
Biologic Enzymes		
B. subtilis	Detergent workers	+
Bromelin	Pharmaceutical industry	+
Flaviastase	Pharmaceutical industry	
Fungal amylase	Manufacturing, bakers	
Pancreatin	Pharmaceutical industry	
Paparin	Laboratory/packing	+
Pepsin	Pharmaceutical industry	+
Trypsin	Plastics/pharmaceutical industry	+
Vegetables		
Gum acacia	Printers	+
Gum tragacanth	Gum manufacturing	
Other		
Crab	Crab processing	+
Hoya	Oyster farming	
Prawn	Prawn processing	+
Silkworm larva	Sericulture	+
Low Molecular Weight Substances		
Anhydrides		
Phthalic anhydride	Plastics/resins	+
Tetrachlorophthalic anhydride	Plastics/resins	+
Trimetallic anhydride	Plastics/resins	+
Diisocyanates		
Diphenylmethane diisocyanate	Foundries	+
Hexamethylene diisocyanate	Spray painting	+
Toluene diisocyanate	Plastics/varnish	+
Drugs		
Amprolium hydrochloride	Poultry feed mixer	+
Cephalosporins	Pharmaceutical	+

TABLE 4. *Continued*

Vectors	Industries	Skin tests
Methyldopa	Pharmaceutical	+
Penicillins	Pharmaceutical	+
Phenylglycine acid chloride	Pharmaceutical	+
Piperazine hydrochloride	Chemists	+
Psyllium	Laxative manufacturing	+
Salbutamol intermediate	Pharmaceutical	+
Spiramycin	Pharmaceutical	+
Sulfone chloramides	Manufacturer, brewer	+
Tetracycline	Pharmaceutical	+
Metals		
Chromium	Tanning	+
Cobalt	Hard metal industry	+
Nickel	Metal plating	+
Platinum	Platinum refinery	+
Tungsten carbide	Hard metal industry	
Vanadium	Hard metal industry	
Other chemicals		
Azodicarbonamide	Plastics/rubber	
Dimethyl ethanolamine	Spray painting	+
Dioazonium salt	Photocopying/dye	+
Ethylene diamine	Photography	+
Formalin	Hospital staff	+
Freon	Refrigeration	+
Furfural alcohol	Foundry mold making	+
Hexachlorophene	Hospital staff	+
Paraphenylene diamine	Fur dying	+
Persulfate salts and henna	Hairdressing	+
Urea formaldehyde	Insulation/resin	+

Modified from Chan-Yeung and Lam, ref. 87, with permission.

neutrophil chemotactic activity in lavage fluid after allergen challenge (355). Patients with Japanese summer-type hypersensitivity pneumonitis have been carefully studied with respect to the generation of chemotactic vectors as well as for the role of cellular immunity in the immunopathogenesis of this disorder (354). In this seasonal disease, *Trichosporon cutaneum*, an arthrospore-forming yeast, appears to represent the offending antigen, since most patients manifest IgA and IgG antibodies against this antigen in their BAL fluids (7, 318). When the BAL fluids from patients in the acute phase of this disease are compared with those in the nonacute phase, the complement component, C5a des Arg, has been found to be significantly elevated in patients in the acute phase (95.0 ± 18.0 ng/ml versus 36.7 ± 4.5 ng/ml) (354). C5a des Arg BAL levels are also significantly higher in acute phase patients than in normal subjects (30.1 ± 3.7 ng/ml). Chemotactic activity has also been measured in the BAL fluids obtained from patients in both the acute and nonacute phases of this hypersensitivity pneumonitis. Polymorphonuclear leukocyte chemotactic activity in the BAL fluids recovered from acute phase patients is 36.2 ± 4.5% of that of zymosan-activated sera chemotactic activity used as a positive control, and such fluids have been shown to be much more chemotactic than BAL fluids from nonacute patients (354). Polymorphonuclear leukocyte chemotaxis in BAL fluids from healthy control subjects is $13.4 \pm 2.2\%$ of that of positive controls, which is similar to that measured in nonacute phase patients (354). Significant correlations ($r = 0.923$) have been found between chemotactic activity, C5a des Arg levels, and elevated polymorphonuclear leukocyte numbers in BAL fluids. Leukotriene B_4, a potent neutrophil chemoattractant, has not been detected in BAL fluids from these patients. Since C5a des Arg is less active as a chemotactic agent than its cleavage product, C5a (161), it has been postulated that the fungal antigens implicated as vectors of Japanese summer-type hypersensitivity pneumonitis may activate alveolar macrophages, which in turn synthesize C5 with subsequent cleavage of this molecule to C5a des Arg by a macrophage enzyme or carboxypeptidase B in the lung (299). Investigations by Japanese researchers have also suggested that BAL fluids from patients with this type of hypersensitivity pneumonitis may contain a mast cell–derived chemotactic factor (294). In support of these speculations concerning complement activation, BAL fluid C1q levels in summer-type hypersensitivity have been shown to be significantly elevated (0.4 to 10 μg/ml) as compared with in healthy controls (<0.02 μg/ml) (317). Further, the ratio of C1q to albumin is much higher in BAL fluids from such patients than the same ratio in serum. BAL fluid C3 levels have also been shown to be elevated in these same patients (7 to 93 μg/ml) as compared with controls (<1.0 μg/ml). Serum C1q levels are not significantly different in hypersensitivity patients and controls, and for this reason, local conditions in the lung are probably responsible for the elevated C1q levels in summer-type hypersensitivity. In addition, BAL C1q levels in these patients have been shown to be correlated with IgA and IgG antibody levels against *T. cutaneum* (317). Such findings suggest that immune complex formation activates the classic pathway of complement.

In addition to the changes in eosinophils and neutrophils mediated by disease-induced chemotactic factors, a significant increase in helper T-lymphocyte numbers in lavage fluids has been documented, and such increments in this cell type persist for at least 96 hours after the allergen challenge (111). Recent studies may require modifications of these findings, since studies of both BAL fluids and peripheral blood cells have clearly demonstrated changes in the total cell numbers in BAL fluids as well as altered ratios in $CD4^+$ and $CD8^+$ cells in acute asthma (65,306).

In hypersensitivity pneumonitis or extrinsic allergic alveolitis, the numbers of cells recovered by BAL have been shown to be increased fivefold when compared with healthy controls (308). This increment in cell numbers is made up predominantly of T lymphocytes. Further, it is primarily the $CD8^+$ T-lymphocyte subset that is increased, with little change in the numbers of $CD4^+$ lymphocytes. Thus, the $CD4^+ : CD8^+$ ratio is significantly lower than normal (0.5 versus 1.6) (308). In addition, there is an increase in $HNK\text{-}1^+$ cells in the BAL fluids from patients with extrinsic allergic alveolitis (308). In patients with asymptomatic extrinsic allergic alveolitis, there is a tendency toward increases in the number of $CD8^+$ cells in BAL fluids, but it is not as significant a change as is observed in symptomatic patients. In order to evaluate these changes in helper/suppressor T lymphocytes, the functions of these cells have been examined using *in vitro* assays. The hypothesis proposed for testing was the concept that helper T lymphocytes correlate with active granuloma formation, whereas suppressor/cytotoxic T cells and natural killer cells are usually associated with regulation and regression of the granulomatous reaction. Recent studies have now shown that symptomatic farmers with extrinsic allergic alveolitis have significant increases in the spontaneous cytotoxicity of their BAL lymphocytes when compared with asymptomatic patients and healthy control subjects (202,307). Further, such cytotoxicity is not restricted to a single-cell type but includes cytotoxic mechanisms of natural killer cells, non–major histocompatibility complex restricted cytotoxic T cells, and lymphokine-activated killer cells (308). Other studies have found different results for patients with hypersensitivity pneumonitis. In these other studies, patients with symptomatic disease appear to have increased *in vitro* suppressor T-cell activity, whereas asymptomatic patients have increased *in vivo* suppressor T-lymphocyte activity (181). In contrast to the studies showing an excess of $CD8^+$ lymphocytes in BAL fluids, these investigations demonstrated higher numbers of $CD4^+$ lymphocytes and a near normal $CD4^+ : CD8^+$ ratio (1.6) (228). The differences in these two studies may be related to the stage of the pathological process, since increased $CD4^+$ lymphocytes may be more characteristic of a chronic process, and those lavages with an excess of $CD8^+$ cells are more likely to represent an acute, active process. Similar changes have been documented in acute summer-type hypersensitivity disease in which $CD8^+$ cells predominate during the acute phase (355).

These recent studies emphasize several points regarding the assessment of hypersensitivity pneumonitis by BAL studies. First, C1q levels seem to be a selective marker for this disorder, since BAL C1q levels are not elevated in sarcoidosis, the prototype of the BAL lymphocyte-predominant disorders. Second, the changes in the numbers of $CD4^+$ and $CD8^+$ lymphocytes may provide a method for assessing disease activity and progression. Third, measurement of excessive numbers of specific cell types in a BAL specimen is not adequate; the function of such cells must also be assessed. Bronchoalveolar lavage seems to hold significant promise as a tool for understanding the pathogenesis of hypersensitivity disorders.

Recent evaluations of peripheral blood lymphocytes in patients with acute asthma may also provide additional suggestions as to the pathogenesis of hypersensitivity disorders. These studies have focused primarily on the state of lymphocyte activation and the levels of substances generated by activated lymphocytes (65). In patients with status asthmaticus, the percentages of $CD4^+$ peripheral blood lymphocytes expressing the activation markers, HLA-DR, Il-2R, and VLA-1 (very late activation antigen) are all significantly elevated in comparison to the percentages observed in patients with mild asthma or chronic obstructive lung disease as well as in healthy controls (65). In contrast to these findings, $CD8^+$ lymphocytes do not show increased percentages of interleukin-2R and VLA-1 positive cells. $CD8^+$ cells do show increased HLA-DR positivity to a degree similar to the $CD4^+$ cells. Interleukin-2 receptor expression on $CD4^+$ lymphocytes appears to decrease as the clinical and laboratory parameters of asthma improve with time. In these same patients with severe asthma, on their first day of hospitalization mean serum concentrations of soluble interleukin-2R and interferon-gamma are elevated at levels of 532 ± 47 U/ml and 1.86 ± 0.16 U/ml, respectively. For the control populations cited previously, levels of interleukin-2R are 307 ± 39 U/ml, 298 ± 31 U/ml, and 296 ± 13 U/ml for patients with chronic obstructive airway disease, mild asthma, and healthy volunteers. As can be seen, these values are all lower than those in patients with severe asthma. The levels of interferon-gamma in these same groups are 1.20 ± 0.07 U/ml, 1.33 ± 0.06 U/ml, and 1.23 ± 0.04 U/ml, respectively. These values are also significantly below those observed in patients with acute asthma. For the most part, the concentrations of these serum components decrease as the disease comes under control clinically. It is of interest to note that activated T lymphocytes are reported to be more common in patients with nonatopic asthma than in those with atopy (65). Since CD4$^+$ lymphocytes are a primary source of granulocyte-macrophage colony stimulating factor and interleukin-5, there is speculation that these mediators contribute to the chemotaxis, prolonged survival, and activation of eosinophils in asthma. Since these changes in T-lymphocyte activation have only been documented in the peripheral blood of subjects with status asthmaticus, it is not certain that similar changes will occur with the asthma associated with hypersensitivity pneumonitis. Nonetheless, these changes provide a basis for mechanistic studies of BAL fluids in such patients.

Macrophage numbers also increase up to 96 hours after airways challenge in patients with seasonal asthma who manifest a positive intradermal skin test to allergen, a positive methacholine challenge, and a positive response to inhaled allergen (111). The lavaged macrophages are primarily peroxidase-negative, suggesting that they are newly arrived from the peripheral blood. The release of mediators from alveolar macrophages after exposure to relevant allergens (mite extract and wheat flour) has also been studied using BAL macrophages obtained before and after such challenges (141). Allergic asthmatics without allergen exposure and normal, healthy volunteers have been used as control subjects for this study. Mean culture media IL-IB concentrations either before or after challenge with allergen in the allergen-sensitive subjects are not significantly different from those in the control groups (203 ± 50 pg/ml and 276 ± 134 pg/ml versus 139 ± 81 pg/ml). In those allergic subjects who develop a late phase response to allergen compared with those who show only an early phase response, there is a significant increase in tumor necrosis factor activity in culture media supernatants ($12,305 \pm 3,862$ pg/ml versus 829 ± 312 pg/ml) (141). Such data suggest that tumor necrosis factor may contribute to the late phase response in allergic asthma. There have also been reports that mast cell numbers are decreased in asthmatics who experience both early and late phase reactions (101). Such findings are supported, in part, by the electron microscopic appearance of the cells recovered by BAL (125). Mast cells recovered after allergen exposure are degranulated, and eosinophils are characterized as "hypodense" because they have lost their crystalline central core that contains an arginine-rich major basic protein (178). Major basic protein has also been found in human basophils (3). Both histamine, the primary mediator of mast cells, and major basic protein have been found in the sputum and blood of asthmatics. When segmental airway lavage with a double-lumen bronchoscope and a balloon-tipped catheter is carried out, significantly elevated levels of histamine ($2,403 \pm 633$ pg/ml) and prostaglandin D_2 (306 ± 62 pg/ml) have been measured in asthmatics compared with non-allergic healthy controls in whom these mediator levels were 184 ± 63 pg/ml and 93 ± 17 pg/ml, respectively (357). In standardized BALs, histamine levels have also been found to be elevated in asthmatics (188 ± 42 pg/ml) compared with controls (11 ± 11 pg/ml) (357). In contrast to these findings, no significant alterations in leukotriene B_4 levels between asthmatics and healthy controls have been detected in these studies. Since leukotriene B_4 (LTB_4) has been implicated in late-onset asthma, the timing of the lavage may have been one reason why changes in LTB_4 between asthmatics and normal subjects in this compound were not determined in this study. Histamine levels have also been correlated with increased airways cholinergic (methacholine) hyperreactivity (47). Leukotrienes have also been measured in pulmonary macrophages obtained from lung tissue removed at surgery for lung cancer (298). Macrophage cultures from such lungs stimulated with anti-IgE and A-23187 release both leukotriene B_4 and leukotriene C_4. Leukotriene B_4 levels were found to be 4.3 ± 2.2 ng/10^7 cells, and leukotriene C_4 levels were 0.6 ± 0.05 ng/10^7 cells after a 5-minute incubation with calcium ionophore. Levels of both leukotrienes are lower after anti-IgE stimulation than those observed after stimulation with A23187. Further, as the time after stimulation increases, the levels of these mediators decrease as a result of the metabolism of these lipid mediators by inflammatory cells. Studies have also been performed on BAL fluids obtained from asymptomatic and symptomatic subjects with asthma (342). Subjects with symptomatic asthma have higher leukotriene B_4 and leukotriene C_4 levels in their BAL fluids than do control subjects (0.58 ± 0.06 pmole/ml and 0.36 ± 0.1 pmole/ml versus 0.36 ± 0.05 pmole/ml and 0.12 ± 0.02 pmole/ml). There is a reasonably good correlation between the leukotriene B_4 levels and the number of neutrophils recovered by BAL. These data suggest that patients with hypersensitivity pneumonitis may also show elevated levels of leukotriene B_4 and leukotriene C_4 in their BAL fluids. Macrophages from asthmatics have also been shown to release decreased quantities of lysosomal enzymes as well as prostaglandins when challenged with specific allergens compared with normal alveolar macrophages (137,329). Such changes have been correlated with the degree of eosinophilia, and it has been suggested that the release of major basic protein by such cells causes damage to the alveolar macrophage (126). In fact, major basic protein can stimulate the release of histamine from human basophils (361).

Eosinophilic cationic protein, an arginine-rich protein associated with human eosinophil granules, has also been determined to be present in BAL fluids obtained from asthmatics after antigen challenge (92). Such changes in eosinophilic cationic protein levels have only been observed in those with early and late responses but not in those manifesting only an early response (104). This eosinophil-derived protein is more potent than major basic protein (216), but its complete biological roles have yet to be established.

In both unchallenged and allergen-challenged asthmatics, there are changes in the permeability of the airways (110,111). In patients with mild asthma, BAL lavage specimens show a decrease in alpha-proteinase inhibitor concentrations and an increase in S-IgA levels compared with specimens obtained from healthy control subjects (111). In the absence of allergen challenge, the levels of albumin, alpha-2-macroglobulin, IgG, IgM, fibrinogen, ceruloplasmin, and transferrin have been reported to be the same as the amounts measured in healthy subjects (111). After antigen challenge, in the asthmatics there is a generalized increase in the levels of proteins in the acellular BAL fluid, with a greater increase in low molecular weight components (alpha-1-proteinase, ceruloplasmin, transferrin, and albumin) than in the levels of high molecular weight substances such as fibrinogen and alpha-2-macroglobulin. Since radiolabeled albumin administered via the bloodstream has been measured in the lavage fluid immediately after instillation of allergen in the airways, such increases in this radiolabeled plasma protein are seen to represent changes in bronchoalveolar permeability induced by antigens (111). Such changes in permeability are confined to the lung segments exposed to the allergen and do not represent a generalized phenomenon. The mechanism by which such permeability changes are mediated is not completely understood.

As might be expected, high molecular weight, heat-stable neutrophil chemotactic activity has been found in the circulation of asthmatics after challenge with specific antigens (9). This chemoattractant has also been measured in asthmatics and is likely to contribute to the influx of neutrophils observed in asthmatic responses of the airways (179,234). This chemotactic agent is found in both early and late phase asthma responses. The release of neutrophil chemotactic activity is not limited to specific types of asthma but has been observed in exercise-induced asthma, aspirin-induced asthma, and milk-induced asthma (168,203,244).

Finally, in the asthmatic populations allergic to high molecular weight substances, specific IgE antibodies have been detected in serum (72,112). The frequency of such IgE antibodies is quite high. For example, in patients who are allergic to laboratory animals, IgE antibodies specific for urinary extracts from such animals have been detected by the radioallergosorbent (RAST) test in more than 50% of workers with such allergies to laboratory animals (32,82,260). In contrast to this finding, only 2% of workers without allergic responses to laboratory animals have been determined to have IgE antibodies reactive to rat urinary proteins (260). Similar frequencies of positive serum tests for IgE antibodies have been found in workers allergic to crabmeat. The latter studies have also shown a significant decrease in the frequency of IgE-specific antibodies after removal from exposure to snow crabs (208). In addition to positive tests for IgE antibodies, skin tests with the antigen have also been found to be positive in a large proportion of allergic patients and have produced an erythematous reaction with a diameter more than 2 mm larger than that of control reactions (60,124,314).

Occupational asthmas resulting from the exposure to low molecular weight chemicals have unique characteristics and should be considered as separate and distinct entities (112). It is also clear that their symptom complex may overlap with that observed in hypersensitivity pneumonitis. The most common offenders of this form of occupational asthma are acid anhydrides such as trimellitic, phthalic, tetrachlorophthalic, and maleic acid anhydrides, isocyanates such as toluene, diphenyl methane, and hexamethylene diisocyanate, and Western red cedar or plicatic acid.

In the case of trimellitic acid, an immediate reaction alone, a late phase reaction, or a dual reaction can be observed, including an early and a late phase response (283,359). The immunological basis of this disorder results from the binding of these acid anhydrides to free amino acids (especially lysine) in proteins to form hapten-protein conjugates, which then become neoantigens (112). Trimellitic acid binds to a number of constituents, including human serum albumin, erythrocytes, and basophils (112,246,248). When trimellitic acid binds to the IgE of basophils, incubation with serum IgG from sensitized individuals releases histamine (4). Trimellitic acid-human serum albumin conjugates also stimulate blood lymphocytes (248). Although these trimellitic–allergic workers show an increase in IgE antibodies specific for trimellitic and protein conjugates, their symptoms have not been analyzed specifically by BAL (249). Such analyses may be significant because there are several other clinical syndromes that occur with trimellitic acid exposure (359, 360). Such syndromes include an immediate irritative reaction, a flu-like illness resembling a hypersensitivity pneumonitis, and the so-called pulmonary anemia syndrome (247). The irritative disorder requires no latent period and presents as rhinorrhea, cough, epistaxis, and wheezing. Such symptoms improve within 8 hours and are not known to be associated with bronchial hypersensitivity reactions. These workers have increased levels of IgG, IgA, and IgM antibodies, which are said to react with trimellitic acid conjugates and to activate the complement cascade (248). Bronchoalveolar lavage in such patients might differentiate this type III reaction from the type I response usually observed with this chemical. The pulmonary anemia syndrome is rare and is said to be a type III hypersensitivity reaction as well (245).

Like exposure to trimellitic acid, exposure to isocyanates also may induce a variety of different respiratory tract reactions (11,34,53,114,209,210,224). It may induce an upper respiratory tract irritation, an acute chemical bronchitis, hypersensitivity pneumonitis, and asthmatic episodes. Like what occurs in exposure to trimellitic acid, an immediate, late, or dual response may be observed (23,38, 54,239,243). Bronchial hyperreactivity frequently accompanies this disorder and may become more severe with isocyanate exposure, but bronchial hyperreactivity is not an absolute finding in all cases of isocyanate-induced asthma (150,210).

The enigma of isocyanate-induced asthma may be related to the reactivity of toluene diisocyanate and its related molecules. Such chemicals react with a wide variety of organic compounds, including hydroxy, amine, and sulfhydryl groups (112). It is also postulated that such isocyanate conjugates are reactive and may polymerize. This broad chemical reactivity makes the task of identifying IgE- or IgG-specific antibodies difficult. Nonetheless, specific IgE antibodies against toluene diisocyanate and diphenylmethanediisocyanate have been recognized when isocyanate antigens have been used that restrict polymerization (10,39,176,188,358).

Bronchoalveolar lavage has been used as a tool to evaluate and differentiate the pathological responses observed with immediate and late responses to toluene diisocyanate (107). The number of neutrophils and eosinophils as well as the albumin concentrations are significantly higher in patients with late phase asthmatic reactions when compared with those with immediate or early phase responses. Interestingly, no differences in these three parameters have been observed between normal healthy volunteers and the early phase asthmatics. These studies suggest that the late phase bronchoalveolar changes observed 8 hours after toluene diisocyanate exposure that can be blocked by glucocorticoids represent inflammatory responses, whereas early phase responses are unaffected by steroids and occur by means of a different mechanism (108). Such findings are consistent with the elevated leukotriene B_4 levels described in late phase asthmatic reactions.

Western red cedar dust is another common cause of occupational asthma in certain geographical areas. Plicatic acid makes up about 50% of the red cedar extract by weight and has been implicated as the stimulus for asthmatic reactions in exposed workers (50). Even though this acid has been shown to activate the classic pathway of complement, IgE-mediated responses appear to be the primary mechanism for the expression of asthma in sensitized workers. Specific IgE antibodies against plicatic acid–human serum albumin conjugates have been detected in 30% to 40% of patients with red cedar dust–induced asthma (242,326). Plicatic acid can induce both immediate and late responses and dual reactions (242). Late responses are far more common than immediate reactions. Bronchoalveolar lavage studies have documented increased levels of albumin and greater numbers of eosinophils in the late phase reactions frequently observed in such patients (192). Such findings implicate an inflammatory response. Total protein and IgG levels are also increased in lavage fluids obtained from patients with red cedar–induced asthma. Even after removal of allergic patients from exposure to red cedar dust, more than 50% have persistent asthmatic symptoms (51). No evaluations of BAL in such patients have been undertaken.

TYPE II HYPERSENSITIVITY DISORDERS

There appears to be an increased frequency of Goodpasture's syndrome after hydrocarbon exposure (21,46,121,182,185,186,235,304). Although Goodpasture's syndrome is a rare disorder, the history of solvent exposure prior to onset of this immune disorder emphasizes the need to evaluate patients with immune glomerulonephritis and pulmonary symptoms for anti–alveolar basement membrane antibodies as well as anti–glomerular basement membrane antibodies. Since it appears that the latter antibodies are more common and in higher titers than anti–alveolar membrane antibodies, such antibodies should be sought in the sera of patients with any form of pulmonary-renal syndrome (121,186). The chemicals implicated in these immune disorders include hydrocarbon solvents, carbon tetrachloride, trichloroethane, and even gasoline after long exposure times in animals. Mercury chloride administered to rats also triggers an immune-mediated glomerulonephritis that appears to be associated with heritable factors (290). No BAL analyses are available from such organic solvent–exposed patients with Goodpasture's syndrome, but comparisons among lavage samples from patients with idiopathic hemosiderosis (320) and solvent-exposed patients might be useful in isolating patients with solvent-induced Goodpasture's syndrome.

TYPE III HYPERSENSITIVITY DISORDERS

As noted previously, the immunopathogenesis of hypersensitivity pneumonitis is incompletely understood. When suitable antigens are characterized, precipitating antibodies against such antigens are almost always detected (251,253). Such reactions may even be observed in BAL fluids (117,226,336). A classic Arthus reaction of the skin after challenge with antigen and the onset of pulmonary symptoms within 8 hours after inhalation challenge strongly implicate soluble immune complexes as the mediators of the pathological response. Together with these data and the description of immunopathological findings of antigen, antibody, and complement in lung specimens should make such disorders immune complex-mediated diseases.

The presence of precipitating antibodies in asymptomatic individuals and the absence of markers of complement consumption in symptomatic individuals cast doubt on this mechanism (113). The infiltration of lymphocytes and macrophages as well as the presence of granulomas suggests a cell-mediated process (266,267). Lymphocytes from such lungs also react with appropriate antigens to produce lymphokines and to trigger antigen-induced lymphoproliferation (300). As might be expected, granuloma formation may be the result of frustrated phagocytosis of immune complexes rather than a sign of cell-mediated reaction. Since hypersensitivity pneumonitis has been classified as a type III hypersensitivity disorder, we have elected to maintain such a classification even though the changes observed may be mediated by more than one immune mechanism. Further, there is substantial evidence that type I hypersensitivity responses are not involved in its pathogenesis. A number of specific antigens have also been identified in these disorders, and they are associated with specific occupations and exposures from such occupations (Table 5). The recognition of such antigens may be useful in the characterization of specific etiological agents.

In such hypersensitivity disorders, significant alterations are observed in BAL fluids, Chronic hypersensitivity pneumonitis shows an increase in the total cell numbers recovered by lavage, with a significant increase in the percentage of T lymphocytes (15,348). The level of IgG is also significantly increased when measured as a function of the albumin concentration. In some cases, the T lymphocytes respond to antigens presumed to play a role in inciting the disease (226). This has been clearly shown for patients with pigeon breeder's lung whose lymphocytes proliferate in response to pigeon antigens (226).

Bronchoalveolar lavage lymphocytosis has also been clearly documented in pa-

TABLE 5. *Etiological vectors of hypersensitivity pneumonitis*

Disease	Occupation	Antigens	Source
Aspergillosis		Various aspergilli	Aspergilli spores
Bagassosis	Sugar cane workers	*Thermoactinomyces sacchari*	Moldy sugar cane
Avian handler's lung	Bird handlers	Proteins from sera, feathers, etc.	Pigeons, parakeets Chickens, turkeys, ducks
Cheese worker's lung	Cheese workers	*Penicillium caseii P. roquefortii*	Cheese molds
Coffee worker's lung	Coffee workers	*Thermoactinomyces* spp.	Coffee bean dust
Detergent worker's lung	Detergent workers	*Bacillus subtilis*	Detergent beads, wood dust
Dry rot disease	Old house inhabitants	*Merulius lacrimans*	Old wood
Farmer's lung	Farmers	*Micropolyspora faeni* *T. vulgaris, T. sacchari*	Moldy hay or grain
Furrier's lung	Furriers	Animal hair protein	Fox fur
Humidifier's lung	Officer workers and others	*T. vulgaris, T. candidus* *M. faeni*	Humidifiers, air conditioners
Horseback rider's lung	Horseback riders	*Sporobolomyces* spp.	Moldy barn straw
Lichen picker's lung	Lichen pickers	*Rhizopus* spp. *Cladosporium* spp. *Penicillium* spp. *Aspergillus* spp.	Moldy lichen
Malt worker's lung	Brewery workers	Various aspergilli	Malt dust
Mushroom worker's lung	Mushroom workers	*Thermoactinomyces vulgaris* *M. faeni*	Compact
Paprika splitter's lung	Paprika splitters	*Mucor stolonifer*	Moldy paprika pods
Pituitary snuff-taker's lung	Snuff producers	Porcine and bovine pituitary protein	Snuff protein
Suberosis	Cork workers	*Penicillium frequentans*	Moldy cork dust
Summer-type pneumonitis	Japanese populations	*Trichosporon cutaneum*	Arthrospore-forming yeast
Wheat weevil's disease	Flour workers	*Sitophilus granarius*	Infected wheat flour
Wood worker's lung	Wood workers	*Cryptostroma corticale*	Moldy maple bark
		Aureobasidium pullulans	Moldy redwood dust
		Graphium spp.	Moldy redwood dust
		Alternaria tenius	Moldy wood pulp
		Saccharomonospora viridis	

tients with farmer's lung, but the surprising fact is that a significant number of asymptomatic patients also have abnormal BAL findings with lymphocytosis to a degree comparable to those symptomatic subjects (63,64). Controversy exists with regard to the lymphocyte subsets in farmer's lung. Some have shown an increase in T-suppressor lymphocytes as compared with T-helper lymphocytes, whereas others have detected no differences in the subsets from the normal ratio (202). Further, some investigations have demonstrated T-cell activation with the expression of HLA-DR and activated T-cell markers such as MLR1-3 (228). Such T-cell activation may signal an ongoing immune alveolitis in such patients. Further, recent studies have detected a marked increase in markers of fibroblast activation (29).

Measurement of hyaluronate and type III procollagen peptide in lavage fluids from normal healthy subjects is always less than 15 μg/ml and 0.2 μg/ml, respectively, whereas in subjects with acute episodes of farmer's lung, the levels are markedly increased within the range of 137 to 1,125 μg/ml for hyaluronate and 2.8 to 19.4 μg/ml for the procollagen peptide. The utility of these markers is that they return to normal as the acute process subsides. Hyaluronate levels have also been proposed as prognostic indicators in sarcoidosis, and as might be predicted, such changes in the BAL composition are nonspecific (148). Nonetheless, T-cell markers alone are not sufficient to document disease-related changes. It is probably essential in these situations to assess the functional capacities of such cells.

Additional cellular and acellular components have also been determined to be altered in hypersensitivity diseases. In patients with extrinsic allergic alveolitis, mast cell numbers are increased in BAL fluids obtained from this population (152–154). Further, it has been suggested that removal of such patients from their exposure source leads to a decrease in mast cell numbers to levels of control subjects. Investigations have also determined that these mast cells are the mucosal T-dependent type of mast cell (153). Patients with increased mast cell numbers do not manifest increased levels of IgE and eosinophils in their BAL fluid, and none are atopic (153). In a few patients, antibodies against antigens believed to play a role in extrinsic allergic asthma have been detected (42,43,157,247,269,336,346). Such antibodies are usually of the IgG or IgA class and have been found in both asymptomatic and symptomatic patients; therefore their role in the pathogenesis of these diseases remains undetermined.

TYPE IV HYPERSENSITIVITY DISORDERS

Silicosis

Silicosis (chronic) is the prototype of type IV hypersensitivity disorders, but berylliosis is probably a better characterized form of this group of disorders. The most important types of crystalline silicon dioxide from a medical aspect are alpha quartz, cristobalite, and tridymite. Alpha quartz is the most common type of silica in commercial use and is the silica to which granite workers, sandblasters, slate workers, and shale miners are exposed.

Despite the prevalence of this disease, there are relatively few data on the characteristics of BAL fluids in humans with silicosis. Studies have been performed on a small number of sandblasters who were exposed to silica between 1 and 12 years prior to lavage (302). In these studies, no differences have been detected between those with silicosis and a healthy control population in the numbers of cells recovered, their viability, their adherence to plastic, and their capacity to phagocytose and kill *Listeria monocytogenes*. Lavages from patients with silicosis do have increased numbers of type II pneumonocytes that have been identified by electron microscopy and distinguished from alveolar macrophages by their characteristic lamellar bodies and the rarity of polyphagolysosomes (302).

In another study of a small group of granite workers (nine subjects), striking differences in BAL immunoglobulin content between healthy controls and silica-exposed workers have been found (41). The mean BAL IgG and IgA concentrations in silica-exposed workers are 10.3 ± 2 μg/ml and 6.63 ± 3.3 μg/ml, respectively, whereas controls are 3.3 ± 0.5 μg/ml and 1.78 ± 0.07 μg/ml, respectively. In addition to these changes, IgM levels are higher than 30 ng/ml in 90% of the exposed group, whereas IgM levels are undetectable in 90% of control populations. When these data are expressed as a fraction of the BAL albumin or total protein concentration, there is no change in such differences. Albumin and total protein concentrations from lavage fluid do not differ between the control and experimental groups. In contrast to BAL immunoglobulin changes, no serum protein variations between control and silica-exposed groups have been observed. Since BAL albumin and total protein concentrations are not different in control and experimental groups, the BAL immunoglobulin changes in silica-exposed subjects suggest that such alterations are related to local immune responses rather than to increased epithelial permeability.

Increased percentages of lymphocytes in BAL fluids obtained from this silica-exposed population have been demonstrated, but the numbers of workers evaluated for these changes are small (41,309). Bronchoalveolar lavage lymphocytes from the silica-exposed group have been shown to represent $15.5 \pm 3.3\%$ of the total cells, whereas in the control group, they are only $5.6 \pm 0.9\%$. As might be expected, the number of alveolar macrophages with intracellular particulate material as measured by polarized light microscopy is significantly higher in the silica-exposed group compared with a control group ($76 \pm 4\%$ versus $6 \pm 1\%$) (41). Such particulate excesses have been confirmed by electron microscopy with x-ray energy spectroscopy. The remainder of the cell count and differential count shows no differences between control and experimental groups.

The striking finding of elevated BAL immunoglobulin in silica-exposed workers without active disease deserves careful confirmation. Silica particles are known to be cytotoxic, and such cytotoxic responses result from the capacity of silica to react with plasma membranes, causing increased permeability and osmotic lysis (5,6, 86,100). These events do not occur when silica is coated with poly-2-vinylpyridine-1-oxide or if serum proteins are present (271). Silica may also increase lipid peroxidation, which can be prevented by free radical scavengers (128). Fibroblast cultures treated with supernatants from silica-exposed human alveolar macrophages show increased collagen synthesis (162). Such changes have also been observed with the supernatants from certain animal macrophages exposed to silica.

Patients with interstitial lung disease associated with chronic inhalation of organic dusts have also been examined by BAL. In one study, no difference was found between control and experimental populations with respect to BAL lymphocyte percentages (22 ± 7 versus 15 ± 2) (275). However, the percentage of neutrophils in lavages from patients with asbestosis, silicosis, and coal worker's pneumoconiosis is significantly different from that of controls (3.3 ± 0.6 versus $1.7 \pm 0.2\%$), but there is no significant difference in the percentage of neutrophils from the lavages within the three disease groups.

Bronchoalveolar lavage inflammatory cells from patients with both asbestosis and silicosis release significantly more superoxide anion (31.4 ± 3.3 nm cytochrome c reduced/10^6 cells-hour) and hydrogen peroxide (6.1 ± 0.8 nm/10^6 cells-hour) compared with controls (16.0 ± 2.2 nm cytochrome c reduced/10^6 cells-hour and 2.4 ± 0.7 nm/10^6 cells-hour respectively) (275). These latter studies have only evaluated the lavage specimens from three patients with silicosis, and such data are biased toward patients with the other two disorders (asbestosis and coal worker's pneumoconiosis) under study.

More recent studies of nonsmoking coal miners with either simple pneumoconiosis or progressive massive fibrosis demonstrated an increased spontaneous and progressive massive fibrosis–stimulated release of superoxide anion from alveolar macrophages recovered by lavage from such workers (340). Even though coal miners can develop progressive massive fibrosis from the inhalation of silica-free carbon (347), such data support the previous findings of Rom and colleagues (275). Further, these recent studies also demonstrate a much greater release of superoxide radical from macrophages obtained from patients with progressive massive fibrosis than from those with simple pneumoconiosis. The findings of increased superoxide release by macrophages suggest that these cells are activated by some mechanism associated with dust and/or silica exposure. They also provide evidence that macrophages may play a role in lung destruction.

Another distinctive feature of progressive massive fibrosis has been elucidated by BAL studies comparing patients with asbestosis and silicosis (293). These studies demonstrated a significant increase in the total protein content and free elastase-like activity in BAL fluids from patients compared with controls. No differences in BAL parameters between patients with simple silicosis (21 patients) and those with progressive massive fibrosis (9 patients) were detected in this study. Similarly, mediators known to induce fibroblast proliferation (fibronectin and alveolar macrophage–derived growth factor) have been found to be elevated in the supernatants from alveolar macrophage cultures of BAL cells recovered from patients with silicosis, coal worker's pneumoconiosis, and asbestosis (275). Fibronectin levels are 6.2 ± 1.6 ng/10^6 cells-hour in the experimental group and 1.1 ± 0.7 ng/10^6 cells-hour in the controls (275). Only five patients with silicosis have been evaluated, and the measurements of two such patients fell within the normal range. Such data are also biased for the other two disorders, for which larger numbers of patients have been examined. In the case of alveolar macrophage–derived growth factor, its levels are also higher in patients with silicosis than in normals, but as noted previously, only 5 persons with silicosis have been examined.

Recent studies have confirmed these changes in fibronectin secretion. In these studies, BAL has been proposed as a method of treatment for silicosis because lung function improved in over one third of such patients after whole lung lavage (325). In 50% of the patients undergoing lavage, approximately 30 to 70 mg of silica have been recovered, and more than 70 mg has been removed by lavage in about 33% of the patients. In these studies from China, BAL fluids show an increase not only in fibronectin levels but also increased angiotensin-converting enzyme activities. About 10% of the patients who underwent BAL also had a factor in the supernatant from their alveolar macrophage cultures that stimulates fibroblast proliferation.

In studies of granite workers in Vermont, both interleukin-1 and tumor necrosis factor-alpha have been measured in supernatant culture media recovered from BAL macrophages (85). No differences between control and experimental levels of supernatant interleukin-1 and tumor necrosis factor-alpha have been detected in lipopolysaccharide-stimulated macrophage cultures. Studies of BAL in nonsmokers with silicosis in North Africa have documented significant alterations in immunoregulatory T-cell subsets through the use of immunofluorescent antibody markers (149). In these studies, a significant increase in BAL lymphocytes has been observed compared with that found in nonsmoker control lavage specimens (17.2 ± 2.9 cells/ml versus 10.8 ± 1.03 cells/ml). Lymphocytes in the lavages from patients with silicosis represent $14 \pm 5.7\%$ as compared with $5.8 \pm 2.7\%$ for controls. These investigations have also demonstrated a significant difference in the lymphocyte subsets obtained by lavage from silicosis patients and controls. Cells with the $CD8^+$ phenotype have been shown to be increased as compared with controls ($39.5 \pm 2.8\%$ versus $2.65 \pm 1.8\%$), whereas those cells with the $CD4^+$ phenotype remain relatively similar in patients with silicosis and controls ($35.2 \pm 3.2\%$ versus $40 \pm 1\%$) (149). Thus, the $CD4^+$ to $CD8^+$ ratio is significantly lower in those with silicosis (0.85 ± 0.2) than in healthy controls (1.48 ± 0.12). The other cell markers in silicosis have been found to be as follows—$CD8^+$/Leu 7 ($17.3 \pm 4.5\%$), CD16 ($5 \pm 2.2\%$), and CD25 ($11.8 \pm 2.2\%$)—whereas percentages in the controls have been determined to be $8.1 \pm 1.31\%$, $2.3 \pm 1.4\%$, and $3.6 \pm 1.51\%$, respectively, for these same markers. Bronchoalveolar lavage T lymphocytes from patients with silicosis have also been shown to produce significantly increased quantities of interferon-gamma in culture (36 UI/ml) compared with controls (5 UI/ml) (149). Similarly, interleukin-2 production has been shown to be increased in BAL lymphocyte cultures as compared with controls (180 ± 44 SI versus 77 ± 30 SI). Bronchoalveolar lavage T lymphocytes from patients with silicosis have also been shown to express activation markers. These changes are said to be present in the peripheral blood, but no data have been published to support such statements.

Little is known about the changes in cell-mediated immunity associated with silicosis in humans. A well-documented increase in the susceptibility to tuberculosis in humans has been documented, and normal delayed hypersensitivity skin tests have been reported in silicosis patients (12,301). No other significant changes in cell-mediated immunity have been recorded in humans. Nonetheless, a variety of changes have been observed in animals. In mice, silicotic lung extracts induce monocyte proliferation, and antigens induce lymphoproliferation as well. Rabbit alveolar macrophage adherence and enzyme content have been reported to be increased after *in vivo* silica exposure, and rat alveolar macrophage killing of *staphylococci* has been shown to be enhanced after *in vivo* silica exposure (86,322). Tolerance to pneumococcal pneumonia has also been reported to be increased in rat macrophages exposed to silica *in vivo* (100). These changes speak to an increase in cell-mediated immunity after *in vivo* silica exposure.

In contrast to these finding, mice exposed *in vivo* to silica appear to be more susceptible to infections with *Neisseria gonorrhoeae* and *Haemophilus influenzae*

(37,356). Murine splenic, pulmonary, and peritoneal macrophages show a decreased phagocytic capacity in mice exposed to silica *in vivo*. Alveolar and splenic macrophage helper function in antibody synthesis is reported to be suppressed in silica-exposed mice (221). These data suggest that silica decreases cell-mediated immunity in animals. In the case of humoral immunity after silica exposure, there appears to be a general augmentation in humans as well as in animals, but some animal studies have also shown a decrease in antibody production after silica exposure.

In summary, few BAL studies have been conducted in workers exposed to silica, and when such evaluations have been undertaken, the numbers of workers studied have been small. Clearly, immunological changes have been described in BAL fluids recovered both from silica-exposed populations without disease and patients with silicosis. More detailed evaluations of the changes in BAL cells and cell-free components need to be performed so that the role of the immune system in the production of silicosis can be understood.

There is also little known about the changes in BAL induced by silicates such as talc ($Mg_3Si_4O_{10}(OH)_2$), vermiculite, micas, kaolinite ($Al_2O_3SiO_2H_2O$), bentonite, feldspar, and Fuller's earth. One recent report has characterized a mica-related pneumoconiosis in a rubber worker (193a). Even though the authors identified the mineral as mica by spectroscopy, the absolute identification as muscovite, phlogopite, or vermiculite was not reported. In this single case, no asbestos fibers or silica particles were identified in the BAL fluid recovered from the patient. BAL fluid also showed an excess of neutrophils (20%), which contained phagocytosed crystalline material within their cytoplasm. The clinical findings in this single patient are consistent with a pneumoconiosis, since they demonstrated restrictive lung function and fine reticular lung fibrosis by chest computed tomographic scan. This interesting patient was seen 30 years after exposure, indicating the insidious onset of this disorder (193a).

A variety of other inorganic dusts have been associated with pneumoconioses, but such exposures have not been examined in detail by clinical, radiographic, and laboratory parameters such as BAL. Slate worker's pneumoconiosis serves to illustrate the problems with these inorganic dusts and disease expression (69,134). Inorganic dusts are mixtures of chemicals. For example, the slate from Wales contains mica, feldspar, and large quantities of crystalline quartz. Workers most likely to be afflicted with this pneumoconiosis are those mining slate for commercial use. Pathological studies of patients with slate worker's pneumoconioses have determined that it is a mixed dust pneumoconiosis expressing some features similar to those of silicosis but others that are different. Other inorganic dusts capable of causing pneumoconioses are also contaminated with quartz. Such dusts include kaolin, diatomite (kieselguhr), gypsum, and some forms of coal dust (71). In addition to quartz contamination, some inorganic dusts contain tremolite fibers, members of the asbestos mineral group. In some mining sites talc and vermiculite are contaminated by tremolite, and mesotheliomas and lung cancers have been shown to be associated with such exposures. Azeolite, called erionite, has also been associated with an increased incidence of mesotheliomas. Human-made fibers that have been manufactured to replace asbestos as insulation are still under study, and their relationships to lung disease need to be more completely defined. Nonetheless, there is sufficient evidence of disease associations, including lung cancer, to warrant careful analyses of populations exposed to all such fibers. Future studies should focus on the bronchoalveolar lavage changes observed in silica-exposed populations and those seen with silicatosis and inhalation of other inorganic dusts so that a better concept of the pathogenic factors can be derived from evaluations of such lung cell populations.

Berylliosis

Probably the most classic form of a type IV hypersensitivity disorder is chronic berylliosis. Beryllium metal or its salts result in acute and chronic changes in the lung (73,190,285). The chemical pneumonitis associated with acute exposures to beryllium probably results from direct tissue injury and does not involve an immune mechanism (190,333). Chronic berylliosis, on the other hand, is associated with an immune-mediated alveolitis resulting in the formation of granulomas (123,285). The pathological picture of chronic berylliosis is comparable to what is observed in chronic delayed-type hypersensitivity reactions.

Observations indicate that more than a simple exposure to beryllium is necessary before chronic berylliosis develops (190). Patch skin tests have been used to detect exposed individuals sensitive to beryllium, but such tests are not sensitive or specific. Further, skin testing may sensitize individuals to beryllium, and there is little correlation between the presence of pulmonary berylliosis and positive test results (78,190). Recently, more specific tests have been developed using sensitized T cells as targets for beryllium. In these tests, either peripheral blood lymphocytes or BAL lymphocytes incubated with beryllium or its salts have been assayed for their production of migration inhibition factor or for their induction of lymphoproliferation (99,147,261,332,351). It is now well documented that BAL lymphocytes are more responsive than peripheral blood lymphocytes (105). In fact, in a small group of patients (14) with berylliosis, mononuclear cells obtained by lavage and then exposed either to beryllium sulfate or to beryllium fluoride (10^{-4}M) responded with significant proliferation in all patients studied (278). Such sensitivity and specificity have been confirmed by other studies, but these studies emphasize the use of elevated concentrations of beryllium salts (100 μM), since some normal subjects respond to lower doses. Thus, lymphoproliferation induced by beryllium salts shows a sensitivity of nearly 100%. Further, none of the small number of samples from healthy subjects or those with non-beryllium lung disease give positive responses. Thus, the test also appears to be specific. Peripheral blood lymphocytes may respond to beryllium salts, but they are far less sensitive to beryllium stimulation than bronchoalveolar lymphocytes. Although tests of sensitivity to beryllium are useful for the identification of patients with beryllium exposure, their role in the detection of active disease is not clear.

Characterization of BAL cells from patients with chronic berylliosis often shows an increase in total cells in the BAL fluids as well as elevated numbers of lymphocytes. Representative data give values for total BAL cells of $33.6 \pm 9.4 \times 10^4$ cells/ml as compared with $6.4 \pm 1.7 \times 10^4$ cells/ml in controls, and the percentages of lymphocytes are 56.8 ± 6.7 in patients with chronic berylliosis and 10.9 ± 2 in controls (277,278). Further, lymphocyte subsets have also been characterized. Most of the BAL lymphocytes are T-helper cells ($67.8 \pm 4.9\%$), and 19.1 ± 3.8 percent are found to be T-suppressor cells. Thus, in chronic berylliosis the helper-to-suppressor-cell ratio is 4.7 ± 0.9 as opposed to a ratio of 1.6 ± 0.53 in control individuals. In some studies, there is a significant decrease in the percentage of total macrophages (40 ± 5 versus 87 ± 2), but other studies have not detected any difference in the percentages of macrophages between controls and those with chronic berylliosis (237,277).

Recent studies have expanded the studies of beryllium in patients with chronic berylliosis (285). The percentage of T cells and helper T cells has been found to be elevated as in previous studies, and in addition, a greater percentage of T lymphocytes is found to be activated as measured by HLA-DR positivity (77,105,277). These studies confirm a dose-response relationship between beryllium salts and lymphocyte proliferation, and they also confirm the increased sensitivity of the lung lymphocytes to beryllium-induced proliferation as compared with peripheral blood lymphocytes (285). In fact, the stimulation index in patients with chronic berylliosis using beryllium sulfate is 103 ± 23 for BAL lymphocytes and 5 ± 3 for peripheral blood lymphocytes (285). These investigations have also determined that purified BAL CD4$^+$ cells proliferate at a significantly higher rate (152 ± 47) when stimulated with beryllium salts than do BAL CD8$^+$ cells (2 ± 1). Such data have been confirmed by evaluating the subsets proliferating by cell cycle fluorescence–activated cell-sorter analysis. Further, the proliferating CD4$^+$ cells are antigen-specific (beryllium) and class II restricted. To prove such a relationship, anti–class II antibodies have been shown to inhibit beryllium-triggered lymphoproliferation, whereas anti–class I antibodies do not (285). Further, phytohemagglutinin-induced T-cell proliferation is not inhibited by anti–class II antibodies. In addition, beryllium-induced proliferation is inhibited by anti–interleukin-2 receptor antibodies to a degree that is almost identical to the inhibition of phytohemagglutinin-induced proliferation by the same antibody. The isolation of T-cell clones from BAL fluids of patients with berylliosis clearly demonstrates the specificity of the beryllium-induced lymphoproliferation, since these clones respond in a dose-dependent fashion to beryllium sulfate but not to other metal salts (285). Further, T-cell clones that are responsive to tetanus toxoid and streptokinase isolated from the BAL fluids recovered from the same patients manifest a proliferative response to their specific antigens but not to beryllium. Beryllium-specific clones do not proliferate in response to tetanus toxoid or streptokinase. These T-cell clones have been determined to be primarily of the CD4$^+$ phenotype ($91 \pm 1\%$).

In summary, these recent studies have conclusively demonstrated that chronic berylliosis is a hypersensitivity disorder. The antigen-specific, class II restricted response of T-helper cells may be a useful screen to characterize susceptibility to the disorder, since only a small percentage of beryllium-exposed individuals develop chronic berylliosis. The primary role of $CD4^+$ T cells in this process indicates the significance of these cells in granuloma formation. On the basis of these cell-mediated responses, chronic berylliosis clearly represents the prototype for type IV hypersensitivity disorders.

Asbestosis

A variety of studies have utilized BAL as a means both of assessing exposure to asbestos and of characterizing disease pathogenesis and progression (130,132, 156,272,352). In most studies, the percentages of neutrophils and eosinophils are increased in BAL specimens obtained from workers exposed to asbestos. Representative BAL data from patients with asbestosis show $7.4 \pm 0.7\%$ neutrophils and $2.2 \pm 0.4\%$ eosinophils in the total cell count obtained by lavage in contrast to $2 \pm 0.5\%$ neutrophils and $0.4 \pm 0.01\%$ eosinophils in controls (272). Thus, asbestosis is a disorder in which neutrophils are found in a higher percentage than normal in BAL fluids. Recent studies have also shown an increase in the percentages of lymphocytes in BAL fluids recovered from asbestos-exposed workers as compared with an age-matched, unexposed population. In asbestos-exposed subjects, the mean percentage of lymphocytes in the lavage fluids is 19.1 ± 2.8 as compared with 9.7 ± 1.6 in the control group (339). The absolute concentration of lymphocytes is also higher in the asbestos-exposed group compared with controls (31.6 $\pm 5.2 \times 10^3$ lymphocytes/ml lavage versus $14.7 \pm 2.5 \times 10^3$ lymphocytes/ml lavage). The lymphocytosis detected in the lavage correlates well in one study with the presence of asbestos-related pleural disease (339). Bronchoalveolar lavage B-lymphocyte, T-lymphocyte (total), and T-helper cell concentrations are also higher in those patients with pleural disease and asbestos exposure than in those with exposures and no pleural disease. T-suppressor cells are not increased, but these findings differ among various studies (132,339). Recently, studies have documented increases in the T4:T8 ratios in lavages from patients with asbestos exposure, and such changes have been attributed to an increase in T4 helper lymphocytes (66,96,339). Other changes in BAL lymphocytes have also been observed in asbestos-exposed patients (155). Some investigators have shown increased interleukin-2 receptor expression on the lymphocytes recovered by lavage from asbestos-exposed subjects (67). Such data implicate T-cell activation. More recent studies have not measured any increase in soluble interleukin-2 receptor levels in BAL fluids from patients with a history of asbestos exposure (96). Unfortunately, these studies have not examined the cell surface expression of such markers; therefore the results of this more recent study are inconclusive as to whether T-cell activation is a component of asbestos exposure or not. Not all patients exposed to asbestos express changes in their BAL lymphocyte population.

In granulomatous lung disorders, such as sarcoidosis, elevated levels of serum antiotensin-converting enzyme have been used as a marker of disease activity (199).

Both elevated and normal levels of serum angiotensin-converting enzyme have been reported in asbestos-exposed subjects (19,96,143,173). In those patients reported to have elevated levels of this enzyme in their BAL fluids, no clinical differences between those with elevated and those with normal enzyme levels have been described (19). Thus, the level of this enzyme does not represent a significant measurement of value for characterizing differences between various clinical expressions in patients exposed to asbestos.

Since inflammatory processes of the lung are found after inorganic dust exposure, including silica and asbestos, evaluation of components of inflammation has been undertaken in patients with such disorders. In both silicosis and asbestosis, there is a significant increase in the BAL levels of total protein, free elastase-like activity, immunoactive alpha-1-proteinase inhibitor, and neutrophil elastase inhibitory capacity (293). Based on measurements of the molar ratio of neutrophil elastase inhibitory capacity and alpha-1-proteinase inhibitor, some investigators have reported mean values for this ratio to be higher in patients with asbestosis than in those with progressive massive fibrosis and silicosis and in controls (293). Such data suggest that patients with asbestosis have greater protection from neutrophil elastase than those with silicosis and that such protective activity does not result from alpha-1-proteinase inhibitor alone.

One of the most significant parameters of asbestos exposure and lung disease has been infrequently addressed—the relationship between asbestosis fiber type and size and the occurrence of disease. In most studies of asbestos exposure, the industry in which the asbestos workers have been engaged is given, but the type and size of asbestos fiber are rarely analyzed in BAL specimens. Since it has been clearly shown that the primary asbestos fiber type is, at times, contaminated by other fiber types, such information becomes critical for assessing relationships between fiber type and disease. This information, and data on what other chemicals are in the work environment, represent important details that need the attention of investigators.

Asbestos fibers are separated into two primary classes: serpentine (chrysotile) and amphibole (70,230). Chrysotile is the most common serpentine fiber, whereas amphiboles represent a wide variety of fibers, including crocidolite, amosite, anthophyllite asbestos, tremolite asbestos, and actinolite asbestos. Since these materials all differ in their chemical and physical properties, it is not surprising to find that their biological properties also vary. Because the mechanisms by which asbestos fibers cause disease are incompletely understood, it may be useful to relate the type of fiber to specific disease processes. Asbestos causes several primary disorders: pulmonary interstitial fibrosis (asbestosis); lung cancer; and mesotheliomas of the serosal surfaces of the pleura, peritoniteum, and pericardium. Cigarette smoking is most usually related to the increased risk of lung cancer in asbestos workers, although cancer does rarely occur in nonsmokers who are unexposed to asbestos (70,230,291). Amphibole asbestos is said to be more commonly associated with lung cancer than are chrysotile fibers (230). It is always important to characterize other occupational exposures in asbestos workers with cancer because such chemicals may act as cocarcinogens or represent the primary carcinogen (230).

In the case of mesotheliomas, the most common type of asbestos associated with mortality has been crocidolite asbestos, but malignant mesothelioma may also occur without any known antecedent asbestos exposure (164,230). More recent data have clearly shown that chrysotile types of asbestos may be highly contaminated with amphibole fibers, and it is the contamination with crocidolite, amosite, and tremolite that has been related to the development of mesotheliomas (55,58,131,164, 194,303,337,338). Thus, amphiboles seem to be more significant inducers of lung disease and cancer than chrysotile. Further, the size of such fibers is related to their carcinogenic potential (323). Long fibers (5 to 8 μm) appear to have a greater carcinogenic potential than short fibers (87,88,230). Chrysotile ($Mg_6Si_4O_{10}(OH)_8$) is also more soluble than crocidolite ($Na_2(Fe^{3+})_2(Fe^{2+})_3Si_8O_{22}(OH)_2$), which is relatively insoluble (231).

Several recent studies are pertinent to the characterization of asbestos fibers in humans. First, the distribution of asbestos fibers has been shown to vary, depending on the lobe selected for lavage. Bronchoalveolar lavage studies show that the right lower lobe has a much higher concentration of asbestos bodies than the right upper or middle lobe, whereas uncoated fibers appear to be in higher concentration in the right upper lobe compared with the right lower lobe (327). Thus, long fibers seem to be preferentially deposited in the lower lobes, whereas short, uncoated fibers find their way to the upper lobes. Thus, BAL of a single lung lobe may provide an inappropriate assessment of the type and size of asbestos fiber deposited. Another study has focused on the misclassification of patients with mesotheliomas (48). Two women thought to have had no exposure to asbestos were found to have been exposed during the repair of sacks used to hold this fiber. Analysis of their lung lesions revealed a mixed exposure in one patient due to tremolite, chrysolite, crocidolite, and amosite, whereas the second patient showed only crocidolite fibers on analysis. This study emphasizes the need for a careful occupational history accompanied by appropriate tissue analyses to avoid misclassification of exposed patients. Finally, a comparison of the degree of lung fibrosis with asbestos fiber concentration and size has characterized the fibrogenic potential of different asbestos fibers (amosite > chrysolite > tremolite). Further, comparisons of asbestos fiber size with the degree of lung fibrosis suggest that short asbestos fibers may be more significant than long fibers in lung fibrosis.

Sophisticated techniques can now distinguish various types of asbestos, and the use of transmission electron microscopy, x-ray diffraction, and energy dispersive x-ray spectroscopy is essential to identify asbestos types in BAL samples (14,27, 79). Such examinations might permit a more relevant evaluation of exposed patients in relation to their risks for specific asbestos-related diseases. Recent studies from Australia have shown that the pattern and severity of the alveolitis observed in crocidolite- and chrysotile-exposed workers do not differ when BAL specimens from those exposed to each of these fibers are compared (272). Unfortunately, these studies only determined the type of fiber exposure by work place history, and no direct evaluation of fiber type in the BAL was undertaken. Other studies have shown that fewer asbestos bodies exist in BAL specimens recovered from subjects whose exposure occurred at times more distant in the past than from those with recent exposures (94). In the future, more careful documentation of asbestos fiber type and disease relationships may be rewarding.

Asbestos bodies have been quantitated in lavage fluids recovered from large populations with asbestosis or other types of interstitial lung disease (26,56,57,93,94, 102,273,350). Asbestos bodies represent asbestos fibers coated with ferroprotein. Such studies have demonstrated that the enumeration of asbestos bodies in bronchoalveolar lavages is useful as a marker of asbestos exposure even when such exposures have occurred 25 to 50 years prior to the procedure. Asbestos body counts are not good markers of disease, even though most patients with asbestos-related disease have been shown to have asbestos bodies in their lavages. Unfortunately, patients with no asbestos-related disease may also have increased numbers of asbestos bodies in their lavage fluid. A better marker of this disease may result from future studies in which the types of asbestos are identified. Such data may provide a more realistic means of risk assessment for exposed populations.

Morphological characterizations of alveolar macrophages recovered by BAL from workers exposed to particulates have been described in some detail (324). Unfortunately, such studies have not delineated any specific alterations related to the various species of inorganic particulates under study. Subjects with a history of exposure to inorganic dusts showed markedly increased levels of cytoplasmic particles in their alveolar macrophages when compared with healthy, unexposed controls. These cytoplasmic particles vary in their morphological appearance when seen by light and transmission electron microscopy, but specific particle composition could not be assessed by these methods. Multinucleated alveolar macrophages are more common in particulate-exposed populations, and alveolar macrophages from such patients also showed increased rufflings, filopodia, pinocytotic vesicles, and subplasmalemmal linear densities when compared with cells from unexposed subjects. On the basis of these morphological changes, it has been concluded that alveolar macrophages from such particulate-exposed populations are activated. Thus, particulate-exposed subjects have nonspecific morphological changes in their alveolar macrophage that are consistent with activation or stimulation. Such changes are not restricted to those exposed to asbestos but may relate to other disorders in which organic dust exposure occurs.

Since neutrophils and eosinophils are found in higher numbers in lavages from asbestos-exposed individuals, the mechanism by which these cells accumulate in the alveolar space comes into question. *In vitro* studies have clearly demonstrated that asbestos fibers can induce the release of neutrophil chemotactic factor from human alveolar macrophages (136,200,240,274,297). More recently, *in vivo* studies have confirmed the release of neutrophil chemotactic factor from alveolar macrophages obtained by lavage from patients with asbestosis (156). In these studies, neutrophil chemotactic factor release has been assayed by utilizing the supernatant recovered from alveolar macrophages obtained by lavage to determine the chemotactic activity of such supernatants. In control subjects, the neutrophil chemotactic factor activity is low (3 ± 1 neutrophils/high power field), whereas in patients with asbestosis there is a striking increase in activity (97 ± 19 neutrophils/high power field). No stimulus is necessary to generate the release of neutrophil chemotactic factor from these macrophages. The quantity of neutrophil chemotactic factor from these macrophages is comparable to what is measured when macrophages are treated with opsonized zymosan. In asbestos-exposed individuals without asbestosis, only those individuals who have increased numbers of neutrophils in their lavage demonstrate an increased spontaneous release of neutrophil chemotactic factor activity (156). In these patients, neutrophil chemotactic factor activity is 93 ± 24 neutrophils per high power field as opposed to 11 ± 7 neutrophils per high power field in those exposed to asbestos without increased neutrophils in their lavage fluids. Such neutrophil chemotactic factor release is also spontaneous, and there is an additional increase in its activity (148 ± 15 neutrophils/high power field) when opsonized zymosan is added. Thus, neutrophil chemotactic factor release appears to mediate, in part, the increased numbers of neutrophils in lavages recovered from subjects with asbestosis as well as those with early changes of an asbestos-induced alveolitis.

Other studies have evaluated the levels of leukotriene B_4, a potent leukocyte chemotaxin, in lavages from patients with asbestosis and asbestos-exposed subjects (130). This mediator is more difficult to assay because it is rapidly hydrolyzed to inactive components by inflammatory cells. Thus, leukotriene B_4 may be released at local sites to mediate neutrophil/eosinophil migration, but elevated levels may not easily be detected as a result of its local degradation. Nonetheless, *in vitro* studies have detected leukotriene B_4 in media derived from alveolar macrophages in culture (211). Using alveolar macrophages from BALs obtained from patients with asbestosis, patients exposed without asbestosis, healthy nonsmoking volunteers, and smokers with early chronic obstructive pulmonary disease, the following results were observed (130). Leukotriene B_4 levels are elevated in the media obtained from macrophage cultures of patients with asbestosis compared with cultures from asbestos-exposed patients without disease, healthy volunteers, or smokers with chronic obstructive pulmonary disease. Further, leukotriene B_4 levels measured after macrophages are stimulated with A-23187 or arachidonate are markedly elevated in patients with asbestosis or asbestos-exposed subjects without disease when compared with such levels in the other two groups. Thus, alveolar macrophages from patients with asbestos exposure seem primed to release larger quantities of leukotriene B_4 than cells obtained from healthy subjects or cigarette smokers with chronic obstructive pulmonary disease. Such changes in leukotriene B_4 may contribute to the leukocyte migration to the lung observed in asbestosis or asbestos-exposed populations. Further, this mediator and other macrophage mediators may serve as immunomodulatory substances.

In recent animal studies, it has been shown that IgG causes a dose-dependent increase in superoxide anion generation by alveolar macrophages exposed to chrysolite asbestos (296). This response appears to be specific as related to both particulate and protein, since other proteins are unable to duplicate this response, and acid-washed silica, crocidolite asbestos, talc, and aluminum microspheres do not induce such changes. Both chrysotile and crocidolite have also been shown to stimulate superoxide anion production by human alveolar macrophages (296). Opsonization of these fibers with IgG enhances their stimulation of superoxide production, but IgA opsonization has no effect. The rank order of potency of immunoglobulin subclasses to enhance superoxide production has been determined to be $IgG_1 > IgG_3 > IgG_2 > IgG_4$. The last subclass actually blocks superoxide anion production. It has been postulated that this process may contribute to the pathogenesis of asbestosis because superoxide radicals may cause tissue damage and mutations.

Measurements of BAL hyaluronate levels have been proposed as a means of differentiating patients with asbestosis from those without specific diagnostic criteria to make the diagnosis of asbestosis (20). Hyaluronate levels of BAL in healthy control subjects are 54 ± 7 ng/ml, and in asbestos-exposed patients without asbestosis, they are 68 ± 9 ng/ml. These values are not significantly different, buy hyaluronate levels in patients with asbestosis are 231 ± 82 ng/ml. This value is significantly different from those of both controls and patients with exposure but without asbestosis. When these measurements are expressed as a fraction of BAL albumin levels, the significant differences between patients with asbestosis and those without active disease persist. Such changes have also been observed in animals exposed to asbestos who have clinical and radiographic findings of asbestosis compared to those with exposure but no symptoms or signs of asbestosis. The measurement of BAL hyaluronate levels has been proposed as an inexpensive means to segregate those patients with asbestosis from those without clinical disease. Since hyaluronate reflects fibroblast activity, it may also be a useful marker of fibrosis. Similar changes between patients with asbestosis exposure and controls have been determined when surfactant-associated protein A is measured in BAL fluids (258). For those with asbestos exposure, the level of this protein is 0.41 ± 0.06 µg/ml, whereas the level in normal healthy volunteers is 1.05 ± 0.22 µg/ml. Since surfactant has been postulated to have an immunomodulatory role, the low level of this surfactant-associated protein in patients with asbestos exposure may signify altered immune function. Thus, it appears that a panel of measurements in BAL specimens might delineate the status of disease activity, and cellular alterations may provide a rationale for appropriate therapeutic interventions.

In summary, since the discovery of disease associated with asbestos more than a half-century ago, recent studies using BAL fluids have begun to unravel the mechanisms for asbestos-related disease and provide a rationale for early recognition and treatment. Continued evaluations need to be undertaken to recognize early markers of disease and to characterize the associated fibers and the biological responses to such fibers in the human lung. It is reasonable to think that in the next decade, methods will be formulated to assess the effects of treatment regimens on specific lung changes associated with asbestos.

HARD METAL LUNG DISEASE

Although progressive interstitial fibrosis of the lung has been observed in workers employed in the hard metal tool industry, few detailed analyses of BAL specimens from these exposed populations have been undertaken. In those patients in whom

BAL has been performed, the changes appear to be related to the type of lung disease elicited by the exposure. Patients who have been exposed to high-speed grinding tools acquire an interstitial lung disease with a fibrosing alveolitis, restrictive functional defects, and a decreased diffusing capacity (98). These workers have increased numbers of cells recovered by lavage, and such lavage cell populations contain numerous multinucleated giant cells, a characteristic feature of this illness (2,13,76). None of the lavages recovered from such patients manifest a lymphocytosis or an excess of neutrophils (90). The macrophages do contain refractile dust particulates. Elemental analyses show many particles of tungsten associated with titanium or cobalt (90). In contrast to these patients, other workers have developed occupational asthma after exposure to cobalt, and such responses are related to the dose of cobalt rather than the duration of exposure (133). High doses are more likely to trigger an asthmatic response associated with rhinitis and chest tightness. Bronchoconstriction is also more likely to occur with poor ventilation and toward the end of the day. Both these characteristics are related to the increased dose of cobalt delivered to the lung under such circumstances. Bronchoconstrictive responses are seen after bronchial provocation with cobalt (90,311). The BAL findings are reported as normal in these patients, but few patients have been fully evaluated. Thus, this disorder remains incompletely characterized from the standpoint of the cellular responses in the bronchoalveolar spaces or the chemical changes associated with such cell alterations. Nonetheless, such analyses are required to determine which factors are involved in the pathogenesis of these two types of lung disease seen with cobalt and hard metal exposures. Further, asthmatic reactions to exposure to a number of metals have been described. Immediate reactions to complex salts of platinum, late asthmatic responses to chromates, nickel sulfate, nickel carbonyl, and vanadium have been characterized as causes of occupational asthma (35,45,214, 252). Antibodies (IgG and IgE) against complexes formed between nickel and human serum albumin have been identified, but other immunological features have not been well characterized in these metal-induced disorders.

OTHER METALS

Exposure to metals may also lead to IgE-mediated acute and late phase reactions that mimic hypersensitivity pneumonitis, but attacks of metal fume fever may also be precipitated by such exposures. The latter disorder is thought to have an immunological basis, but proof remains elusive. Whether metal fume fever with its flu-like symptoms and the occasional associated asthma represents a single entity with variation over time or different responses to the same component remains to be resolved.

Metal fume fever is the most common reaction observed after the inhalation of metal oxides. Zinc is an especially common offender, but the oxides of aluminum, selenium, antimony, cadmium, iron, magnesium, nickel, silver, and tin have all been reported to cause metal fume fever (109). Typically, such metal oxides induce a delayed response in workers that occurs 4 to 12 hours after exposure and is manifested by rigors, myalgias, arthralgias, diaphoresis, and dyspnea. These constitutional symptoms may also be accompanied by fever, lung rales, and wheezing. Chest x-ray findings are usually normal, but arterial hypoxemia is present with a peripheral blood leukocytosis. In cases in which the exposure dose is high, a pneumonitis or pulmonary edema may be seen.

Recently, a single patient has been reported with recurring zinc fume fever who was studied by inhalation challenge both with methacholine and zinc (335). Methacholine challenge was characterized in this patient by low-grade, nonspecific bronchial hyperreactivity. Zinc exposure testing was performed in association with BAL and measurements of blood zinc levels. Blood zinc levels were found to be elevated after zinc fume challenges, and BAL specimens revealed a striking increase in the total lavage cell count (94×10^6 cells/ml versus a control of 7.3×10^6 cells/ml) with a marked increase in polymorphonuclear leukocytes. After 7 weeks without zinc exposure, the patient's total lavage cell count had returned to normal, but pleomorphic changes in alveolar macrophages still existed. Such results are consistent with what has been observed in the alveoli of cats and guinea pigs after exposure to zinc fumes (103,330) and probably represent a chemical pneumonitis.

As noted previously, the pathogenesis of metal fume fever is incompletely understood. Some investigators believe that the symptoms result from the release of endogenous pyrogens from leukocytes (254), whereas others believe that these metal oxides catalyze oxidative reactions in the lung (227). Still others postulate that metal proteinates formed between inhaled metals and tissue components act as neoantigens that generate antibodies, and the resultant antigen-antibody complexes cause disease expression (215). Bronchoalveolar lavage studies in the single patient cited previously seem to suggest that the alveolar response is similar to what has been observed early in the course of hypersensitivity pneumonitis (118,331). However, accompanying the neutrophil alveolitis of hypersensitivity pneumonitis is a marked lymphocytosis, and this BAL abnormality was absent in the patient with metal fume fever. This finding casts doubt on the concept that metal fume fever is a form of hypersensitivity pneumonitis. It does emphasize the need for additional studies with metal challenges and BAL to characterize the possible immunopathogenesis of this disorder.

Acute and late phase pulmonary responses, similar to IgE-mediated reactions, have been recorded in the literature (109,177,206). All these reports suggest that occupational asthma may occur as a result of zinc fume exposure. Two patients with zinc fume-induced asthma have documented hyperresponsiveness to either histamine or methacholine. No BAL evaluations were performed, but one patient underwent a zinc fume challenge that resulted in a recurrence of asthma. Thus, it would appear that zinc fumes, like those of cobalt and chromium (224,279), can be the cause of occupational asthma in rare instances.

A third type of pulmonary disease is associated with zinc exposure—a chemical pneumonitis secondary to the inhalation of zinc chloride (175,212). These patients often succumb to a progressive lung disorder characterized by extensive mucosal edema and ulceration with interstitial pneumonia. Autopsy studies have confirmed these responses to be produced by chemical injury. The most common setting in which this occurs is accidental exposure from the fumes of smoke accumulation bombs that consist primarily of zinc chloride (166).

Such clinical findings in humans have not been accompanied by studies investigating the pathogenesis of these disorders, but some data exist as to the effects of zinc on specific cellular functions (52,59,77a). Zinc dietary supplementation in healthy males results in a significant decrease both in neutrophil migration toward a chemotactic agent and in bacteria ingestion (52) at levels of plasma zinc higher than normal (83.0 ± 9.2 mg/dl versus 199.7 ± 18.5 µg/dl). Further, under these conditions, there is a precipitous decrease in peripheral blood lymphocyte proliferation to phytohemagglutinin when plasma zinc levels reach 181.5 ± 21.1, and such a suppression of lymphocyte proliferation persists at plasma zinc levels of 199.7 ± 18.5 µg/dl. Recovery of phytohemagglutinin responsiveness is observed at plasma zinc levels of 167.4 ± 20.3 µg/dl and attains near normal responsiveness at levels of 90.3 ± 10.0 µg/dl. Other studies have examined the *in vitro* effects of zinc on human B cells (77a). These studies demonstrate that zinc is a B-cell mitogen. Zinc added to peripheral blood mononuclear cell cultures triggers a polyclonal response that results in the generation of plaque-forming cells. Other investigations have shown that zinc triggers the proliferation of both human and murine peripheral blood lymphocytes (22,281,282). Such responses are monocyte-dependent (281). The effects on peripheral blood neutrophil function have also been evaluated (59). Oxygen consumption of latex-activated dog neutrophils is reduced by 50% at a zinc concentration of 33 µM. Further reductions are observed in a dose-response fashion at higher levels of zinc. No effect on oxygen consumption was observed with resting neutrophils. Yeast particle phagocytosis by dog granulocytes is also significantly reduced by zinc in a dose-response fashion (59). Bactericidal activity is not significantly altered by zinc despite the reduction in phagocytosis. Zinc has also been shown to inhibit the *in vitro* release of histamine from mast cells (180). The contributions of these *in vitro* studies to the possible immunopathogenesis of zinc toxicity in humans remain to be determined.

Recently, guinea pigs exposed to various levels of zinc oxide (0 to 12.1 mg/m^3 for 3 hours $\times$ 3 consecutive days) have been examined by lavage to determine markers of injury (62,68). In these studies, 2.3 mg/m^3 zinc oxide was shown to have no effect on the guinea pig lung, whereas higher levels of zinc oxide caused significant changes in lavage constituents. The most sensitive markers of injury were found to be lactate dehydrogenase and alkaline phosphatase activities and the increment in BAL neutrophils. In addition to these parameters, lavage fluid abnormalities were also correlated with the lung damage found by morphological analyses. These data are more suggestive of an inflammatory response than an immunological disorder. Intratracheal instillation of zinc chloride in rats (0.15 ml/100 g body weight of 0.5 mg/ml zinc chloride) results in an acute inflammatory reaction associated with an increase in BAL neutrophils, eosinophils, and macrophages. Bronchoalveolar lavage albumin levels increase 15-fold and hemoglobin levels increase 5-fold. Alveolar macrophage phagocytic capacity decreases for several weeks after zinc chloride instillation. These preliminary animal studies clearly document an inflammatory response to zinc chloride, but no data have been derived to address the possibility of an immunological process.

Recent studies have evaluated human exposures to zinc oxide fumes in an attempt to model the changes observed in metal fume fever (30). These volunteers have been exposed to zinc at levels between 23 and 171 mg/m^3 for 15 to 30 minutes in an exposure chamber. Two subjects exposed to the highest levels of zinc developed a syndrome like metal fume fever with chills, fever, and myalgias, although the other five subjects had no such symptoms. The BAL cellular content from these subjects has documented an increase in neutrophils, macrophages, and helper T lymphocytes. Further, the increments in BAL macrophages and neutrophils have been correlated with zinc fume concentrations (r = 0.89 and r = 0.90). In all subjects, BAL neutrophils have been shown to represent an increased percentage of the cells recovered by lavage, with a mean percentage of 31% and a range of 18% to 48%. Zinc concentrations also correlated well with activated and helper T lymphocytes (r = 0.98 and r = 0.94). Thus, zinc oxide fumes trigger inflammatory and immune responses in the lung, but the actual mechanisms by which such responses occur remain to be determined.

As suggested previously, a variety of metals can cause asthma. The complex halide salts of platinum are probably the best example of IgE-mediated hypersensitivity (24,232,250). Such patients also frequently have elevated IgE levels (232). Nickel, chromium, cobalt, and *perhaps* aluminum are also reported to trigger asthmatic attacks (31,83,90,133,151,165,183,191,207,224,238,279,295,311,313). More attention needs to be focused on these metals because it is more than likely that such exposure-induced causes of asthma are underrecognized and incompletely identified. Additional associations between metals and pulmonary diseases have been reviewed (236), and this comprehensive review should be consulted to determine the state of the art regarding metal exposures and lung diseases, including cancer.

OZONE

Studies of human volunteers exposed to ozone have evaluated both nasal and pulmonary inflammatory and immune cell changes (142,305). Bronchoalveolar lavage cell counts obtained from sham-treated (room air) and ozone-treated (0.4 to 0.6 ppm for 2 hours) volunteers 3 hours after the termination of the ozone exposure have been examined, and ozone-treated humans demonstrate a striking increase in the mean percentage of neutrophils as well as a significant increase in the mean percentage of monocytes and macrophages (305). The absolute numbers of monocytes and macrophages are not altered by ozone, and the differences between the total numbers of cells recovered by lavage are not significant when the results from sham- and ozone-treated humans are tabulated. In addition, significant changes in lymphocyte, eosinophil, or epithelial cell numbers calculated as mean percentages have not been observed between these two groups.

Ozone exposure does increase airway responsiveness to methacholine, which is associated with significant increases in prostaglandin E_2, thromboxane B_2, and prostaglandin $F_{2\alpha}$ levels in lavage fluids obtained 2 hours after methacholine challenge (305). Bronchial hyperactivity to histamine has also been documented in healthy adults exposed to 0.6 ppm ozone for 2 hours (139). The increments in cyclooxygenase products after ozone exposure may contribute to the changes in airways responsiveness to methacholine. This argument has been reinforced by studies of ozone-treated dogs in which cyclooxygenase activity and the production of its mediators was blocked (106). Increments in airways responsiveness are prevented by this pharmacological manipulation.

Ozone-induced lower airways inflammation has been examined in humans by BAL, and mediators/modulators of inflammation and immunity have been measured in the fluid recovered (189). In these studies, humans have been exposed to 0.4 ppm ozone for 2 hours and lavage fluid obtained 18 hours later. A significant increase in neutrophils and a significant decrease in percentage of macrophages have been observed. Total cell numbers do not change between sham- and ozone-treated subjects nor does the percentage of lymphocytes. The increase in neutrophils is much greater than the decrease in macrophages. Immunoreactive neutrophil elastase is also increased both in the cell-free lavage fluid and in lavage neutrophils. Since assays for elastase using methoxy-Suc-Ala-Ala-Pro-Val-pNA show no elastase activity, it has been suggested that immunoreactive elastase is coupled to an antiprotease (189). Such increments in elastase activity are partially the result of the neutrophil influx. Elevated levels of protein, albumin, and IgG have also been demonstrated in the lavage fluid obtained from ozone-treated humans, which suggests that a change in vascular permeability has occurred with the transudation of plasma proteins.

To determine the mediators of inflammatory cell influxes associated with ozone exposure, several investigators have examined lavage fluids for chemotactic agents. In ozone-exposed humans only small but significant increments in C3a have been measured (189). No increase in the inflammatory cell chemotaxins, C5a or leukotriene B_4, has been detected. However, the levels of prostaglandin E_2, an immunomodulatory substance, are twofold higher in ozone-exposed lavage fluids than in controls, and fibronectin, a fibroblast chemotaxin, is significantly elevated in lavage fluid from ozone-exposed humans (189).

Recent investigations have also demonstrated that human nasal lavages reflect the increases in neutrophils observed in ozone-exposed humans (142). In these studies, 0.5 ppm ozone is administered for 4 hours on two occasions separated by 12 hours. Nasal lavages performed immediately after the first exposure show a striking increase in neutrophils (5.03×10^4 versus 1.54×10^4 per milliliter of lavage fluid recovered). Neutrophil numbers increased to 12.38×10^4 per milliliter by 12 hours after the initial ozone exposure, and neutrophil numbers are still elevated 22 hours following the second exposure.

Little evidence exists to suggest that ozone exposure is responsible for an increase in either viral or bacterial infections in humans. In an epidemiological examination of commercial airline flight crews exposed to high altitudes and increased ozone levels, symptoms of respiratory tract irritation were documented to be significantly different from those flight crews flying at lower altitudes or for shorter times at high altitudes, but no evidence of increased respiratory tract infections was noted (263). Further, no difference in the course of rhinovirus infections has been observed between human volunteers exposed to 0.3 ppm ozone for 6 hours per day after nasal inoculation with virus and control subjects exposed to room air under the same conditions (159). Serial nasal lavage viral titers did not differ between controls and ozone-treated subjects. Ozone exposure has been shown not to alter the response of nasal mucosa to neutrophil invasion from that observed in control subjects, and no changes in interferon production have been measured between the control and experimental groups. Serum neutralizing antibody levels against rhinovirus are similar in ozone-exposed and unexposed volunteers, and no difference in the response of peripheral blood lymphocytes to *Candida albicans* or rhinovirus antigens has been observed between ozone-exposed and unexposed volunteers (159). Further, these same two groups show no difference between their levels of circulating T lymphocytes, as measured by the numbers of E rosettes. Thus, humans exposed to a moderate dose of ozone appear to respond to rhinovirus infection in a manner identical to that of normal subjects not exposed to ozone. *In vitro* studies of the virucidal capacity of ozone have shown that poliovirus, vesicular stomatitis virus, encephalomyocarditis virus, coxsackievirus, echovirus, and adenovirus are inactivated by ozone, but the *in vitro* concentrations used in such experiments are several magnitudes greater than the ozone concentrations that would occur with environmental or industrial exposures (36,184,205,316).

In the late 1970's, studies demonstrated deficiencies in peripheral blood immune cells from humans exposed to ozone (255,257,292). One such study examined the numbers of rosette-forming T and B lymphocytes in peripheral blood samples obtained from healthy males exposed to 0.4 ppm ozone for 4 hours. The results of these studies showed a significant depression in the capacity of B lymphocytes to form rosettes with sensitized human erythrocytes when preozone blood samples were compared with postozone samples in the same subject. No change in the number of T-cell rosettes was observed in these subjects. The deficiencies in B-cell rosettes were most significant in samples drawn immediately after ozone exposure, and there was a modest recovery toward preozone exposure numbers at 72 hours and 2 weeks after ozone exposure (292). The authors speculated that ozone had disrupted B-cell receptors, resulting in an alteration in rosette formation. Another study examined the response of peripheral blood lymphocytes to phytohemagglutinin at concentrations of 2 and 20 µg/ml after an *in vivo* exposure to 0.4 ppm ozone for 4 hours (256). The mean lymphocyte response to 2 µg/ml phytohemagglutinin evaluated immediately after ozone exposure was suppressed but did not attain statistical significance, whereas with 20 µg/ml of phytohemagglutinin the response was also suppressed but attained statistical significance. Two weeks after ozone exposure, the lymphocyte response in all subjects had returned to normal. These authors compare their results with the mechanisms operative in ultraviolet irradiation–induced immunosuppression and speculate that free radicals generated by ozone are the mediators of such changes. Since immunosuppression is associated with a higher incidence of malignancy (140), chronic ozone exposure could contribute to the expression of tumors in humans. Investigations have confirmed the suppression of T-lymphocyte proliferation to phytohemagglutinin in ozone-exposed humans used as their own controls and extended these observations to show that ozone does not alter lymphocyte responses to concanavalin A, pokeweed mitogen, or *Candida albicans* antigen (257). Further, no significant differences in the number of T lymphocytes forming spontaneous rosettes with sheep erythrocytes have been observed. The authors propose that lymphocyte responses to phytohemagglutinin could serve as markers of ozone exposure.

Peripheral blood leukocytes from humans exposed to ozone (0.3 to 0.4 ppm for 4 hours) show a significant decrease in phagocytic and bactericidal activities, and such effects have been postulated to result from changes in cell membranes, opsonization functions, or interference in intracellular enzyme synthesis (255). However, there is little evidence to support an increased frequency of infection after ozone exposure.

More recently the *in vitro* functions of mononuclear cells exposed to 1 ppm ozone for 4 hours have been examined (18). Such studies reconfirm the suppression of phytohemagglutinin-induced (1 µg/ml) lymphocyte proliferation and extend these observations to include suppression of lymphocyte proliferation after stimulation with pokeweed mitogen (1:1000 dilution of Gibco Stock solution) and concanavalin A (15 µg/ml). Time-dependent increases in the suppression of proliferation have been observed at 2, 4, and 6 hours of ozone exposure, and a severe depression of lymphocyte proliferative responses to these mitogens is observed after 6 hours of ozone exposure. Pokeweed mitogen–induced proliferation is more sensitive to suppression by ozone than is phytohemagglutinin- or concanavalin A-induced proliferation. These investigators also exposed lymphocytes and monocytes separately and subsequently combined ozone-treated lymphocytes with untreated monocytes or ozone-treated monocytes with untreated lymphocytes to assess differences in the proliferative responses to these same mitogens. Such experiments show that proliferative responses are suppressed when either lymphocytes or monocytes are exposed to ozone. Since exposure of both cell types to ozone gives the greatest degree of suppression, the authors suggest that the effects of ozone on lymphocytes and monocytes are additive in their inhibition of mononuclear cell proliferation. Ozone-exposed (1 ppm for 6 hours) and untreated monocytes show no difference in their capacity to release interleukin-1 after lipopolysaccharide treatment (1 µg/ml) for 24 hours (18). On the other hand, lipopolysaccharide-induced HLA-DR expression is reduced by 40% in ozone-exposed monocytes. These results suggest that monocyte-dependent, class II restricted immune responses might be altered after ozone exposure.

To evaluate the mechanism by which concanavalin A and pokeweed mitogen decrease lymphocyte proliferation, levels of interleukin-2, a lymphocyte growth factor, and interleukin-2 receptors have been measured in ozone-exposed lymphocytes and unexposed cells (18). After ozone exposure, interleukin-2 levels are significantly reduced in pokeweed mitogen–stimulated lymphocyte culture supernatants. Further, the number of interleukin-2 receptors on concanavalin A and pokeweed mitogen–stimulated lymphocytes is the same on ozone-exposed lymphocytes and unexposed cells, whereas the number of cells expressing interleukin-2 receptors is reduced in the ozone-exposed lymphocyte populations. The authors conclude from these studies that ozone caused a selective effect on immune cells, since ozone reduces monocyte HLA-DR expression and T lymphocyte interleukin-2 production but does not affect interleukin-1 production or the numbers of interleukin-2 receptors.

In addition to these mechanisms of ozone-induced cell-mediated toxicity, significant increases in prostaglandins in lung lavages in association with neutrophil influxes have been observed in ozone-exposed humans. Both prostaglandin E_2, prostaglandin $F_{2\alpha}$, and thromboxane B_2 levels are increased in these BAL fluids (189,305). These prostaglandins are not only vasoactive compounds but prostaglandin E_2 is an immunomodulatory agent that has the capacity to suppress immune responses (49). Thus, the release of these mediators may represent another mechanism by which ozone alters immune responses.

In summary, human immune assessment after ozone exposure clearly demonstrates a reduction in lymphocyte proliferation using samples obtained from the peripheral blood. Since the recovery of lymphocytes is low in lavage fluids obtained from human volunteers, appropriate assessments of the effects of ozone on lung lymphocyte behavior have not been performed. The clinical role of these deficiencies in ozone-induced immune dysfunction in humans remains to be determined. The *in vitro* studies of ozone-exposed mononuclear cells provide data concerning the mechanism of these ozone-induced changes, but it is difficult to extrapolate the ozone dose from such *in vitro* studies to the *in vivo* state.

NITROGEN OXIDES

Recent investigations have addressed the question of human respiratory infection (viral) and nitrogen dioxide (NO_2) exposure (138). Unfortunately, the results of these studies in which healthy human volunteers were exposed to 2 ppm NO_2 for 2 hours on 3 consecutive days in the first year, 3 ppm in the second year with the same time schedule, and 1 to 2 ppm in the third year are inconclusive. Groups exposed to NO_2 show neither a significant increase in the recovery of virus nor a fourfold or greater increase in influenza-specific antibody titers in serum or nasal washes when compared with control groups not exposed to NO_2. In the third year of the study, the sample size was increased and there was a trend toward more infections in the NO_2-exposed group (91%) than in the control group (71%), but the data did not attain statistical significance (138). These studies examined the effects of NO_2 on a viral infection, but studies of bacterial infections have not been done in humans.

A number of human studies have demonstrated increased sensitivity of airways to bronchoconstrictors in both normal and asthmatic subjects. The earliest investigations of humans with asthma exposed to NO_2 under controlled conditions showed a moderate degree of bronchial obstruction in the central airways and a very significant increase in bronchial sensitivity to carbachol (241). In these studies, NO_2 exposures varied between 210 $\mu g/m^3$ and 488 $\mu g/m^3$ for 1 hour, which represents about 0.1 to 0.2 ppm of NO_2. Sensitivity to NO_2 varied from individual to individual, and no consistent dose-response relationships were observed. Although not all the asthmatics exposed to NO_2 in this study showed changes in bronchial responsivity, more than half of the study group did, and these results led to the conclusion that humans vary in their sensitivity to NO_2. Subsequent investigations have confirmed these results and show that NO_2 exposure also enhances both exercise-induced bronchospasm in asthmatics and airway hyperreactivity after cold air provocation (16). When assessing bronchial hyperreactivity after NO_2 exposure, several parameters need to be emphasized. There is no single pulmonary function test to assess responses to NO_2. Since this pollutant has its primary effect on terminal bronchioles, a strong case can be made for employing pulmonary function tests that detect changes in the peripheral deposition of NO_2 and using exercised subjects to increase the chance for delivery of this pollutant to peripheral sites. Selection of subjects is also an important parameter that may significantly influence experimental results. Some investigators believe that differences in responses to NO_2 may result from the selection of asthmatics who have no resting airway obstruction or no bronchial hyperreactivity (16). Using isocapneic cold air hyperventilation assures investigators that their asthmatic subjects are hyperreactive before they undergo NO_2 exposure. In one study in which bronchial hyperreactivity and peripheral airways obstruction were observed after NO_2 administration at levels comparable to the peak levels in urban areas (0.3 ppm NO_2 for 30 minutes), both resting airway obstruction and bronchial hyperactivity were determined to be present in the asthmatics under study before exposing them to NO_2 (16). Other investigators have shown similar responses to NO_2 at doses in the same range (510 $\mu g/m^3$ for 30 minutes on four separate days) but failed to measure any change in airway resistance or breathing patterns at significantly higher doses (1,000 $\mu g/m^3$) under the same conditions noted previously (40). No explanation has been provided for the absence of a change in airway resistance at 1,000 $\mu g/m^3$ of NO_2, but defense mechanisms have been proposed as contributors to preventing injury to the airways. Thus, NO_2 causes increased airways resistance in asthmatics as well as hyperreactivity to various bronchoconstrictors and cold air. More consistent changes are observed if the subjects selected demonstrate hyperreactivity before NO_2 exposure and have abnormalities in pulmonary function that are indicative of asthma prior to their exposure to pollutants.

A number of studies have also evaluated the response of healthy subjects (without asthma) to NO_2. With few exceptions, most of the early studies showed minimal, if any, effect on airway resistance after NO_2 exposure (91,116,146). Such negative results have even been observed with NO_2 doses as high as 4 ppm for 1.25 hours with heavy exercise (204). Other studies appear to complement these findings, since they also show no changes in lung volumes, flow rates, or respiratory symptoms in normal healthy volunteers but do demonstrate a significant increase in airway reactivity to methacholine when nonsmoking subjects are exposed to 2 ppm NO_2 for 1 hour (222). Thus, increased airway responsiveness is observed after NO_2 exposure without associated bronchoconstriction.

Recent investigations of *in vitro* influenza virus infection have evaluated human alveolar macrophage functions in cells obtained by lavage from human volunteers exposed to 0.6 ppm of NO_2 for 3 hours (120). Cells exposed to NO_2 under these conditions show a tendency to inactivate influenza virus less efficiently than air-exposed control cells, and these same cells with diminished viral inactivation activity secrete increased quantities of interleukin-1. Macrophages exposed to NO_2 that do not manifest a change in viral inactivation show decreased interleukin-1 production. The results of these studies in a small number of human subjects are inconclusive, but they do suggest that BAL may be a useful tool in assessing the effects of pollutants on macrophage functions.

Further, *in vitro* cell exposure systems have been used to evaluate alveolar macrophage responses to oxidants (262a). Using this methodology, human alveolar macrophages have been exposed to 5 or 15 ppm of NO_2 for 3 hours *in vitro* while measuring the release of neutrophil chemotactic factor and interleukin-1, potent mediators of inflammation. When compared with air-exposed macrophage cultures, no differences in cell viability or neutrophil chemotactic factor or interleukin-1 release could be detected after NO_2 exposure (259). Thus, despite the capacity of NO_2 to induce an inflammatory response in the lower respiratory tract of humans and animals, neutrophil chemotactic factor and interleukin-1 production by alveolar macrophages does not appear to be the primary mediator of such a reaction at these doses of NO_2.

Other studies have shown a 45% decrease in the functional activity of alpha-1-protease inhibitor in NO_2-exposed humans with no change in the quantity of immunoreactive alpha-1-protease inhibitor between healthy nonsmokers and nonsmoking humans exposed to NO_2 (3 or 4 ppm) for 3 hours with intermittent exercise (223). This protease defect observed in BAL fluids from NO_2-exposed humans has not been accompanied by any changes in neutrophil quantities or elastase-like activity. Thus, short exposures of humans to NO_2 cause a reduction in alpha-1-protease inhibition, a factor known to protect human tissues from proteolytic attack. Subsequent studies, using low level exposures of NO_2 (0.6 to 1.5 ppm), have shown transient but significant (47%) increases in alpha-2-macroglobulin levels in lavages from healthy, nonsmoking human volunteers (119) exposed continuously to 0.6 ppm NO_2. Here again, these changes were not associated with an influx of inflammatory cells and were not accompanied by any changes in lavage proteins signifying an altered epithelial barrier. What role such alpha-2-macroglobulin changes play in the host defense against oxidants is unknown. Furthermore, continuous NO_2 exposure to higher doses (1.5 ppm) did not result in any alterations in macroglobulin levels in the lavage fluids recovered from this experimental group. Thus, the changes in alpha-2-macroglobulin remain incompletely understood, as do the health effects of NO_2 in humans.

A recent paper provides provocative data on the changes in BAL cell composition after low-dose NO_2 exposures and suggests that animals may not be good models for humans (286). In these studies, young healthy males were exposed to 7 mg NO_2/m^3 for 20 minutes, and BAL specimens were obtained 4, 8, 24, and 72 hours after exposure for comparison with preexposure lavage specimens. The exposure concentration (4 ppm) was selected because it was comparable to NO_2 concentrations that occur outdoors and in certain industries but at a level below the exposure limits for the work place (5.5 ppm or 10 mg NO_2/m^3). Significant increases in BAL mast cell numbers are observed at 72 hours after exposure. No changes in BAL lymphocyte numbers are observed at 72 hours. Further, no change in T-cell subsets (helper/cytotoxic) are observed with the increment in lymphocytes. There is a modest increase (not statistically significant) in lysozyme-positive macrophages, but the total macrophage numbers are not altered by NO_2 exposures. These latter findings are in contrast to those observed after human sulfur dioxide (SO_2) exposures, where there is a significant increase in BAL macrophage numbers (286). Such differences may be related to the differences in lung deposition between water-insoluble NO_2 and water-soluble SO_2. There was no change in BAL neutrophil numbers in these human NO_2 exposure studies, which is in contrast to the significant neutrophilia observed in NO_2-exposed rats (135).

This provocative study of healthy humans exposed to NO_2 raises several important questions that may have an impact on the relevance of studies of environmental pollutants. This study also illustrates the importance of using specific mast cell stains to detect changes in the number of these cells and focuses attention on the role of these cells in the pathogenesis of lung changes that may occur in association with NO_2 exposures. The role of lymphocyte and mast cell chemotaxins and the biological roles of these cells must certainly be investigated if we are to understand such NO_2-induced changes in humans. Finally, the differences between the cell changes observed in BAL fluids from rats and from humans emphasize the need to reexamine species differences in the response to pollutants. Such differences may explain why the immunotoxic effects observed in animals have frequently not been seen in humans.

In summary, human exposure to NO_2 has provided inconsistent data bases. An increased rate of infection after NO_2 exposure may occur, particularly in the most susceptible groups such as children. Further, there is sufficient evidence to suggest that increased airway reactivity occurs both in normal healthy subjects and in asthmatics. As with ozone, the focus of studies concerned with immunopathogenesis of NO_2 must emphasize hypersensitivity reactions, alveolar macrophage functions, and other immunoprotective functions, but few such studies have been performed in humans. Animal studies still remain as the primary published sources of results regarding the health effects of NO_2.

SULFUR DIOXIDE

Human volunteers exposed to 5 and 13 ppm sulfur dioxide (SO_2) for 10 to 30 minutes manifest a significant increase in pulmonary flow resistance. Such exposures also show a dose-response relationship, with the most significant alterations observed at doses of 13 ppm of SO_2 (122). Subsequent investigations have observed changes in expiratory flow rates with SO_2 concentrations of 1 ppm when the pollutant is delivered by mouth only and nasal breathing has been blocked (315). These data are perfectly consistent with the fact that scrubbing of this pollutant takes place, in large part, by moist nasal passages (319).

Since SO_2 induces bronchoconstriction, studies have been undertaken to determine the sensitivity of patients with asthma and seasonal rhinitis. Studies in which human volunteers breathed 1, 3, or 5 ppm SO_2 for 10 minutes demonstrate that asthmatics are much more sensitive to SO_2 than are normal healthy volunteers and subjects with atopic rhinitis (310). Since the nose and nasopharynx can efficiently remove SO_2, exposures have been restricted to the oral route. Atropine blocks the SO_2-induced bronchoconstrictor responses and for this reason, a role for parasympathetic pathways and muscarinic receptors as the ultimate mediators of this response to SO_2 has been proposed.

It should not be surprising to find that exercise induces bronchoconstrictor responses in asthmatic subjects, and exposure to SO_2 at doses as low as 0.5 ppm with exercise for 10 minutes also causes bronchoconstriction. These data all suggest that SO_2 could contribute to the proposed link between air pollutants and the increased morbidity from asthma. Indeed, ozone, a well-characterized air pollutant, causes an increase in the sensitivity of asthmatics to SO_2 (187), whereas low exposures of NO_2 do not (280).

The effects of pharmacological agents on SO_2-induced bronchoconstriction have also been evaluated. Disodium cromoglycate inhibits SO_2-induced bronchoconstrictor responses (233,310a,310b). Since this agent is primarily known for its capacity to block the degranulation of mast cells, these studies give credence to the hypothesis that cromolyn might affect neurogenic-mediated bronchoconstrictor responses by mechanisms quite separate from its effects on mast cells. Cromolyn inhibition of SO_2-induced bronchoconstriction is a dose-dependent response (233). Since cromolyn has the capacity to inhibit neural activity, it could be concluded that SO_2-induced bronchoconstriction is entirely dependent on neurogenic mechanisms without any involvement of the immune system. Nonetheless, the data published to date do not exclude the possibility that more than one mechanism is responsible for the observed bronchoconstrictor responses to SO_2. This possibility takes on more significance when the increments in lymphocytes and mast cells in the BAL fluid obtained after the administration of SO_2 to humans are considered (287–289).

In addition to increments in lymphocytes and mast cells, lavage fluids from SO_2-exposed humans also manifest an increased number of alveolar macrophages, including more lysozyme-positive macrophages than is normally observed. Since the total number of macrophages is not always increased after SO_2 exposure, such an increase in lysozyme-positive cells probably indicates macrophage activation (28,61,201). The cell increments in BAL fluids obtained after SO_2 exposure peaked at 24 hours and returned to normal by 72 hours (287). No increase in albumin has been measured in BAL fluids after SO_2 exposures, indicating the absence of any change in bronchial epithelial permeability. Bisulfite ions or SO_2 gas but not sulfite ions appears to be the active mediator of bronchoconstriction. Subsequent studies should evaluate sulfite as a more potent trigger of changes in BAL fluids.

It has been shown that exposure to 0.3 ppm NO_2 for 30 minutes, as noted previously, did not potentiate SO_2-induced airways responses over a dose range of 0.25 to 4 ppm for short time periods (less than 10 minutes). On the other hand, patients with allergic asthma have been evaluated after exposures during moderate exercise to the following two regimens: air for 45 minutes followed by 100 ppb SO_2 for 15 minutes; or 129 ppb ozone for 45 minutes followed by 120 ppb SO_2. In these experiments, ozone significantly increases bronchial hyperresponsiveness in these allergic patients, such that they respond to SO_2 doses below the threshold for responsiveness to this pollutant. Such results clearly indicate that interactions between some airborne pollutants do occur and that such interactions may contribute to the pathogenesis of asthma in susceptible populations (323a).

CONCLUSION

There should be no question that BAL studies in humans have made significant contributions to our understanding of the pulmonary response to environmental and chemical pollutants. Nonetheless, such studies are far from complete. The cellular responses to the most common environmental pollutants have been reasonably well defined, but the functional capacities of such BAL cells have been less completely evaluated, and the molecular basis of the lung injuries mediated by pollutants remains, for the most part, poorly characterized. In large part, organic chemical exposures have also been incompletely evaluated with respect to their potential to cause lung and respiratory tract damage, despite the fact that inhalation still remains a major portal of entry for such agents. Further, xenobiotic metabolism by lung cells remains to be examined in more detail, and greater emphasis is needed on the use of BAL cells and their functions as biomarkers of exposure, susceptibility, and effect. Bronchoalveolar lavage holds promise as a valuable adjunct for the early diagnosis of environmentally induced lung damage, for the characterization of the pathogenesis of such exposures, and perhaps even for the assessment of therapeutic initiatives to alter lung and respiratory functions in a positive fashion.

REFERENCES

1. Abboud, R. T., Fera, T., Richter, A., Tabona, M. Z., and Johal, S. (1985): Acute effect of smoking on the functional activity of alpha$_1$-protease in bronchoalveolar lavage fluid. *Am. Rev. Respir. Dis.*, 131:79–85.
2. Abraham, J. L. (1986): Lung pathology in 22 cases of giant cell interstitial pneumonia (GIP) suggests GIP is pathognomonic of cobalt (hard metal) disease. 3rd International Conference on Environmental Lung Disease, Montreal.
3. Ackerman, S. J., Kephart, G. M., Habermann, T. M., Greipp, P. R., and Gleich, G. J. (1983):

Localization of eosinophil granule major basic protein in human basophils. *J. Exp. Med.*, 158:946–961.

4. Akiyama, K., Pruzansky, J. J., and Patterson, R. (1984): Hapten-modified basophils: A model of human immediate hypersensitivity that can be elicited by IgG antibody. *J. Immunol.*, 133:3286–3290.

5. Allison, A. C. (1977): Mechanisms of macrophage damage in relation to the pathogenesis of some lung disease. In Lung Biology in Health and Disease, edited by J. D. Brain, D. F. Proctor, and L. M. Reid. Marcel Dekker, Inc., New York.

6. Allison, A. C., Harrington, J. S., and Birbeck, M. (1966): An examination of the cytotoxic effects of silica on macrophages. *J. Exp. Med.*, 124:141–153.

7. Ando, M., Yoshida, K., Soda, K., and Araki, S. (1986): Specific bronchoalveolar lavage IgA antibody in patients with summer-type hypersensitivity pneumonitis induced by *Trichosporon cutaneum*. *Am. Rev. Respir. Dis.*, 134:177–179.

8. Armstrong, J. T. (1978): Methods of quantitative analysis of individual micro-particles with electron beam instruments. *Scanning Electron Microsc. Proc.*, 1:455–467.

9. Atkins, P. C., Norman, M., Weiner, M., and Zweimann, B. (1977): Release of neutrophil chemotactic activity during immediate hypersensitivity reactions in humans. *Ann. Intern. Med.*, 86:415–418.

10. Avery, S. B., Stetson, D. M., Pan, P. M., and Matthews, K. P. (1969): Immunological investigation of individuals with toluene diisocyanate asthma. *Clin. Exp. Immunol.*, 4:585–596.

11. Axford, A. T., McKerrow, C. B., Parry Jones, A., and Le Quesne, P. M. (1976): Accidental exposure to isocyanate fumes in a group of firemen. *Br. J. Ind. Med.*, 33:65–71.

12. Bailey, W. C., Brown, M., Buechner, H. A., Weill, H., Ichinose, H., and Ziskind, M. (1974): Silico-mycobacterial disease in sandblasters. *Am. Rev. Respir. Dis.*, 110:115–125.

13. Balmes, J. R. (1987): Respiratory effects of hard-metal dust exposure. *Occup. Med. State of the Art Rev.*, 2:327–344.

14. Barbers, R. G., and Abraham, J. L. (1989): Asbestosis occurring after brief inhalational exposure: Usefulness of bronchoalveolar lavage in diagnosis. *Br. J. Ind. Med.*, 46:106–110.

15. Bascom, R., Kennedy, T. P., Levitz, D., and Zeiss, C. R. (1985): Specific bronchoalveolar lavage IgG antibody in hypersensitivity pneumonitis from diphenylmethane diisocyanate. *Am. Rev. Respir. Dis.*, 131:463–465.

16. Bauer, M. A., Utell, M. J., Morrow, P. E., Speers, D. M., and Gibb, F. R. (1986): Inhalation of 0.30 ppm nitrogen dioxide potentiates exercise-induced bronchospasm in asthmatics. *Am. Rev. Respir. Dis.*, 134:1203–1208.

17. Baughman, R. P., Bosken, C. H., Loudon, R. G., Hurtubise, P., and Wesseler, T. (1983): Quantitation of bronchoalveolar lavage with methylene blue. *Am. Rev. Respir. Dis.*, 128:266–270.

18. Becker, S., Jordan, R. L., Orlando, G. S. (1989): In vitro ozone exposure inhibits mitogen-induced lymphocyte proliferation and IL-2 production. *J. Toxicol. Environ. Health*, 26:469–483.

19. Begin, R., Cantin, A., Berthiaume, Y., Boileau, R., Bisson, G., Lamoureaux, G., Rola-Pleszczynski, M., Drapeau, G., Masse, S., and Boctor, M. (1985): Clinical features to stage alveolitis in asbestos workers. *Am. J. Ind. Med.*, 8:521–536.

20. Begin, R., Cantin, A., Martel, M., and Fabi, D. (1990): Pulmonary accumulation of hyaluronate in asbestosis. *Am. Rev. Respir. Dis.*, 141:A241.

21. Beirne, G. J., and Brennan, J. T. (1972): Glomerulonephritis associated with hydrocarbon solvents. *Arch. Environ. Health*, 25:365–369.

22. Berger, N. A., and Skinner, A. M., Sr. (1979): Characterization of lymphocyte transformation induced by zinc ions. *J. Cell Biol.*, 61:45–55.

23. Bernstein, I. L. (1982): Isocyanate-induced pulmonary disease: A current perspective. *J. Allergy Clin. Immunol.*, 70(Suppl.):24–31.

24. Biagini, R. E., Bernstein, I. L., Gallagher, J. S., Moorman, W. J., Brooks, S., and Gann, P. H. (1985): The diversity of reaginic immune responses to platinum and palladium metallic salts. *J. Allergy Clin. Immunol.*, 76:794–802.

25. Bice, D. E. (1985): Methods and approaches for assessing immunotoxicity of the lower respiratory tract. In Immunotoxicology and Immunopharmacology, edited by J. Dean, pp. 145–157. Raven Press, New York.

26. Bignon, J. (1979): Possibilities offertes par l'etude des particules minerals dans le lavage bronchoalveolaire. *Rev. Fr. Med. Respir.*, 7:291–294.

27. Bignon, J., Sebastien, P., Gandichet, A., and Jourand, M. C. (1980): Biological effects of al-

tapulgite. In Biological Effects of Mineral Fibres (vol. 1), edited by J. C. Wagner, pp. 163–181. International Agency for Research on Cancer, Scientific Publications, Lyon.

28. Bjermer, L., Back, O., Roos, G., and Thunell, M. (1986): Mast cells and lysozyme positive macrophages in bronchoalveolar lavage from patients with sarcoidosis. *Acta Med. Scand.*, 220:161–166.

29. Bjermer, L., Engstrom-Laurent, A., Lundgren, R., Rosenhall, L., and Hallgren, R. (1987): Hyaluronate and type III procollagen peptide concentrations in bronchoalveolar lavage fluid as markers of disease activity in farmer's lung. *Br. Med. J.*, 295:803–806.

30. Blanc, P. D., Bigby, B., Bernstein, M. S., Wong, H., and Boushey, H. A. (1990): The role of lung inflammation in metal fume fever. *Am. Rev. Respir. Dis.*, 141:A594.

31. Block G. Y., and Yeung, M. (1982): Asthma induced by nickel. *J.A.M.A.*, 247:1600–1602.

32. Bothman, P. A., Davis, G. E., and Teasdale, E. L. (1987): Allergy to laboratory animals: A prospective study of its incidence and of the influence of atopy in its development. *Br. J. Ind. Med.*, 44:627–632.

33. Brody, A. R., Roe, M. W., Evans, J. N., and Davis, G. S. (1980): Use of backscattered electron imaging to quantify the distribution of inhaled crystalline silica. In Scanning Electron Microscopy, pp. 301–306. IITR, Chicago.

34. Brooks, S. M. (1977): Bronchial asthma of occupational origin. *Scand. J. Work Environ. Health*, 3:53–72.

35. Browne, R. C. (1955): Vanadium poisoning from gas turbines. *Br. J. Ind. Med.*, 12:57–59.

36. Burleson, G. R., Murray, T. M., and Pollard, M. (1975): Inactivation of viruses and bacteria by ozone, with and without sonication. *Appl. Microbiol.*, 29:340–344.

37. Burrell, R. (1981): Immunological aspects of silica. In Health Effects of Synthetic Silica Particulates, p. 82. American Society for Testing Materials, Philadelphia.

38. Butcher, B. T. (1979): Inhalation challenge testing with toluene diisocyanate. *J. Allergy Clin. Immunol.*, 64:655–657.

39. Butcher, B. T., Salvaggio, J. E., O'Neil, C. E., Weill, H., and Gang, O. (1976): Toluene diisocyanate pulmonary disease. Immunopharmacologic and mecholyl challenge studies. *J. Allergy Clin. Immunol.*, 59:223–227.

40. Bylin, G., Hedenstierna, G., Lindvall, T., and Sundin, B. (1988): Ambient nitrogen dioxide concentrations increase bronchial responsiveness in subjects with mild asthma. *Eur. Respir. J.*, 1:606–612.

41. Calhoun, W. J., Christman, J. W., Ershler, W. B., Graham, W. G. B., and Davis, G. S. (1986): Raised immunoglobulin concentrations in bronchoalveolar lavage fluid of healthy granite workers. *Thorax*, 41:266–273.

42. Calvanico, N. J., Ambegaonkar, S. P., Schlueter, D. P., and Fink, J. M. (1980): Immunoglobulin levels in bronchoalveolar lavage fluid from pigeon breeders. *J. Lab. Clin. Med.*, 96:129–140.

43. Campbell, J. A., Kryda, M. D., Treuhaft, M. W., Marx, J. J., and Roberts, R. C. (1983): Cheese worker's hypersensitivity pneumonitis. *Am. Rev. Respir. Dis.*, 127:495–496.

44. Cantrell, E. T., Warr, G. A., Busbee, D. L., and Martin, R. R. (1973): Induction of aryl hydrocarbon hydroxylase in human pulmonary alveolar macrophages by cigarette smoking. *J. Clin. Invest.*, 52:1881–1884.

45. Card, W. I. (1935): A case of asthma sensitivity to chromates. *Lancet*, 2:1348–1349.

46. Carlier, B., Schroeder, E., and Mahieu, P. (1980): A rapidly and spontaneously reversible Goodpasture's syndrome after carbon tetrachloride inhalation. *Acta Clin. Belg.*, 35:193–198.

47. Casale, T. B., Wood, D., Trapp, S., Rickerson, H., Metzger, W. J., and Hunninghake, G. W. (1986): Bronchoalveolar lavage fluid (BAL) histamine levels in normals, allergic rhinitis and asthmatics. *J. Allergy Clin. Immunol.*, 77:182.

48. Case, B. W., McCaughey, W. T. E., Harrigan, M., and Sebastien, P. (1990): Exposure misclassification for mesothelioma in a chrysotile mining district. *Am. Rev. Respir. Dis.*, 141: A242.

49. Ceuppens, J. L., and Goodwin, J. S. (1984): Prostaglandins as modulators of T- and B-lymphocyte function. In Immune Modulation Agents and Their Mechanisms, edited by R. L. Fenichel, and M. A. Chirigos, vol. 25, pp. 627–648. Marcel K. Dekker, Inc., New York.

50. Chan-Yeung, M., Barton, G. M., and MacLean, L. (1973): Occupational asthma and rhinitis due to western red cedar (*Thuja plicata*). *Am. Rev. Respir. Dis.*, 108:1094–1102.

51. Chan-Yeung, M., MacLean, L., and Paggario, P. L. (1987): Follow-up study of 232 patients with

occupational asthma caused by western red cedar (*Thuja plicata*). *J. Allergy Clin. Immunol.*, 79:792–796.

51a. Chan-Yeung, M. and Lam S. (1986): Occupational Asthma. *Am. Rev. Respir. Dis.*, 133:686–703.

52. Chandra, R. K. (1984): Excessive intake of zinc impairs immune responses. *J.A.M.A.*, 252:1443–1446.

53. Charles, J., Bernstein, A., Jones, B., Jones, D. J., Edwards, J. H., Seal, R. M. E., and Seaton, A. (1976): Hypersensitivity pneumonitis after exposure to isocyanate. *Thorax*, 31:127–136.

54. Chester, E. H., Martinez-Catinchi, F. L., Schwartz, H. J., Fleming, G. M., and McDonald, E. W. (1979): Patterns of airway reactivity to asthma produced by exposure to toluene diisocyanate. *Chest*, 755:229–231.

55. Churg, A. (1988): Chrysotile, tremolite, and malignant mesothelioma in man. *Chest*, 93:621–628.

56. Churg, A., and Warnock, M. L. (1977): Correlation of quantitative asbestos body counts and occupation in urban patients. *Arch. Pathol. Lab. Med.*, 101:629–634.

57. Churg, A., Warnock, M. C., and Green, N. (1979): Analysis of the cores of ferruginous (asbestos) bodies from the general population. II. True asbestos bodies and pseudoasbestos bodies. *Lab. Invest.*, 40:31–38.

58. Churg, A., Wiggs, B., Depaoli, L., Kampe, B., and Stevens, B. (1984): Lung asbestos content in chrysotile workers with mesothelioma. *Am. Rev. Respir. Dis.*, 130:1042–1045.

59. Chvapil, M., Stankova, L., Zukoski, C., IV, and Zukoski, C., III (1977): Inhibition of some functions of polymorphonuclear leukocytes by zinc. *J. Lab. Clin. Med.*, 89:135–146.

60. Cockcroft, A., Edwards, J., McCarthy, P., and Anderson, N. (1981): Allergy in laboratory animal workers. *Lancet*, 1:827–830.

61. Cohn, J. R., Buckley, C. E., Hohl, C. A., Tyson, G., and Neish, D. D. (1983): Persistent cutaneous cellular immune responsiveness in a nursing home population. *J. Am. Geriatr. Soc.*, 31:261–265.

62. Conner, M. W., Flood, W. H., Rogers, A. E., and Amdur, M. O. (1988): Lung injury in guinea pigs caused by exposures to ultrafine zinc oxide: Changes in pulmonary lavage fluid. *J. Toxicol. Environ. Health*, 25:57–69.

63. Cormier, Y., Belanger, J., Beaudoin, J., Laviolette, M., Beaudoin, R., and Hebert, J. (1984): Abnormal bronchoalveolar lavage in asymptomatic dairy farmers. Study of lymphocytes. *Am. Rev. Respir. Dis.*, 130:1046–1049.

64. Cormier, Y., Belanger, J., Leblanc, P., and Laviolette, M. (1986): Bronchoalveolar lavage in farmer's lung disease: Diagnostic and physiological significance. *Br. J. Ind. Med.*, 43:401–405.

65. Corrigan, C. J., and Kay, A. B. (1990): CD_4 T-lymphocyte activation in acute severe asthma. Relationship to disease severity and atopic status. *Am. Rev. Respir. Dis.*, 141:970–977.

66. Costabel, U., Bross, K. J., Huck, E., Guzman, J., Matthys, H. (1987): Lung and blood lymphocytes in asbestosis and in mixed dust pneumoconiosis. *Chest*, 91:110–112.

67. Costabel, U., Bross, K. J., Reuter, C., Ruhle, K-H, and Matthys, H. (1986): Alterations in immunoregulatory T-cell subsets in cigarette smokers. A phenotypic analysis of bronchoalveolar and blood lymphocytes. *Chest*, 90:39–44.

68. Conner, M. W., Flood, W. H., Rogers, A. E, and Amdur, M. O. (1988): Lung injury in guinea pigs caused by multiple exposures to ultrafine zinc oxide: Changes in pulmonary lavage fluid. *J. Toxicol. Environ. Health*, 25:57–69.

69. Craighead, J. E., and Emerson, R. J. (1986): Slateworker's pneumoconiosis: Lung disease due to a mixture of slate and silicate dust. In Silica, Silicosis and Cancer: Controversy in Occupational Medicine. Cancer Research Monographs, edited by D. F. Goldsmith, D. M. Winn, and G. M. Shy, p. 533. Praeger Publishers, New York.

70. Craighead, J. E., and Mossman, B. T. (1982): The pathogenesis of asbestos-associated diseases. *N. Engl. J. Med.*, 306:1446–1455.

71. Craighead, J. E., Kleinerman, J., Abraham, J. L., Gibbs, A. R., Green, F. H. Y., and Juliano, E. B. (1988): Diseases associated with exposure to silica and nonfibrous silicate minerals. Silicosis and silicate disease committee. *Arch. Pathol. Lab. Med.*, 112:673–720.

72. Crimi, E., Scordamalglia, A., Crimi, P., Zupo, S., and Barocci, S. (1983): Total and specific IgE in serum, bronchial lavage, and bronchoalveolar lavage of asthmatic patients. *Allergy*, 38:553–559.

73. Cruz, R. (1987): Chronic beryllium disease in a precious metal refinery. Clinical epidemiologic and immunologic evidence for continuing risk from exposure to low level beryllium fume. *Am. Rev. Respir. Dis.*, 135:201–208.

74. Crystal, R. G., Gadek, J. E., Ferrans, V. J., Fulmer, J. D., Line, B. R., and Hunninghake, G. W. (1981): Interstitial lung disease: Current concepts of pathogenesis, staging and therapy. *Am. J. Med.*, 70:542–568.
75. Crystal, R. G., Reynolds, H. Y., and Kalica, A. R. (1986): Bronchoalveolar lavage. The report of an international conference. *Chest*, 90:122–131.
76. Cugell, D. W., Morgan, W. K. C., Perkins, D. G., and Rubin, A. (1990): The respiratory effects of cobalt. *Arch. Intern. Med.*, 150:177–183.
77. Cullen, M. R., Kominsky, J. R., Rossman, M. D., Cherniak, M. G., Rankin, J. A., Balmes, J. R., Kern, J. A., Daniele, R. P., Palmer, L., Naegel, G. P., McManus, K., and Cruz, R. (1987): Chronic beryllium disease in a precious metal refinery. Clinical epidemiologic and immunologic evidence for continuing risk from exposure to low level beryllium fume. *Am. Rev. Respir. Dis.*, 135:201–208.
77a. Cunningham-Rundles, S., Cunningham-Rundles, C., Dupont, B., and Good, R. A. (1980): Zinc-induced activation of human B lymphocytes. *Clin. Immunol. Immunopathol.*, 16:115–122.
78. Curtis, G. H. (1959): The diagnosis of beryllium disease with special reference to the patch test. *Arch. Industr. Hyg.*, 19:150.
79. Damiano, V. V., Daniele, R. P., Tucker, H. T., and Dauber, J. H. (1982): Quantification of silica uptake by alveolar macrophages—an empirical scanning electron microprobe method. In Fortieth Annual Proceedings of Electron Microscopy Society of America, edited by G. W. Bailey, pp. 332–333. Electron Microscopy Society, Washington, D.C.
80. Daniele, R. P., Dauber, J. H., Altose, M. D., Rowlands, D. T., Jr., and Gorenberg, D. J. (1977): Lymphocyte studies in asymptomatic cigarette smokers. A comparison between lung and peripheral blood. *Am. Rev. Respir. Dis.*, 116:997–1005.
81. Daniele, R. P., Elias, J. A., Epstein, P. E., and Rossman, M. D. (1985): Bronchoalveolar lavage: Role in the pathogenesis, diagnosis, and management of interstitial lung disease. *Ann. Intern. Med.*, 102:93–108.
82. Davies, G. E., Thompson, A. V., Niewola, Z., Burrows, G. E., Teasdale, E. L., Bird, D. J., and Phillips, D. A. (1983): Allergy to laboratory animals: A retrospective and a prospective study. *Br. J. Ind. Med.*, 40:442–449.
83. Davies, J. E. (1986): Occupational asthma caused by nickel salts. *J. Soc. Occup. Med.*, 36:29–31.
84. Davis, G. S. (1986): Bronchoalveolar lavage and the technological dilemma. *Am. Rev. Respir. Dis.*, 133:181–183.
85. Davis, G. S., Christman, J. W., Hill-Eubanks, L., and Pfeiffer, L. M. (1990): Interleukin-1 and tumor necrosis factor-secretion by alveolar macrophages from Vermont granite workers. *Am. Rev. Respir. Dis.*, A247.
86. Davis, G. S., Hemenway, D. R., Evans, J. N., Lapenas, D. J., and Brody, A. R. (1981): Alveolar macrophage stimulation and population changes in silica exposed rats. *Chest*, 80:85–105.
87. Davis, J. M. G. (1989): In Non-Occupational Exposure to Mineral Fibers, edited by J. Bignon, J. Peto, and R. Saracci, pp. 33–45. International Agency for Research on Cancer, Lyon.
88. Davis, J. M. G., Addison, J., Bolton, R. E., Donaldson, K., Jones, A. D., and Smith, T. (1986): The pathogenicity of long versus short fibre samples of amosite asbestos administered to rats by inhalation and intraperitoneal injection. *Br. J. Exp. Pathol.*, 67:415–430.
89. Davis, R. (1981): Effects of synthetic silicas on mouse peritoneal macrophages in vitro. In Health Effects of Synthetic Silica Particulates, edited by D. D. Dunnon, p. 67. American Society for Testing Materials, Philadelphia.
90. Davison, A. G., Haslam, P. L., Corrin, B., Coutts, H., Dewar, A., Riding, W. D., Studdy, P. R., and Newman-Taylor, A. J. (1983): Interstitial lung disease and asthma in hard-metal workers: Bronchoalveolar lavage, ultrastructural, and analytical findings and the results of bronchial provocation tests. *Thorax*, 38:119–128.
91. Dawson, S. V., and Schenker, M. B. (1979): Health effects of inhalation of ambient concentrations of nitrogen dioxide. *Am. Rev. Respir. Dis.*, 120:281–292.
92. De Monchy, J. G., Kauffman, H. F., Venge, P., Koeter, G. H., Jansen, H. M., Sluiter, H. J., and De Vries, K. (1985): Bronchoalveolar eosinophilia during allergen-induced late asthmatic reactions. *Am. Rev. Respir. Dis.*, 131:373–376.
93. De Vuyst, P., Dumortier, P., Moulin, E., Yourassowsky, N., and Yernault, J. C. (1987): Diagnostic value of asbestos bodies in bronchoalveolar lavage. *Am. Rev. Respir. Dis.*, 136:1219–1224.
94. De Vuyst, P., Jedwab, J., Dumortier, P., Vandermoten, G., Vande Weyer, R., and Yernault, J. C. (1982): Asbestos bodies in bronchoalveolar lavage. *Am. Rev. Respir. Dis.*, 126:972–976.

95. Delafuente, J. C. (1985): Immunosenescence: Clinical and pharmacologic considerations. *Med. Clin. North Am.*, 69:475–486.

96. Delcos, G. L., Flitcraft, D. G., Brousseau, K. P., Windsor, N. T., Nelson, D. L., Wilson, R. K., and Lawrence, E. C. (1986): Bronchoalveolar lavage analysis, gallium-67 lung scanning and soluble interleukin-2 receptor levels in asbestos exposure. *Am. Rev. Respir. Dis.*, 134:A195.

97. Demarest, G. B., Hudson, L. D., and Altman, L. C. (1979): Impaired alveolar macrophage chemotaxis in patients with acute smoke inhalation. *Am. Rev. Respir. Dis.*, 119:279–286.

98. Demedts, M., Gheysens, B., Nagel, J., Verbeken, E., Lauweryns, J., van den Eeckhout, A., Lahaye, D., and Gyselen, A. (1984): Cobalt lung in diamond polishers. *Am. Rev. Respir. Dis.*, 130:130–135.

99. Denham, S., and Hall, J. G. (1988): Studies on the adjuvant action of beryllium. III. The activity in the plasma of lymph efferent from nodes stimulated with beryllium. *Immunology*, 64:345–351.

100. deShazo, R. D. (1982): Current concepts about the pathogenesis of silicosis and asbestosis. *J. Allergy Clin. Immunol.*, 70:41–49.

101. Diaz, P., Galleguillos, F. R., Gonzalez, M. C., Pantin, C. F., and Kay, A. B. (1984): Bronchoalveolar lavage in asthma: The effect of disodium chromoglycate (cromolyn) on leukocyte counts, immunoglobulins, and complement. *J. Allergy Clin. Immunol.*, 74:41–48.

102. DiMenza, L., Hirsch, A., Sebastien, P., Gandichet, A., and Bignon, J. (1980): Assessment of part asbestos exposure in patients: Occupational questionnaire versus monitoring in broncho-alveolar lavage. In Biological Effects of Mineral Fibres, edited by J. C. Wagner, pp. 609–614. IARC, Lyon.

103. Drinker, K. R., and Drinker, P. (1928): Metal fume fever; results of the inhalation by animals of zinc and magnesium oxide fumes. *J. Ind. Hyg.*, 10:56–70.

104. Durham, S. R., and Kay, A. B. (1985): Eosinophils, bronchial hyperreactivity and late-phase asthmatic reactions. *Clin. Allergy*, 15:411–418.

105. Epstein, P. E., Dauber, J. H., Rossman, M. D., and Daniele, R. P. (1982): Bronchoalveolar lavage in a patient with chronic berylliosis: Evidence for hypersensitivity pneumonitis. *Ann. Intern. Med.*, 97:213–216.

106. Fabbri, L. M., Aizawaka, H., O'Bryne, P. M., Bethel, R. A., Walters, E. H., Holtzman, M. J., and Nadel, J. A. (1985): An anti-inflammatory drug (BW755C) inhibits airway hyperresponsiveness induced by ozone in dogs. *J. Allergy Clin. Immunol.*, 76:162–166.

107. Fabbri, L. M., Boschetto, P., Zocca, E., Milani, G., Pivirotto, F., Plebani, M., Burlina, A., Licata, B., and Mapp, C. E. (1987): Bronchoalveolar neutrophilia during late asthmatic reactions induced by toluene diisocyanate. *Am. Rev. Respir. Dis.*, 136:36–42.

108. Fabbri, L. M., Chiesura, P., Dal Vecchio, L., Di Giacomo, G. R., Zocca, E., De Marzo, N., Maestrelli, P., and Mapp, G. E. (1985): Prednisone inhibits late asthmatic reactions and the associated increase in airway responsiveness induced by toluene-diisocyanate in sensitized subjects. *Am. Rev. Respir. Dis.*, 132:1010–1014.

109. Farrell, F. J. (1987): Angioedema and urticaria as acute and late phase reactions to zinc fume exposure, with associated metal fume fever-like symptoms. *Am. J. Ind. Med.*, 12:331–337.

110. Fink, R. B. Jr., Metzger, W. J., Richerson, H. B., Zavala, D. C., Moseley, P. L., Schoderbek, W. E., and Hunninghake, G. W. (1987): Increased bronchovascular permeability following allergen exposure in sensitive asthmatics. *J. Appl. Physiol.*, 63:1147–1155.

111. Fink, R. B. Jr., Richerson, H. B., Zavala, D. C., and Hunninghake, G. W. (1987): Bronchoalveolar lavage in allergic asthmatics. *Am. Rev. Respir. Dis.*, 135:1204–1209.

112. Fine, J. M., and Balmes, J. R. (1988): Airway inflammation and occupational asthma. *Clin. Chest Med.*, 9:577–590.

113. Fink, J. N. (1973): Hypersensitivity pneumonitis. *J. Allergy Clin. Immunol.*, 52:309–317.

114. Fink, J. N., and Schlueter, D. P. (1978): Bathtub refinisher's lung: An unusual response to toluene diisocyanate. *Am. Rev. Respir. Dis.*, 118:955–959.

115. Finley, T. N., and Ladman, A. J. (1972): Low yield of pulmonary surfactant in cigarette smokers. *N. Engl. J. Med.*, 286:223–227.

116. Folinsbee, L. J., Horvath, S. M., Bedi, J. F., and Delehunt, J. C. (1978): Effect of 0.62 ppm NO_2 on cardiopulmonary function in young male nonsmokers. *Environ. Res.*, 15:199–205.

117. Fournier, E. C., Santarro, F., Aerts, C., Laboute, C., and Viosin, C. (1983): Study of bronchoalveolar lavage before and after the inhalation challenge test in bird fancier's disease. Deduction about immunological mechanisms involved. In Sarcoidosis and Other Granulomatous Disorders. Ninth International Conference, pp. 578–583. Pergamon Press, Paris.

118. Fournier, E., Tonnel, A. B., Gosset, P. H., Wallaert, B., Ameisen, J., and Voisin, C. (1985):

Early neutrophil alveolitis after antigen inhalation hypersensitivity pneumonitis. *Chest*, 88:563–566.

119. Frampton, M. W., Finkelstein, J. N., Roberts, N. J., Jr., Smeglin, A. M., Morrow, P. E., and Utell, M. J. (1989): Effects of nitrogen dioxide exposure on bronchoalveolar lavage proteins in humans. *Am. J. Respir. Cell Mol. Biol.*, 1:499–505.

120. Frampton, M. W., Smeglin, A. M., Roberts, N. J., Jr., Finkelstein, J. N., Morrow, P. E., and Utell, M. J. (1989): Nitrogen exposure in vivo and human alveolar macrophage inactivation of influenza virus in vitro. *Environ. Res.*, 48:179–192.

121. Franchini, I., Cavatorta, A., Falzoi, M., Lucertini, S., and Mutti, A. (1983): Early indicators of renal damage in workers exposed to organic solvents. *Int. Arch. Occup. Environ. Health*, 52:1–9.

122. Frank, N. R., Amdur, M. O., Worcester, J., and Whittenberger, J. L. (1962): Effects of acute controlled exposure to SO_2 on respiratory mechanics in healthy male adults. *J. App. Physiol.*, 17:252–258.

123. Freiman, D. G., and Hardy, H. L. (1970): Beryllium disease: The relation of pulmonary pathology to clinical course and prognosis based on a study of 130 cases from the U.S. Beryllium Case Registry. *Hum. Pathol.*, 1:25–44.

124. Frew, A. J., and Kay, A. B. (1988): The pattern of late-phase skin reactions to extracts of aeroallergens. *J. Allergy Clin. Immunol.*, 81:1117–1121.

125. Friedman, M. M., and Kaliner, M. A. (1987): Symposium on mast cells and asthma. Human mast cells and asthma. *Am. Rev. Respir. Dis.*, 135:1157–1164.

126. Frigas, E., Loegering, D. A., and Gleich, G. J. (1980): Cytotoxic effects of guinea pig eosinophil major basic protein on tracheal epithelium. *Lab. Invest.*, 42:35–43.

127. Fulmer, J. D. (1982): Bronchoalveolar lavage. *Am. Rev. Respir. Dis.*, 126:961–963.

128. Gabor, S. Z., Anca, Z., Zugravu, E., Cingudeance, M., and Bohm, B. (1980): In vitro and in vivo quartz-induced lipid peroxidation. In The In Vitro Effects of Mineral Dusts, edited by R. C. Brown, M. Chamberlain, R. Davies, and I. D. Gormley, p. 131. Academic Press, New York.

129. Gadek, J. E., Fells, G. A., and Crystal, R. G. (1979): Cigarette smoking induces functional antiprotease deficiency in the lower respiratory tract of humans. *Science*, 206:1315–1316.

130. Garcia, J. G. N., Griffith, D. E., Cohen, A. B., and Callahan, K. S. (1989): Alveolar macrophages from patients with asbestos exposure release increased levels of leukotriene B_4. *Am. Rev. Respir. Dis.*, 139:1494–1501.

131. Gardner, M. J., Winter, P. D., Paunett, B., and Powell, C. A. (1986): Follow-up study of workers manufacturing chrysotile asbestos cement products. *Br. J. Ind. Med.*, 43:726–732.

132. Gellert, A. R., Langford, J. A., Winter, R. J. D., Uthayakumar, S., Sinha, G., and Rudd, R. M. (1985): Asbestosis: Assessment by bronchoalveolar lavage and measurement of pulmonary epithelial permeability. *Thorax*, 40:508–514.

133. Gheysens, B., Auwerx, J., van den Eeckhout, A., and Demedts, M. (1985): Cobalt-induced bronchial asthma in diamond polishers. *Chest*, 88:740–744.

134. Gibbs, A., Craighead, J. E., and Pooley, F. (1986): The pathology of slateworkers pneumoconiosis in Wales and Vermont. In Inhaled Particles, pp. 273–276, Pergamon Press, London.

135. Glasgow, J. E., Pietra, G. G., Abrams, W. R., Blank, J., Oppenheim, D. M., and Weinbaum, G. (1987): Neutrophil recruitment and degranulation during induction of emphysema in the rat by nitrogen dioxide. *Am. Rev. Respir. Dis.*, 135:1129–1136.

136. Glassroth, J. L., Bernardo, J., Lucey, E. C., Center, D. M., Jung-Legg, Y., and Snider, G. L. (1984): Interstitial pulmonary fibrosis induced in hamsters by intratracheally administered chrysotile asbestos. *Am. Rev. Respir. Dis.*, 130:242–248.

137. Godard, P., Chaintreuil, J., Damon, M., Coupe, M., Flandre, O., Paulet, A. C., and Michel, F. B. (1982): Functional assessment of alveolar macrophages: Comparison of cells from asthmatics and normal subjects. *J. Allergy Clin. Immunol.*, 70:88–93.

138. Goings, S. A. J., Kulle, T. J., Bascom, R., Sauder, L. R., Green, D. J., Hebel, J. R., Clements, M. L. (1989): Effect of nitrogen dioxide exposure on susceptibility to influenza A virus infection in healthy adults. *Am. Rev. Respir. Dis.*, 139:1075–1081.

139. Golden, J. A., Nadel, J. A., and Boushey, H. A. (1978): Bronchial hyperirritability in healthy subjects after exposure to ozone. *Am. Rev. Respir. Dis.*, 118:287–294.

140. Good, R. A. (1972): Relations between immunity and malignancy. *Proc. Natl. Acad. Sci. U.S.A.*, 69:1026–1032.

141. Gosset, P., Tsicopoulos, A., Tonnel, A. B., and Capron, A. (1990): Induction of TNF release by alveolar macrophages after allergen challenge in asthmatics: Correlation with the late phase reaction. *Am. Rev. Respir. Dis.*, 141:A677.

142. Graham, D., Henderson, F., and House, D. (1988): Neutrophil influx measured in nasal lavages of humans exposed to ozone. *Arch. Environ. Health* 43:228–233.

143. Gronhagen-Riska, C., Kurppa, K., Fyhrquist, F., Jhingran, S. G., and Selroos, O. (1978): Angiotensin-converting enzyme and lysozyme in silicosis and asbestosis. *Scand. J. Respir. Dis.*, 59:228–231.

144. Gross, N. J. (1980): Allergy to laboratory animals: Epidemiologic, clinical and physiologic aspects, and a trial of cromolyn in its management. *J. Allergy Clin. Immunol.*, 66:158–165.

145. Gutowski, J. K., Innes, J. B., Weksler, M. E., and Cohen, S. (1986): Impaired nuclear responsiveness to cytoplasmic signals in lymphocytes from elderly humans with depressed proliferative responses. *J. Clin. Invest.*, 78:40–43.

146. Hackney, J. D., Thiede, F. C., Linn, W. S., Pedersen, E. E., Spier, C. E., Law, D. C., and Fischer, D. A. (1978): Experimental studies on human health effects of air pollutants. IV. Short-term physiological and clinical effects of nitrogen dioxide exposure. *Arch. Environ. Health* 33:176–181.

147. Hall, J. G. (1984): Studies on the adjuvant action of beryllium. I. Effects on individual lymph nodes. *Immunology*, 53:105–113.

148. Hallgren, R., Eklund, A., Engstrom-Laurent, A., and Schmekel, B. (1985): Hyaluronate in bronchoalveolar lavage fluid: A new marker in sarcoidosis reflecting pulmonary disease. *Br. Med. J.*, 290:1778–1781.

149. Hamzaoui, A., Kamel, A., Hamzaoui, K., Chabbou, A., and El-Gharbi, B. (1990): Alterations in immunoregulatory T cell subsets in silicosis. *Am. Rev. Respir. Dis.*, 141:A245.

150. Hargreave, R. E., Ramsdale, E. H., and Pugsley, S. O. (1984): Occupational asthma without bronchial hyperresponsiveness. *Am. Rev. Respir. Dis.*, 130:513–515.

151. Hartmann, A., Wicthrich, B., and Bolognini, G. (1982): Berufsbedingte Lungenkrankheiten bei der Hartmetallproduktion und -bearbeitung. Ein allergisches Geschehen? *Schweiz. Med. Wochenschr.*, 112:1137–1141.

152. Haslam, P. L. (1987): Bronchoalveolar lavage in extrinsic allergic alveolitis. *Env. J. Resp. Dis.*, 71.

153. Haslam, P. L., Dewar, A., Butchers, P., Primett, Z. S., Newman-Taylor, A., and Turner-Warwick, M. (1987): Mast cells, atypical lymphocytes, and neutrophils in bronchoalveolar lavage in extrinsic allergic alveolitis. Comparison with other interstitial lung diseases. *Am. Rev. Respir. Dis.*, 135:35–47.

154. Haslam, P. L., Dewar, A., Butchers, P., and Turner-Warwick, M. (1982): Mast cells in bronchoalveolar lavage fluids from patients with extrinsic allergic alveolitis (synonym: hypersensitivity pneumonitis). *Am. Rev. Respir. Dis.*, 125(Suppl.):51.

155. Haslam, P. L., Turoszek, A., Merchant, J. A., and Turner-Warwick, M. (1978): Lymphocyte responses to phytohemagglutinin in patients with asbestosis and pleural mesothelioma. *Clin. Exp. Immunol.*, 31:178–188.

156. Hayes, A. A., Rose, A. H., Musk, A. W., and Robinson, B. W. S. (1988): Neutrophil chemotactic factor release and neutrophil alveolitis in asbestos-exposed individuals. *Chest*, 94:521–525.

157. Hebert, J., Beaudoin, J., Laviolette, M., Beaudoin, R., Belanger, J., and Cormier, Y. (1985): Absence of correlation between the degree of alveolitis and antibody levels to *Micropolysporum faeni. Clin. Exp. Immunol.*, 60:572–578.

158. Helmers, R. A., Dayton, C. S., Floerchinger, C., and Hunninghake, G. W. (1989): Bronchoalveolar lavage in interstitial lung disease: Effect of volume of fluid infused. *J. Appl. Physiol.*, 67:1443–1446.

159. Henderson, F. W., Dubovi, E. J., Harder, S., Seal, E., Jr., and Graham, D. (1988): Experimental rhinovirus infection in human volunteers exposed to ozone. *Am. Rev. Respir. Dis.*, 137:1124–1128.

160. Henderson, R. F., Benson, J. L., McClellan, R. O., and Pickrell, J. A. (1985): New approaches for the evaluation of pulmonary toxicity: Bronchoalveolar lavage fluid analysis. *Fund. Appl. Toxicol.*, 5:451–458.

161. Henson, P. M., McCarthy, K., Larsen, G. L., Webster, R. O., Gielas, P. C., Dreisin, R. B., King, T. E., and Shaw, J. O. (1979): Complement fragments, alveolar macrophages, and alveolitis. *Am. J. Pathol.*, 97:93–110.

162. Heppleston, A. G. (1981): The macrophage in fibrogenesis by quartz. In Health Effects of Synthetic Silica Particulate, edited by D. D. Dunnom, p. 62. American Society for Testing Materials, Philadelphia.

163. Hill, J. O., Bice, D. E., Harris, D. L., Muggenburg, B. A. (1983): Evaluation of the pulmonary immune response by analysis of bronchoalveolar fluids obtained by serial lung lavage. *Int. Arch. Allergy Appl. Immunol.*, 71:173–177.

164. Hirsch, A., Brochard, P., DeCremoux, H., Erkan, L., Sebastien, P., DiMenza, L., and Bignon, J. (1982): Features of asbestos-exposed and unexposed mesothelioma. *Am. J. Ind. Med.*, 3:413–422.

165. Hjortsberg, U., Nise, G., Orbalk, P., Soes-Petersen, U., and Arborelius, M., Jr. (1986): Bronchial asthma due to exposure to potassium aluminum tetrafluoride. *Scand. J. Work Environ. Health*, 12:223.

166. Hjortso, E., Qvist, J., Bud, M. I., Thomsen, J. L., Andesen, J. B., Wiberg-Jorgensen, F., Jensen, N. K., Jones, R., Reid, L. M., and Zapol, W. M. (1988): ARDS after accidental inhalation of zinc chloride smoke. *Intensive Care Med.*, 14:17–24.

167. Hoidal, J. R., Fox, R. B., LeMarbe, P. A., Perri, R., and Repine, J. E. (1981): Altered oxidative metabolic responses in vitro of alveolar macrophages from asymptomatic cigarette smokers. *Am. Rev. Respir. Dis.*, 123:85–89.

168. Hollingsworth, H. M., Downing, E. T., Braman, S. S., Glassroth, J., Binder, R., and Center, D. M. (1984): Identification and characterization of neutrophil chemotactic activity in aspirin-induced asthma. *Am. Rev. Respir. Dis.*, 130:373–379.

169. Hoogsteden, H. C., vanHal, P. Th. W., Wijkhuijs, J. M., te Velde, A. A., Figdor, C. G., and Hilvering, C. (1990): Alveolar macrophages with immature and mature morphology exhibit a distinct immunologic phenotype. *Am. Rev. Respir. Dis.*, 141:A675.

170. Hook, W. A., Powers, K., and Siraganian, R. P. (1984): Skin tests, and blood leukocyte, histamine release of patients with allergies to laboratory animals. *J. Allergy Clin. Immunol.*, 73:457–465.

171. Hughes, D. A., Haslam, P. L., Townsend, P. J., and Turner-Warwick, M. (1985): Numerical and functional alterations in circulatory lymphocytes in cigarette smokers. *Clin. Exp. Immunol.*, 61:459–466.

172. Hunninghake, G. W., Gadek, J. E., Kawanami, O., Ferrans, V. J., and Crystal, R. G. (1979): Inflammatory and immune processes in the human lung in health and disease: Evaluation by bronchoalveolar lavage. *Am. J. Pathol.*, 97:149–206.

173. Huuskonen, M. S., Javisilo, J., Koskinen, H., and Kivisto, H. (1986): Serum angiotensin-converting enzyme and lysosomal enzymes in asbestosis. *Lung*, 164:165–171.

174. Janoff, A., Raju, L., and Dearing, R. (1983): Levels of elastase activity in bronchoalveolar lavage fluids of healthy smokers and nonsmokers. *Am. Rev. Respir. Dis.*, 127:540–544.

175. Johnson, F. A., and Stonehill, R. B. (1961): Chemical pneumonitis from inhalation of zinc chloride. *Dis. Chest*, 40:619–624.

176. Karol, M. H., Ioset, H. H., Yves, C. A., Alarie, Y. C. (1978): Tolyl-specific IgE antibodies in workers with hypersensitivity to toluene diisocyanate. *Am. Ind. Hyg. Assoc.*, 39:454–458.

177. Kawane, H., Soejima, R., Limeki, S., Niki, Y. (1988): Metal fume fever and asthma. *Chest*, 93:1116–1117.

178. Kay, A. B. (1985): Eosinophils as effector cells in immunity and hypersensitivity disorders. *Clin. Exp. Immunol.*, 62:1–12.

179. Kay, A. B., Lee, T. H., and Durham, S. R. (1984): Mediators of hypersensitivity and inflammatory cells in early- and late-phase asthmatic reactions. In Asthma: Physiology, Immunopharmacology, and Treatment, edited by K. F. Austin, and L. M. Lichenstein, pp. 211–227. Academic Press, London.

180. Kazimierczak, W., and Maslinski, C. (1974): The effects of zinc ions on selective and nonselective histamine release in vitro. *Agent Action*, 4:1–6.

181. Keller, R. H., Schwartz, S., Schlueter, D. P., Bar-Sela, S., and Fink, J. N. (1984): Immunoregulation in hypersensitivity pneumonitis: Phenotypic and functional studies of bronchoalveolar lavage lymphocytes. *Am. Rev. Respir. Dis.*, 130:766–777.

182. Keogh, A. M., Ibels, L. S., Allen, D. H., and Isbister, J. P. (1984): Exacerbation of Goodpasture's syndrome after inadvertent exposure to hydrocarbon fumes. *Br. Med. J.*, 288:188.

183. Keskinen, H., Kalliomaki, P. L., and Alanko, K. (1980): Occupational asthma due to stainless steel welding fumes. *Clin. Allergy*, 10:151–159.

184. Kessel, J. F., Allison, D. K., Moore, F. J., and Kaime, M. (1943): Comparison of chlorine and ozone and virucidal agents of poliomyelitis virus. *Proc. Soc. Exp. Biol. Med.*, 53:71–73.

185. Klavis, G., and Drommer, W. (1970): Goodpasture-syndrome and benzineinwirkung. *Arch. Toxicol.*, 26:40–50.

186. Kleinknecht, D., Morel-Maroger, L., Callard, P., Adhemar, J-P, and Mahieu, P. (1980): Antiglomerular basement membrane nephritis after solvent exposure. *Arch. Intern. Med.*, 140:230–232.

187. Koenig, J. Q., Covert, D. S., Hanley, Q. S., Van Belle, G., and Pierson, W. E. (1990): Prior exposure to ozone potentiates subsequent response to sulfur dioxide in adolescent asthmatic subjects. *Am. Rev. Respir. Dis.*, 141:377–380.

188. Konzen, R. B., Croft, B. F., Scheel, L. D., and Gorski, C. H. (1966): Human response to low concentrations of p,p-diphenylmethane diisocyanate (MDI). *Am. Ind. Hyg. Assoc. J.*, 27:121–127.

189. Koren, H. S., Devlin, R. B., Graham, D. E., Mann, R., McGee, M. P., Horstman, D. H., Kozumbo, W. J., Becker, S., House, D. E., McDonnell, W. F., and Bromberg, P. A. (1989): Ozone-induced inflammation in the lower airways of human subjects. *Am. Rev. Respir. Dis.*, 139:407–415.

190. Kriebel, D., Brain, J. D., Sprince, N. L., and Kazemi, H. (1988): The pulmonary toxicity of beryllium. *Am. Rev. Respir. Dis.*, 137:464–473.

191. Kusaka, Y., Yokoyama, K., Sera, Y., Yamamoto, S., Sone, S., Kyono, H., Shirakawa, T., and Goto, S. (1986): Respiratory diseases in hard metal workers: An occupational hygienic study in a factory. *Br. J. Ind. Med.*, 43:474–485.

192. Lam, S., Chan-Yeung, M., LeRiche, J., Kijek, K., and Phillips, D. (1985): Cellular changes in bronchial lavage fluids following late asthmatic reactions in patients with red cedar asthma. *Am. Rev. Respir. Dis.*, 131:A42.

193. Lam, S., Leriche, J. C., Kijek, K., and Phillips, D. (1985): Effect of bronchial lavage volume on cellular and protein recovery. *Chest*, 88:856–859.

193a. Landas, S. K., and Schwartz, D. A. (1990): Mica pneumoconiosis. A case report using energy-dispersive spectroscopy. *Am. Rev. Respir. Dis.*, 141:A247.

194. Langer, A. M., and Nolan, R. P. (1989): In Non-Occupational Exposure to Mineral Fibres, edited by J. Bignon, J. Peto, R. Saracci, pp. 330–335. International Agency for Research on Cancer, Lyon.

195. Laughter, A. H., Martin, R. R., and Twomey, J. J. (1977): Lymphoproliferative responses to antigens mediated by human pulmonary alveolar macrophages. *J. Lab. Clin. Med.*, 89:1326–1332.

196. Laviolette, M., Chang, J., and Newcombe, D. S. (1984): Human alveolar macrophages: A lesion in arachidonic acid metabolism in cigarette smokers. *Am. Rev. Respir. Dis.*, 124:397–401.

197. Laviolette, M., Coulombe, R., Picard, S., Braquet, P., and Borgeat, P. (1986): Decreased leukotriene B_4 in smokers' alveolar macrophages in vitro. *J. Clin. Invest.*, 77:54–60.

198. Lawrence, E. C. (1988): Cellular immune responses of the lung. In Immunology and Immunologic Diseases of the Lung, edited by R. P. Daniele, pp. 97–114. Blackwell Scientific Publications, Boston.

199. Lawrence, E. C., Teague, R. B., Gottlieb, M. S., Jhingran, S. G., and Liebermann, J. (1983): Serial changes in markers of disease activity with corticosteroid treatment in sarcoidosis. *Am. J. Med.*, 74:747–756.

200. Le Maho, S., Bignon, J., Lambre, C., Jaurand, M. C., and Masse, R. (1984): Early cellular and biochemical alveolar responses following tracheal inoculation with low dose of asbestos and quartz. *Arch. Immunol. Ther. Exp.*, 32:85–98.

201. Leakes, E. S., and Myrvik, Q. N. (1968): Changes in the morphology and lysozyme content of free alveolar cells after intravenous injection of killed BCG in oil. *J. Reticuloendoth. Soc.*, 5:33–53.

202. Leatherman, J. W., Michael, A. F., Schwartz, B. A., and Hoidal, J. R. (1984): Lung T cells in hypersensitivity pneumonitis. *Ann. Intern. Med.*, 100:390–392.

203. Lee, T. H., Nagakura, T., Papageorgiou, N., Iikura, Y., and Kay, A. B. (1983): Exercise-induced late asthmatic reactions with neutrophil chemotactic activity. *N. Engl. J. Med.*, 308:1502–1505.

204. Linn, W. S., Solomon, J. C., Trim, S. C., Spier, C. E., Shamoo, D. A., Venet, T. G., Avol, E. L., and Hackney, J. D. (1985): Effects of exposure to 4 ppm nitrogen dioxide in healthy and asthmatic volunteers. *Arch. Environ. Health*, 40:234–239.

205. Majumdar, S., Ceckler, W. H., and Sproul, O. J. (1973): Inactivation of poliovirus in water by ozonation. *J. Water Pollut. Control Fed.*, 45:2433–2443.

206. Malo, J-L., and Cartier, A. (1987): Occupational asthma due to fumes of galvanized metal. *Chest*, 92:375–377.

207. Malo, J-L, Cartier, A., Doepner, M., Nieboer, E., Evans, S., and Dolovich, J. (1982): Occupational asthma caused by nickel sulfate. *J. Allergy Clin. Immunol.*, 69:55–59.
208. Malo, J-L, Cartier, A., Ghezzo, H., Lefrance, M., McCants, M., Lehrer, S. B. (1988): Patterns of improvement in spirometry, bronchial hyperresponsiveness, and specific IgE antibody levels after cessation of exposure in occupational asthma caused by snow-crab processing. *Am. Rev. Respir. Dis.*, 138:807–812.
209. Mapp, C. E., Dal Vecchio, L., Boschetto, P. (1986): Toluene diisocyanate-induced asthma without airway hyperresponsiveness. *Eur. J. Respir. Dis.*, 68:89–95.
210. Mapp, C. E., Polato, R., Maestrelli, P., Hendrick, D. J., and Fabbri, L. M. (1985): Time course of the increase in airway responsiveness associated with late asthmatic reactions to toluene diisocyanate in sensitized subjects. *J. Allergy Clin. Immunol.*, 75:568–572.
211. Martin, T. R., Altman, L. C., Albert, R. K., and Henderson, W. R. (1984): Leukotriene B_4 production by the human alveolar macrophage. *Am. Rev. Respir. Dis.*, 129:106–111.
212. Matarese, S. L., and Matthews, J. I. (1986): Zinc chloride (smoke bomb) inhalation lung injury. *Chest*, 89:308–309.
213. McCombs, C. C., Michalski, J. P., Westerfield, B. T., and Light, R. W. (1982): Human alveolar macrophages suppress the proliferative response of peripheral blood lymphocytes. *Chest*, 82:266–271.
214. McConnell, L. H., Fink, J. N., Schleuter, D. P., and Schmidt, M. G. (1973): Asthma caused by nickel sensitivity. *Ann. Intern. Med.*, 78:888–890.
215. McCord, C. P. (1960): Metal fume fever as an immunological disease. *Int. Med. Surg.*, 29:101–107.
216. McLaren, D. J., Olsson, J. R., McKean, J. R., Venges, P., and Kay, A. B. (1981): Morphological studies on the killing of schistosomula of *Schistosoma mansoni* by human eosinophil and neutrophil cationic proteins in vitro. *Parasite Immunol.*, 33:359–373.
217. Merrill, W. W., Goodenberger, D., Strober, W., Matthay, R. A., Naegel, G. P., and Reynolds, H. Y. (1980): Free secretory component and other proteins in human lung lavage. *Am. Rev. Respir. Dis.*, 122:156–161.
218. Merrill, W. W., Goodman, M., Matthay, R. A., Naegel, J. P., Van Devoorde, Myl, A. D., and Reynolds, H. Y. (1981): Quantitation of carcinoembryonic antigen in lung lining fluid of normal smokers and nonsmokers. *Am. Rev. Respir. Dis.*, 123:29–31.
219. Merrill, W. W., Naegel, G. P., Olchowski, J. J., and Reynolds, J. J. (1985): Immunoglobulin G subclass proteins in serum and lavage fluid of normal subjects. Quantitation and comparison with immunoglobulin A and E. *Am. Rev. Respir. Dis.*, 131:584–587.
220. Metzger, W. J., Zavala, D., Richerson, H. B., Moseley, P., Iwamota, P., Monick, M., Sjverdsma, K., and Hunninghake, G. (1989): Local allergen challenge and bronchoalveolar lavage of allergic asthmatic lungs: Description of the model and local airway inflammation. *Am. Rev. Respir. Dis.*, 135:433–440.
221. Miller, S. D., and Zarkower, A. (1974): Alterations of murine immunologic responses after silica dust inhalation. *J. Immunol.*, 113:1533–1543.
222. Mohsenin, V. (1988): Airway responses to 2.0 ppm nitrogen dioxide in normal subjects. *Arch. Environ. Health*, 43:242–246.
223. Mohsenin, V., and Gee, J. B. L. (1987): Acute effect of nitrogen dioxide exposure on the functional activity of alpha-1-protease inhibitor in bronchoalveolar lavage fluid of normal subjects. *Am. Rev. Respir. Dis.*, 136:646–650.
224. Moller, D. R., Brooks, S. M., Bernstein, D. I., Cassedy, K., Enrione, M., and Bernstein, I. L. (1986): Delayed anaphylactoid reaction in a worker exposed to chromium. *J. Allergy Clin. Immunol.*, 77:45–46.
225. Moller, D. R., McKay, R. T., and Bernstein, I. L. (1986): Persistent airways disease caused by toluene diisocyanate. *Am. Rev. Respir. Dis.*, 134:175–176.
226. Moore, V. L., Pederson, G. L., Hauser, W. C., and Fink, J. N. (1980): A study of lung lavage materials in patients with hypersensitivity pneumonitis: In vitro response to mitogen and antigen in pigeon breeder's disease. *J. Allergy Clin. Immunol.*, 65:365–370.
227. Mori, T., Akashi, S., and Nukada, A. (1975): Effects of the inhalation of catalytically active metallic oxide fumes on rabbits. *Int. Arch. Occup. Environ. Health*, 36:29–39.
228. Morneux, J., Cordier, G., Pages, J., Vergnon, J. M., Lefevre, R., Brune, J., and Revillard, J. P. (1984): Activated lung lymphocytes in hypersensitivity pneumonitis. *J. Allergy Clin. Immunol.*, 74:719–727.

229. Morrison, H. M., and Stockley, R. A. (1988): The many uses of bronchoalveolar lavage. *Br. Med. J.*, 296:1758.

230. Mossman, B. T., Bignon, J., Corn, M., Seaton, A., and Gee, J. B. L. (1990): Asbestos: Scientific developments and implications for public policy. *Science*, 247:294–301.

231. Mossman, B. T., and Gee, J. B. L. (1989): Asbestos-related diseases. *N. Engl. J. Med.*, 320: 1721–1730.

232. Murdoch, R. D., Pepys, J., and Hughes, E. G. (1986): IgE antibody responses to platinum group metals: A large scale refinery survey. *Br. J. Ind. Med.*, 43:37–43.

233. Myers, D. J., Bigby, B. G., and Boushey, H. A. (1986): The inhibition of sulfur dioxide-induced bronchoconstriction in asthmatic subjects by cromolyn is dose-dependent. *Am. Rev. Respir. Dis.*, 133:1150–1153.

234. Nagy, L., Lee, T. H., and Kay, A. B. (1982): Neutrophil chemotactic activity in antigen-induced late asthmatic reactions. *N. Engl. J. Med.*, 306:497–501.

235. Nathan, A. W., and Toseland, P. A. (1979): Goodpasture's syndrome and trichloroethane intoxication. *Br. J. Clin. Pharmacol.*, 8:284–286.

236. Nemery, B. (1990): Metal toxicity and the respiratory tract. *Eur. Respir. J.*, 3:202–219.

237. Newman, L. S., Kreiss, K., King, T. E., Jr., Seay, S., and Campbell, P. A. (1989): Pathologic and immunologic alterations in early stages of beryllium disease. Re-examination of disease definition and natural history. *Am. Rev. Respir. Dis.*, 139:1479–1486.

238. Novey, H. S., Habib, M., and Wells, I. D. (1983): Asthma and IgE antibodies induced by chromium and nickel salts. *J. Allergy Clin. Immunol.*, 72:407–412.

239. O'Brien, M., Harries, M. G., Burge, P. S., and Pepys, J. (1979): Toluene diisocyanate induced asthma. I. Reactions to TDI, MDI, HDI and histamine. *Clin. Allergy*, 9:1–6.

240. Oberdoerster, G., Ferin, J., Marcello, N. L., and Meinhold, S. H. (1983): Effects of intrabronchially instilled amosite on lavagable lung and pleural cells. *Environ. Health Perspect.*, 51:41–48.

241. Orehek, J., Massari, J. P., Gayrard, G. C., Grimand, C., and Charpin, J. (1976): Effect of short-term, low level nitrogen dioxide exposure on bronchial sensitivity of asthmatic patients. *J. Clin. Invest.*, 57:301–307.

242. Paggiaro, P. L., and Chan-Yeung, M. (1987): Patterns of specific airway response in asthma due to western red cedar (*Thuja plicata*): Relationship with length of exposure and lung function measurements. *Clin. Allergy*, 17:333–339.

243. Paggiaro, P. L., Iunocenti, A., Bacci, E., Rossi, O., and Talini, D. (1986): Specific bronchial reactivity to toluene diisocyanate (TDI): Relationship with baseline clinical findings. *Thorax*, 41:279–282.

244. Papageorgiou, N., Lee, T. H., Nagakura, T., Cromwell, O., Wraith, D. G., and Kay, A. B. (1983): Neutrophil chemotactic activity in milk-induced asthma. *J. Allergy Clin. Immunol.*, 72:75–82.

245. Patterson, R., Addington, W., Banner, A. S., Byron, G. E., Franco, M., Herbert, F. A., Nicotra, M. B., Pruzansky, J. J., Rivera, M., Roberts, M., Yawn, D., and Zeiss, C. R. (1979): Antihapten antibodies in workers exposed to trimellitic anhydride fumes: A potential immunopathogenetic mechanism for the trimellitic anhydride pulmonary disease-anemia syndrome. *Am. Rev. Respir. Dis.*, 120:1259–1267.

246. Patterson, R., Suszko, I. M., Zeiss, C. R., and Pruzansky, J. J. (1981): Characterization of hapten-human serum albumins and their complexes with specific human antisera. *J. Clin. Immunol.*, 1:181–185.

247. Patterson, R., Wang, J. L. F., Fink, J. N., Calvanico, N. J., and Roberts, M. (1979): IgA and IgG antibody activities of serum and bronchoalveolar fluid from symptomatic and asymptomatic pigeon breeders. *Am. Rev. Respir. Dis.*, 120:1113–1118.

248. Patterson, R., Zeiss, C. R., and Pruzansky, J. J. (1982): Immunology and immunopathology of trimellitic anhydride pulmonary reactions. *J. Allergy Clin. Immunol.*, 70:19–23.

249. Patterson, R., Zeiss, C. R., Roberts, M., Pruzansky, J. J., Wolkonsky, P., and Chacon, R. (1978): Human antihapten antibodies in trimellitic anhydride inhalation reactions. Immunoglobulin classes of anti-trimellitic anhydride antibodies and hapten inhibition studies. *J. Clin. Invest.*, 62:971–978.

250. Pepys, J. (1982): Occupational asthma: An overview. *J. Occup. Med.*, 24:534–538.

251. Pepys, J. (1966): Pulmonary hypersensitivity disease due to inhaled organic antigens. *Ann. Intern. Med.*, 64:943–948.

252. Pepys, J., Pickering, C. A. C., and Hughes, E. G. (1972): Asthma due to inhaled chemical agents-complex salts of platinum. *Clin. Allergy*, 2:391–396.
253. Pepys, J., Riddell, R. W., Citron, K. M., and Clayton, M. (1962): Precipitins against extracts of hay and molds in the serum of patients with farmer's lung, aspergillosis, asthma and sarcoidosis. *Thorax*, 17:366–374.
254. Pernis, B., Vigliani, E. C., Cavagna, C., and Finulli, M. (1960): Endogenous pyrogen in the pathogenesis of zinc-fume fever. *Med. Lav.*, 51:579–586.
255. Peterson, M. L., Harder, S., Rommo, N., and House, D. (1978): Effect of ozone on leukocyte function in exposed human subjects. *Environ. Res.*, 15:485–493.
256. Peterson, M. L., Rummo, N., House, D., and Harder, S. (1978): In vitro responsiveness of lymphocytes to phytohemmagglutinin. *Arch. Environ. Health*, 33:59–63.
257. Peterson, M. L., Smialowicz, R., Harder, S., Ketcham, B., and House, D. (1981): The effect of controlled ozone exposure on human lymphocyte function. *Environ. Res.*, 24:299–308.
258. Phelps, D. S., Ginns, L. C., Sprince, N. L., and Oliver, L. C. (1990): Changes in surfactant-associated protein A resulting from asbestos exposure. *Am. Rev. Respir. Dis.*, 141:A243.
259. Pinkston, P., Smeglin, A., Roberts, N. J., Jr., Gibb, F. R., Morrow, P. E., and Utell, M. J. (1988): Effects of in vitro exposure to nitrogen dioxide on human alveolar macrophage release of neutrophil chemotactic factor and interleukin-1. *Environ. Res.*, 47:48–58.
260. Platt-Mills, T. A. E., Heymann, P. W., Longbottom, J., and Wilkins, S. R. (1987): Airborne allergens associated with asthma: Particle sizes carrying dust mite and rat allergens measured with a cascade impactor. *J. Allergy Clin. Immunol.*, 77:850–857.
261. Price, C. D., Williams, W. J., Pugh, A., and Joynson, D. H. (1977): Role of in vitro and in vivo tests of hypersensitivity in beryllium workers. *J. Clin. Pathol.*, 30:24–28.
262. Rankin, J. A., Naegel, G. P., and Reynolds, H. Y. (1986): Use of a central laboratory for analysis of bronchoalveolar lavage fluid. *Am. Rev. Respir. Dis.*, 133:186–190.
262a. Rasmussen, R. E. (1984): In vitro systems for exposure of lung cells to NO_2 and O_3. *J. Toxicol. Environ. Health*, 13:397–411.
263. Reed, D., Glaser, S., and Kaldor, J. (1980): Ozone toxicity symptoms among flight attendants. *Am. J. Ind. Med.*, 1:43–54.
264. Rennard, S., Basset, G., Lecossier, D., O'Donnell, K., Martin, P., and Crystal, R. G. (1986): Estimation of volume of extravascular lung water recovered by lavage using urea as a marker of dilution. *J. Appl. Physiol.*, 60:532.
265. Rennard, S. I., Ghafouri, M., Thompson, A. B., Linder, J., Vaughan, W., Jones, K., Ertl, R. F., Christensen, K., Prince, A., Stahl, M. G., and Robbins, R. A. (1990): Fractional processing of sequential bronchoalveolar lavage to separate bronchial and alveolar samples. *Am. Rev. Respir. Dis.*, 141:208–217.
266. Reynolds, H. Y. (1987): Bronchoalveolar lavage. *Am. Rev. Respir. Dis.*, 135:250–263.
267. Reynolds, H. Y. (1978): The importance of lymphocytes in pulmonary health and disease. *Lung*, 155:225–242.
268. Reynolds, H. Y., and Chretien, J. (1984): Respiratory tract fluids: Analysis of content and contemporary use in understanding lung disease. *DM*, 30:1–103.
269. Reynolds, H. Y., Fulmer, J. D., Kazmierowski, J. A., Roberts, W. C., Frank, M. M., and Crystal, R. G. (1977): Analysis of cellular and protein components of bronchoalveolar lavage fluid from patients with idiopathic pulmonary fibrosis and hypersensitivity pneumonitis. *J. Clin. Invest.*, 59:165–175.
270. Reynolds, H. Y., and Newball, H. H. (1974): Analysis of proteins and respiratory cells obtained from human lungs by bronchial lavage. *J. Lab. Clin. Med.*, 84:559–573.
271. Rios, A., and Simmons, R. (1972): Poly-2-vinylpyridine N-oxide reverses the immunosuppressive effects of silica and carrageenan. *Transplant*, 13:343–345.
272. Robinson, B. W. S., Rose, A. H., James, A., Whitaker, D., and Musk, A. W. (1986): Alveolitis of pulmonary asbestosis. Bronchoalveolar lavage studies in crocidolite- and chrysotile-exposed individuals. *Chest*, 90:390–402.
273. Roggli, V. L., Greenberg, S. D., McLarty, J. W., Hurst, G. A., Hieger, L. R., Farley, M. L., and Mabry, L. C. (1980): Comparison of sputum and lung asbestos body counts in former asbestos workers. *Am. Rev. Respir. Dis.*, 122:941–945.
274. Rola-Pleszcynski, M., Gonin, S., and Begin, R. (1984): Asbestos-induced lung inflammation: Role of local macrophage-derived chemotactic factors in accumulation of neutrophils in the lungs. *Inflammation*, 8:53–62.

275. Rom, W. N., Bitterman, P. B., Cantin, A., Crystal, R. G., and Rennard, S. I. (1987): Characterization of the lower respiratory tract inflammation of nonsmoking individuals with interstitial lung disease associated with chronic inhalation of inorganic dusts. *Am. Rev. Respir. Dis.*, 136:1429–1434.
276. Rossi, G. A., Sacco, O., Vassallo, F., Degli Innocenti, L., and Ravazzoni, C. (1988): Bronchoalveolar lavage during fiberoptic bronchoscopy: What has it brought to pulmonary medicine? *Respiration*, 54(Suppl. 1):49–58.
277. Rossman, M. D. (1988): Chronic beryllium disease. In Immunology and Immunologic Diseases of the Lung, edited by R. P. Daniele, pp. 351–359. Blackwell Scientific Publications, Boston.
278. Rossman, M. D., Kern, J. A., Elias, J. A., Cullen, M. R., Epstein, P. E., Preuss, O. P., Markham, T. N., and Daniele, R. P. (1988): Proliferative response of bronchoalveolar lymphocytes to beryllium. A test for chronic beryllium disease. *Ann. Intern. Med.*, 108:687–693.
279. Roto, P. (1980): Asthma, symptoms of chronic bronchitis and ventilatory capacity among cobalt and zinc production workers. *Scand. J. Work Environ. Health*, 6(Suppl. 1):1–49.
280. Rubenstein, I., Bigby, B. G., Reiss, T. F., and Boushey, H. A., Jr. (1990): Short-term exposure to 0.3 ppm nitrogen dioxide does not potentiate airway responsiveness to sulfur dioxide in asthmatic subjects. *Am. Rev. Respir. Dis.*, 141:381–385.
281. Ruhl, H., and Kirchner, H. (1977): Monocyte-dependent stimulation of human peripheral T cells by zinc. *Fed. Proc.*, 36:1284.
282. Ruhl, H., Kirchner, H., and Bochert, G. (1971): Kinetics of the Zn^{++} stimulation of human peripheral lymphocytes *in vitro*. *Proc. Soc. Exp. Biol. Med.*, 137:1089–1092.
283. Sale, S. R., Roach, D. E., Zeiss, C. R., and Patterson, R. (1981): Clinical and immunologic correlations in trimellitic anhydride airway syndromes. *J. Allergy Clin. Immunol.*, 68:188–193.
284. Saltini, C., Hance, A. J., Ferrans, V. J., Basset, F., Bitterman, P. B., and Crystal, R. G. (1984): Accurate quantification of cells recovered by bronchoalveolar lavage. *Am. Rev. Respir. Dis.*, 130:650–658.
285. Saltini, C., Winestock, K., Kirby, M., Pinkston, P., and Crystal, R. G., (1989): Maintenance of alveolitis in patients with chronic beryllium disease by beryllium-specific helper T cells. *N. Engl. J. Med.*, 320:1103–1109.
286. Sandstrom, T., Andersson, M. C., Kolmodin-Hedman, B., Stjernberg, N., and Angstrom, T. (1990): Bronchoalveolar mastocytosis and lymphocytosis after nitrogen dioxide exposure in man. A time-kinetic study. *Eur. Respir. J.*, 3:138–143.
287. Sandstrom, T., Stjernberg, N., Andersson, M-C, Kolmodin-Hedman, B., Lindstrom, K., and Rosenhall, L. (1989): Cell response in bronchoalveolar lavage fluid after sulfur dioxide exposure. *Scand. J. Work Environ. Health*, 15:142–146.
288. Sandstrom, T., Stjernberg, N., Andersson, M-C, Kolmodin-Hedman, B., Lundgren, R., and Angstrom, T. (1989): Is the short term limit value for sulfur dioxide safe? Effects of controlled chamber exposure investigated with bronchoalveolar lavage. *Br. J. Ind. Med.*, 46:200–203.
289. Sandstrom, T., Stjernberg, N., Andersson, M-C., Kolmodin-Hedman, B., Lundgren, R., Rosenhall, L., and Angstrom, T. (1989): Cell response in bronchoalveolar lavage fluid after exposure to sulfur dioxide: A time-response study. *Am. Rev. Respir. Dis.*, 140:1828–1831.
290. Sapin, C., Druet, E., and Druet, P. (1977): Induction of anti-glomerular basement membrane antibodies in the Brown-Norway rat by mercuric chloride. *Clin. Exp. Immunol.*, 28:173–179.
291. Saracci, R. (1987): The interactions of tobacco smoking and other agents in cancer etiology. *Epidemiol. Rev.*, 9:175–193.
292. Savino, A., Peterson, M. L., House, D., Turner, A. G., Jeffries, H. E., and Baker, R. (1978): The effect of ozone on human cellular and humoral immunity: Characterization of T and B lymphocytes by rosette formation. *Environ. Res.*, 15:65–69.
293. Scharfman, A., Hayem, A., Davril, M., Marko, D., Hannothiaux, M. H., and Lafitte, J. J. (1989): Special neutrophil elastase inhibitory activity in BAL fluid from patients with silicosis and asbestosis. *Eur. Respir. J.*, 2:751–757.
294. Schenkel, E., Atkins, P. C., Yost, R., and Zweiman, B. (1982): Antigen-induced neutrophil chemotactic activity from sensitized lung. *J. Allergy Clin. Immunol.*, 70:321–325.
295. Scherrer, M., and Maillard, J. M. (1982): Hartmetall-pneumopathien. *Schweiz. Med. Wochenschr.*, 112:198–207.
296. Scheule, R. K., and Holian, A. (1989): IgG specifically enhances chrysotile asbestos-stimulated superoxide anion production by the alveolar macrophage. *Am. J. Respir. Cell Mol. Biol.*, 1:313–318.

297. Schoenberger, C. I., Hunninghake, G. W., Kawanami, O., Ferrans, V. J., Crystal, R. G. (1982): Role of alveolar macrophages in asbestosis: Modulation of neutrophil migration to the lung after acute asbestos exposure. *Thorax*, 37:803–809.

298. Schonfeld, W., Schluter, B., Hilger, R., and Honig, W. (1988): Leukotriene generation and metabolism in isolated human macrophages. *Immunology*, 65:529–536.

299. Schorlemmer, H. U., Edwards, J. H., Davies, P., and Allison, A. C. (1977): Macrophage responses to mouldy hay dust, *Micropolyspora faeni* and zymosan, activators of complement by the alternative pathway. *Clin. Exp. Immunol.*, 27:198–207.

300. Schuyler, M., Thigpen, T., and Salvaggio, J. E. (1978): Local pulmonary immunity in pigeon breeder's disease. *Ann. Intern. Med.*, 88:355–358.

301. Schuyler, M., Ziskind, M., and Salvaggio, J. (1977): Cell-mediated immunity in silicosis. *Am. Rev. Respir. Dis.*, 116:147–151.

302. Schuyler, M. S., Gaumer, H. R., Stankus, R. P., Kaimal, J., Hoffman, E., and Salvaggio, J. E. (1980): Bronchoalveolar lavage in silicosis. Evidence of type II cell hyperplasia. *Lung*, 157:95–102.

303. Sebastien, P., McDonald, J. C., McDonald, A. D., Case, B., and Hartley, R. (1989): Respiratory Cancer in Chrysotile Textile and Mining Industries: Exposure Inferences from Lung Analysis. *Br. J. Ind. Med.*, 46:180–187.

304. Seeliger, K., and Huland, H. (1973): Kasuistischer beitrag zur atiologie des Goodpasture-Syndrome. *Med. Klin.*, 68:437–440.

305. Seltzer, J., Bigby, B. G., Stulbarg, M., Holtzman, M. J., Nadel, J. A., Ueki, I. F., Leikauf, G. D., Goetzl, E. J., and Boushey, H. A. (1986): O_3-induced change in bronchial reactivity to methacholine and airway inflammation in humans. *J. Appl. Physiol.*, 60:1321–1326.

306. Semenzato, G. (1988): Current concepts on bronchoalveolar lavage cells in extrinsic allergic alveolitis. *Respiration*, 54(Suppl. 1):59–65.

307. Semenzato, G., Agostini, C., Zambello, R., Trentin, L., Chilosi, M., Pizzolo, G., Marcer, G., and Cipriani, A. (1986): Lung T cells in hypersensitivity pneumonitis: Phenotypic and functional analyses. *J. Immunol.*, 137:1164–1172.

308. Semenzato, G., Trentin, L., Zambello, R., Agostini, C., Cipriani, A., and Marcer, G. (1988): Different types of cytotoxic lymphocytes are involved in the cytolytic mechanisms taking place in the lung of patients with hypersensitivity pneumonitis. *Am. Rev. Respir. Dis.*, 137:70–74.

309. Sharma, S. K., Pande, J. N., and Verma, K. (1988): Bronchoalveolar lavage fluid (BALF) analysis in silicosis. *Ind. J. Chest Dis. Allied Sci.*, 30:257–261.

310. Sheppard, D., Wong, W. S., Uehara, C. F., Nadel, J. A., and Boushey, H. A. (1980): Lower threshold and greater bronchomotor responsiveness of asthmatic subjects to sulfur dioxide. *Am. Rev. Respir. Dis.*, 122:873–878.

310a.Sheppard, D., Nadel, J. A. and Boushey, H. A. (1981): Inhibition of sulfur dioxide-induced bronchoconstriction by sodium chromoglycate in asthmatic subjects. *Am. Rev. Respir. Dis.*, 124:257–259.

310b.Sheppard, D., Saisho, A., Nadel, J. A. and Boushey, H. A. (1981): Exercise increases sulfur dioxide-induced bronchoconstriction in asthmatic subjects. *Am. Rev. Respir. Dis.*, 123:486–491.

311. Shirakawa, T., Kusaka, Y., Fujimura, N., Goto, S., Kato, M., Heki, S., and Morimoto, K. (1989): Occupational asthma from cobalt sensitivity in workers exposed to hard metal dust. *Chest*, 95:29–37.

312. Sibelle, Y., and Reynolds, H. Y. (1990): Macrophages and polymorphonuclear neutrophils in lung defense and injury. *Am. Rev. Respir. Dis.*, 141:471–501.

313. Simonsson, B. G., Sjoberg, A., Rolf, C., and Haeger-Aronson, B. (1985): Acute and long-term airway hyperactivity in aluminum-salt exposed workers with nocturnal asthma. *Eur. J. Respir. Dis.*, 66:105–118.

314. Slovak, A. J. M., and Hill, R. N. (1987): Does atopy have any predictive value for laboratory animal allergy? A comparison of different concepts of atopy. *Br. J. Ind. Med.*, 44:129–132.

314a.Slovak, A. J. M. and Hill, R. N. (1981): Laboratory Animal Allergy: A Clinical Survey of an Exposed Population. *Br. J. Ind. Med.*, 38:38–41.

315. Snell, R. E., and Luchsinger, P. C. (1969): Effects of sulfur dioxide on expiratory flow rates and total respiratory resistance in normal human subjects. *Arch. Environ. Health*, 18:693–698.

316. Snyder, J. E., and Chang, P. W. (1974): Relative resistance of eight human enteric viruses to ozonation in Sangatucket River water. In Proceedings of the IOI Workshop on Aquatic Applications of Ozone, pp. 82–99. International Ozone Institute, Boston.

317. Soda, K., Ando, M., Sakata, T., Sugimoto, M., Nakashima, H., and Araki, S. (1988): C_{1q} and C_3 in bronchoalveolar lavage fluid from patients with summer-type hypersensitivity pneumonitis. *Chest*, 93:76–80.

318. Soda, K., Ando, M., Shimazu, K., Sakata, T., Yoshida, K., and Araki, S. (1986): Different classes of antibody activities to *Trichosporon cutaneum* antigen in summer-type hypersensitivity pneumonitis by enzyme-linked immunosorbent assay. *Am. Rev. Respir. Dis.*, 133:83–87.

319. Speizer, F. E., and Frank, N. R. (1966): The uptake and release of SO_2 by the human nose. *Arch. Environ. Health*, 12:725–728.

320. Sprecace, G. A. (1963): Idiopathic pulmonary hemosiderosis. Personal experience with six adults treated within a ten-month period, and a review of the literature. *Am. Rev. Respir. Dis.*, 88:330–337.

321. Springmeyer, S. C. (1987): The clinical use of bronchoalveolar lavage. *Chest*, 92:771–772.

322. Stankus, R. P., and Salvaggio, J. F. (1981): Bronchopulmonary humoral and cellular enhancement in experimental silicosis. *J. Reticuloendoth. Soc.*, 29:153–161.

323. Stanton, M. F., Layard, M., Tegeris, A., Miller, E., May, M., and Kent, E. (1977): Carcinogenicity of fibrous glass. Pleural response in the rat in relation to fiber dimension. *J. Natl. Cancer Inst.*, 58:587–603.

323a.Stjernberg, N., Eklund, A., Nystrom, L., Rosenhall, L., Emmelin, A. and Stromqvist, L-H., (1985): Prevalence of bronchial asthma and chronic bronchitis in a community in northern Sweden; relation to environmental and occupational exposure to sulfur dioxide. *Eur. J. Respir. Dis.*, 67:41–49.

324. Takemura, T., Rom, W. N., Ferrans, V. J., and Crystal, R. G. (1989): Morphologic characterization of alveolar macrophages from subjects with occupational exposure to inorganic particles. *Am. Rev. Respir. Dis.*, 140:1674–1685.

325. Tan, G-X, Huan, Y-Z., and Hu, S. (1990): Whole lung lavage as an effective treatment of silicosis. *Am. Rev. Respir. Dis.*, 141:245.

326. Tse, K. S., Chan, H., and Chan-Yeung, M. (1982): Specific IgE antibodies in workers with occupational asthma due to western red cedar. *Clin. Allergy*, 12:249–258.

327. Teschler, H., Friedrichs, K. H., Ramin, C., Konietzko, N., and Costabel, U. (1990): BAL asbestosis burden: Topographic changes from upper to lower lobe? *Am. Rev. Respir. Dis.*, 141:A240.

328. Thompson, A. B., and Rennard, S. I. (1988): Assessment of airways inflammation utilizing bronchoalveolar lavage. *Clin. Chest Med.*, 9:635–642.

329. Tonnel, A. B., Gosset, P., Joseph, M., Fourmier, E., and Capron, A. (1983): Stimulation of alveolar macrophages in asthmatic patients after local provocation test. *Lancet*, 1:1406–1408.

330. Turner, J. A., and Thompson, L. R. (1926): Health hazards of brass foundries: 1. Field investigations of the health hazards of the brass-foundry industry. 2. Laboratory studies relating to the pathology of brass foundreymen's ague (Bulletin 157). Public Health Service.

331. van den Bosch, J. M. M., Heye, C., Wagenaar, S. S., and van Velzen-Blad, H. C. (1986): Bronchoalveolar lavage in extrinsic allergic alveolitis. *Respiration* 49:45–51.

332. Van Ganse, W. F., Oleffe, J., Van Hove, W., and Groetenbriel, C. (1972): Lymphocyte transformation in chronic pulmonary berylliosis. *Lancet*, 1:1023.

333. van Ordstrand, H. S., Hughes, R., and Carmody, M. G. (1943): Chemical pneumonia in workers extracting berryllium oxide. *Cleve. Clin. Q.*, 10:10–18.

334. Villager, B., Broekelmann, T., Kelley, D., Heymach, G. J., and McDonald, J. A. (1981): Bronchoalveolar fibronectin in smokers and nonsmokers. *Am. Rev. Respir. Dis.*, 124:652–654.

335. Vogelmeier, C., Konig, G., Bencze, K., and Fruhmann, G. (1987): Pulmonary involvement in zinc fumc fever. *Chest*, 92:946–948.

336. Voisin, C., Tounel, A. B., Lahoute, C., Robin, H., Lebas, J., and Aerts, C. (1981): Bird fancier's lung: Studies of bronchoalveolar lavage and correlations with inhalation provocation tests. *Lung*, 159:17–22.

337. Wagner, J. C., Berry, G., and Pooley, F. D. (1982): Mesotheliomas and asbestos type in asbestos textile workers: A study of lung contents. *Br. Med. J.*, 285:603–606.

338. Wagner, J. C., Newhouse, M. L., Corrin, B., Rossiter, C. E. R., Griffiths, D. M., Lyons, J., Sheers, G., and Moncrieff, C. B. (1988): Correlation between fibre content of the lung and disease in east London asbestos factory workers. *Br. J. Ind. Med.* 45:305–308.

339. Wallace, J. M., Oishi, J. S., Barbers, R. G., Batra, P., and Aberle, D. R. (1989): Bronchoalveolar lavage cell and lymphocyte phenotype profiles in healthy asbestos-exposed shipyard workers. *Am. Rev. Respir. Dis.*, 139:33–38.

340. Wallaert, B., Lassalle, P., Fortin, F., Aerts, C., Bart, F., Founier, E., and Voisin, C. (1990):

Superoxide anion generation by alveolar inflammatory cells in simple pneumoconiosis and in progressive massive fibrosis of nonsmoking coal workers. *Am. Rev. Respir. Dis.*, 141:129–133.

341. Walters, E. N., Duddridge, M., and Gardner, P. V. (1989): Bronchoalveolar lavage: Its place in diagnosis and research. *Respir. Med.*, 83:457–458.

342. Wardlaw, A. J., Hay, H., Cromwell, O., Collins, J. V., and Kay, A. B. (1989): Leukotrienes, LTC$_4$ and LTB$_4$, in bronchoalveolar lavage in bronchial asthma and other respiratory diseases. *J. Allergy Clin. Immunol.*, 84:19–26.

343. Warr, G. A., and Martin, R. R. (1973): In vitro migration of human alveolar macrophages: Effects of cigarette smoking. *Infect. Immunol.*, 8:222–227.

344. Warr, G. A., and Martin, R. R. (1974): Chemotactic responsiveness of human alveolar macrophages: Effects of cigarette smoking. *Infect. Immunol.*, 9:769–771.

345. Warr, G. A., and Martin, R. R. (1977): Immune receptors of human alveolar macrophages. Comparison between smokers and nonsmokers. *J. Reticuloendoth. Soc.*, 22:181–187.

346. Warren, D. P. W., and Tse, K. S. (1974): Extrinsic allergic alveolitis owing to hypersensitivity to chickens—significance of sputum precipitins. *Am. Rev. Respir. Dis.*, 109:672–677.

347. Warson, A. J., Black, J., Doig, A. T. and Nagelschmidt, G. (1959): Pneumoconiosis in carbon electrode workers. *Br. J. Ind. Med.*, 16:274–285.

348. Weinberger, S. E., Kelman, J. A., Elson, N. A., Young, R. C., Jr., Reynolds, H. Y., Fulmer, J. D., and Crystal, R. G. (1978): Bronchoalveolar lavage in interstitial lung disease. *Ann. Intern. Med.*, 89:459–466.

349. White, E. W., Denney, P. J., and Irving, S. M. (1966): Quantitative microprobe analysis of microcrystalline powders. In The Electron Microprobe, pp. 791–804. John Wiley, New York.

350. Whitehall, F., Scott, J., and Grimshaw, M. (1977): Relationship between occupations and asbestos-fibre content of the lungs in patients with pleural mesothelioma, lung cancer, and other diseases. *Thorax*, 32:377–386.

351. Williams, W. R., and Williams, W. J. (1982): Development of beryllium lymphocyte transformation tests in chronic beryllium disease. *Int. Arch. Allergy Appl. Immunol.*, 67:175–180.

352. Xaubet, A., Rodriguez-Roison, R., Bombi, J. A., Marin, A., Roca, J., and Agusti-Vidal, A. (1986): Correlation of bronchoalveolar lavage and clinical and functional findings in asbestosis. *Am. Rev. Respir. Dis.*, 133:848–854.

353. Yamada, M., Tamura, N., Shirai, T., and Kira, S. (1986): Flow cytometric analysis of lymphocyte subsets in the bronchoalveolar lavage fluid and peripheral blood of healthy volunteers. *Scand. J. Immunol.*, 24:559–565.

354. Yoshizawa, Y., Nomura, A., Ohdama, S., Tanaka, M., Morinari, H., and Hasegawa, S. (1988): The significance of complement activation in the pathogenesis of hypersensitivity pneumonitis: Sequential changes of complement components and chemotactic activities in bronchoalveolar lavage fluids. *Int. Arch. Allergy*, 87:417–423.

355. Yoshizawa, Y., Ohdama, S., Tanone, M., Tanaka, M., Ohtsuka, M., Uteke, K., and Hosegawa, S. (1986): Analysis of BAL cells and fluids in patient with hypersensitivity pneumonitis: Possible role of chemotactic factors in the pathogenesis of disease. *Int. Arch. Allergy Appl. Immunol.*, 80:376–382.

356. Zarkower, A., Scheuchenzuber, W. J., and Burns, C. A. (1979): Effect of silica dust inhalation on susceptibility of mice to influenza. *Arch. Environ. Health*, 34:372–376.

357. Zehr, B. B., Casale, T. B., Wood, D., Floerchinger, C., Richerson, H. B., and Hunninghake, G. W. (1989): Use of segmental airway lavage to obtain relevant mediators from the lumps of asthmatic and control subjects. *Chest*, 95:1059–1063.

358. Zeiss, C. R., Kanellakes, T. M., Bellone, J. D., Levitz, D., Pruzansky, J. J., and Patterson, R. (1980): Immunoglobulin E-mediated asthma and hypersensitivity pneumonitis with precipitating anti-hapten antibodies due to diphenylmethane diisocyanate (MDI) exposure. *J. Allergy Clin. Immunol.*, 65:346–352.

359. Zeiss, C. R., Patterson, R., Pruzansky, J. J., Miller, M. M., Rosenberg, M., and Levitz, D. (1977): Trimellitic anhydride-induced airway syndromes: Clinical and immunologic studies. *J. Allergy Clin. Immunol.*, 60:96–103.

360. Zeiss, C. R., Wolkonsky, P., Chacon, R., Tuntland, P. A., Levitz, D., Pruzansky, J. J., and Patterson, R. (1983): Syndromes in workers exposed to trimellitic anhydride. *Ann. Intern. Med.*, 98:8–12.

361. Zheutlin, L. M., Ackerman, S. J., Gleich, G. J., and Thomas, L. L. (1984): Stimulation of basophil and rat mast cell histamine release by eosinophil granule-derived cationic proteins. *J. Immunol.*, 133:2180–2185.

Clinical Immunotoxicology, edited by
D. S. Newcombe, N. R. Rose, and J. C. Bloom.
Raven Press, Ltd., New York © 1992.

16

Recent Studies of the Human Immunotoxic Effects of 2,3,7,8-Tetrachlorodibenzo-*p*-Dioxin

Richard E. Hoffman

Colorado Department of Health, Denver, Colorado

This chapter discusses human health effects of exposure to one type of halogenated aromatic hydrocarbon, 2,3,7,8-tetrachlorodibenzo-*p*-dioxin (TCDD) commonly known as dioxin. The epidemiological studies reviewed here were a combined effort of St. Louis University School of Medicine, the Centers for Disease Control (CDC), and the Missouri Department of Health. The studies were funded by the Agency for Toxic Substances and Disease Registry, an agency created by CERCLA (the Superfund law), which is associated with CDC.

The topics presented include (a) a brief history of how dioxin contamination occurred and became recognized in Missouri; (b) a summary of animal immunotoxicological studies of dioxin; (c) an overview of the immunological findings from two published epidemiological studies of health effects of persons exposed to TCDD in Missouri; and (d) an update of studies currently in progress for which the data are still preliminary.

Dioxin contamination in Missouri came to the attention of public health officials in August 1971 following the report of the hospitalization of a 6-year-old girl with hemorrhagic cystitis in St. Louis (7). Bacterial and viral culture results of the child's urine were negative. The girl had been playing in the soil of a horse arena near St. Louis, where numerous horses, dogs, cats, mice, and birds in the arena had died during the 3 months prior to her illness. The animal deaths followed the spraying of a show ring in April and May 1971 with an oil mixture used to control dust. Autopsies of seven horses revealed oral ulcers, ascites, gastric ulcers, hyperkeratosis, nephritis, and, in one case, cystitis. The horses most probably had acute TCDD toxicity with onset days to weeks after initial exposure and with progression over a period of weeks. The girl eventually recovered. At least five other persons who had contact with sprayed horse arena soils had medical complaints, including headaches and skin lesions. Initially the illnesses and animal deaths were postulated to be caused by organophosphate poisoning, but in 1974 TCDD was identified in a soil

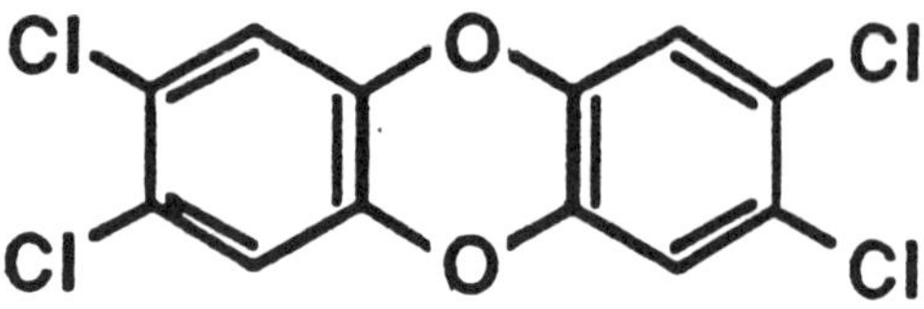

2,3,7,8-tetrachlorodibenzo-p-dioxin

FIG. 1.

specimen that had been collected in 1971; the concentration was 30 parts per million. Investigations conducted by the United States Environmental Protection Agency and the Missouri Department of Natural Resources in the period from 1971 to 1983 ultimately identified 42 sites of contamination with TCDD soil levels of 1 ppb or greater. The TCDD originated in a trichlorophenol production facility in Verona, a town in the southwestern corner of the state. It was mixed with waste oil and transported to eastern parts of the state by a firm that sprayed the mixture on roads, parking lots, and horse arenas in a number of places, the best known of which was Times Beach.

Figure 1 shows the structure of 2,3,7,8-tetrachlorodibenzo-*p*-dioxin, and it is thought that the positions of the four chlorine atoms are responsible for this isomer's extreme toxicity (2).

For example, a pentachlorinated dibenzodioxin isomer with chlorine in the 1,2,3,7,8 positions has a lower median lethal dose (LD_{50}) than a pentachlorinated dibenzodioxin without chlorine in the 2,3,7,8 positions (2). There is known to be species variability in susceptibility to acute TCDD toxicity in the guinea pig, which has an LD_{50} about two orders of magnitude lower than that of certain strains of mice. Dioxin is called a probable carcinogen (2). In animal studies of the effects of TCDD on the immune system, the pathological findings vary, depending on the species, dose, and duration of exposure. A consistent finding, however, has been thymic atrophy (12). Cortical thymic depletion is observed, and in other organs, such as the spleen and lymph nodes, there is depletion of T-dependent areas (1, 13). In animal models, a number of alterations of cell-mediated immune function have been observed, including depressed delayed type hypersensitivity reactions, reduced ability to reject allografts, and increased susceptibility to both endotoxin-producing infectious agents such as *Salmonella* and non–endotoxin-producing bacteria such as *Listeria monocytogenes* (4). *In vitro* studies have corroborated these findings, revealing depressed mitogen-stimulated lymphoproliferation (5) and depressed generation of cytotoxic T lymphocytes (1). The effects appear to be more intense when the chemical is administered during the pre- and postnatal periods than when it is administered solely in postnatal life. Dioxin may affect humoral immune responses in animals but apparently requires higher doses than those inducing defects in cell-mediated immunity (12). Despite the evidence of endotoxin sensitivity following TCDD treatment, little evidence of macrophage functional defects has been observed. The exact mechanism of immunosuppression is not known, but it has been postulated that the initial event in the toxic action of TCDD is mediated through a TCDD receptor in the cytosol; such a receptor has been found in hepatocytes (9a).

In January 1983, the CDC and the Missouri Department of Health initiated a pilot epidemiological study (11). The aforementioned animal studies led the investigators to include evaluation of immune function as part of the medical protocol. Although human exposures to TCDD have occurred numerous times in the past 40 years, none have been exactly analogous to the situation in Missouri, in which the toxin was part of an oil mixture absorbed in soil in residential settings and in which the general population was potentially exposed on a daily basis for periods of months to years. These circumstances made it difficult to extrapolate to the Missouri situation from occupational studies or studies of persons acutely exposed to TCDD in Seveso, Italy. Exposed participants in the pilot study were selected on the basis of living or working at sites with TCDD levels above 100 ppb for at least 6 months or above 20 ppb for at least 2 years.

The pilot study included 66 persons at high risk of exposure and 36 at low to no risk of TCDD exposure. Exposure was assessed by personal interviews and environmental soil sampling. Most of the participants were from Times Beach; a few were exposed at the horse arenas and a few others at two residential sites called the Minker and Stout sites. Over 250 comparisons between groups were made, but only five statistically significant differences were found. The only statistically significant result involving the immune system was a decreased frequency of palpable axillary nodes in the high-risk group (1.7% versus 15.2%, $p < 0.05$, Fisher's exact two-tailed test). Marked depression of lymphocyte proliferation (not defined by the investigators) and T4/T8 ratios less than 1.0 were observed more frequently in the high-risk group (24.3% versus 15.0%, depressed lymphocyte proliferation; 13.2% versus 6.1%, low T4/T8 ratio) (8). The mean response to seven antigens in the Merieux CMI system for testing cutaneous delayed-type hypersensitivity as measured in millimeters of induration was slightly lower in the high-risk group (13.4 mm versus 14.8 mm).

Although it could have been concluded that the results of the study were negative and no further work needed to be done, because of relatively low statistical power and possible exposure misclassification, the investigators decided instead that there needed to be a larger, more epidemiologically rigorous study. The Quail Run Mobile Home site was selected, and this study was conducted from November 1984 through January 1985. Instead of 104 participants, 309 persons (154 exposed and 155 unexposed) were enrolled (6). The level of TCDD soil contamination in this site was, in general, higher than at Times Beach, the peak soil concentration measured being 2,200 ppb at Quail Run versus approximately 1,200 ppb at Times Beach. At Quail Run, interior dust samples with values of TCDD greater than 1 ppb were found in 21 of 31 trailers tested. No home interior specimens were collected in Times Beach. None of the 132 Environmental Protection Agency priority pollutants besides TCDD were found at Quail Run. In the Quail Run study, the exposed group lived an average of 2.8 years at the site and had last resided at the site 3.9 years prior to the examination. The unexposed group consisted of people who lived in mobile home parks where the soil was tested for TCDD and no detectable levels were found. As in the pilot study, a variety of examinations were performed on each participant, with the entire test period lasting about 5 hours. None of the participants gave a history of any immune disorder that could be documented from medical records. The Merieux CMI skin test was applied by one nurse and read at 48 to 72 hours by one of four readers at the participant's home, work, or school. The reader was not told the exposure status of the participant. Tables 1 through 4 show *in vitro* immune system test results from this study. An abnormal test was defined as greater than two standard deviations from the arithmetic mean of the unexposed group. All statistical tests comparing the groups were controlled for age, sex, and socio-economic status. Note that the mean total lymphocyte count is slightly higher in the exposed group (Table 1). B cells were not directly measured, and the non–T-cell count, arbitrarily calculated as the total lymphocyte count minus the number of peripheral T cells with the T11 surface marker, was found to be higher in the exposed group ($p<0.05$). Although the percentages of T3 and T4 cells were significantly lower in the exposed group, the absolute number of cells with these surface markers was not significantly different. The lower percentage of T3 and T4 subsets was attributed to the increased numbers of non–T cells in the exposed group. The

TABLE 1. *T-cell surface marker analyses in the Quail Run Dioxin Study, Missouri, 1984–1985*

Parameter	Exposed (n = 136)		Unexposed (n = 142)	
	Mean (SD)	Abnormal[a]	Mean (SD)	Abnormal
T-cell subset populations:				
T3 (cells/mm^3)	1,698 (519)	1.5	1,673 (493)	1.4
T3 (%)	72 (8)[b]		74 (7)	
T4 (cells/mm^3)	1,021 (353)	0.7	1,033 (346)	0.0
T4 (%)	44 (9)[b]		46 (8)	
T8 (cells/mm^3)	592 (223)	1.5	578 (198)	0.0
T8 (%)	25 (6)		26 (6)	
T11 (cells/mm^3)	1,801 (550)	2.4	1,796 (493)	2.1
T11 (%)	78 (7)[b]		80 (6)	
T4/T8 ratio	1.9 (0.8)	8.2	1.9 (0.6)	6.3
Non–T cell count	540 (289)[b]	H:6.4	445 (198)	H:4.3
		L:0.8		L:0.0
Total lymphocyte count (cells/mm^3)	2,465 (724)	H:0.0	2,311 (634)	H:0.0
		L:2.0		L:0.7

[a]Defined as less than two standard deviations below the mean in the unexposed group for all parameters except T4/T8 ratio defined as abnormal if less than 1.0.

[b]Significantly different from unexposed group ($p<0.05$) with analysis of covariance adjusting for sex, age, and socioeconomic status.

TABLE 2. In vitro *analyses of T-cell function in the Quail Run Dioxin Study, Missouri, 1984–1985*

Parameter	Exposed (n = 135) Mean (SD)	% Abnormal[a]	Unexposed (n = 142) Mean (SD)	% Abnormal
Lymphoproliferative responses (counts per minute):				
Phytohemagglutinin	46,882 (15,112)	3.0	49,266 (17,678)	3.5
Concanavalin A	44,679 (18,104)	3.0	43,630 (16,901)	2.9
Pokeweed mitogen	38,370 (10,696)[b]	H:3.0	34,921 (12,855)	H:1.4
		L:0.0[c]		L:5.6
Tetanus toxoid	25,062 (17,535)	3.0	23,975 (15,038)	0.7
Allogeneic T-cell cytotoxicity (% activity):				
	26 (14)	5.9	28 (15)	4.2

[a]Defined as less than two standard deviations below the mean in the unexposed group for all parameters except for tetanus toxoid stimulation index less than 3.0, and pokeweed mitogen ± two standard deviations from the unexposed group mean.

[b]Significantly different from unexposed group ($p<0.05$) using analysis of covariance to adjust for sex, age, and socioeconomic status.

[c]Significantly different from unexposed group ($p<0.05$). Fisher's exact two-tailed test.

mean serum immunoglobulin G level was not statistically different for the groups. With regard to results of lymphocyte proliferation tests and allogeneic T-cell cytotoxicity, the mean response to pokeweed mitogen was higher in the exposed group. Otherwise, there were no statistically significant differences (Table 2). The comparisons were performed using absolute values; when the values were logarithmically converted to normalize the data, the mean cytotoxicity response was significantly lower in the exposed than in the unexposed group (19.2% versus 23.8%) ($p<0.03$) as well as in the adult (>19 years) (22.8% versus 26.3%) and adult female (21.9% versus 25.1%) subgroups. Table 3 shows the percentage of participants displaying anergy. Anergy was defined as less than 2 mm average induration in response to each of the seven recall antigens. Six (11.8%) of the exposed subjects versus one (1.1%) of the unexposed subjects displayed anergy. Two of the six exposed anergic subjects were less than 20 years of age. There were also differences between groups

TABLE 3. *Frequency of cutaneous anergy and relative anergy in the Quail Run Dioxin Study, Missouri, 1984–1985*

	Exposed n	Anergic	% Relative anergic	Unexposed n	Anergic	% Relative anergic
Total	51	11.8[a]	35.3[a]	93	1.1	11.8
Adults[b]	35	11.4[a]	28.6[a]	71	1.4	11.3
Children	16	12.5	50.0[a]	22	0.0	13.7

[a]Different from unexposed group, $p<0.05$.
[b]Age more than 19 years.

TABLE 4. *Average induration and mean number of positive cutaneous delayed type hypersensitivity responses in the Quail Run Dioxin Study, Missouri, 1984–1985*

	Exposed			Unexposed		
	n	Mean no. positive antigens	Average induration (mm)	n	Mean no. positive antigens	Average induration (mm)
Total	51	2.3[a]	10.1	93	3.1	12.9
Adults[b]	35	2.5	11.0	71	3.2	13.3
Children	16	1.9[a]	8.1	22	2.9	11.4

[a]Different from unexposed group, $p < 0.05$, analysis of covariance adjusted for age, sex, socio-economic status, and date of examination.
[b]Age more than 19 years.

in the proportion of persons displaying relative anergy, which was defined as a positive response to either none or one of the seven antigens. Relative anergy was observed in 35.3% of the exposed group versus 11.8% in the unexposed group. Mean induration and mean number of positive antigens were smaller and fewer in the exposed group (Table 4). However, there were apparent problems with two of the skin test readers. Two readers observed higher than expected rates of anergy in the unexposed group, i.e., 15% and 40%. Based on comparisons with previously published studies of the Merieux CMI test, it was decided to exclude their readings. This excluded 46% of the total group—61% of the exposed and 32% of the unexposed subjects. If their readings were included, the rates of anergy and relative anergy in the exposed and unexposed groups were 16.7% versus 8.1% and 37.9% versus 19.9%, respectively. Using only the data on subjects examined by the two "reliable" readers, no clustering of immune systems defects was found, i.e., clustering of anergy or relative anergy with abnormal *in vitro* tests. Using all subjects, the exposed group had a significantly greater frequency of anergy with at least one *in vitro* abnormality, which tended to be an abnormal absolute T-cell subset count. The investigators' recommendations were as follows:

1. Follow immune function in anergic or relatively anergic individuals, and
2. Study immune function in individuals with known body burdens of TCDD.

Reports of three subsequent studies are presented in order to bring the story of the Missouri TCDD investigations up to July 1991.

First, Quail Run study participants demonstrating anergy or relative anergy, regardless of reader, were contacted 14 to 17 months after their initial examination (3). Twenty-eight of 50 eligible exposed and 15 of 27 unexposed individuals were enrolled in a follow-up medical evaluation, which took place in March and April of 1986. This group represented 56% of the individuals in the original Quail Run study with anergy or relative anergy. No participant had anergy on retesting, and two subjects (one exposed and one unexposed) demonstrated relative anergy. A comparison of *in vitro* initial and follow-up test results indicated that exposed participants had a lower mean T4/T8 ratio on retesting and a higher frequency (17% versus 0%), with a T4/T8 ratio less than 1 than unexposed participants. In the initial study for this subgroup, 24% (6 of 25) of the exposed versus 7% (1 of 15) of the unexposed subjects had T4/T8 ratios less than 1. It must be emphasized that drawing inferences about the effects of TCDD on the immune system from this sample is tenuous—the follow-up was intended to provide medical evaluation for persons with potentially significant immune suppression. The principal investigators considered several possible explanations for the change in the response to the skin tests: (a) differences in test application technique; (b) differences in the potency of antigens; (c) differences in reading the skin tests; (d) sensitization to the antigens on the first application followed by a booster effect on the second application; (e) recovery from immunosuppressive effects of TCDD; and (f) occurrence of chance. The investigators concluded that the most plausible explanations were sensitization to the antigens by the first test and weak potency of the initial skin tests. Interviews with the participants at the time of follow-up evaluation about the skin tests applied in the Quail Run study corroborated the readers' findings—the participants denied induration or erythema at the site where the skin test was applied.

Second, serum collected in 1984 to 1985 from 199 of the Quail Run participants was removed from frozen storage in 1986 for the purpose of measuring levels of thymosin alpha-1 (10). As mentioned earlier, animal studies have not elucidated the exact mechanism of TCDD-induced immune suppression. One hypothesis questioned whether or not there could be a defect in T-cell maturation. Paul Naylor of the Department of Biochemistry of George Washington University performed the measurements of thymosin alpha-1 using a newly developed N-terminal radioimmunoassay. This sample of 199 (94 exposed, 105 unexposed persons) had an increased frequency of anergy in both the exposed group and the subgroup of the 199 who had delayed type hypersensitivity reaction skin tests read by reliable readers; therefore, this indicated that the sample was probably representative of the total group of 309 in the Quail Run study. The mean thymosin level was found to be significantly lower in the exposed group (9.73 ± 304.1 pg/ml versus 1148.7 ± 482.1 pg/ml, $p < 0.01$). Also observed was a statistically significant trend of decreasing thymosin alpha-1 levels with increasing number of years of residence in the TCDD-contaminated area. However, the thymosin alpha-1 levels were not associated with other measures of immune function in the exposed group.

Last, from July 1985 through the fall of 1986, potentially exposed persons from all Missouri sites were asked to undergo abdominal adipose tissue biopsies. Dioxin is lipophilic and is stored in adipose tissue. An interim report describing the TCDD adipose tissue levels in 39 exposed and 57 unexposed persons showed very different distributions of the two groups (9). Six of the 39 exposed persons had levels higher than 100 ppt. The mean TCDD level for the unexposed persons was 7.4 ppt, considerably lower than mean level for persons with residential (21.1 ppt), recreational (90.8 ppt), or occupational (136.2 ppt) TCDD exposures. Persons with recreational exposure rode horses at the contaminated arenas; persons with occupational exposures either worked at the trichlorophenol-producing facility in Verona or worked at contaminated truck terminals in St. Louis. The ranking of the means in these categories is as expected. In the fall of 1986, blood was obtained from 41 persons exposed to TCDD who had previously undergone biopsies; the blood was tested for hematological, liver, and immune functions (14). The analyses were adjusted for age and sex. Statistically significant ($p<0.05$) positive correlations with TCDD levels in adipose tissue were found for both the absolute number and percentage of T8 cells, the percentage of T3, T4, and T11 cells, and serum IgG levels. Nine of the 41 subjects had ratios less than 1.2, and seven of these persons had TCDD levels higher than 60 ppt; one had a TCDD level between 20 and 60 ppt, and the remaining subjects had levels of less than 20 ppt. No correlation of delayed-type hypersensitivity skin test results with TCDD levels was observed. It must be pointed out that a few points at the extremes have a potentially great impact on the correlations. It is unfortunate that a serum TCDD test was not available when the Quail Run study was conducted.

In conclusion, it is difficult to discern a pattern in the Missouri studies of the effects of TCDD on human immune system function. If human immunotoxicity occurs from living near TCDD contaminated soil, it does not appear to have resulted in clinical illness thus far; all immune system findings associated with TCDD exposure in Missouri appear to be subclinical. On the other hand, there is a concern that a potential liver carcinogen could also be modulating immune function.

ACKNOWLEDGMENTS

The author gratefully acknowledges the assistance of John Andrews, M.D., John Bagby, Ph.D., Luther DeWeese, R. Gregory Evans, Ph.D., Henry Falk, M.D., David Forney, Bruce Gibson, Cindy Kempker, Alan Knutsen, M.D., Tina Luebhering, Robert Miller, Ph.D., Larry Needham, Ph.D., Donald Patterson, Ph.D., James Pirkle, M.D., Daryl Roberts, M.Ed., Eric Sampson, Ph.D., Wayne Schramm, M.A., Jeff Staake, M.P.A., Paul Stehr-Green, Dr.PH., Karen Webb, M.D., Pat Willie, R.N., and Matthew Zack, M.D. in the collection and generation of data and analyses for this report.

REFERENCES

1. Clark, D. A., Gauldie, J., Szewczuk, M. R., et al. (1981): Enhanced suppressor cell activity as a mechanism of immunosuppression by 2,3,7,8-tetrachlorodibenzo-p-dioxin (41275). *Proc. Soc. Exp. Biol. Med.*, 168:290–299.
2. Esposito, M. P., Tiernan, T. O., and Dryden, F. E. (1980): Dioxins, pp. 187–229. U.S. Environmental Protection Agency, Cincinnati.
3. Evans, R. G., Webb, K. B., Knutsen, A. P., et al. (1988): A medical follow-up of the health effects of long-term exposure to 2,3,7,8-tetrachlorodibenzo-p-dioxin. *Arch. Environ. Health*, 43:273–278.
4. Faith, R. E., and Luster, M. I. (1979): Investigations on the effects of 2,3,7,8-tetrachlorodibenzo-p-dioxin (TCDD) on parameters of various immune functions. *Ann. N.Y. Acad. Sci. U.S.A.*, 320:564–571.
5. Faith, R. E., Luster, M. I., and Moore, J. A. (1978): Chemical separation of helper cell function and delayed hypersensitivity responses. *Cell. Immunol.*, 40:275–284.

6. Hoffman, R. E., Stehr-Green, P. A., et al. (1986): Health effects of long-term exposure to 2,3,7,8-tetrachlorodibenzo-p-dioxin. *J.A.M.A.*, 255:2031–2038.
7. Kimbrough, R. D., Carter, C. D., et al. (1977): Epidemiology and pathology of a tetrachlorodibenzodioxin poisoning episode. *Arch. Environ. Health*, 32:77–86.
8. Missouri Division of Health, Centers for Disease Control, St. Joseph Hospital of Kirkwood, St. Louis University School of Medicine (1983): Missouri Dixon Health Studies Progress Report, p. 68, Jefferson City, Missouri.
9. Patterson, D. G., Hoffman, R. E., et al. (1986): 2,3,7,8-Tetrachlorodibenzo-p-dioxin levels in adipose tissue of exposed and control persons in Missouri: An interim report. *J.A.M.A.*, 256:2683–2686.
9a. Poland, A., Glover, E., Kende, A. S. (1976) Sterospecific, high affinity binding of 2,3,7,8-tetrachlorodibenzo-p-dioxin by hepatic cytosol. Evidence that the binding species is receptor for induction of aryl hydrocarbon hydroxylase. *J. Biol. Chem.*, 251:4936–4945.
10. Stehr-Green, P. A., Naylor, P. H., and Hoffman, R. E. (1989): Diminished thymosin alpha-1 levels in persons exposed to 2,3,7,8-tetrachlorodibenzo-p-dioxin. *J. Toxicol. Environ. Health*, 28:285–295.
11. Stehr, P. A., Stein, G. F., et al. (1986): A pilot epidemiologic study of possible health effects associated with 2,3,7,8-TCDD contaminations in Missouri. *Arch. Environ. Health*, 41:16–22.
12. Vos, J. G., Faith, R. E., and Luster, M. I. (1980): Immune alterations. In Halogenated Biphenyls, Terphenyls, Naphthalenes, Dibenzodioxins and Related Products, edited by R. D. Kimbrough, pp. 248–254. Elsevier Science Publishers, Amsterdam.
13. Vos, J. G., Moore, J. A., and Zinkl, J. G., (1974): Toxicity of 2,3,7,8-tetrachlorodibenzo-p-dioxin (TCDD) in C57B1/6 mice. *Toxico. Appl. Pharmacol.*, 29:229–241.
14. Webb, K. B., Evans, R. G., Knutsen, A. P., et al. (1989): Medical evaluation of subjects with known body levels of 2,3,7,8-tetrachlorodibenzo-p-dioxin. *J. Toxicol. Environ. Health*, 28:183–193.

Clinical Immunotoxicology, edited by
D. S. Newcombe, N. R. Rose, and J. C. Bloom.
Raven Press, Ltd., New York © 1992.

17

Immunotoxicity of Organophosphorus Compounds

David S. Newcombe* and Ahmed H. Esa†

Department of Environmental Health Sciences, Johns Hopkins University, School of Hygiene and Public Health, Baltimore, MD; †Bone Marrow Transplantation Unit, Oncology Center, Johns Hopkins University, School of Medicine, Baltimore, MD

Organophosphorus compounds are widely used for commercial, household, and industrial purposes. Their commercial applications are diverse and include use as leveling agents for various industrial coatings and surfaces; flame retardants for plastics, synthetic rubber, and fabrics; hydraulic fluids and other lubricants; and stabilizers for rubber and plastics; insecticides; and herbicides (1–5). In addition to obvious industrial exposures, humans may come in contact with organophorphorus compounds from their use of these chemicals as pesticides and weed killers in the home environment (6). Obviously, farmers and others in the agricultural industry are at higher risk for organophosphorus exposure than the general population. In fact, it was found that 6.9×10^6 kg of malathion, a commonly used pesticide, was distributed equally among government, agricultural, and household use in the United States in 1978 (7,8), and today 637×10^6 kg of chemicals per year are sprayed on grains and food (9). Since malathion, like other pesticides, has been consistently detected as a contaminant in food, tobacco, tobacco smoke, fruits, fish, and tissue samples from animals, opportunity for exposure is widespread (7,10–13). Such chemicals and their residues have also been found in air, ground water, and sediments. In addition to the portals of entry of these compounds through the skin and lungs, ingestion of organophosphorus compounds may occur more commonly than might be expected, since ground water is a primary source of drinking water for approximately half the population of the United States (9).

On the basis of the widespread distribution of organophosphorus compounds, there is an increasing focus on determining whether organophosphorus-mediated health effects are observed in humans. Most analyses of the human health effects of these compounds have emphasized the well-characterized anticholinergic actions of this class of chemicals, which are observed either in cases of accidental acute poisonings or as a result of ingestion in suicide attempts (6). The clinical expression of such exposures is primarily that resulting from the inhibition of cholinesterase, which causes elevated blood and tissue levels of acetylcholine and triggers the associated organ dysfunctions resulting from these elevated acetylcholine levels (6).

Recently, noncholinergic mechanisms of organophosphorus activity have been identified and leave open the possibility that organ and tissue dysfunctions may result from such mechanisms, especially after subacute or chronic exposures (14). Such noncholinergic effects of organophosphorus compounds may result from altered nucleic acid metabolism, enzyme phosphorylation with concomitant modulation of enzyme activity, changes in cell membrane fluidity, or altered membrane phospholipid:cholesterol ratios. Since cell membranes are the site of biologically significant receptors, changes in cell membrane fluidity and/or lipid structure have the potential to disrupt normal protein:lipid relationships, which may cause distinct changes in cell function. These changes would seem to be especially critical for immune cell functions, since many of these parameters are membrane-dependent.

The immunotoxic effects of organophosphorus compounds are reviewed here with the assumption that such effects are most likely mediated by noncholinergic mechanisms. Since few epidemiological data exist to evaluate the immunotoxicity of these chemicals in humans, experimental results derived from the study of animals exposed to organophosphorus compounds are included to demonstrate the potential for immunotoxicity of this chemical class. These animal studies are discussed with the assumption that reasonable and useful extrapolations may be made between animal and human data.

The focus on organophosphorus compounds as putative immunotoxic chemicals began in the 1970's when both scientists and lay authors alerted the public to the potential toxic effects of pesticides (15,16). In fact, soon after the suspected immunotoxicity of the organochlorine pesticide, 1,1,-bis (p-chlorophenyl) 2,2,2-trichloroethane (DDT) was reported in animals, organophosphate pesticides were investigated for their potential immunotoxic effects. Animal studies quickly documented changes in the lymphatic organs in rabbits treated with methylparathion (1.5 mg/kg/day), which included cortical atrophy of the thymus and a reduction in the number of germinal centers in the spleen (17). Tuberculin skin reactivity in methylparathion-treated rabbits showed variable effects, and inconclusive evidence for an effect on tuberculin sensitivity has been derived from the published data (17). Both Desi and Fan were able to demonstrate a decrease in the protective responses to *Salmonella typhimurium* challenge in mice following malathion and methylparathion exposure (18,19). Vijay showed that rats formed reaginic antibodies after immunization with malathion (20). Despite evidence that certain organophosphate pesticides decreased hemagglutination titers, complement levels, and the size of splenic lymphoid follicles (21,22), Koller and colleagues found no effect of leptophos treatment (0 to 500 ppm for 12 weeks) on mouse antibody synthesis in response to sheep red blood cells (23). These workers concluded that each organophosphorus compound had to be evaluated separately, and general conclusions could not be drawn from the study of a single compound. Other investigators have suggested that multiple treatments with diisopropyl phosphorofluoridate decreased the number of plaque-forming cells as well as hemolysin and complement titers

(24). Studies with 0,0-dimethyl S-(N-methylcarbomoylmethyl) phosphorodithioate in rats and mice showed an acute decrease in peripheral blood lymphocytes after a single dose (75 mg/kg), and antibody titers against sheep red blood cells in treated mice were suppressed for approximately 10 days after a single dose (75 mg/kg) of the same chemical (25). More detailed studies of the primary antibody response in the presence of parathion (16 mg/kg) have been performed in mice using sheep red blood cells as the antigen (26). On the basis of these studies, both the time course and the quantitative response of immunoglobulin M (IgM) to sheep red blood cells were observed to be altered after acute exposures to parathion. The peak IgM response was delayed, and the total number of plaque-forming cells was reduced. These authors speculated on the mechanisms by which parathion might mediate its immunosuppressive effects and postulated the following: (a) acetylcholine receptors on lymphocytes and monocytes responding to increased cholinergic activity secondary to organophosphorus-mediated cholinesterase inhibition altered the immune response, (b) organophosphorus-induced increased plasma corticosteroid levels resulted in a steroid-dependent immunosuppression, and (c) membrane-associated esterase inhibition by organophosphorus compounds may cause immunosuppressive effects. Despite the different hypotheses postulated as the mechanism by which organophosphorus compounds alter immune responses, most animal experiments used pesticide doses that cause cholinesterase inhibition. Thus, the role of cholinesterase inhibition in the mediation of immunosuppression remains a viable question.

Few investigations have been performed in animals with respect to organophosphorus-induced hypersensitivity reactions of the skin. In a well-documented study, Magnusson and Kligman demonstrated that malathion was a skin sensitizer when administered to guinea pigs either intradermally in 5% to 10% solutions or topically as 10% solutions (27). Sensitization to this compound was not elicited with the Draize procedure. Malathion was a weak skin sensitizer in guinea pigs but had no effect in BALB/c mice. Additional data have been acquired from human studies. Allergic dermatitis has been observed in many agricultural workers, and the sensitizing agents have been identified as organophosphorus, organochlorine, or carbamate compounds (28). Malathion is the most common organophosphorus compound to which individuals have become sensitized (29).

Even though histamine is not implicated as a primary mediator of the pathological skin response observed in contact dermatitis, there is evidence that the alkylphosphate, pinacolyl methylphosphonofluoridate (soman), causes histamine release from rat peritoneal cells (30). This effect of soman was observed both *in vivo* and *in vitro* and was inhibited by disodium cromoglycate. Diisopropyl fluorophosphate also induced histamine release at 10^{-3} M doses; higher concentrations of diisopropyl fluorophosphate (10^{-2} M) inhibited histamine release both by compound 48/80, a histamine secretagogue, and soman. Soman causes a relatively rapid release of histamine (5 to 10 minutes) when administered *in vitro; in vitro* release reaches a maximum at 30 to 45 minutes. Thus, histamine is an important mediator of soman-induced pathophysiological responses in the rat. The role of histamine release in immunological responses induced by organophosphorus compounds has not been investigated, but it may contribute to the hypersensitivity responses observed with this class of chemicals.

The most detailed animal data concerned with the immunological effects of organophosphorus compounds have come from the laboratories of Imamura and colleagues (31–34). These investigators have focused on O,O,S-trimethyl phosphorothioate (OOS-TMP), an impurity formed during the manufacture and storage of certain pesticides at high temperatures. Such trialkylphosphorothioates have been identified in malathion, fenitrothion, and acephate (35,36). These contaminants are not only toxic but also prevent the metabolism of their parent pesticides by inhibiting carboxylesterase activity (37). Imamura and others have also observed a variety of specific immunotoxic effects of OOS-TMP in C57B1/6 (female) mice and rats treated with various doses of this chemical (0.5 to 80 mg/kg). These findings include (a) a transient decrease in thymus size and total lymphocyte number (38), (b) a dose-dependent inability to generate cytotoxic T lymphocytes (30), (c) a dose-dependent suppression of antibody-secreting cells after challenge with sheep red blood cells (31), (d) an increased nonspecific esterase activity associated with resident peritoneal macrophages from OOS-TMP-treated mice (10 mg/kg) (32), (e) an increase in thymic lymphocyte numbers, thymic weight, response to mitogens, humoral immune responses, and interleukin-2 production after low-dose OOS-TMP treatment (0.5 mg/kg) (31), (f) decreased antigen presentation by OOS-TMP-treated (10 mg/kg) splenic macrophages (40), (g) decreased Ia antigen expression on splenic macrophages of OOS-TMP-treated mice (10 mg/kg) (40), and (h) the release of cytostatic macrokines from OOS-TMP-treated mice (10 mg/kg) (40).

Almost all the investigations of immunotoxic effects in humans have been performed *in vitro*. Lee and colleagues were the first to draw attention to the possible effects of pesticides on human leukocyte function (41). These workers demonstrated in *in vitro* experiments that lymphocyte proliferation to phytohemagglutin was decreased in the presence of organophosphate pesticides (trithion, methyl parathion, ruelene) (41). The degree of suppression was minimal (10% to 19%), and only trithion showed a statistically significant effect ($p<0.025$). Dose-response curves for malathion suppression of tritiated thymidine uptake by lymphocytes showed that a concentration of 3.5×10^{-5} M was required for 50% inhibition. In addition to the effects of these pesticides on lymphocyte proliferation, methyl parathion (10 μM) significantly decreased neutrophil chemotaxis, whereas carbophenothion and ruelene showed lesser degrees of suppression. Subsequently, studies by Hermanowicz and Kossman demonstrated a marked impairment ($p<0.001$) in neutrophil chemotaxis in workers exposed to organophosphates in the manufacturing process (42). In their studies, workers were subdivided into three groups, depending on whether they were employed directly in the production of the pesticides, operated machines to package the final product, or had contact with industrial waste as cleaners. In each worker group, chemotaxis was significantly suppressed, but those directly involved in production showed the greatest suppression of chemotactic activity when compared with unexposed controls. No suppression of chemotaxis to zymosan-activated serum was observed if cells were activated with lipopolysaccharide. A significant decrease in neutrophil adhesion was also observed in all worker groups. Enhancement of neutrophil random migration ($p<0.001$) was observed only in those groups exposed during pesticide production and packaging. Spontaneous nitroblue tetrazolium reduction was significantly increased in these same two groups ($p<0.001$) when compared with controls (no exposure). These functional leukocyte parameters were compared with the incidence of infections in employees, and a significant increase in upper respiratory tract infections (tonsillitis and bronchitis) was documented. Further, the increased prevalence of infection was more significant in those workers who had been employed for the longest times; infections were much more frequent in employees who had been working for more than 10 years compared with those employed for only 2 years or less. No correlations were found between the changes in neutrophil parameters examined and the subjects who manifested an increased frequency of infection. Cholinesterase activity was suppressed in all the groups examined, but the rate of infection did not correlate with the degree of suppression of cholinesterase activity. Further, neither phagocytosis nor the generation of chemotactic factor from workers' sera was impaired, suggesting that a defect in the complement receptor might account for the observed defect in chemotaxis.

Preliminary studies from our laboratories indicate that organophosphorus compounds may cause defects in monocyte complement receptors. Our studies showed a significant decrease in the number of monocytes expressing C3bi receptors as well as the number of receptors on each cell after exposure to triphenyl phosphate (10 μM). When corrected for nonspecific fluorescence, there was a 78% decrease in the number of cells expressing C3bi receptors (Fig. 1).

On the other hand, organophosphates may affect nonimmunological mechanisms, producing an increased susceptibility to infection that may be unrelated to phagocyte dysfunction. For example, organophosphates could impair the function of the mucociliary escalator through alterations in ciliary action or mucus production, which in turn could result in a decrease in the clearance of infectious agents from the tracheobronchial tree. Since cholinesterase activity was decreased in the workers studied, there remains the possibility that altered cholinesterase function might be involved in the regulation of host defense functions. Finally, these studies suggest that the bronchoalveolar macrophage system may be altered by pesticides. Such a hypothesis is not inconsistent with the pulmonary toxicity reported in animals exposed to the malathion impurity, OOS-TMP (43,44).

Recent studies concerned with the mechanism of immunosuppression by an oral gold preparation, triethylphosphine gold (auranofin), evaluated the effects of this compound on natural killer cell activity (45). In these studies, human natural killer cell activity against the human leukemia cell line K562 was enhanced at low concentrations of auranofin (0.005 to 0.075 mg/ml), whereas high concentrations (2.5 to 10 mg/ml) caused a marked suppression of natural killer cell activity. Investigations to determine the mechanism of inhibition of natural killer cell activity determined that the response was not monocyte-dependent and was not abolished by the addition of interferon-gamma or interleukin-2 to the cultures. Further, recognition,

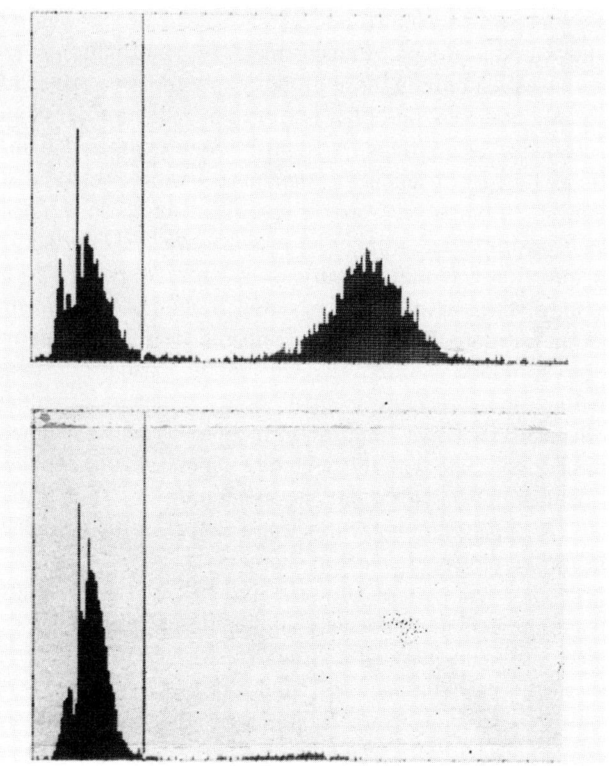

FIG. 1. Analysis of human monoctye C3bi receptor. Pure human peripheral blood monocytes isolated by Ficol-Hypaque and counterflow centrifugation were incubated with a fluorescent-labeled monoclonal antibody Mo1 (CD 16) against human C3bi, and monocyte fluorescence was measured by flow cytometry. Nonspecific fluorescence (6%) was determined by incubating monocytes with an irrelevant monoclonal antibody. **A** shows the results of cells incubated in the absence of organophosphorus compounds, and **B** shows the results of cells incubated with triphenyl phosphate (10 μM). In these diagrams, monocyte cell numbers are plotted on the ordinate and fluorescence intensity is plotted on the abscissa.

adhesion, and conjugation between natural killer cells and their target cells were unaffected by auranofin. Thus, the authors concluded that triethylphosphine gold affected cellular events after binding between the natural killer cell and its target had occurred (45). Unfortunately, these authors did not examine the effects of triethylphosphine on natural killer cell activity. Since some investigations have suggested that the pharmacological activity of auranofin may not be dependent on its gold content, triethylphosphine could represent the active pharmacological component in the mediation of the suppression of natural killer cell activity. Many of the effects of auranofin on inflammatory and immune responses have used triethylphosphine oxide as a control and have observed no significant effect with this compound when compared with auranofin (46). On the other hand, triethylphosphine was not used in natural killer cell experiments, and as far as we know, its effects on this system are unknown (45,47). Even though triethylphosphine is an aliphatic phosphine oxide, it has gross structural similarities to triphenyl phosphate in that both have a trisubstituted phosphoryl moiety. Therefore, it might affect antigen presentation and/or natural killer cell activity. Since serine esterases have been proposed as candidates for the mediation of natural killer cell cytotoxicity (47), a reasonable hypothesis for the effect of triethylphosphine would be the alkylation of serine esterase by either triethylphosphine or a metabolite that would significantly decrease serine esterase activity and suppress esterase-mediated cytotoxicity. This hypothesis does not explain, of course, the documented enhancement of natural killer cell activity at low auranofin concentrations, but it is reasonable to speculate that other pharmacological parameters may be operating at low auranofin concentrations.

Studies from our laboratory have clearly shown that some organophosphorus compounds suppress human natural killer cell activity (Fig. 2). Tetra-o-cresylpiperazinyl diphosphoamidate, triphenylphosphate, and tertiary butyl triphenylphosphate at 20 µM concentrations resulted in a significant suppression of natural killer cell activity ($p<0.001$). Triphenylphosphine oxide and triphenylthiophosphate did not show natural killer cell activity significantly different from that of control values.

In the course of our studies on the immunotoxic effects of organophosphorus

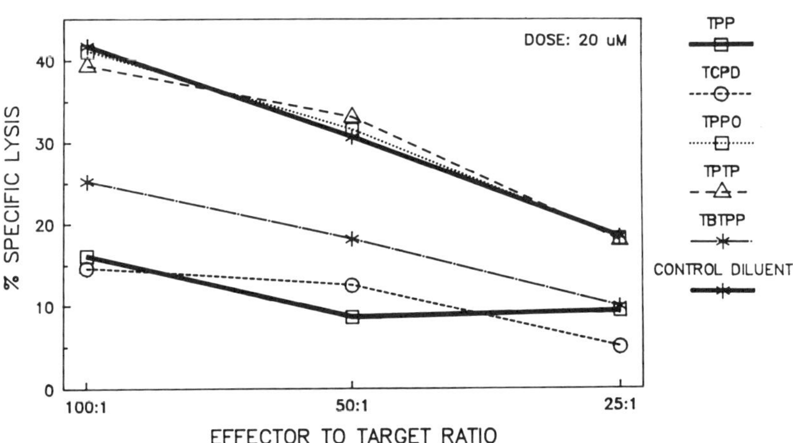

FIG. 2. Effect of organophosphorus compounds on natural killer cell activity. Peripheral blood lymphocytes were isolated by standard procedures and incubated for 1 hour in the presence or absence of organophosphorus compounds. K562 cells were labeled for 1 hour with ^{51}Cr, and graded doses of organophosphorus-treated or control peripheral blood lymphocytes were exposed to target cells for 4 hours. Target cell lysis was measured by the release of radiolabeled chromium after corrections were made for nonspecific release. TPP, triphenyl phosphate; TCPD, tetra-o-cresylpiperazinyl diphosphoamidate; TPPO, triphenylphosphine oxide; TPTP, triphenylthiophosphate; and TBTPP, tertiary butyl triphenylphosphate.

compounds, we sought to identify the primary cellular target for their toxic effects (48). Our data show that those functions less critically dependent on monocytes (mitogenesis) are not as markedly suppressed by organophosphorus compounds as are monocyte-dependent processes such as antigen presentation and antigen (tetanus)-specific lymphoproliferation (48). Experiments designed to evaluate whether the depression in lymphoproliferation is lymphocyte- or monocyte-dependent clearly showed that no significant suppression was observed if lymphocytes were pretreated with tricresylpiperazinyl disphosphoamidate, whereas significant suppression was seen when monocytes were pretreated with the same compound (48). Thus, it appears that the suppression of antigen-specific proliferative responses observed in our studies is a monocyte-specific effect. At present, studies are being performed to determine the mechanisms by which these organophosphorus-mediated alterations in antigen presentation occur. Preliminary data suggest that the expression of class II major histocompatibility complex antigens is not markedly affected by organophosphorus compounds. The effect of organophosphorus compounds was dose-dependent over the range of concentrations tested (0.1 to 20 μM). Further, at 10 μM concentrations, monocyte-nonspecific esterase was significantly inhibited. Even though esterase inhibition has been observed in our studies, we have no direct evidence to implicate this enzyme in the mechanisms by which antigen presentation is impaired. Since the concentrations of organophosphorus compounds causing 50% inhibition of monocyte esterase activity have been determined to be in the range between 1.0 and 10 μM (48), it can be assumed that exposed workers who show a decrease in monocyte esterase activity most likely have circulating concentrations of organophosphorus compounds within this concentration range (49,50). Thus, the esterase inhibition observed *in vitro* provides a reasonable approximation of the *in vivo* dose in exposed work forces (49). A variety of chemicals have been reported to have specific effects on monocyte-dependent accessory cell functions, including leucine methyl ester, gold sodium thiomalate, and 4-aminoquinolones, which are suspected of altering monocyte function either by their lysosomotropic properties or by other more fundamental biochemical parameters (51–53). On the basis of our present data, we suggest that the suppressed, organophosphorus-induced antigen presentation observed by us is probably mediated by a defect in antigen processing that may be related to altered lysosomal activity.

More recent *in vitro* studies have documented diminished spontaneous human monocyte cytotoxicity toward the erythroleukemic K562 cell line in the presence of the organophosphorus agent, bis(4-nitrophenyl)-phosphate (54). These same studies found no alterations in monocyte adhesion, spreading, or phagocytosis after preincubation of human monocytes for 30 minutes with 2.0 mM concentrations of bis(4-nitrophenyl)-phosphate. Spontaneous monocyte cytotoxicity and monocyte binding to K562 cells were shown to be inhibited when high concentrations (10 mM) of bis(4-nitrophenyl)-phosphate were used, whereas lower concentrations (1.0 mM) only impaired cytotoxicity. These studies suggest that monocyte-specific alpha-naphthyl acetate esterases play a role in the spontaneous cytotoxicity of monocytes toward tumor cells. These same investigators were unable to detect any changes in the natural cytotoxicity of lymphocytes toward K562 cells in the presence of bis(4-nitrophenyl)-phosphate. Such findings are in contrast to the data presented here from our laboratories, but the reasons for the differences between our findings and theirs are not clear unless they could be attributed to methodology or effector-to-target ratios. We have now confirmed the impairment of monocyte spontaneous cytotoxicity by organophosphorus compounds other than bis(4-nitrophenyl)-phosphate (55).

To further characterize one monocyte target of organophosphorus agents, we have purified human monocyte carboxylesterase to homogeneity and determined some of its kinetic properties (56). Under nondenaturing conditions, the enzyme was determined to have a molecular weight of approximately 200,000 Daltons, and the pure enzyme protein migrated as a single band on SDS-PAGE with a molecular weight of 60,000 Daltons. Existing data support the concept that the enzyme is a trimer consisting of three monomeric units with estimated molecular weights of 60,000 Daltons each. By isoelectric focusing gel electrophoresis, the enzyme was shown to consist of four isoenzymes with pI values between 7.5 and 7.8. Pure human monocyte carboxylesterase hydrolyzed alpha-naphthyl, ortho-nitrophenyl, and para-nitrophenyl esters, but amide esters and thioesters were not hydrolyzed by the enzyme. Short-chain alcohols (*n*-propanol, *n*-butanol) caused enzyme activation, and organophosphorus compounds, diphenyl carbonate, sodium fluoride, and phenylmethylsulfonyl fluoride inhibited the enzyme. Organophosphorus compounds tested as inhibitors were shown to act in a competitive fashion with enzyme substrates, whereas diphenyl carbonate was found to be a noncompetitive inhibitor. Diisopropyl fluorophosphate bound covalently to the enzyme, whereas the other organophosphorus compounds tested (triphenyl phosphate and tetraphenyl resor cinol diphosphate) did not show covalent bonding but formed tight hydrophobic bonds to the enzyme's active site. On the basis of these findings, we believe monocyte carboxylesterase to be a serine protease with either a serine or a threonine at its active site. We also can document the fact that some organophosphorus compounds do not bind covalently to the enzyme through such amino acids as threonine and serine and that organophosphorus-exposed individuals do not store these compounds through covalent binding to monocyte esterase enzymes.

Our laboratory has also identified at least two membrane localized organophosphorus binding proteins in human monocytes (Fig. 3); one of these binding sites has a molecular weight of 60,000 Daltons and probably represents the monomer of monocyte carboxylesterase, whereas the other has a molecular weight of 25,000 Daltons and its function is unknown. Human lymphocytes also contain diisopropyl fluorophosphate binding sites under the conditions of our experiments (Fig. 3). Such data are consistent with the fact that organophosphorus agents have specificity both for monocyte and lymphocyte functions. In addition, the presence of diisopropyl fluorophosphate binding sites in human neutrophils (Fig. 3) lends credence to the work of Hermanowicz and Kossman (42). Others have characterized

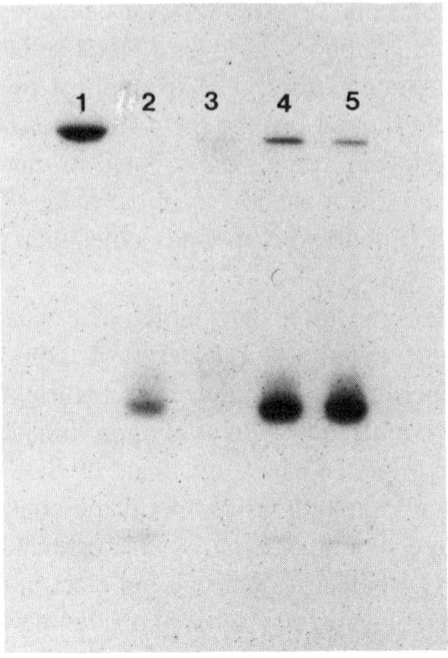

FIG. 3. SDS-polyacrylamide gel electrophoresis (SDS-PAGE) autoradiograph of pure human monocyte carboxylesterase and human neutrophil, lymphocyte, small monocyte, and large monocyte homogenates labeled with [^{3}H] diisopropylfluorophosphate. Human monocyte carboxylesterase (4 μg) was incubated with 1×10^5 cpm of diisopropylfluorophosphate (DFP) for 30 minutes at room temperature. Each cellular homogenate (60 μg) was incubated with 5×10^5 cpm of DFP for 30 minutes at room temperature. The samples were then electrophoresed through SDS-PAGE slabs (12% acrylamide). The gel was fixed, dried, and examined by autoradiography. Exposure time was 5 days. Lane 1 shows the binding activity of pure human monocyte carboxylesterase (60,000 M.W.). Lanes 2,3,4, and 5 show the [^{3}H]-DFP binding for human neutrophil, lymphocyte, small and large monocyte, respectively.

additional organophosphorus-binding proteins in animal macrophages (57). Identification of the function of these organophosphorus-binding proteins is essential to understanding the pathophysiological reactions of this class of chemicals at the cellular level.

These data all suggest that cellular esterases may play an important role in host defense functions. It has recently been shown that serine esterases in large granular lymphocytes (natural killer cells) and cytotoxic T lymphocytes are essential for the killing function of such cells (58–64). Further, organophosphorus compounds such as diisopropyl fluorophosphate have been shown to bind covalently to these serine esterase enzymes, and such binding inhibits the capacity of these cells to perform their killing function (58–64). These data also provide a rational basis for concluding that some esterases play a significant role in the mechanisms by which cells kill other cells.

Since immunosuppression is associated with an increased frequency of certain cancers (65–68), one significant question with respect to the immunosuppression observed with this class of chemicals remains to be answered, namely, the potential mutagenic and/or carcinogenic effects of organophosphorus compounds. Inconclusive results were drawn from the International Agency for Research on Cancer that evaluated the carcinogenic potential of malathion, methyl parathion, parathion, tetrachlorvinphos, and trichlorfon (69). This task force concluded that *little* evidence existed to classify these pesticides as potent mammalian mutagens or carcinogens. Nonetheless, two separate reviews of the carcinogenic properties of malathion and malaoxon have drawn diametrically opposed conclusions regarding the carcinogenicity of these pesticides in rats (70,71). Large numbers of studies in the last decade have been undertaken to evaluate the genotoxic effects of organophosphorus chemicals (72–84) using a variety of test systems, and no clear pattern of mutagenicity or carcinogenicity has emerged. There is no question, however, that specific organophosphorus compounds are carcinogenic and that their metabolites are potent mutagens (73,75). Further, similar studies have been conducted on workers exposed to organophosphorus without conclusive evidence for mutagenicity or carcinogenicity being derived from the data (85–89). Nonetheless, there still remains the potential for mutagenesis and carcinogenesis provoked by organophosphorus compounds, and more direct approaches may be useful, either by seeking DNA or RNA adducts or by documenting significant and prolonged immunosuppression. Particular attention must be directed to careful analyses of population groups, since few epidemiological data are available for migrant workers who are not only exposed to a variety of pesticides but also may be poorly nourished with an associated diet-induced immunosuppression. These occupational settings clearly raise questions concerning possible interactive effects among diet, drugs (steroids), and occupational exposures and mandate that these important scientific initiatives be investigated.

In addition to any direct effects organophosphorus compounds *might* have on the causation of cancer, there is a real possibility that metabolites of parent organophosphorus could contribute to the expression of a carcinogenic response. This fact emphasizes the need for studies of organophosphorus metabolism in humans; such studies are especially relevant to those organophosphorus compounds such as triphenyl phosphate that may be hydrolyzed with the resultant formation of phenol. We have shown that phenol is converted to hydroquinone by human hepatic microsomes (55), and it has been clearly established that both hydroquinone and its closely related byproduct, benzoquinone, can form adducts with DNA (90). Such adduct formation may set the stage for mutations and possibly for the onset of unregulated cell proliferation.

In summary, there is increasing evidence that organophosphorus compounds exert immunosuppressive effects on human as well as animal cell systems. Several important scientific questions remain unanswered, including the clinical expression of individuals exposed to these immunoactive chemicals, the long-term clinical consequences of low-dose, chronic exposures, the possible additive or synergistic effects of these chemicals with pharmacotherapy and/or dietary intake, and most significantly the mechanisms by which these agents cause alterations of the immune system. Although such studies are often looked upon with fear by employer and employee alike, there is the real possibility that some agents in this chemical class may be relatively nontoxic, specific immunoactive agents. In the long term, careful study and evaluation of the immunotoxic potential of these chemicals may unravel their mechanisms of action and facilitate the formulation of nonimmunotoxic derivatives.

REFERENCES

1. Kirk-Othmer Encyclopedia of Chemical Technology (1980): 10:407.
2. Kirk-Othmer Encyclopedia of Chemical Technology (1980): 18:130.
3. Federal Register (1983): 48:57453.
4. Vicedo, J. L., Pellin, M., and Vilanova, E. (1983): Phthalates and organophosphorus compounds as cholinesterase inhibitors in fractions of industrial hexane impurities. *Arch. Toxicol.*, 57:46–52.
5. Laham, S., Long, G. W., and Broxup, B. R. (1985): Subchronic oral toxicity of tributoxyethyl phosphate in the Sprague-Dawley rat. *Arch. Environ. Health*, 40:12–17.
6. Organophosphorus Insecticides: A General Introduction (1986): World Health Organization, Geneva.
7. IARC Working Group (1983): IARC Monographs on the Evaluation of the Carcinogenic Risk of Chemicals to Humans, pp. 103–129. International Agency for Research on Cancer. Lyons, France.
8. Savage, E. P., Keefe, T. J., Wheeler, H. E., et al. (1981): Household pesticide usage in the United States. *Arch. Environ. Health*, 36:304–309.
9. Baltimore Morning Sun (1988 Sept 18): Pesticide silence.
10. U.S. Environmental Protection Agency (1980): Protection of the Environment, pp. 540–541. Code Federal Regulation, Title 40, part 180.11.
11. U.S. Environmental Protection Agency (1980): Malathion: Tolerance and Exemptions from Tolerances for Pesticides Chemicals in or on Agricultural Commodities. Federal Register, 45:76145, 76146.
12. U.S. Food and Drug Administration (1980): Food and Drugs, pp. 374–375, U.S. Code Federal Register, Title 21, part 193.260; part 193.520.
13. U.S. Food and Drug Administration (1980): Food and Drugs, p. 518. U.S. Code Federal Regulation, Title 21, part 561.270.
14. Marquis, J. K. (1985): Noncholinergic mechanisms of insecticide toxicity. *Trends Pharmacol. Sci.*, 6:59–60.
15. Carson, R. (1962): Silent Spring. Boston, Houghton-Mifflin.
16. Ercegovich, C. D. (1973): Relationships of pesticides to immune responses. *Fed. Proc.*, 32:2010–2016.
17. Street, J. C., and Sharma, R. P. (1975): Alteration of induced cellular and humoral immune responses by pesticides and chemicals of environmental concern: Quantitative studies of immunosuppression by DDT, aroclar 1254, carboryl, carbofuran, and methylparathion. *Toxicol. Appl. Pharmacol.*, 32:587–602.
18. Desi, I., Varga, L. and Farkas, I. (1976): Studies on the immunosuppressive effect of organochlorine and organophosphoric pesticides in subacute experiments. *J. Hyg. Epidemiol. Microbiol. Immunol.*, 22:115–127.
19. Street, J. C. (1981): Pesticides and the immune system. In Immunological Considerations in Toxicology, edited by R. P. Sharma, pp. 46–66. CRC Press, Inc., Boca Raton, Florida.
20. Vijay, H. M., Mendoza, C. E., and Lavergne, G. (1978): Production of homocytotropic antibodies (IgE) to malathion in rats. *Toxicol. Appl. Pharmacol.*, 44:137–142.
21. Dinoeva, S. K. (1974): Dynamics of changes in the immune structure of lymphatic follicles of the spleen during pesticide poisoning. *Gig. Sanit.*, 3:85–87.
22. Shtenberg, A. I., Khovaeva, L., and Zavarzin, M. V. (1974): Effect of chlorophos and methylnitrophos on the immune reactions of the organism against the background of protein deficient nutrition. *Vopr. Pitan.*, 4:35–42.
23. Koller, L. D., Exon, J. H., and Roan, J. G. (1976): Immunological surveillance and toxicity in mice exposed to organophosphate pesticide, leptophos. *Environ. Res.*, 12:238–242.
24. Lis, T., and Mierzejewski, J. (1980): Inhibition of immune response by diisopropyl phosphorofluoridate. *Arch. Toxicol. Suppl.*, 4:151–155.

25. Tiefenbach B., and Lange, P. (1980): Studies on the action of dimethoate on the immune system. *Arch. Toxicol. Suppl.*, 4:167–170.

26. Casale, G. P., Cohen, S. D., and DiCapua, R. A. (1984): Parathion-induced suppression of humoral immunity in inbred mice. *Toxicol. Lett.*, 23:239–247.

27. Magnusson, B., and Kligman, A. M. (1970): Allergic Contact Dermatitis in the Guinea Pig. Charles C. Thomas, Springfield, Illinois.

28. Bainova, A. (1982): Dermal absorption of pesticides. In Health Aspects of Chemical Safety, pp. 41–53. Interim Document 9. Toxicology of Pesticides, World Health Organization, Copenhagen.

29. Milby, T. H., and Epstein, W. L. (1964): Allergic contact sensitivity to malathion. *Arch. Environ. Health*, 9:434–437.

30. Newball, H. H., Donlon, M. A., Procell, L. R., et al. (1986): Organophosphate-induced histamine release from mast cells. *J. Pharmacol. Exp. Ther.*, 238:839–845.

31. Rodgers, K. E., Imamura, T., and Devens, B. H. (1985): Effects of subchronic treatment with O,O,S-trimethyl phosphorothioate on cellular and and humoral immune response systems. *Toxicol. Appl. Pharmacol.*, 81:310–318.

32. Rodgers, K. E., Imamura, T., and Devens, B. H. (1985): Investigations into the mechanisms of immunosuppression caused by acute treatment with O,O,S-trimethyl phosphorothioate. I. Characterization of the immune cell population affected. *Immunopharmacology*, 10:171–180.

33. Devens, B. H., Grayson, M. H., Imamura, T., and Rodgers, K. E. (1985): O,O,S-trimethyl phosphorothioate effects on immunocompetence. *Pestic. Biochem. Physiol.*, 24:251–259.

34. Rodgers, K. E., Grayson, M. H., Imamura, T., and Devens, B. H. (1985): *In vitro* effects of malathion and O,O,S-trimethyl phosphorothioate on cytotoxic T lymphocyte responses. *Pestic. Biochem. Physiol.*, 24:260–266.

35. Miles, J. W., Maint, D. L., Starger, M. A., and Teeters, W. R. (1979): S-methyl isomer content of stored malathion and fenitrothion water-dispensable powders and its relationship to toxicity. *J. Agric. Food Chem.*, 27:421–425.

36. Umetsu, N., Grose, F. H., Allahgari, R., et al. (1977): Effect of impurities on mammalian toxicity of technical malathion and acephate. *J. Agric. Food Chem.*, 25:946–953.

37. Mallipudi, N. M., Talcott, R. E., Ketterman, A., and Fukuto, T. R. (1980): Properties and inhibition of rat malathion carboxyesterases. *J. Toxicol. Environ. Health*, 6:585–596.

38. Hammond, P. S., Braunstein, H., Kennedy, J. M., et al. (1982): Mode of action delayed toxicity of O,O,S-trimethyl phosphorothioate in the rat. *Pestic. Biochem. Physiol.*, 18:77–82.

39. Rogers, K. E., Leung, N. Imamura, T., and Ware, C. F. (1986): Time-course study of immune modulation following acute O,S,S-trimethyl phosphorothioate (OSS-TMP) administration. *Fed. Proc.*, 45:329.

40. Rodgers, K. E., Imamura, T., and Devens, B. H. (1985): Investigations into the mechanism of immunosuppression caused by acute treatment with O,O,S-trimethyl phosphorothioate. II. Effect on the ability of murine macrophages to present antigen. *Immunopharmacology*, 10:181–189.

41. Lee, T. P., Moscati, R., and Park, B. H. (1979): Effects of pesticides on human leukocytes functions. *Res. Commun. Chem. Pathol. Pharmacol.*, 23:597–609.

42. Hermanowicz, A., and Kossman, S.: Neutrophil function and infectious disease in workers occupationally exposed to phosphoorganic pesticides: Role of mononuclear-derived chemotatic factor for neutrophils. *Clin. Immunol. Immunopathol.*, 33:13–22.

43. Imamura, T., and Thomas, I. K.: Alterations of alveolar macrophage function and level of bronchopulmonary protease inhibitors in O,O,S-trimethyl phosphorothioate-induced lung injury. *Toxicology*, 37:79–89.

44. Aldridge, W. N., and Nemery, B. (1984): Toxicology of trialkylphosphorothioates with particular reference to lung toxicity. *Fund. Appl. Toxicol.*, 4:5215–5223.

45. Pedersen, B. K., and Abom, B. (1986): Characterization of the in vitro effect of triethylphosphine gold (auranofin) on human NK cell activity. *Clin. Exp. Rheumatol.*, 4:249–253.

46. Walz, D. T., Dimartino, J. J., Griswold, D. E., et al. (1983): Biological actions and pharmokinetic studies of auranofin. *Am. J. Med.*, 75:90–108.

47. Russel, A. S., Davis, P., and Miller, C. (1982): The effect of a new antirheumatic drug, triethylphosphine gold (auranofin) on in vitro lymphocyte and monocyte cytotoxicity. *J. Rheumatol.*, 9:30–35.

48. Esa, A. H., Warr, G. A., and Newcombe, D. S. (1988): Immunotoxicity of organophosphates: Modulation of cell-mediated responses mediated through inhibition of monocyte accessory functions. *Clin. Immunol. Immunopathol.*, 49:41–52.

49. Emmett, E. A., Lewis, P. G., Tamaka, F., et al. (1985): Industrial exposure to organophosphorus compounds: Studies of a group of workers with a decrease in esterase staining monocytes. *J. Occup. Med.*, 27:905–914.

50. Levine, M., Fox, N., Thompson, W., et al. (1986): Inhibition of esterase activity and an undercounting of circulating monocytes in a population of production workers. *J. Occup. Med.*, 28:207–211.

51. Thiele, D. L. (1983): Phenotype of the accessory cell for mitogen-stimulated T and B cell responses in human peripheral blood: Delineation by its sensitivity to the lysosomotropic agent, L-leucine methyl ester. *J. Immunol.*, 131:2282–2290.

52. Salmeron, G., and Lipsky, P. E. (1983): Immunosuppressive potential of antimalarials. *Am. J. Med.*, 75:19–24.

53. Lipsky, P. E., and Ziff, M. (1977): Inhibition of antigen- and mitogen-induced human lymphocyte proliferation by gold compounds. *J. Clin. Invest.*, 59:455–466.

54. Oertel, J., Hagner, G., Kastner, M., and Huhn, D. (1985): The relevance of alphanaphthyl acetate esterases to various monocyte functions. *Br. J. Haematol.*, 61:717–726.

55. Newcombe, D. S. (1990): Unpublished observations.

56. Saboori. A. M., and Newcombe, D. S. (1990): Human monocyte carboxylesterase. Purification and kinetics. *J. Biol. Chem.*, 265:19792–19799.

57. Heck, Louis W., Remold-O'Donnell, E., and Remold, H. G. (1978): DFP-sensitive polypeptides of the guinea pig peritoneal macrophage. *Biochem. Biophys. Res. Commun.*, 83:1576–1583.

58. Hameed, A., Lowrey, D. M., Lichtenheld, M., and Podack, E. R.: Characterization of three serine esterases isolated from human IL-2 activated killer cells. *J. Immunol.*, 141:3142–3147.

59. Masson, D., Nabholz, M., Estrade, C., and Tschapp, J. (1986): Granules of cytolytic T-lymphocytes contain two serine esterases. EMBO J., 5:1595–1600.

60. Simon, M. M., Haschutzky, H., Fruth, U., Simon, H-G, and Kramer, M. D. (1986): Purification and characterization of a T cell specific serine proteinase (TSP-1) from a cloned cytolytic T lymphocyte. EMBO J., 5:3267–3274.

61. Young, J. D-E., Leong, L. G., Liu, C-C., Damiano, A., Wall, D. A., and Cohn, Z. A. (1986): Isolation and characterization of a serine esterase from cytolytic T cell granules. *Cell*, 47:183–194.

62. Hudig, D., Redelman, D., and Minning, L. L. (1984): The requirement for proteinase activity for human lymphocyte-mediated natural cytotoxicity (NK): Evidence that the proteinase is serine dependent and has aromatic amino acid specificity of cleavage. *J. Immunol.*, 133:2647–2654.

63. Pasternak, M. S., and Eisen, H. N. (1985): A novel serine esterase expressed by cytotoxic T lymphocytes. *Nature*, 314:743–745.

64. Young, J. D.-E, and Liu, C-C (1988): Multiple mechanisms of lymphocyte-mediated killing. *Immunol. Today*, 9:140–144.

65. Penn, I. (1978): Malignancies associated with immunosuppressive or cytotoxic therapy. *Surgery*, 83:492–502.

66. Penn, I. (1978): Tumors arising in organ transplant recipients. In Advances in Cancer Research, vol. 28, edited by G. Klein and S. Weinhouse. Academic Press, New York.

67. Penn, I. (1982): The occurrence of cancer in immune deficiencies. *Curr. Probl. Cancer*, 6:1–64.

68. Penn, I. (1985): Neoplastic consequences of immunosuppression. In Immunotoxicology and Immunopharmacology, edited by J. H. Dean, M. I. Luster, A. E. Munson, and H. Amos. Raven Press, New York.

69. International Agency for Research on Cancer (1983): Miscellaneous chemicals. Monographs on the Carcinogenic Risk of Chemicals to Humans, vol. 30. Lyons, International Agency for Research on Cancer.

70. Huff, J. E., Bates, R., Estis, S. L., et al. (1985): Malathion and malaoxon: Histopathology reexamination of the National Cancer Institute's carcinogenesis studies. *Environ. Res.*, 37:154–173.

71. Reuber, M. D. (1985): Carcinogenicity and toxicity of malathion and malaoxon. *Environ. Res.*, 37:119–153.

72. Georgian, L. (1975): The comparative cytogenic effects of aldrin and phosphamidon. *Mut. Res.*, 31:103–108.

73. Rocchi, P., Perocco, P., Alberghini, W., et al. (1980): Effect of pesticides on scheduled and unscheduled DNA synthesis of rat thymocytes and human lymphocytes. *Arch. Toxicol.*, 45:101–108.

74. Chen, H. H., Hsueh, J. L., Sirianni, S. R., and Huang, C. C. (1981): Induction of sister-chromatid exchanges and cell cycle delay in cultured membrane cells treated with eight organophosphorus pesticides. *Mut. Res.*, 88:307–316.

75. Sobti, R. C., Krishan, A., and Pfaffenberger, C. D. (1982): Cytokinetic and cytogenetic effects of some agricultural chemicals on human lymphoid cells in vitro: Organophosphates. *Mut. Res.*, 102:89–102.
76. Degraeve, N., and Montschen, J. (1984): Genetic and cytogenetic effects induced in the mouse by an organophosphorus insecticide: Malathion. *Environ. Res.*, 34:170–174.
77. Holme, J. A., Soderlund, E. J., Hongslo, J. K., et al. (1983): Comparative genotoxicity studies of the flame retardant Tris (2,3-dibromopropyl) phosphate and possible metabolites. *Mut. Res.*, 124:213–224.
78. Grover, I. S., and Malhi, P. K. (1985): Genotoxic effects of some organophosphorus pesticides. I. Induction of micronuclei in bone marrow cells in rat. *Mut. Res.*, 155:131–134.
79. Soderlund, E. J., Dybing, E., Holme, J. A., et al. (1985): Comparative genotoxicity and nephrotoxicity studies of two halogenated flame retardants Tris (1,3-dichloro-2-propyl) phosphate and Tris (2,3-dibromopropyl) phosphate. *Acta Pharmacol. Toxicol.*, 56:20–29.
80. Imamura, T., and Talcott, R. E. (1985): Mutagenic and akylating activities of organophosphate impurities of commercial malathion. *Mut. Res.*, 155:1–6.
81. Tzoneva, M., Kappas, A., Georgieva, V., et al. (1985): On the genotoxicity of the pesticides. Endodan and Kilicar in 6 different test systems. *Mut. Res.*, 157:13–22.
82. Nelson, S. D., Omichinski, J. G., Iyer, L., et al. (1984): Activation mechanism of Tris (2,3,-dibromopropyl) phosphate to the potent mutagen, 2-bromoacrolein. *Biochem. Biophys. Res. Commun.*, 121:213–219.
83. Prival, M. J., McCoy, E. C., Gutter, B., and Rosenkranz, H. S. (1977): Tris (2,3-dibromopropyl) phosphate: Mutagenicity of a widely used flame retardant. *Science*, 195:76–78.
84. Soderlund, E. J., Nelson, S. D., and Dybing, E. (1979): Mutagenic activation of tris (2,3-dibromopropyl) phosphate: The role of microsomal oxidative metabolism. *Acta Pharmacol. Toxicol.*, 45:112–121.
85. Dulont, F. N., Pastori, M. C., Olivero, O. A., et al. (1985): Sister-chromatid exchanges and chromosomal aberrations in a population exposed to pesticides. *Mut. Res.*, 143:237–244.
86. Van Bao, T., Szabo, I., Ruzicska, P., and Czeize, A. (1974): Chromosome aberrations in patients suffering acute organic phosphate insecticide intoxication. *Hum. Genet.*, 24:33–57.
87. Stocbo, R. de C., Becak, W., Gaeta, R., and Rabello-Gay, M. N. (1982): Cytogenetic studies of workers exposed to methyl parathion. *Mut. Res.*, 103:71–76.
88. Kiraly, J., Szentesi, I., Ruzicska, M., and Czeize, A. (1979): Chromosone studies in workers producing organophosphate insecticides. *Arch. Environ. Contam. Toxicol.*, 8:309–319.
89. Yoder, J., Watson, M., and Benson, W. W. (1973): Lymphocyte chromosome analysis of agricultural workers during extensive occupational exposure of pesticides. *Mut. Res.*, 21:335–340.
90. Jowa, L., Winkle, S., Kalf, G., Witz, G., and Snyder, R. (1986): Deoxyguanosine adducts formed from benzoquinone and hydroquinone. *Adv. Exp. Med. Biol.*, 197:825–832.

Clinical Immunotoxicology, edited by
D. S. Newcombe, N. R. Rose, and J. C. Bloom.
Raven Press, Ltd., New York © 1992.

18

Environmental Chemicals with Immunotoxic Properties

Ali M. Saboori and David S. Newcombe

*Department of Environmental Health Sciences, Johns Hopkins University,
School of Hygiene and Public Health, Baltimore, MD*

INTRODUCTION

The immune system is an extremely complex organization of cells and organs designed to provide host defenses against infectious organisms, toxic foreign substances, and altered cells. The immunity developed against these harmful agents may be either inherited (natural immunity) or acquired. Further, acquired immunity may be based either on antibodies (humoral immunity) or dependent on T-cell–mediated reactions (cell-mediated immunity).

Although organs such as the spleen, thymus, liver, and lymphatic system play a major role in immune functions, it is the bone marrow, with its pluripotent cells, and the peripheral blood leukocytes that are the primary targets of immunotoxic agents, and the most well-characterized effects of such agents are on the surface membranes of immune cells essential for the recognition and elimination of foreign substances threatening to the host. Immunosuppression has been the major effect of environmental chemicals, but autoimmune and hypersensitivity responses are also known to occur in association with exposure to environmental chemicals.

Most studies evaluating the sensitivity of the immune system to environmental chemicals have been performed in animals. Human immunotoxic effects are incompletely documented at the present time, but the potential for damage to the human immune system remains a serious environmental problem. Animal studies remain as useful models to determine under what conditions human immunotoxicity might occur. Further, host defense functions are much more readily evaluated in animals than in humans. Animals that are either congenitally immunodeficient or depleted of specific blood cell types are easily challenged with infectious organisms or tumor cells and monitored for the development of disease. Such immunoaltered animals can also be exposed to environmental chemicals and subsequently challenged with microorganisms or tumor cells to assess the time and dose effects of such chemicals. Further, animal models permit the development of defined test panels to assess immunosuppression and immune enhancement such as have been devised by the National. Toxicology Program.

In reviewing the immunotoxic potential of environmental chemicals, it may be useful to read the early reviews describing their immunosuppressive effects of environmental chemicals (1,2) and to understand the mechanisms by which immunosuppressive agents can be correlated with the loss of a specific subpopulation of immune cells and/or their functions (3,4).

In this chapter, we review those environmental chemicals known to be immunotoxic in animals and their mechanism of action, when known. We also characterize human immunotoxic responses to environmental chemicals in selected instances in which sufficient experimental data exist.

Aromatic Hydrocarbons

The aromatic hydrocarbons represent a most important class of commercial and environmental chemicals, since they are produced in large volume and the possibilities for exposure are widespread. Further, the prototypic molecule for this group, benzene, is a known human leukemogen. In 1980, more than 5×10^6 tons of benzene were produced in the United States, and more than 2×10^6 workers were exposed to this toxic chemical. Human exposures from personal activities such as active and passive smoking, use of consumer products containing benzene, and exposure to motor vehicle exhaust appear to be equally important sources of benzene exposure as those well-characterized occupational exposures from pumping gasoline, employment in chemical plants, and other commercial sources. Even food, water, and other beverages may contain benzene, as the recent Perrier water contamination illustrates. The highest public health priority in relation to benzene is the control of exposure, so that a clear reduction in occupationally related and incidental exposure completely erases those cancers associated with this simple organic molecule. Leukemia, aplastic anemia, multiple myeloma, lymphoma, and perhaps lung cancer have all been implicated as diseases that can be associated with benzene exposures. Since immunotoxicity may play a role in the development of cancer, the toxic effects and mechanism of action of benzene and toluene on the immune system take on added significance.

Benzene is the simplest aromatic hydrocarbon, and it occurs naturally in petroleum, fruits, fish, vegetables, nuts, dairy products, beverages, eggs, cooked chicken, and heat-treated or canned beef (5,6). Benzene levels between 150 and 204 mg/m^3 of cigarette smoke have been reported as a byproduct of cigarette smoking (7). This simple aromatic ring compound is used as an intermediate in the manufacture of other chemicals, and it has also been used as a solvent to increase the octane rating of unleaded gasoline. Benzene has also been used in industry for the preparation of benzene ring derivatives, including polymers, detergents, pesticides, and other intermediates for use in chemical and pharmaceutical processes such as the preparation of chlorinated solvents, the manufacture of rubber cements, adhesives, and printing inks, and as a degreasing and cleaning agent (8). Because of its lipophilic properties and its production of biologically reactive intermediates through metabolic biotransformations (9,10), benzene poses a significant health problem for both the general public and industrial workers.

Benzene exposure in rabbits, rats, and mice results in anemia, hypoplastic bone marrow, and lymphocytopenia. Benzene metabolism, which is required for its toxicity, occurs predominantly in the liver, but bone marrow can also metabolize benzene. In the liver, the major metabolite of benzene, phenol, is converted to secondary metabolites, hydroquinone and catechol (11,12). Phenol and hydroquinone can be transported from the liver to the bone marrow, where they may be metabolized by a peroxidase-mediated pathway (13,14) to form p-benzoquinone via the semiquinone radical (15).

Benzene at a dose of 440 mg/kg body weight for 3 days reduces antibody production to bacterial antigens in both rabbits and C57Bl/6 mice (16). In mice, cell-mediated immunity is enhanced at a low dose (31 mg/L) of benzene but suppressed at high doses (166 to 790 mg/L) of benzene (17). Lymphocytes are particularly sensitive to benzene toxicity via inhalation. Benzene inhalation (300 ppm) results in a significant depression in the number of B lymphocytes in the bone marrow and spleen of C57Bl/6 mice (18). Benzene increases the permeability of lymphocyte lysosomal membranes, which releases lysosomal enzymes into the cytoplasm, causing a decrease in the number of both B and T lymphocytes (18,19). Benzene (300 ppm) also reduces the number of T lymphocytes in the thymus and spleen of C57Bl/6 mice (18). Proliferation and maturation of lymphocyte progenitor cells are regulated by polypeptide lymphokines, which are produced both *in vivo* and *in vitro* by T lymphocytes. Benzene, if metabolized in lymphocytes to intermediates such as p-benzoquinone could inhibit the production of lymphokines. Exposure to p-benzoquinone completely inhibits the proliferation of mouse T cell and the production of T-cell lymphokines by concanavalin A-stimulated lymphocytes (20).

In the bone marrow, benzene or its metabolites are cytotoxic for hematopoietic progenitor and stromal cells. This may be a significant factor in benzene-induced myelosuppression (21). Benzene and its metabolites have been shown to inhibit both nuclear and mitochondrial replication and transcription. DNA synthesis is also inhibited in hematopoietic cells from mice exposed to a single dose of 3,000 ppm benzene (22). In *in vitro* experiments, DNA replication in rabbit bone marrow mitochondria is inhibited in a dose-dependent manner by the benzene metabolites hydroquinone, p-benzoquinone, and 1,2,4-benzenetriol, as evidence by the inhibition of [³H]dTTP incorporation into the characteristic mitochondrial replication intermediates (23). *In vitro* transcription of mouse lymphocytes (20) and macrophages (24) is inhibited, in a dose-dependent manner, by the benzene metabolites phenol, hydroquinone, and p-benzoquinone. Translation is also inhibited subsequent to the inhibition of RNA synthesis. Phenol is further metabolized in macrophages by a peroxidase to a reactive species that inhibit RNA synthesis and covalently bind to macromolecules. Benzene also inhibits RNA synthesis by infiltrating the plasma membrane and preventing the transport of uridine into the cells (25). Thus, the immunosuppressive effects of benzene and its metabolites occur by inhibiting lymphocyte DNA, RNA, and protein synthesis.

Epidemiological studies have shown that workers exposed to benzene have lower levels of serum complement, IgG, and IgA but not IgM when compared to nonexposed individuals (26). These data provide suggestive clinical evidence that the immune system is altered in humans exposed to benzene.

In summary, the main toxicological targets of benzene are hematopoietic cells. Benzene suppresses humoral and cell-mediated immunity and reduces the number of B and T cells in the bone marrow, thymus, and spleen. On the basis of animal studies, bone marrow function as well as humoral and cell-mediated immune responses should be carefully monitored in humans exposed to benzene.

Toluene is another commonly used aromatic hydrocarbon. It is produced in large quantities and is used primarily as a solvent. Toluene is present in gasoline, and it is also used in the production of benzene and other chemicals such as benzoic acid, nitrotoluenes, dyes, pharmaceuticals, food additives, and plastics. Besides being present in organic chemicals, toluene is also used in many consumer products, including household aerosols, paints, varnishes, rust preservatives, adhesives, glue, flame-retardant chemicals, and solvent-based cleaning and sanitizing agents (27). Hence, such broad industrial and home applications increase the risk of toluene exposure to both industrial workers and the general public.

Toluene exposure at a dose of 4,000 ppm is reported to produce a variety of symptoms in humans and experimental animals, such as kidney and liver damage and various neurological disorders (28,29). In addition, toluene at a dose of 1,000 mg/m^3 has been shown to be embryotoxic in rats, mice, and rabbits (30,31).

The immunosuppressive effects of toluene are somewhat less than those of benzene, and only high concentrations of toluene (105 mg/kg/day) for 4 weeks suppress antibody production in mice (32). Treatment of mice with toluene at this high dose level also reduces interleukin-2 production by T lymphocytes. Since interleukin-2 is produced by helper T cells following stimulation with mitogens, toluene suppresses the function of T-helper cells (32). Low concentrations of toluene (17 mg/L) administered in drinking water for 4 weeks suppress murine cell-mediated immunity.

Toluene immunotoxicity, like benzene immunotoxicity, has been attributed to the formation of various reactive intermediates. *In vivo* and *in vitro* studies have indicated that toluene via oxidation of its aromatic ring is activated to give reactive intermediates that bind to biological macromolecules (33). Cresol is such an intermediate formed by the aromatic oxidation of toluene through an arene oxide intermediate that binds to biomacromolecules. Other reactive intermediates of toluene are superoxide anions that are produced during the oxidation of cresol to form secondary metabolites such as semiquinones and quinones. Benzene metabolites such as phenol also bind to biomacromolecules (24). The covalent binding capacity of toluene intermediates to biomacromolecules is much lower than what is observed with benzene intermediates, and this difference might explain the immunosuppressive effect of toluene, which is lower than that of benzene.

In summary, toluene suppresses humoral immunity, cell-mediated immunity, and interleukin-2 production by T lymphocytes at lower doses than those that cause nephrotoxicity, liver damage, and embryotoxicity in the experimental animals. On the basis of animal studies, humoral and cell-mediated immune responses as well as interleukin-2 production by T-helper cells should be monitored in toluene-exposed populations.

Polyhalogenated Aromatic Hydrocarbons

Polyhalogenated aromatic hydrocarbons are commonly used as heat transfer media in transformers as well as in the formulation of pesticides and fire retardants. They are also generated during the manufacture of phenols and biphenyls and occur as byproducts of incineration. Isomers of polyhalogenated hydrocarbons manifest a variety of toxic responses, including carcinogenicity, hepatotoxicity, teratogenicity, neurotoxicity, and immunotoxicity. Immunotoxic effects are observed with chlorinated dibenzo-*p*-dioxins, dibenzofurans, polychlorinated biphenyls (PCBs), polybrominated biphenyls (PBBs), and hexachlorobenzene. These same groups of compounds are also carcinogenic.

Polychlorinated Dibenzo-*p*-Dioxins and Polychlorinated Dibenzofurans

Polychlorinated dibenzo-*p*-dioxins (PCDDs) and polychlorinated dibenzofurans (PCDFs) are tricyclic aromatic compounds with multiple positional isomers, since the number of halogen atoms can vary between one and eight. The structures of two representative molecules of each chemical class are shown in Fig. 1. These complex chlorinated or brominated molecules are stable even with heating to high temperatures (700°C). In polar solutions, the solubility and volatility of these compounds increase as the number of halogen substitutions decreases. The most extensively studied PCDD is 2,3,7,8-tetrachlorodibenzo-*p*-dioxin (TCDD). TCDD is an extraordinarily potent teratogen (34) and carcinogen (35). It also serves as the prototype for a large series of halogenated aromatic hydrocarbon stereoisomers, all of which produce similar toxic effects and elicit common biochemical responses (36). 2,3,7,8-Tetrachlorodibenzofuran (TCDF) is a PCDF that shares the same magnitude of toxicity as TCDD.

PCDDs and PCDFs are commonly detected in the emissions from the combustion of municipal and industrial wastes and are components of the exhaust emissions from diesel and petrol-fueled vehicles (37). No matter what the source of these compounds, they are often found with other substances such as PBBs, chlorinated phenols, and polychlorinated tetraphenyls as well as phenoxyacetic acid herbicides. Very small amounts of PCDDs and PCDFs have also been detected in cigarette smoke and charcoal-grilled steaks (38), and they are produced as unwanted byproducts from the manufacture of a number of commercially available industrial and agricultural chemicals such as chlorophenols used as fungicides, herbicides, slimicides, and chlorinated aromatic hydrocarbons. TCDD is also a contaminant in

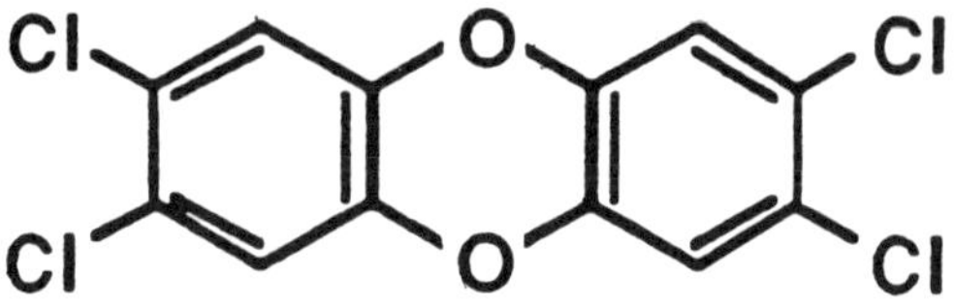

2,3,7,8-tetrachlorodibenzo-p-dioxin

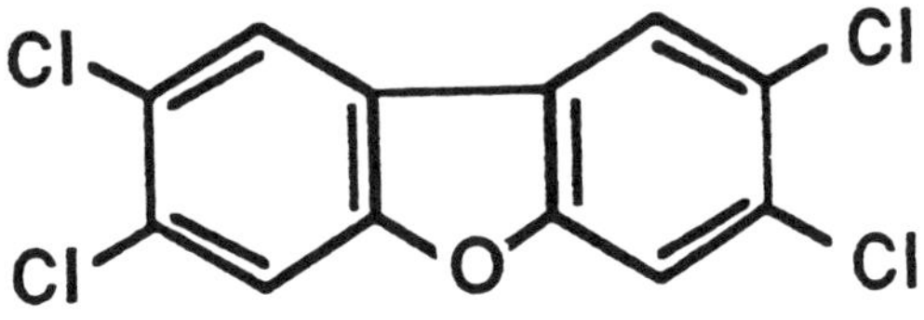

2,3,7,8-tetrachlorodibenzofuran

FIG. 1. Representative polychlorinated dibenzo-p-dioxins and polychlorinated dibenzofurans compounds.

the production of 2,4,5-trichlorophenoxyacetic acid, a herbicide, which has been associated with occupational chloracne in workers employed in the manufacture of these compounds (39). PCBs (commercial Aroclors) also contain high levels of PCDFs (40).

In animals, the adsorption of 2,3,7,8-TCDD via the gastrointestinal tract and skin is dependent on the carrying agent (41). This compound is concentrated in the fat stores, muscle, and skin in monkeys and guinea pigs, but the liver is the primary site of TCDD deposition in other animals (42). Liver concentrations of PCDDs and PCDFs are dependent on the degree of chlorination. Increasing chlorination causes greater hepatic concentration. In general metabolites of these compounds are less toxic than the parent compound.

Acute TCDD toxicity is manifested by weight loss, thymic atrophy, and gastrointestinal hemorrhage (43). The thymic atrophy primarily affects the cortex of the gland, and death caused by TCDD usually occurs a month or more after the initial exposure. The LD_{50} values for animals receiving 2,3,7,8-TCDD by gavage ranges from 0.6 μg kg^{-1} in Hartley guinea pigs (the most susceptible species) to about 5 mg kg^{-1} in the golden Syrian hamster (41).

Subacute TCDD toxicity has been studied in Sprague Dawley rats who have received this chemical by gavage in various doses (0.01 μg kg^{-1} day^{-1} to 1 μg kg^{-1} day^{-1}, administered 5 days/week) for 13 weeks (44). No effect is observed with a total dose of 0.65 μg kg^{-1}, whereas the highest dose levels cause weight loss, hepatic abnormalities, increased urinary porphyrin levels, and thymus involution. Females are more sensitive to the effect of TCDD than are males. Lesions similar to the chloracne observed in humans after dioxin exposure have been produced in the skin of hairless mice and in the ears of rabbits exposed to TCDD (34,45).

Chronic toxicity of PCDDs results primarily in hepatic dysfunctions in rodents, whereas in monkeys, chronic TCDD administration leads to a hypocellular bone marrow with its attendant hematological manifestations, widespread epithelial hypertrophy, skin abnormalities, and gastritis and ulceration (46). Thus, immune dysfunctions may be a part of acute, subacute, and chronic TCDD toxicity. In acute and subacute toxicity, thymus involution and its associated immunological defects account for TCDD-induced immunotoxicity, whereas in chronic TCDD toxicity, hypocellular bone marrow and its accompanying pancytopenia are likely to compromise host defense functions.

The detection of increased urinary porphyrins is a key biomarker of halogenated hydrocarbon exposure, since TCDD, hexachlorobenzene, and other compounds in this chemical family inhibit hepatic uroporphyrinogen decarboxylase activity (47,48). This metabolic alteration creates a clinical syndrome like porphyria cutanea tarda. Two major epidemics of environmentally induced porphyria have been documented. One occurred after the ingestion of wheat contaminated with the fungicide, hexachlorobenzene, and the other was the result of TCDD contamination of an industrial factory producing 2,4,5-tri-phenoxytrichloroacetic acid (48). Unfortunately, immunological parameters were not examined in either of these exposed populations, and therefore no correlations can be drawn between the induction of a toxic porphyria and immune dysfunction. Nonetheless, halogenated hydrocarbon exposures can often be monitored by measurements of urinary porphyrins, and *in vitro* and *in vivo* immune assessment can readily be undertaken in such populations if the opportunity arises.

Thymic involution/atrophy is one of the most consistent immunotoxic expressions of TCDD and related compounds. Such changes are especially pronounced in the cortex of the gland and are associated with the depletion of lymphocytes. As might be expected with such alterations, both humoral and cell-mediated immune dysfunctions result from such exposures. For the most part, the immunotoxic effects of PCDDs parallel the affinity of such compounds for the Ah receptor and for aryl hydrocarbon hydroxylase inducibility. Such a rationale has been derived from experiments in which Ah-responsive and Ah-unresponsive mice strains were shown to express differences in the numbers of hemolytic plaque-forming cells (49). In Ah-responsive mice (C3H/HeN and C57BL/6), the number of plaque-forming cells produced after TCDD administration (1 to 2 µg/kg/day for 7 days) was significantly reduced. A much higher dose of TCDD (30 µg/kg/day) was required to elicit the same response in nonresponsive (DBA/2) mice. TCDF (180 µg/kg) also reduces humoral immune responses in C57BL/6 mice but not in DBA/2 mice. Depressed antibody responses and suppressed cell-mediated immunity have also been observed in guinea pigs after TCDD and TCDF treatment (50,51). The dose of TCDF required to elicit such responses is tenfold higher than that used to induce identical changes with TCDD. Such altered immune responses are detected in the absence of overt signs of generalized toxicity, which makes monitoring of immune responses in exposed populations essential if correlations between health effects and exposure are to be documented.

TCDD and related halogenated aromatic hydrocarbons such as TCDF produce a pattern of toxic responses similar to that observed with polyaromatic hydrocarbons through the induction of a variety of enzymes, including aryl hydrocarbon hydroxylase. These aromatic hydrocarbons bind reversibly with high affinity to a cytosolic protein (dioxin or Ah receptor) that is the receptor for this inductive response. The ligand-receptor complex is then passed through the nuclear membrane and binds to DNA (52). Binding of this complex to DNA alters the rate of gene translation of enzyme protein and other macromolecules, possibly in the promoter and inhibitor regions (53), which are ultimately responsible for the enhanced expression of these enzymes. These regulatory sequences are called enhancer sequences. Nucleotide fragments with such properties are termed xenobiotic regulatory elements or drug regulatory elements (54–57). The physical properties of the steroid receptor and those of the TCDD receptor are similar, since both receptors interact with polyanions and their cytoplasmic components are linked to heat shock proteins (58–63). Some have even suggested that TCDD receptors belong to the family of genes associated with steroid receptors (64). Such an association may link steroid activity, TCDD receptors, and immunoregulation. TCDD also acts on selected targets within the immune system to produce thymic atrophy, suppressed cellular immunity, and inhibition of antibody production to T-lymphocyte–dependent antigens. The number of Ah receptors in murine liver, kidney, thymus, lung, and heart has been measured, and the thymus and lung have been found to express the highest concentrations of this receptor (65). This suggests that these tissues may be the most sensitive to TCDD. TCDD also alters murine thymic epithelial cells, which causes defective thymus-dependent maturation of T-lymphocyte precursors. This response is mediated through cell-cell contacts between thymocytes and thymic epithelial cells (66).

The mediation of the effects of TCDD and related compounds by the Ah receptor and the subsequent modification of gene expression represent a mechanism similar to that observed with steroid hormones whose cell receptor and ligand receptor complexes trigger altered gene expression. Since the effects of TCDD on the thymus are indistinguishable from those observed with glucocorticoid treatment, investigations have been undertaken to determine whether TCDD induces its immunotoxicity by a glucocorticoid-dependent process.

Glucocorticoids are known to induce programmed cell death in immature thymocytes by activating an endogenous nuclear endonuclease that splits the host DNA into oligonucleosome-sized fractions, resulting in cell death (67,68). Such glucocorticoid-induced fragmentation of DNA is dependent on elevated intracellular calcium concentrations that appear to be rate-limiting in this process of programmed cell death (69). TCDD treatment of intact animals results in the disappearance of those thymocytes sensitive to glucocorticoid-induced programmed cell death (70). Thus, both glucocorticoid-induced and TCDD-induced thymocyte cell death are dependent on a subpopulation of immature thymocytes. Indeed, TCDD potentiates glucocorticoid-induced thymocyte depletion and death. Since calcium ionophores also stimulate thymocyte subpopulation cell death by a glucocorticoid-independent pathway (71–73), experiments have been done to determine whether TCDD alters the sensitivity to calcium ionophore treatment. TCDD treatment has been found to deplete both glucocorticoid- and A23187-sensitive thymocytes. Further, TCDD treatment potentiates glucocorticoid-induced DNA fragmentation. Experiments also show that depletion of extracellular calcium or blocking of intracellular calcium mobilization prevents thymocyte fragmentation (69,74). TCDD potentiated glucocorticoid-induced DNA fragmentation but did not potentiate A23187-induced changes. Such data suggest that TCDD-induced thymocyte effects are mediated by a receptor-dependent rather than a receptor-independent process. Further, since cell selection of lymphocyte precursors occurs in the thymus, it has been suggested that TCDD may alter the pool of mature T lymphocytes in the peripheral blood.

Other studies have been designed to evaluate and compare the effects of TCDD and dexamethasone on lymphocyte function (75). Since some animal studies demonstrated that TCDD affected both humoral and cell-mediated immunity, B-cell activities have also been evaluated in TCDD-treated B-cell cultures. In those studies, the late events in B-cell maturation are altered in TCDD-treated mice, giving rise to decreased numbers of antibody-producing cells (75). These studies also demonstrate that phosphoinositol turnover, surface Ia antigen expression, nucleotide incorporation, and cell cycle kinetics are not affected by TCDD. Thus, the transition from G_0 to G_1 or G_{1B} or S, after treatment of cell cultures with anti-Ig, remains intact. Early events in B-cell activation, such as phospholipase C–mediated hydrolytic activity and surface Ia antigen expression, are unimpaired by TCDD and provide proof that TCDD does not diminish early events in B-cell activation. Nonetheless, TCDD does block immunoglobulin secretion by B cells in response to T-cell–replacing factor, B-cell growth factor, and anti-Ig stimulation. Further, TCDD decreases the expression of an antigen expressed exclusively on plasma cells. Such data suggest that TCDD alters late events in B-cell maturation, probably by affecting steps in the transition to G_2 and M in the cell cycle. TCDD does not inhibit lipopolysaccharide-stimulated immunoglobulin secretion, and such data suggest that either lipopolysaccharide stimulates a TCDD-refractory B-cell subset or the receptor-mediated T-cell derived lymphokine signal for B-cell immunoglobulin secretion is an essential factor for TCDD inhibitory activity. The absence of a need for this lymphokine with lipopolysaccharide stimulation could account for refractoriness to TCDD in this setting.

In contrast to the effects of TCDD on late events in B-cell maturation, corticosteroids (dexamethasone) affect multiple events in B-cell maturation, including early events. Dexamethasone blocks the phosphoinositide signal transduction pathway, as manifested by a decreased accumulation of inositol phosphate and surface Ia antigen expression. B cells are thus prevented from entering the cell cycle (the transition to G_0). In addition to the decrease in Ia antigen expression, dexamethasone treatment also diminishes the expression of the interleukin-2 receptor.

Although dexamethasone alters both early and late events in B-cell maturation, its primary effects are on early events in B-cell maturation, in contrast to the effects of TCDD, which alter late events in the maturation of B cells. The detailed experiments demarcating the effects of TCDD and corticosteroids on B cells have been described by Luster and colleagues (75).

Additional studies have shown that the suppressive effects of TCDD on antibody production by the B cell and that adherent cells (macrophages) and nonadherent T cells are not likely contributors to TCDD-induced suppression of antibody production (76). There is speculation that the effect of TCDDs on B cells may be mediated by alterations in tyrosine kinase–mediated phosphorylation of B-cell proteins (75,76).

Evidence for these TCDD effects on monocytes and B cells has clearly been demonstrated in animal studies. In C57BL/6 mice, TCDD (1 μg/kg/week intraperitoneally for 4 weeks) lowers the cellular content of the thymus gland by 50%, and at a higher dose (25 μg/kg/week) it also reduces the cellularity of the spleen and deceases the number of peripheral blood lymphocytes (77). The number of spleen plaque-forming cells produced in response to sheep erythrocytes (T-dependent antigen) or trinitrophenol-conjugated *Brucella abortus* is significantly reduced 6 days after immunization in animals treated with TCDD (10 μg/kg/week) by the intraperitoneal route. Serum IgM, IgG, and IgA levels are also reduced in these animals. Such responses have been shown not to be attributable to the reduction of T-helper cells but have been proposed to be caused by T-suppressor cell activation. More recent data implicate a mechanism related to B-cell dysfunction for such decrements in serum antibody levels.

The production of cytotoxic T lymphocytes in response to the injection of 2×10^7 P-815 irradiated tumor cells (a source of H-2^d alloantigen) has been measured 6 or 7 days after immunization with spleen cell suspensions from TCDD-treated (0.1 μg/kg/week or higher doses) and untreated animals. TCDD-treated cells produce fewer cytotoxic T cells than control cells. On the basis of these results, immune surveillance mechanisms, including those regulating the expression of virus-altered cells and perhaps malignant cells, may be altered by TCDD.

TCDD severely affects the developing immune system in animals. Pre- and postnatal exposure to TCDD at doses of 5 μg/kg in F344 rats suppresses both delayed hypersensitivity and lymphoproliferative responses (77,78). Thus, newborns may be particularly sensitive to TCDD exposures. The thymic mechanisms discussed previously emphasize the significance of TCDD-induced immune responses in the perinatal period.

The recent controversies regarding the role of dioxin as an agent responsible for specific health effects, including increased frequencies of soft tissue sarcomas and melanomas in exposed populations, focus on the need for ongoing investigations related to the immune system and other TCDD-mediated health effects (79–83). This is further emphasized by studies that failed to confirm the depression of delayed type hypersensitivity in the Quail Run, Missouri, mobile home park residents who had significant exposures to TCDD (81). Initial studies of this population showed that a significant number of these subjects were anergic to a battery of antigens, but follow-up studies did not confirm this finding. To account for the follow-up results, the authors proposed that either the initial skin test antigens were weak or the initial skin tests sensitized the recipients to the antigens. Nonetheless, these results raise the question of the effect of TCDD on the human immune system. The prolonged half-life of TCDD in human tissues and the newer methods to measure low levels of this chemical in fat stores provide the appropriate tools to correlate exposure dose with health effects and should resolve these issues (84–86).

In summary, TCDDs and TCDFs are generated by natural and manmade combustion of waste products as well as being present as unwanted byproducts of industrial processes. These chemicals have been demonstrated in body tissues such as liver, skin, and fat stores of apparently healthy animals and humans. They exert an immunotoxic effect at doses comparable to those causing carcinogenic, teratogenic, and neurotoxic responses. On the basis of animal studies, humoral and cell-mediated immune responses and cytotoxic T-cell functions should be carefully monitored in individuals exposed to PCDDs and PCDFs. Greater morbidity from viral infections might be expected in such exposed populations.

Polychlorinated Biphenyls

Polychlorinated biphenyls (PCBs) are inert chemicals that are resistant to biological and chemical degradation. These compounds have many desirable physical and chemical properties (low volatility, water solubility, thermostability, nonflammability, high dielectric constant, and solubility in most organic solvents) that make them suitable for many industrial applications, including use as plasticizers, heat transfer fluids, organic diluents, wax extenders, adhesives, fire retardants, dielectric fluids for capacitors and transformers, paints and printing inks, and pesticide extenders (87,88). In 1968, PCB poisoning occurred in a Japanese population. Later studies showed that the poisoning resulted from the contamination of edible rice bran oil with PCBs that had been used as coolants in the manufacturing process (89). A second incident of contamination of rice with PCBs occurred in western central Taiwan in 1979 (90). This incident claimed more than 2,000 victims. Thus, chemical contamination of foods may lead to disastrous results for human populations.

The degree of PCB toxicity depends on the chloride content of the compound; the higher the degree of chlorination, the more toxic the compound (91). Studies with individual PCB congeners have demonstrated that the most toxic PCB congeners contain five or six chloride groups/biphenyl. Exposure of female Sherman rats to Aroclor 1260, which has on the average about 6.3 chloride molecules per mole, at a dose of 100 ppm in their diet for approximately 21 months, resulted in hepatocellular carcinomas and neoplastic nodules in the liver in more than 14% and 78% of animals, respectively. Less than 0.6% of control animals showed such lesions. These data confirm the potent carcinogenic properties of these molecules (92).

The immunotoxic effects of PCBs in animals include cortical atrophy of the thymus, a reduction in the numbers of germinal centers in the spleen and lymph nodes, and a reduction in the number of circulating lymphocytes. Feeding mice 167 μg PCB/g body weight for 3 weeks also leads to decreased serum immunoglobulin concentrations (93). Similar effects occur in monkeys given 2.5 to 5 ppm PCB for 6 months (94), and such effects are reported in other animal species as well (95,96). Thus, humoral immunity appears to be altered by these compounds. PCBs also inhibit both primary and secondary antibody responses to sheep red blood cells and memory cell functions in mice. The diminished antibody production in PCB-poisoned animals is more likely related to a decrease in T-helper cells (90) than to a defect in B cells (87), but such mechanisms need further evaluation. Serum immunoglobulin (IgM and IgA) levels in patients who have been exposed to PCB are lower than the level observed in unexposed individuals (97), but serum IgG concentrations are unaffected.

PCBs also suppress cell-mediated immunity in experimental animals. Feeding PCBs to guinea pigs (98) and rabbits at a dose of 32 g/kg results in a decreased delayed type hypersensitivity response to tuberculin (99). PCBs also affect phagocytic cells of experimental animals and humans. Exposure of mice to PCBs enhances their susceptibility to endotoxin shock (94), and this increased susceptibility might result in the impairment of macrophage function. Individuals exposed to PCBs also show impaired cell-mediated immune responses when they are tested by the subcutaneous injection of a solution containing streptokinase and streptodornase. About 40% of PCB-exposed individuals have a positive response, whereas of the normal healthy volunteers tested, 80% had a positive response (100). However, careful delayed type hypersensitivity testing with multiple antigens has not been undertaken in such populations. The mean percentages of polymorphonuclear cells and monocytes containing Fc and complement receptors on the cell surface are lower in samples obtained from PCB-exposed patients compared with samples obtained from normal healthy volunteers (101). This observed decrease in the percentage of receptor-bearing cells characterizes an impairment of the cellular functions of professional phagocytes with a possible increase in the risk of infections.

PCBs are metabolized by various enzymes in animal species. The major metabolic products are phenolic compounds, but dihydroxy, dihydrodiol, and thioether metabolites have also been identified (102). *In vivo* and *in vitro* studies have shown that PCBs undergo metabolic activation and alkylate cellular macromolecules such as protein, RNA, and DNA (103). PCBs also affect leukocytes directly. PCBs, dissolved in dimethyl sulfoxide and added to leukocytes *in vitro* at a final concentration of 10^{-5} M, suppress a variety of leukocyte functions such as lymphocyte mitogenic response as well as glycolysis, glucose uptake, and intracellular adenosine triphosphate concentrations (104).

In summary, polychlorinated biphenyls have carcinogenic and immunotoxic properties in both humans and experimental animals. Immunotoxic effects require PCB doses lower than those necessary for the induction of cancer. On the basis of animal and human studies, humoral immune responses, B- and T-cell functions, phagocytic cell responses, and cell-mediated immune responses should be monitored in PCB-exposed individuals.

Polybrominated Biphenyls

Polybrominated biphenyls (PBBs) are components of FireMaster BP-6 and FF-1, chemical mixtures commonly used as fire retardants. In 1973, PBBs were accidentally substituted for magnesium oxide, a livestock supplement, and widespread pollution of the food chain occurred in Michigan over a period of 7 months (105). This poisoning also led to human exposure through the consumption of PCB-tainted beef. Workers employed in industries manufacturing the fire retardants were also found to represent another exposed population group.

PBBs have been measured in human adipose tissue, blood, and breast milk of exposed workers as well as in individuals residing on PBB-exposed farms and in the general population of Michigan. The median adipose tissue concentration of PBB in production workers (n = 7) at one Michigan chemical plant was 46.9 ppm, whereas nonproduction workers (n = 20) exhibited significantly lower levels (2.49 ppm) (106). Since PBBs have been detected in human milk samples (107) and appear to be readily excreted by this route, nursing newborns have also been exposed to these chemicals while breast feeding.

PBBs have a chemical structure similar to that of PCBs. They are fat-soluble and stored in the thymus gland, liver, brain, and adipose tissues, where they persist for long periods of time. The toxic effects of PBBs on the liver, kidney, thyroid, thymus, and lymphocytes of various animals have been reported (105). PBB ingestion has caused preneoplastic changes, microsomal enzyme induction, and thyroid hyperplasia in experimental animals. Exposure of dairy cattle to PBBs at 500 ppm causes porphyria with accumulation of porphyrins in the liver, kidneys, and other organs. At a dose of 300 to 500 ppm in rats, PBBs cause liver and microsomal enzyme induction; they have also been shown to be tumor promoters. PBB and several (purified) isomers are known to inhibit metabolic cooperation between 6-thioguanine-sensitive and -resistant Chinese hamster V79 cells in a manner similar to that of phorbol esters (108). Thus, PBBs have properties similar to those of other polyhalogenated aromatic hydrocarbons. Their capacity to induce enzymes and alter porphyrin metabolism may serve as exposure biomarkers.

Mice exposed to PBBs at doses between 3.0 and 30 mg/kg body weight and rats exposed to 30 mg/kg manifest impaired cell-mediated immune functions, as evidenced by a reduction in mitogenic stimulation by the polyclonal T-cell activators, phytohemagglutinin and concanavalin A (109). In addition, murine and rodent lymphoid organ weights are reduced in animals treated with 30 mg/kg of PBBs. Although PBBs primarily affect cell-mediated (T-cell) immunity, humoral immune functions are also suppressed in mice at 30 mg/kg doses. Statistically significant decreases in *in vitro* mitogenic responses to the polyclonal B-cell activator, lipopoylsaccharide, as well as decreases in serum IgG and IgM levels and a slight reduction in spleen weight and primary antibody response to sheep red blood cells have been observed at this dose. Such data lead to the suspicion that this chemical may also affect B-cell maturation in a manner similar to TCDD (75,76). However, serum IgG, IgM, and IgA levels have been determined to be slightly higher in residents of Michigan who were exposed to PBB in 1973 when compared to unexposed individuals (108). Peripheral blood lymphocytes from 18 of 45 Michigan farmers showed impaired cell-mediated immune responses and decreased numbers of T and B lymphocytes (110).

The exact mechanism of toxicity of PBBs in experimental animals is not fully understood. The commercial PBB, FireMaster, is a mixed-type inducer of rat hepatic drug-metabolizing enzymes (111). PBBs also induce drug-metabolizing enzymes in both hepatic and extrahepatic tissues of several other animal species (112,113). In fact, the degree of enzyme induction triggered by PBBs in mice (114) and quail (112) is similar to that observed for PCBs.

In summary, PBBs are tumor promoters and inducers of liver enzymes in experimental animals and potential immunotoxins in humans and experimental animals. PBBs primarily affect cell-mediated immunity, but humoral immunity may also be altered. As occurs with PCBs, immune alterations are found with PBB doses lower than those necessary to induce generalized toxicity. Some experiments suggest that PBBs may act by mechanisms similar to those of TCDD. On the basis of human and animal studies, cell-mediated and humoral immune responses should be monitored in PBB-exposed individuals, even in the absence of overt signs of toxicity.

Hexachlorobenzene

Hexachlorobenzene (HCB) is a polychlorinated hydrocarbon that is an intermediate used in several industrial processes; it also has been extensively used as a fungicide. It is also a contaminant of various pesticide products and of municipal waste incineration (115). A recent conference on HCB has highlighted the worldwide concern regarding this compound and its potentially adverse effects on humans (116).

HCB (100 ppm for 90 weeks) is a potent carcinogen in rats, causing thyroid and liver tumors (117), and it also induces hepatic porphyria in humans and experimental animals through its inhibition of uroporphyrinogen decarboxylase (118). Many of the effects of HCB, including hepatic porphyria, resemble those of TCDD and related halogenated aromatic hydrocarbons (116). Recently, it has been shown that HCB also binds to the Ah receptor for TCDD (119). Therefore, it is possible that the toxicological effects of HCB may be similar to those of TCDD, since they both bind to the same receptor.

HCB (167 ppm) affects both humoral and cell-mediated immune responses in the adult mouse (120). It significantly depresses the production of antibody-forming cells, delayed type hypersensitivity, mixed lymphocyte responses, and T- and B-cell–specific mitogen blastogenesis. Immunomodulating effects of HCB vary with the species under study. Although HCB depresses humoral responses in mice, it enhances humoral immune responses to tetanus toxin in rats (121). *In utero* exposure of BALB/c mice to HCB (0.5 or 5.0 mg/kg/day throughout gestation) results in a depression of delayed-type hypersensitivity responses to oxazolone (122). HCB at the highest dose (5.0 mg/kg) causes a significant decrease in mixed lymphocyte response of the HCB-exposed animals. HCB may also affect the development or maturation of the immune response in mice. A significant increase in the relative distribution of splenic T cells (increase in T-suppressor cells and decrease in T-helper cells) and a decrease in splenic B cells has been documented in the offspring of the HCB-treated female mice.

Thus, HCB is carcinogenic and immunotoxic in experimental animals, but its potential for such responses in humans has yet to be completely defined. HCB binds to the TCDD receptor (Ah receptor) in rat liver and may induce toxic effects similar to those observed with TCDD. Immune alterations require doses of HCB lower than those seen with induction of cancer. On the basis of animal studies, humoral and cell-mediated immune responses and T-cell functions should be carefully monitored in HCB-exposed individuals.

In summary, polyhalogenated aromatic hydrocarbons commonly cause thymic atrophy, which is particularly prominent in the cortex of the gland where the most primitive T-lymphocyte precursors reside. In humans, the thymus attains its maximal growth *in utero* and is largest at birth. From this point onward, the gland begins to undergo a gradual involution until it becomes a residual organ in adulthood and has only a fine rim of cortex left in contrast to large cortical expression in neonates. Removal of the thymus in neonatal life leads to a dramatic alteration in the immunological response of the host, especially in the T-dependent processes of cell-mediated immunity. In contrast, thymectomy in adults leads to little apparent change in immunological capacity. Thus, exposure to polyhalogenated aromatic hydrocarbons may have disastrous consequences in the prenatal or neonatal infant, whereas exposure in adulthood may have little or no effect on the functions of the immune system.

The thymus gland is extremely sensitive to stress, and corticosteroids cause dramatic cortical atrophy of the gland. These findings bring to mind the comparisons between the TCDD receptors and steroid receptors, and such relationships may provide the impetus to seek further biochemical connections between steroids, polyhalogenated aromatic hydrocarbons, and the immune system.

Although there are some data to support the concept that polyhalogenated aromatic hydrocarbons mediate an immunotoxic effect in humans, little hard evidence is forthcoming regarding any long-term effects on the immune system. Even though there appears to be sufficient evidence that polyhalogenated aromatic hydrocarbons are carcinogenic and behave as tumor promoters, the linkage between polyhalogenated aromatic hydrocarbon exposure, immune dysfunction, and tumorigenesis needs to be explored more carefully to determine whether subtle changes in the host's immune system may contribute to the chemical-induced carcinogenesis observed with this class of chemicals.

Polycyclic Aromatic Hydrocarbons

Polycyclic aromatic hydrocarbons (PAHs) are annulated benzene ring compounds formed from the incomplete combustion of organic matter such as fossil fuel. Human portals of entry to complex mixtures of these chemicals are primarily by the following routes: (a) the gastrointestinal tract from the ingestion of contaminated water (123) or broiled, smoked, or otherwise processed foods (124); (b) the respiratory tract from tobacco smoke (125) and/or the inhalation of air polluted with soot, coke, or automobile exhaust fumes (126); and (c) the skin from direct contact exposures in the work place (127).

As the aromatic hydrocarbon content of cigarette smoke indicates, some PAHs are common environmental pollutants, and the potent carcinogenic properties of these chemicals have focused attention on these agents (128). In fact, Sir Percivall Pott in 1775 first diagnosed scrotal cancer in chimney sweeps exposed to soot and coal tar, and the active agents were identified as PAHs over a century later. Surprisingly, PAHs shown to have carcinogenic activity are also immunosuppressive (129), and these findings have provided suggestive evidence that the risk of cancer may be associated with their immunosuppressive activity. As has been well established by other studies, the risk of cancer is greater in individuals who manifest an immunocompromised state. This association of cancer and immunosuppression is well documented in patients who have undergone renal transplantation and post-transplantation immunosuppression to avoid organ rejection and who also have an increased frequency of neoplastic disorders. Further, children with inborn deficiencies of their immune system also have a high incidence of malignant tumors. The immunotoxicity and carcinogenic properties of three major PAHs, 7,12-dimethylbenzanthracene, benzo[a]pyrene, and 3-methylcholanthrene, have been well studied (130), but few studies evaluating immunosuppression and the occurrence of cancer have been performed in individuals exposed to PAHs.

Dimethylbenzanthracene (0.75 mg/kg body weight) administered to mice by gavage for two doses at 14-day intervals causes lung tumors, and a 0.2% solution applied to the skin of mice daily for 6 to 8 weeks also results in skin tumors (131,132). In rats, dimethylbenzanthracene (6 mg/kg body weight) administered by intravenous injection causes mammary gland tumors (133). Methylcholanthrene, when applied to the skin of mice at a single dose of 26 mg/kg body weight, causes skin tumors. Dimethylbenzanthracene also causes this effect at a single dose of 2.5 mg/kg body weight when applied to the skin (134). Benzo[a]pyrene, when applied to the skin once a week over a 2-week period at the very low dose of 5 μg, causes skin tumors in mice (135). This chemical also causes lung tumors in mice at a dose of 3 mg/kg body weight when added to the diet twice (2 hours apart) with the same treatment repeated 6 weeks later (135). In humans exposed to these agents, malignancies of the skin, bowel, bladder, and lung have been observed with increased frequency (136,137). After a long latent period (10 to 20 years), keratotic papillomas occur in exposed areas of skin in coal tar workers. Such lesions are premalignant, and a few patients develop squamous cell carcinoma with malignant degeneration of these papillomas. Trauma and exposure to ultraviolet light appear to be cofactors in the generation of coal tar–induced cancers.

These three agents also suppress antibody production to both T-dependent and T-independent antigens (138–140). The immunosuppressive effects of dimethylbenzanthracene-treated mice lasts for 2 months, suggesting the possibility that such an effect might be the result of a maturation or functional arrest of a cell essential for antibody formation. The finding of a decrease in the number of progenitor B cells provides further evidence of a PAH-mediated B-cell defect rather than an isolated T-cell abnormality. In mice treated with benzo[a]pyrene (400 mg/kg body weight administered subcutaneously for 10 days over a 2-week period), B-lymphocyte maturation to antibody-producing cells is inhibited (141). When dimethylbenzanthracene is administered by ten subcutaneous injections over a 2-week period at a dose of 10 mg/kg body weight, the generation of a B-cell precursor is blocked (26,138). Mice treated with methylcholanthrene at a single dose of 50 mg/kg body weight show an increase in the number of T-suppressor cells in the spleen (142). In neonatal mice, dimethylbenzanthracene, at a single dose of 60 µg dissolved in trioctanoin and injected subcutaneously, suppresses both primary (IgM) and secondary (IgG) immune responses to sheep red blood cells (130). Benzo[a]pyrene also impairs the production of interleukin-1, a factor essential for T-cell proliferation and lymphokine production as well as for B-cell proliferation and differentiation. Interleukin-1 also activates natural killer cells and macrophages, with a resultant increase in their cytocidal activity. Thus, the immunosuppressive effects of dimethylbenzanthracene, benzo[a]pyrene, and methylcholanthrene appear to act primarily by altering B-cell maturation or function, but defects in T-cell regulation cannot be completely excluded as contributors to the suppression of humoral immunity. In general, the doses of these agents believed to cause immunosuppression are comparable to doses that induce tumors.

The pathogenesis of tumor formation from polycyclic hydrocarbon exposure may be a multifactorial process. In humans, chromosomal aberrations (sister chromatid exchanges) have been observed in peripheral blood lymphocytes recovered from patients undergoing treatment with coal tar applications to their skin for psoriasis (143). Such patients also excrete PAHs in their urine, and urinary PAH levels and chromosomal aberrations can be correlated with the dose of coal tar. These measurements may be useful as biomarkers of PAH exposure in industrial settings as well. Although such chromosomal abnormalities represent rearrangements of cellular DNA, their relationship to carcinogenesis and immunosuppression remains incompletely understood.

Since cell-mediated immunity probably also contributes to host defenses against tumor formation, suppression of these parameters might also contribute to the increased expression of tumors in exposed animals or humans. Both methylcholanthrene and benzo[a]pyrene suppress cytotoxic T-cell activity in mice exposed *in vivo* (142). In dimethylbenzanthracene-treated mice, cytotoxic T-cell function can be restored by the addition of interleukin-2 or CD4 cells to lymphocyte cultures (144,145). Thus, the CD4 cell may be the primary target rather than the cytotoxic T cell *per se*. This would suggest that the cytotoxic T cells affected by PAHs are class II restricted CD4$^+$ cytotoxic T cells. Dimethylbenzanthracene, benzo[a]pyrene, and methylcholanthrene also suppress natural killer cell activity (142). These immunosuppressive effects would clearly result in the inability of the PAH-treated host to destroy virus-infected cells and could also result in defective host defenses against tumor cell recognition and destruction. The effect of benzo[a]pyrene on interleukin-1 production and the resultant alteration in T-cell proliferation as well as natural killer cell and macrophage activation could also contribute to defective host defenses against tumor cell growth. As noted previously, ultraviolet light acts as a cofactor in the development of PAH-associated skin cancer. Such cofactor activity raises the intriguing question of the relationships between the immunotoxicity of PAHs and ultraviolet light. Ultraviolet light is known to cause the activation of suppressor T cells and to impair antigen presentation in mice. It has been postulated that these suppressor T cells may play a role in tumor susceptibility.

Since mice treated with dimethylbenzanthracene are more susceptible to infections with *Listeria monocytogenes*, the defective cell-mediated immunity observed in these mice causes a functional abnormality that appears to implicate an alteration in macrophage function (138). Activated macrophages are the primary effector cells involved in the destruction of this bacterium, and infections with *Listeria monocytogenes* are often observed in immunocompromised hosts. Thus, immune mechanisms may be affected that may increase susceptibility to both tumors and infections.

Knowledge about the basic mechanisms by which these compounds cause immunosuppression remains incomplete, but the induction of cell transformation by reactive diol-epoxides has been postulated as one possible mechanism. For example, the activation of benz[a]pyrene is a multistep process, including the oxidation across aromatic double bonds by the action of the mammalian cytochrome P-450 enzyme system. Such oxidative reactions result in the formation of simple epoxides and the subsequent formation of dihydrodiols by the action of epoxide hydrolases. A second round of cytochrome P-450–mediated oxidation at a site of olefinic double bonds results in the formation of reactive diol-epoxides. The activated diol-epoxide binds primarily to the exocyclic amino groups of deoxyguanine to form DNA adducts and thus induces cell transformations. Immune cells that are continually undergoing proliferation and differentiation could well be sensitive to the effect of such PAH metabolites. The metabolism of methylated PAHs (dimethylbenzanthracene and methylcholanthrene) might also result in the formation of a reactive methylene carbonium ion that binds to DNA (146). Another mechanism for the immunosuppressive effects of PAHs might be the induction of aryl hydrocarbon hydroxylase (147). The binding of PAHs to Ah receptors could activate the Ah complex, which induces cytochrome P-450 isoenzymes (148). These enzymes then could generate the PAH metabolites noted previously.

In summary, PAHs are carcinogenic and immunosuppressive. The immunotoxic effects of these compounds may contribute to their carcinogenic action. These compounds, by inhibiting the immune cells required for tumor resistance such as cytotoxic T cells, natural killer cells, and cytocidal macrophages, could permit the growth of acquired or spontaneously arising tumors. PAHs induce malignant transformation at doses that are immunotoxic in animals. On the basis of animal studies, humoral immune responses and cell-mediated immunity such as cytotoxic T- and natural killer cell functions should be monitored in individuals exposed to PAHs and correlated with the urinary levels of PAH metabolites. Further, characterization and measurement of DNA adducts from peripheral blood cells might lead to useful dose-response data. The role of the effects of ultraviolet light on the immune system and its apparent cofactor activity in PAH-induced skin carcinogenesis requires further evaluation.

Urethane

Urethane (ethyl carbamate) is a low molecular weight organic ester that is soluble in water, alcohol, ether, and oils. It is used commercially as a solubilizer and cosolvent for pesticides, fumigants, and cosmetics and as an intermediate in the synthesis of other organic chemicals (149,150). Low concentrations of urethane (0.1 mg/ml or less) are also found in wine, beer, orange juice, and other soft drinks, resulting from the presence of diethyl pyrocarbonate (151,152).

In mice, rats, and hamsters, the primary toxicological expression of urethane and its metabolites is carcinogenesis (153). The agent is an active carcinogen by oral, inhalation, subcutaneous, or intraperitoneal routes and produces a variety of different tumors, including lymphomas, lung adenomas, melanomas, angiosarcomas, and hepatomas (154–162). Tumor-producing doses range from 0.5 mg/kg body weight to 25 mg/kg body weight of the test animal. In mice, urethane combined with irradiation causes leukemia (163), and some workers have suggested this effect requires the presence of thymic immaturity, bone marrow damage, and viral release (164). The metabolic products of urethane have been identified in rats, rabbits, and humans (165,166). In the urine, free urethane, N-hydroxy urethane, acetyl-N-hydroxy urethane, ethyl mercapturic acid, and N-acetyl-S-ethoxy carbonylcysteine have been identified, and some of these metabolites also have carcinogenic activity. They may also be immunoactive if their chemical properties are similar to those properties of urethane that mediate their activity against immune functions.

Urethane alters certain immune functions. A dose of 4 mg urethane/g body weight in mice ($B_6C_3F_1$) results in thymic atrophy with an associated loss of cortical lymphocytes (167). Splenic lymphoctye proliferation to the stimulating effect of concanavalin A is significantly depressed in urethane-treated mice when compared with untreated mice. The response of splenic lymphocytes to PHA in urethane-treated mice is not different from the response observed in untreated mice. Mixed lymphocyte reactions are also unchanged from those of control mice. Similarly, delayed type hypersensitivity responses, as measured by the radiometric ear assay, are not altered in mice treated with 4 mg urethane/g body weight (167).

Humoral immune responses measured by enumerating the number of plaque-forming cells generated against sheep red blood cells are significantly reduced (40%) in urethane-treated mice (4 mg/g urethane). Further, antibody response to the T-independent antigen, lipopolysaccharide, is also significantly reduced (>50%). Phagocytosis and bacterial killing by peritoneal macrophages from urethane-treated and untreated mice show no differences. At doses of 1 mg/g, 2 mg/g, and 4 mg/g body weight, macrophages from urethane-treated mice demonstrate increased tumor cytostasis when compared with controls. Thus, macrophage functions remain relatively intact in urethane-treated mice (167).

Urethane significantly decreases the proliferative responses of spleen colony-forming units and granulocyte-macrophage progenitor cells in the absence of changes in bone marrow cellularity.

Luster and colleagues have interpreted the capacity of urethane to inhibit rapidly proliferating cells, such as progenitor cells of the bone marrow and B lymphocytes as the primary effect of the urethane's immunotoxic responses (167). Urethane has no effect on cell-mediated immunity, but it does alter humoral immunity (antibody production). The most striking effect of urethane on peripheral blood cells is its dramatic suppression of natural killer cell activity (167–169). This effect was mouse strain–specific, and when present, it varied in its degree of suppression from strain to strain. These data suggest a genetic factor may influence natural killer cell suppression.

The mechanisms for the immune system activities of urethane are not well characterized, but some facts permit speculation about possible mechanisms. It is known that urethane is a mutagen that induces sister chromatid exchanges in human lymphocytes (170). Further, an electrophilic urethane metabolite has been identified that is bound to nucleic acids in tissues in which urethane induces tumors (171,172). Urethane also suppresses rapidly dividing cells, and myelotoxicity appears to be essential for the induction of leukemia observed with ionizing radiation (167).

In summary, it is likely that urethane alters primarily humoral immune functions as well as those specific host defense functions mediated by natural killer cells. Immune alterations require urethane doses higher than those seen in the induction of cancer. It cannot be predicted with certainty what actual human immunotoxic responses might be observed in urethane-exposed populations, but on the basis of the studies in mice, it would appear that bone marrow function, humoral immune responses, and natural killer cell functions such as the killing of virus-infected cells should be monitored.

Phorbol Diesters

Phorbol esters represent a group of complex chemicals originally extracted from the seeds of a plant species called *Croton tiglium L.* in the *Euphorbiaceae* family. The *Euphorbiaceae* family includes common house plants that contain irritants, but little else is known about the nature of irritants with the exception of croton oil, from which the tumor promoter, phorbol ester, has been characterized. Croton oil has been used as a purgative in veterinary medicine, but its toxicity has led to its discontinuance. Humans have ingested small amounts of croton oil (20 drops) with subsequent fatality. Thus, the acute toxicity of croton oil and phorbol esters is well known. Subsequently, 12-0-tetra-decanoyl-phorbol-13-acetate (TPA) has been shown to be a tumor promoter. Although a selective population of health professionals have used this compound to investigate tumorigenesis and cell differentiation, no human immunotoxicity has been reported. Further, these compounds are now manufactured and made available commercially from small specialized chemical firms, and to date no immunotoxic responses have been reported from their manufacturers and vendors. However, it is doubtful that careful occupational surveys have been conducted to document such potential toxic effects.

Phorbol myristate acetate, PMA or TPA, represents a biologically active substance that potentiates the action of carcinogens in inducing epidermoid tumors of mouse skin (173). TPA stimulates cell division in cells that either are or have become growth inhibited. TPA stimulates 3T3 cell proliferation at a very low concentration (174). The dose for half maximal effect (ED_{50}) is 6 to 9 ng/ml. TPA induces a transient inhibition of DNA synthesis preceding its stimulatory action. For example, TPA treatment of primary cultures at a dose of 0.1 µg/ml of mouse epidermal cells for 1 hour initially inhibits [^{3}H]-thymidine incorporation into DNA, when it is measured at 24 hours. After this inhibition, incorporation of [^{3}H]-thymidine is stimulated to levels four to seven times that observed in controls up to 96 hours (175). TPA is also a mitogen for blood cells. At a concentration of 10^{-7} M, TPA stimulates bovine lymph node lymphocytes (about twofold) if such cells are exposed immediately after isolation from animals (176). TPA also stimulates mouse spleen lymphocytes (about fivefold) and human peripheral blood lymphocytes (about 20-fold) at a concentration of 10^{-6} M (177,178).

In general, TPA suppresses T-lymphocyte more than B-lymphocyte production. Treatment of mice with 40 mg/kg TPA results in a reduction of splenic T and B lymphocytes by 50% and 18%, respectively (179). This leads to suppression of lymphoproliferative responses to the mitogens (phytohemagglutinin, Concanavalin A) and reduces the ability of mice to generate an immune response to both T- and B-dependent mitogens. Natural killer cell activity in mice is also suppressed by TPA at a concentration of 20 mg/kg.

The mitogenic effect of TPA on human T lymphocytes appears to occur by the direct induction of a T-cell growth factor, interleukin-2 (180). Under certain conditions, TPA appears to stimulate T-suppressor cell activity, since treatment of cultured human T-lymphoid (CEM) leukemia cells with TPA at a dose of 16 nM results in the appearance of cells phenotypically similar to mature suppressor T cells. These cells express differentiation antigens reactive with OKT3 monoclonal antibody and suppress [^{3}H]-thymidine incorporation into phytohemagglutinin-activated peripheral blood lymphocytes (181).

Phorbol esters enhance chemotactic activity and activate phagocytosis by polymorphonuclear leukocytes. TPA at a dose of 1 ng/ml causes a twofold response over controls in assays of polymorphonuclear leukocyte chemotaxis (182). Bacterial chemotactic factor caused a 4.5-fold increment in chemotaxis, and the combination of TPA and bacterial chemotactic factor leads to 32-fold increase of this response. TPA increases the number of intracellular vacuoles in human polymorphonuclear leukocytes (183). These changes always occur after a 5-minute exposure of cells to 100 ng or more of TPA. Cytochemical observations show that TPA, at concentrations between 5 and 20 ng/ml, causes the release from polymorphonuclear leukocytes of 22% and 33% of the total cellular lysozyme content (184), which reaches a plateau within 20 minutes. TPA also causes the release of 41% of the total alkaline phosphatase activity from these cells within 15 minutes of exposure. Phorbol diester also causes platelet aggregation at a dose of 20 nM (185).

TPA also stimulates macrophages. This compound, at a dose of 10^{-7} M, has been found to stimulate mouse peritoneal macrophages to produce large quantities (200-fold) of plasminogen activator in low plasminogen activator–producing cells (186). The ED_{50} for TPA is between 5×10^{-9} M and 5×10^{-8} M, and stimulation of the plasminogen activator activity decreases at TPA concentrations higher than those inducing optimal release.

Many of the actions of TPA and related phorbol esters on immune function are receptor-mediated. TPA receptors have been detected in peritoneal macrophages (187), human peripheral blood lymphocytes (188), lymphoid cell lines (189), and the human monoblast cell line, U937 (190). Binding of TPA to its receptor triggers a series of biochemical responses. These include increased phagocytosis by U937 cells, increased turnover of phospholipids (191), increased production and metabolism of arachidonic acid (192), enhancement of cellular transport processes (193), alteration in cyclic nucleotide metabolism (194), and direct activation of protein kinase C (195). Such receptors are not likely to have been developed for TPA *per se*, but they are the binding sites for other important physiological substances such as diacylglycerol.

In summary, TPA enhances phagocytosis of polymorphonuclear leukocytes, stimulates macrophages to produce plasminogen activator, and causes platelet aggregation at doses that also cause proliferation of epidermal cells. TPA suppresses cell-mediated immunity and natural killer cell activity at doses higher than those causing the proliferation of epidermal cells. These *in vitro* studies mandate that cell-mediated immunity, T-cell function, natural killer cell activity, and neutrophil and macrophage functions should be monitored in humans exposed to phorbol esters and compounds with similar activities.

Organotins

Organotin compounds have a variety of industrial applications, including use as heat stabilizers, catalytic agents, antifungal or antimicrobial agents, industrial and agricultural biocides (e.g., in wood preservatives), and as components of antifouling paints. Dibutyltin compounds are primarily utilized as stabilizers for polyvinylchloride plastics and other chlorine-containing materials (196), and small amounts (0.5% to 3.0%) of this stabilizer combine with the hydrochloric acid released from the polymer during its high temperature manufacturing process to prevent degradation of plastics (197). Small quantities of dialkyltin compounds are extracted from bottles constructed of polyvinylchloride into fluids stored in such containers. Tributyltin compounds are also used as biocides (197), and such derivatives, which are toxic to gram-positive bacteria, are mixed with gram-negative bactericides to be used as disinfectants for hospital floors and sports arenas (198). The oxides of tributyltin are effective biocidal preservatives for wood, cotton, textiles, paper, and stains (197,199). Tributyltin oxide is also added to marine paints as an antifouling agent. Furthermore, food chain accumulation and bioconcentration of tributyltin oxide have been reported in crabs, oysters, and salmon (200–202). Its broad use in the industrial and home environments makes exposure to organotins relatively common, but such exposures are usually in low doses.

Organotin compounds produce four major types of toxicity in experimental animals: neurotoxicity, hepatotoxicity, cutaneous toxicity, and immunotoxicity. Rats exposed to 20 ppm of triethyltin hydroxide via the dietary route exhibit impaired hind limb movement within 9 days of exposure as a manifestation of neurotoxicity (203). In general, di- and tributyltins appear to be less potent neurotoxicants than trimethyltin and triethyltin compounds. The bile ducts in rats and mice are the primary site of toxic injury from exposure to dibutyltin chloride and several other dialkyltin compounds (204). A single oral dose of dibutyltin dichloride at 50 mg/kg produces inflammation of the bile duct in rats (205) and serves to illustrate the hepatotoxic properties of these compounds. Necrosis, edema, and inflammation of the skin are observed in rats after topical exposure to dipropyltin dichloride, di-isopropyltin dichloride, or diethyltin dichloride at 80 mg/kg per day for 5 consecutive days (204).

Organotins also appear to alter multiple components of the animal inflammatory and immune systems, and in some experimental settings, certain effects of these agents are species-specific. Despite probable human exposures, no known examples of human immunotoxicity have been reported to date. In rats exposed via the dietary route to low doses (20 ppm) of dibutyltin dichloride or dioctyltin dichloride, significant thymus atrophy occurs within 2 weeks of exposure (206). In weaning rats, ingestion of 50 to 150 ppm of these compounds for 2 weeks reduces the thymus weight to 50% to 80%. This compound also reduces the spleen and lymph node weights of these animals but has no effect on other organs. However, the thymus atrophy is completely reversible within 2 weeks after the termination of exposure.

The oxides of tributyltin at doses of 80 ppm for 4 weeks also induce thymus atrophy in rats. This response is associated with reduced peripheral lymphocyte counts, increased serum IgM levels, and decreased serum IgG levels (207). Tributyltin oxide, at a dose of 120 or 80 ppm in the diet for 6 weeks, inhibits T-cell mitogen-induced incorporation of [^{3}H]-thymidine into thymocyte DNA, and 80 ppm of this same chemical inhibits this reaction in spleen cells. The total number of T cells in the affected spleens is reduced by 50% to 60%, and such reductions are characterized by a decrease in the number of both T-helper and T-suppressor cells.

More recent studies have elucidated the effects of di-*n*-butyltin dichloride on thymus atrophy in rats (208). As is known, organotin induces cortical thymic atrophy in rats, and no atrophy is observed in the medulla (208). In a time-dependent fashion, thymocyte subpopulations are reduced in association with dibutyltin administration. CD2-positive and CD8-positive cells are significantly diminished on days 3 and 4 after treatment. CD4-positive and CD5-positive cells are maximally decreased on day 5. From days 2 through 5, OX44-positive cells have been observed in increased numbers. Since these OX44-positive cells do not carry macrophage markers, it has been concluded that dibutyltin blocks the maturation of prothymocyte-like cells (OX44) and their subsequent differentiation into more mature thymocytes (208,209). The authors could not exclude the possibility of OX44-positive cells migrating from the medullary area of the thymus to the depleted cortical areas of the gland. Nonetheless, there is speculation that dibutyltin interferes with the interactions between thymocytes and thymus epithelial cells (208).

Cell-mediated immune responses, including delayed type hypersensitivity reactions to tuberculin, skin allograft rejection, and T-cell mitogen-induced stimulation of mitotic activity in thymocytes, spleen cells, and peripheral lymph nodes, are diminished in rats fed 50 to 150 ppm dibutyltin dichloride or 150 ppm dioctyltin dichloride for 6 weeks (210,211). In contrast to rats, mice and other animal species appear to be resistant to the thymolytic action of alkyltin compounds (206). For example, dibutyltin dichloride, at a dose of 150 ppm for 4 weeks, does not have any adverse effects on mice (210).

Tributyltin oxide at a dose of 20 or 80 ppm for 6 weeks suppresses the natural cytotoxic activity of rat peritoneal macrophages, as assessed by their *in vitro* activity against murine YAC lymphoma cells. Furthermore, this compound, at a dose of 80 ppm, suppresses the capacity of natural killer cells to destroy the murine YAC lymphoma cells (212). It has been postulated that the suppression of these animal immune responses by tributyltin oxide may cause an increased incidence of neoplastic disease as well as infection (212). With respect to the latter, chemotaxis of rabbit neutrophils in response to formyl-methionyl-leucyl-phenylalanine is inhibited *in vitro* in a concentration-dependent manner by exposure to 0.1 to 10 μM of tributyltin chloride, dibutyltin dichloride, or triphenyltin chloride (213). Tributyltin chloride (1 μM) or triphenyltin chloride or 50 μM triethyltin chloride *in vitro* also inhibits the phagocytic and exocytotic activities of rabbit polymorphonuclear leukocytes (214).

The mechanisms for these toxic responses are incompletely understood, but some investigations have begun to probe the intracellular effects of this chemical class. Organotins inhibit pyruvate and alpha-ketoglutarate dehydrogenase activity in rat thymocytes, which results in the inhibition of the tricarboxylic acid cycle. Dimethyltin, diethyltin, dibutyltin, and dioctyltin derivatives all inhibit *in vitro* oxygen uptake and pyruvate accumulation in tissues and isolated mitochondria. These compounds may also inhibit oxidation of alpha-ketoacid by interaction of these dialkyltin compounds and dithiol groups of either lipoic acid, a cofactor of the alpha-ketoacid dehydrogenase system, or lipoyl dehydrogenase, which is another component of this enzyme system (215,216). Dibutyltin dichloride at a dose of 10 μM (which does not affect cell viability) reduces mitogen-stimulated DNA synthesis and basal DNA, RNA, and protein synthesis in rat and murine thymocytes (217,218). In such experiments, reduced oxygen consumption and elevated pyruvate production are accompanied by the stimulation of glycolysis, which generates optimal adenosine triphosphate levels in these alkyltin-exposed thymocytes. This might indicate that the reduction of energy supply in such cells is not caused by the inhibition of macromolecular synthesis. Such dibutyltin dichloride exposures also decrease intracellular cyclic adenosine monophosphate levels without affecting adenosine triphosphate concentrations, suggesting that the antiproliferating action of dialkyltins might be due to subtle changes in cell metabolism. These dialkyltins at low concentrations may also interact with sulfhydryl groups of the plasma membrane or cytoskeleton of these cells to produce an antiproliferative action. At high concentrations, these compounds may reduce the viability of thymocytes in culture (219).

Trialkyltin derivatives, in contrast to the dialkyltin compounds, have little affinity for sulfhydryl groups (216). Inhibition of oxygen uptake by tissues and cell homogenates incubated *in vitro* with trialkyltins is accompanied by a decrease in pyruvate production (216,220,221). Low concentrations of trialkyltin derivatives may pass through the outer mitochondrial membrane, where they act as Cl^-/OH^- exchangers to produce uncoupling of oxidative phosphorylation by reducing the pH on the inner side of the outer mitochondrial membrane. In addition, trimethyltin, triethyltin, tributyltin, tripropyltin, and other triorganotins, may produce an oligomycin-like inhibition of oxidative phosphorylation by binding to mitochondria of these cells (222,223). Low concentrations of triethyltin chloride, tributyltin chloride, tripropyltin chloride, and trihexyltin chloride, which do not have any effect on cell viability, decrease cellular adenosine triphosphate content by inhibiting energy metabolism in isolated thymocytes and increase lactate production in these cells. Further, these cells exhibit decreased RNA, DNA, and protein synthesis (224,225). Hence the antiproliferative action of trialkyltin compounds, unlike that of the dialkyltin derivatives, might occur by inhibition of oxidative phosphorylation. On the other hand, tributyltin compounds, at high concentrations, damage the plasma membrane of thymocytes and are cytotoxic to these cells (214,225,226).

In summary, organotin compounds are used primarily as stabilizers for polyvinylchloride plastics and other chlorine-containing materials and as biocides and antifouling agents in marine paints. These compounds produce immunotoxicity in experimental animals. Such immune alterations require organotin at doses similar to those necessary to produce other organ-specific forms of toxicity. The mechanisms for these immunotoxic responses are incompletely understood, but these substances induce thymic atrophy and cause a reduction in spleen and lymph node weights in experimental animals by disrupting energy metabolism of plasma membrane integrity. No human immunotoxic responses to these chemicals have been documented, but on the basis of the animal studies reported, humoral and cell-mediated immune responses as well as natural killer cell and macrophage functions should be monitored in human populations exposed to these compounds. Further, the association between cancer and immunosuppression requires that careful consideration be given to the possibility that an increased frequency of cancer may result from organotin exposures and subtle immunosuppressive responses.

CONCLUDING REMARKS

Environmental chemicals present in food chains, consumer products, or released into the environment as byproducts of other compounds may be either carcinogenic or immunosuppressive. They usually exert their immunotoxic effects at doses lower than or comparable to those necessary for the induction of cancer. Binding of these chemicals to DNA, RNA, and membrane proteins (receptors) results in the alteration of cellular gene expression and metabolism.

The carcinogenic properties of polyhalogenated biphenyls have recently been reviewed (227). Metabolites of polychlorinated and polybrominated biphenyls as well as benzene and toluene bind to cellular components (such as RNA, DNA, and proteins) and alter either transcription or translation in the cells. PBBs, TCDD and related halogens, HCB, and metabolites of methylated polyaromatic hydrocarbons (dimethylbenzanthracene and methylcholanthrene) all bind to a cytosolic protein (Ah receptor), which results in the induction of a large number of cellular enzymes such as Ah protein (aryl hydrocarbon hydroxylase).

The physical properties of TCDD and steroid receptors are similar, which suggests that the TCDD receptors may be related to steroid receptors. Since TCDD and related halogenated hydrocarbons are immunosuppressive, the similarity of TCDD and steroid receptors may link steroid activity, TCDD receptors, and immunoregulation.

The clinical symptoms associated with human exposure to these chemicals may be very subtle. Experimental data, using *in vivo* animal models and *in vitro* leukocyte cultures, have helped to clarify the mechanism of immunosuppressive effects of these chemicals. Further epidemiological studies are required to investigate the toxic effect of these chemicals on the immune system of occupationally or incidentally exposed human populations. It is hoped that such data may further define safety standards for these chemicals.

REFERENCES

1. Vos, J. G. (1977): Immune suppression as related to toxicology. *CRC Crit. Rev. Toxicol.* 5:67–101.
2. Koller, L. D. (1979). Effects of environmental contaminants on the immune system. *Adv. Vet. Sci. Comp. Med.*, 23:267–295.
3. Dean, J. H., Luster, M. I., Boorman, G. A., Leubke, R. W., and Lauer, L. D. (1980): The effect of adult exposure to diethylstilbestrol in the mouse: Alterations in tumor susceptibility and host resistance parameters. *J. Reticuloendothel. Soc.*, 28:571–583.
4. Dean, J. H., Luster, M. I., Boorman, G. A., Padarathsingh, M. L., Luebke, R. W., and Clements, M. E. (1981): Host resistance models as endpoints of assessing immune alterations following chemical exposure: Studies with diethylstilbestrol, cyclophosphamide and 2,3,7,8-tetrachlorodibenzo-p-dioxin. In The Biological Relevance of Immune Suppression As Induced by Genetic Therapeutic and Environmental Factors, edited by J. H. Dean and M. I. Padarathsingh, pp. 233–258. Van Nostrand and Reinhold Company, New York.
5. Chang, S. S., and Peterson, R. J. (1977): Symposium: The basis of quality in muscle food. Recent developments in the flavor of meat. *J. Food Sci.*, 42:298–305.

6. U.S. Environmental Protection Agency (1980): Ambient Water Quality Criteria for Benzene (EPA-440/ 5-80-018), pp. C1–C8, C16–C35, C67–C100. Washington, D.C.

7. Lauwerys, R. R. (1979): Industrial Health and Safety, Human Biological Monitoring of Industrial Chemicals. Benzene, CEC Report EUR 6570/11979. Commission of the European Communities, Luxembourg.

8. Brief, R. S., Lynch, J., Bernath, T., and Scala, R. A. (1980): Benzene in the workplace. *Am. Ind. Hyg. Assoc. J.*, 41:616–623.

9. Irons, R. D. (1985): Quinones as toxic metabolites of benzene. *J. Toxicol. Environ. Health*, 16:673–678.

10. Gisela, W., Latriano, L., and Goldstein, B. D. (1989): Metabolism and toxicity of trans, trans-muconaldehyde, an open-ring microsomal metabolite of benzene. *Environ. Health Perspect.*, 82:19–22.

11. Sammett, D., Lee, E W., Kocsis, J. J., and Snyder, R. (1979): Partial hepatectomy reduces both metabolism and toxicity of benzene. *J. Toxicol Environ. Health*, 5:785–792.

12. Tunek, A., Platt, K. L., Przybylski, M., and Oesch, F. (1980): Multi-step metabolic activation of benzene. Effect of superoxide dismutase on covalent binding to microsomal macromolecules, and identification of glutathione conjugates using high pressure liquid chromatography and field desorption mass spectrophotometry. *Chem. Biol. Interact.*, 33:1–17.

13. Rickert, D. E., Baker, T. S., Bus, J. S., Barrow, C. S., and Irons, R. D. (1979): Benzene disposition in the rat after exposure by inhalation. *Toxicol. Appl. Pharmacol.*, 49:417–423.

14. Sawahata, T., Rickert, D. E., and Greenlee, W. F. (1985): Metabolism of benzene and its metabolites in bone marrow. In Toxicology of the Blood and Bone Marrow, edited by R. D. Irons, pp. 141–148. Raven Press, New York.

15. Rusch, G. M., Leong, B. K. J., and Laskin, S. (1977): Benzene metabolism. *J. Toxicol. Environ. Health* (Suppl. 2):23–36.

16. Wierda, D., Irons, R. D., and Greenlee, W. F. (1981): Immunotoxicity in C57BL/6 mice exposed to benzene and Aroclor 1254. *Toxicol. Appl. Pharmacol.* 60:410–417.

17. Hsieh, G. C., Sharma, R. P., and Parker, R. D. R. (1988): Subclinical effects of groundwater contaminants I: Alteration of humoral and cellular immunity by benzene in CD-1 mice. *Arch. Environ. Contam. Toxicol.*, 17:151–158.

18. Rozen, M. G., and Snyder, C. A. (1985): Protracted exposure of C57Bl/6 mice to 300 ppm benzene depresses B- and T-lymphocyte numbers and mitogen responses. Evidence for thymic and bone marrow proliferation in response to the exposures. *Toxicology*, 37:13–26.

19. Moszczynsky, P., and Lisiewicz, J. (1984): Occupational exposure to benzene, toluene, and xylene and the T lymphocyte functions. *Haematologia*, 17:449–453.

20. Post, G. B., Snyder, R., and Kalf, G. F. (1985): Inhibition of RNA synthesis and interleukin-2-production in lymphocytes *in vitro* by benzene and its metabolites hydroquinone and p-benzoquinone. *Toxicol. Lett.*, 29:161–167.

21. Gaido, K. W., and Wierda, D., (1986): Hydroquinone suppression of bone marrow stromal cells supported hematopoiesis *in vitro* is associated with prostaglandin E2 production. *Toxicologist*, 6:286.

22. Lee, E. W. (1985): Effect of benzene of DNA synthesis in mouse hemopoietic cells following exposure by inhalation. *Toxicologist*, 5:146.

23. Schwartz, C. S., Snyder, R., and Kalf, G. F. (1985); The inhibition of mitochondrial DNA replication *in vitro* by the metabolites of benzene, hydroquinone and p-benzoquinone. *Chem. Biol. Interact.*, 53:327–350.

24. Post, G. B., Snyder, R., and Kalf, G. F. (1986): Metabolism of benzene in macrophages *in vitro* and the inhibition of RNA synthesis by benzene metabolites. *Cell Biol. Toxicol.*, 2:231.

25. Kalf, G. F. (1987): Recent advances in the metabolism and toxicity of benzene. *CRC Crit. Rev. Toxicol.*, 18:141–159.

26. Dean, J. H., Murray, M. J., and Ward, E. C. (1986): Toxic responses of the immune system. In Casarett and Doull's Toxicology, the Basic Science of Poisons, edited by C. D. Klaassen, M. O. Amdur, and J. Doull, pp. 245–285. Macmillan Publishing Company, New York.

27. Fishbein, L. (1985): An overview of environmental and toxicological aspects of aromatic hydrocarbons: II. Toluene. *Sci. Total Environ.*, 42:267–288.

28. Benignus, V. A. (1981): Neurobehavioral effects of toluene. A review. *Neurobehav. Toxicol. Teratol.*, 3:407–415.

29. Hayden, J. W., Peterson, R. J., and Bruckner, J. V. (1977): Toxicology of toluene (methyl-benzene): Review of current literature. *Clin. Toxicol.*, 11:549–559.

30. Courtney, K. D., Andrews, J. E., Springer, J., Menache, M., Williams, T., Dalley, L., and Graham, J. A. (1986): A perinatal study of toluene in CD-1 mice. *Fundam. Appl. Toxicol.*, 6:145–154.

31. Ungvary, G., and Tatrai, E. (1985): On the embryotoxic effects of benzene and its alkyl derivatives in mice, rats, and rabbits. *Arch. Toxicol. Suppl.*, 8:425–430.

32. Hsieh, G. C., Sharma, R. P., and Parker, R. D. (1989): Immunotoxicological evaluation of toluene exposure via drinking water in mice. *Environ. Res.*, 49:93–103.

33. Pathiratne, A., Puyear, R. L., and Brammer, J. D. (1986): Activation of ^{14}C-toluene to covalently binding metabolites by rat liver microsomes. *Drug Metab. Dispos.*, 14:386–391.

34. Schwetz, B. A., Norris, J. M., Sparschu, G. L., Rowe, V. K., Gehring, P. J., Emerson, J. L., and Gehbig, C. G. (1973): Toxicology of chlorinated dibenzo-p-dioxins. *Environ. Health Perspect.*, 5:87–99.

35. Kociba, R. J., Keyes, D. G., Beyer, J. E., Carreon, R. M., Wade, C. E., Dittenber, D. A., Kalnins, R. P., Frauson, L. E., Park, C. N., Barnard, S. D., Hummel, R. A., and Humiston, C. G. (1978): Results of a two year chronic toxicity and oncogenicity study of 2,3,7,8-tetra-chlorodibenzo-p-dioxin (TCDD) in rats. *Toxicol. Appl. Pharmacol.*, 46:279–303.

36. Poland, A., Greenlee, W. F., and Kende, A. S. (1979): Studies on the mechanism of action of the chlorinated dibenzo-p-dioxins and related compounds. *Ann. N.Y. Acad. Sci.*, 320:214–230.

37. Ballschmiter, K., Buchert, H., Niemczyk, R., Munder, A., and Swerev, M. (1986): Automobile exhausts versus municipal-waste incineration as sources of the polychloro-dibenzodioxins (PCDDs) and -furans (PCDFs) found in the environment. *Chemosphere*, 15:901–915.

38. Esposito, M. P., and Watkins, D. R. (1980): Airborne dioxins. The problem in review. Presentation given at the 73rd Annual Meeting of the Air Pollution Control Association, June 22–27, 1980, Montreal, Quebec.

39. Kimmig, V. J., and Schulz, K. H. (1957): Berufliche Akne (Sog Chlorakne) durch Chlorierte Aromatische Zykliche Ather. *Dermatologica*, 115:540–546.

40. Vos, J. G., Koeman, J. H., Van Der Maas, H. L., ten Noever De Braaw, M. C., and de Vos, R. H. (1970): Identification and toxicological evaluation of chlorinated dibenzofuran and chlori-nated naphthalene in two commercial polychlorinated biphenyls. *Food Cosmet. Toxicol.*, 8:625–633.

41. U.S. Environmental Protection Agency (1984): Health Assessment document for PCDDs, Parts 1 and 2: External Review Draft, PB 84-220268, Washington, D.C.

42. Van Miller, J. P., Matlar, R. J., and Allen, J. R. (1976): Tissue distribution and excretion of tritiated TCDD in nonhuman primates and rats. *Food Cosmet. Toxicol.*, 14:31–41.

43. Skene, S. A., Dewhurst, I. C., and Greenberg, M. (1989): Polychlorinated dibenzo-p-dioxins and polychlorinated dibenzofurans: The risks to human health. A review. *Hum. Toxicol.*, 8:173–203.

44. Kociba, R. J., Keeler, P. A., Park, C. N., and Gehring, P. J. (1976): 2,3,7,8-Tetra-chlorodibenzo-p-dioxin (TCDD): Results of a 13-week oral toxicity study in rats. *Toxicol. Appl. Pharmacol.*, 35:553–574.

45. Puhvel, S. M., Sakamoto, M., Ertl, D. C., and Reisner, R. M. (1982): Hairless mice as a model for chloracene: A study of cutaneous changes induced by topical application of established chlorac-negenes. *Toxicol. Appl. Pharmacol.* 64:492–503.

46. Allen, J. R., Barsotti, D. A., Van Miller, J. P., Abrahamson, L. J., and Lalich, J. J. (1977): Morphological changes in monkeys consuming a diet containing low levels of 2,3,7,8-tetra-chlorodibenzo-p-dioxin. *Food Cosmet. Toxicol.*, 15:401–410.

47. Nebert, D. W., and Weber, W. W. (1990): Pharmocogenetics. In Principles of Drug Action. The Basis of Pharmacology, edited by W. B. Pratt and P. Taylor, 3rd ed., pp. 469–531. Churchill Livingstone, London.

48. Poland, A., and Glover, E. (1973): 2,3,7,8-Tetrachlorodibenzo-p-dioxin: A potent inducer of δ-aminolevulinic acid synthetase. *Science*, 179:476–477.

49. Vecchi, A., Sironi, M., Canegrati, M. A., Recchia, M., and Garattini, S. (1983): Immunosup-pressive effects of 2,3,7,8-tetrachlorodibenzo-p-dioxin in strains of mice with different suscep-tibility to induction of aryl hydrocarbon hydroxylase. *Toxicol. Appl. Pharmacol.*, 68:434–441.

50. Vos, J. G., Moore, J. A., and Zinkl, J. G. (1973): Effects of 2,3,7,8-tetrachlorodibenzo-p-dioxin on the immune system of laboratory animals. *Environ. Health Perspect.*, 5:149–162.

51. Luster, M. I., Faith, R. E., and Lawson, L. D. (1979): Effects of 2,3,7,8-tetrachlorodibenzofuran (TCDF) on the immune system in guinea pigs. *Drug Chem. Toxicol.*, 2:49–60.
52. Greenlee, W. F., and Poland, A. (1979): Nuclear uptake of 2,3,7,8-tetrachlorodibenzo-p-dioxin in C57Bl/6J and DBA/2J mice. *J. Biol. Chem.*, 254:9814–9821.
53. Jones, P. B. C., Galeazzi, D. R., Fisher, J. M., and Whitlock, J. P. Jr. (1985): Control of cytochrome P_1-450 gene expression by dioxin. *Science*, 227:1499–1502.
54. Sogawa, K., Fujisawa-Sehara, A., Yemane, M., and Fujii-Kuriyama, Y. (1986): Location of regulatory elements responsible for drug induction in the rat cytochrome p-450c gene. PNAS, U.S.A., 83:8044–8048.
55. Gonzalez, F. J., and Nebert, D. W. (1985): Autoregulation plus upstream positive and negative control regions associated with transcriptional activation of the mouse P_1-450 gene. *Nucleic Acids Res.*, 13:7269–7288.
56. Denison, M. S., Fisher, J. M., and Whitlock, J. P. Jr. (1988): Inducible, receptor-dependent protein-DNA interactions at a dioxin-responsive transcriptional enhancer. PNAS, U.S.A., 85:2528–2532.
57. Fujisawa-Sehara, A., Yamane, M., and Fujii-Kuriyama, Y. (1988): A DNA-binding factor specific for xenobiotic responsive elements of P-450c gene exists as a cryptic form in cytoplasm: Its possible translocation to nucleus. PNAS, U.S.A., 85:5859–5863.
58. Denison, M. S., Fisher, J. M., and Whitlock, J. P. Jr. (1988): The DNA recognition site for the dioxin-Ah receptor complex. *J. Biol. Chem.*, 263:17221–17224.
59. Gustafsson, J. A., Carlstedt-Duke, J., Poellinger, L., Okret, S., Wikstrom, A. C., Bronnegard, M., Gillner, M., Dong, Y., Fuxe, K., Cintra, A., Harfstrand, A., and Agnati, L. (1987): Biochemistry, molecular biology, and physiology of the glucocorticoid receptor. *Endocrinol. Rev.*, 8:185–234.
60. Wilhelmsson, A., Wikstrom, A. C., and Poellinger, L. (1986): Polyanionic-binding properties of the receptor for 2,3,7,8-tetrachlorodibenzo-p-dioxin. A comparison with the glucocorticoid receptor. *J. Biol Chem.*, 261:13456–13463.
61. Cuthill, S., and Poellinger, L. (1988): DNA binding properties of dioxin receptors in wild-type and mutant mouse hepatoma cells. *Biochemistry*, 27:2978–2982.
62. Perdew, G. H. (1988): Association of the Ah receptor with the 90-kDa heat shock protein. *J. Biol. Chem.*, 263:13802–13805.
63. Denis, M., Cuthill, S., Wikstrom, A. C., Poellinger, L., and Gustafsson, J. A., (1988): Association of the dioxin receptor with the M_r 90,000 heat shock protein: A structural kinship with the glucocorticoid receptor. *Biochem. Biophys. Res. Commun.*, 155:801–807.
64. Evans, R. M. (1988): The steroid and thyroid hormone receptor superfamily. *Science*, 240:889–895.
65. Silkworth, J. B., and Vecchi, A. (1985): Role of Ah receptor in halogenated aromatic hydrocarbon immunotoxicity. In Immunotoxicology and Immunopharmacology, edited by J. H. Dean, M. I. Luster, A. E. Munson, and H. Amos, pp. 263–275. Raven Press, New York.
66. Greenlee, W. F., Dold, K. M., Irons, R. D., and Osborne, R. (1985): Evidence for direct action of 2,3,7,8-tetrachlorodibenzo-p-dioxin (TCDD) on thymic epithelium. *Toxicol. App. Pharmacol.*, 79:112–120.
67. Wyllie, A. H., Kerr, J. F. R., and Currie, A. R. (1980): Cell death: A significance of apoptosis. *Int. Rev. Cytol.*, 68:251–306.
68. Wyllie, A. H. (1980): Glucocorticoid-induced thymocyte apoptosis is associated with endogenous endonuclease activation. *Nature* (London), 284:555–556.
69. McConkey, D. J., Hartzell, P., Duddy, S. K., Hakansson, H., and Orrenius, S. (1988): 2,3,7,8-Tetrachlorodibenzo-p-dioxin kills immature thymocytes by Ca^{2+}-mediated endonuclease activation. *Science* 242:256–259.
70. McConkey, D. J., and Orrenius, S. (1989): 2,3,7,8-Tetrachlorodibenzo-p-dioxin (TCDD) kills glucocorticoid-sensitive thymocytes *in vivo. Biochem. Biophys. Res. Commun.*, 160:1003–1008.
71. McConkey, D. J., Hartzell, P., Nicotera, P., and Orrenius, S. (1989): Calcium activated DNA fragmentation kills immature thymoctyes. *FASEB J.*, 3:1843–1849.
72. Smith, C. A., Williams, G. T., Kingston, R., Jenkinson, E. J., and Owen, J. J. T. (1989): Antibodies to CD3/T-cell receptor complex induce death by apoptosis in immature T cells in thymic cultures. *Nature* (London), 337:181–184.
73. Wyllie, A. H., Morris, R. G., Smith, A. L., and Dunlop, D. (1984): Chromatin cleavage in

apoptosis: Association with condensed chromatin morphology and dependence on macromolecular synthesis. *J. Pathol.*, 142:67–77.

74. McConkey, D. J., Nicotera, P., Hartzell, P., Bellomo, G., Wyllie, A. H., and Orrenius, S. (1989): Glucocorticoids activate a suicide process in thymocytes through an elevation of cytosolic Ca^{2+} concentration. *Arch. Biochem. Biophys.*, 269:365–370.

75. Luster, M. I., Germolec, D. R., Clark, G., Wiegand, G., and Rosenthal, G. J. (1988): Selective effects of 2,3,7,8-tetrachlorodibenzo-p-dioxin and corticosteroid on *in vitro* lymphocyte maturation. *J. Immunol.*, 140:928–935.

76. Dooley, R. K. and Holsapple, M. P. (1988): Elucidation of cellular targets responsible for tetrachlorodibenzo-p-dioxin (TCDD)-induced suppression of antibody responses: I. The role of the B lymphocyte. *Immunopharmacology*, 16:167–180.

77. Clark, D. A., Gauldie, J., Szewczuk, M. R., and Sweeney, G. (1981): Enhanced suppressor cell activity as a mechanism of immunosuppression by 2,3,7,8-tetrachlorodibenzo-p-dioxin. *Proc. Soc. Exp. Biol. Med.*, 168:290–299.

78. Faith, R. E., and Moore, J. A. (1977): Impairment of thymus-dependent immune function by exposure of the developing immune system to 2,3,7,8-tetrachlorodibenzo-p-dioxin (TCDD). *J. Toxicol. Environ. Health*, 3:451–464.

79. Bertazzi, P. A., Zocchetti, C., Pesatori, A. C., Guercilena, S., Sanarico, M., and Radice, L. (1989): Ten-year mortality study of the population involved in the Seveso incident in 1976. *Am. J. Epidemiol.*, 129:1187–1200.

80. Bond, G. G., McLaren, E. A., Lipps, T. E., and Cook, R. R. (1989): Update of mortality among chemical workers with potential exposure to the higher chlorinated dioxins. *J. Occup. Med.*, 31:121–123.

81. Evans, R. G., Webb, K. B., Knutsen, A. P., Roodman, S. T., Roberts, D. W., Gagby, J. R., Garrett, W. A. Jr., and Andrews, J. S. (1988): A medical follow-up of the health effects of long-term exposure to 2,3,7,8-tetrachlorodibenzo-p-dioxin. *Arch. Environ. Health*, 43:273–278.

82. Blair, A. (1990): Herbicides and non-Hodgkin's lymphoma: New evidence from a study of Saskatchewan farmers. *J. Natl. Cancer Inst.*, 82:544–545.

83. Wigle, D. T., Semenciw, R. M., Wilkins, K., Riedel, D., Ritter, L., Morrison, H. I., and Mao, Y. (1990): Mortality study of Canadian male farm operators: Non-Hodgkin's lymphoma mortality and agricultural practices in Saskatchewan. *J. Natl. Cancer Inst.*, 82:575–582.

84. CDC Veterans Health Studies (1988): Serum 2,3,7,8-tetrachlorodibenzo-p-dioxin levels in U.S. Army Vietnam-era veterans. *J.A.M.A.* 260:1249–1254.

85. Kahn, P. C., Gochfeld, M., Nygren, M., Hansson, M., Rappe, C., Velez, H., Ghent-Guenther, T., and Wilson, W. P. (1988): Dioxins and dibenzofurans in blood and adipose tissue of Agent Orange-exposed Vietnam veterans and matched controls. *J.A.M.A.*, 259:1661–1667.

86. Pirkle, J. L., Wolfe, W. H., Patterson, D. G., Needham, L. L., Michalek, J. E., Miner, J. C., Peterson, M. R., and Phillips, D. L. (1989): Estimates of the half-life of 2,3,7,8-tetrachlorodibenzo-p-dioxin in Vietnam veterans of operation ranch hand. *J. Toxicol. Environ. Health*, 27:165–171.

87. Fishbein, L. (1974): Toxicity of chlorinated biphenyls. *Ann. Rev. Pharmacol.*, 14:139–156.

88. World Health Organization (1976): Environmental Health Criteria. 2: Polychlorinated Biphenyls and Terphenyls. WHO, Geneva.

89. Tsukamoto, H. (1969): Group of chemical studies on Yusho. The chemical studies on detection on toxic compounds in the rice bran oils used by the patients of Yusho. *Fukuoka Acta Med.*, 60:497.

90. Lee, T. P., and Chang, K. J. (1985): Health effects of polychlorinated biphenyls. In Immunotoxicology and Immunopharmacology, edited by J. H. Dean, M. I. Luster, A. E. Munson, and H. Amos, pp. 415–422. Raven Press, New York.

91. Safe S. (1984): Polychlorinated biphenyls (PCBs) and polybrominated biphenyls (PBBs): Biochemistry, toxicology and mechanism of action, *CRC Crit. Rev. Toxicol.*, 13:319–395.

92. Kimbrough, R. D., Squire, R. A., Linder, R. E., Strandberg, J. D., Montali, R. J., and Burse, V. W. (1975): Induction of liver tumors in Sherman strain female rats by polychlorinated biphenyls (Aroclor 1260). *J. Natl. Cancer Inst.*, 55:1453–1459.

93. Loose, L. D., Silkworth, J. B., Pittman, K. A., Benitz, K. F., and Mueller, W. (1978): Impaired host resistance to endotoxin and malaria in polychlorinated biphenyls and hexachlorobenzene-treated mice. *Infect. Immunol.*, 20:30–35.

94. Thomas, P. T., and Hindsdill, R. D. (1978): Effects of polychlorinated biphenyls on the immune responses of rhesus monkeys and mice. *Toxicol. Appl. Pharmacol.*, 44:41–51.

95. Koller, L. D., and Thigpen, J. E., (1973): Reduction of antibodies to pseudorabies virus in PCB exposed rabbits. *Ann. J. Vet. Res.*, 34:1605–1606.

96. Vos, J. G., and De Roij, T. H. (1972): Immunosuppressive activity of a polychlorinated biphenyls preparation on the humoral immune response in guinea pigs. *Toxicol. Appl. Pharmacol.*, 21:549–555.

97. Chang, K. J., Hsieh, K. H., Lee, T. P., Tang, S. Y., and Tung, T. C. (1981): Immunologic evaluation of patients with PCB-poisoning: Determination of lymphocyte subpopulations. *Toxicol. Appl. Pharmacol.*, 61:58–53.

98. Vos, J. G., and Van Driel-Grootenhuis, L. (1972): PCB-induced suppression of humoral and cell-mediated immunity in guinea pigs. *Sci. Total Environ.*, 1:289–302.

99. Street, J. C., and Sharma, R. P. (1975): Alteration of induced cellular and humoral responses by pesticides and chemicals of environmental concern: Quantitative studies of immunosuppression by DTT, Aroclor 1254, carbaryl, carbofuran, and methylparathion. *Toxicol. Appl. Pharmacol.*, 32:587–602.

100. Chang, K. J., Hsieh, K. H., Tang, S. Y., Tung, T. C., and Lee, T. P. (1982). Immunological evaluation of patients with polychlorinated biphenyl poisoning: Evaluation of delayed-type skin hypersensitive response and its relation to clinical studies. *J. Toxicol. Environ. Health*, 9:217–223.

101. Chang, K. J., Hsieh, K. H., Lee, T. P., and Tung, T. C. (1982): Immunologic evaluation of patients with polychlorinated biphenyl poisoning: Determination of phagocytes and Fc and complement receptors. *Environ. Res.*, 28:329–334.

102. Matthews, H. B., and Dedrick, R. L. (1984): Pharmacokinetics of PCBs, *Annu. Rev. Pharmacol. Toxicol.*, 24:85–103.

103. Morales, N. M., and Matthews, H. B., (1979): *In vivo* binding of 2,3,6,2′,3′,6′-hexachloro-biphenyl and 2,4,5,2′,4′,5′-hexachlorobiphenyl to mouse liver macromolecules. *Chem.-Biol. Interact.*, 27:99–110.

104. Lee, T. P., and Park, B. H. (1980): Effects of Aroclor 1254 on leukocyte glucose uptake. *J. Toxicol. Environ. Health*, 6:607–611.

105. Kay, K. (1977): Polybrominated biphenyls (PBB) environmental contamination in Michigan, 1973–1976. *Environ. Res.*, 13:74–93.

106. Wolff, M. S., Anderson, H. A., Camper, F., Nikaido, M. N., Daum, S. M., Haymes, N., and Seilkoff, I. J. (1979): Analysis of adipose tissue and serum from PBB (polybrominated biphenyl)-exposed workers. *J. Environ. Pathol. Toxicol.*, 2:1397–1411.

107. Barr, M. Jr. (1980): Pediatric aspects of the Michigan polybrominated biphenyl contamination. *Environ. Res.*, 21:255–274.

108. Bekesi, J. G., Roboz, J., Fischbein, A., Roboz, J. P., Solomon, S., and Greaves, J., (1985): Immunological, biological, and clinical consequences of exposure to polybrominated biphenyls. In Immunotoxicology and Immunopharmacology, edited by J. H. Dean, M. I. Luster, A. E. Munson, and H. Amos, pp. 393–406. Raven Press, New York.

109. Luster, M. I., Faith, R. E., and Moore, J. A. (1978): Effects of polybrominated biphenyls (PBB) on immune response in rodents. *Environ. Health Perspect.*, 23:227–232.

110. Beski, J. G., Holland, J. F., Anderson, H. A., Fischbein, A. S., Room, W., Wolff, M. S., and Selikoff, I. J. (1978): Lymphocyte function of Michigan dairy farmers exposed to polybrominated biphenyls. *Science*, 199:1207–1209.

111. Dent, J. G., Elcombe, C. R., Netter, K. J., and Gibson, J. E. (1978): Rat hepatic microsomal cytochrome(s) P-450 induced by polybrominated biphenyls. *Drug Metab. Dispos.*, 6:96–101.

112. Babish, J. G., Gutenmann, W. H., and Stoewsand, G. S. (1975): Polybrominated biphenyls: Tissue distribution and effect on hepatic microsomal enzymes in Japanese quail. *J. Agric. Food Chem.*, 23:879–882.

113. Gupta, B. N., McConnell, E. E., Goldstein, J. A., Harris, M. W., and Moore, J. A. (1983). Effects of polybrominated biphenyl mixture in the rat and mouse. I. Six-month exposure. *Toxicol. Appl. Pharmacol.*, 68:1–18.

114. Ahotupa, M., and Aitio, A. (1978): Effect of polybrominated biphenyls on drug metabolizing enzymes in different tissue of C57 mice. *Toxicology*, 11:309–314.

115. Tobin, P. (1985): Known and potential sources of hexachlorobenzene. In Hexachlorobenzene: Proceedings of an International Symposium, edited by C. R. Morris and J. R. P. Cabral, pp. 3–11. International Agency for Research on Cancer (IARC Science Publication, No. 77), Lyon.

116. Hexachlorobenzene: Proceedings of an International Symposium, Lyon, (1985): edited by C. R.

Morris and J. R. P. Crabral. International Agency for Research on Cancer, (IARC Science Publication, No. 77), Lyon.

117. Smith, A. G., and Cabral, J. R. P. (1980): Liver-cell tumors in rats fed hexachlorobenzene. *Cancer Lett.*, 11:169–172.

118. Strik, J. J. T., Debets, W. A., Debets, F. M. H., and Koss, G. (1980): Chemical porphyria. In Halogenated Biphenyls, Terphenyls, Naphthalenes, Dibenzodioxins and Related Products, edited by R. D. Kimbrough, pp. 191–239. Elsevier/North-Holland, Amsterdam.

119. Hahn, M. E., Goldstein, J. A., Linko, P., and Gasiwicz, T. A. (1989): Interaction of hexachlorobenzene with the receptor for 2,3,7,8-tetrachlorodibenzo-p-dioxin *in vitro* and *in vivo*. *Arch. Biochem. Biophys.*, 270:344–355.

120. Loose, L. D., Pittman, K. A., Silkworth, J. B., Mueller, W., and Coulston, F. (1978): Environmental chemical-induced immune dysfunction. *Ecotoxicol. Environ. Safety*, 2:173–178.

121. Vos, J. G., Van Logten, M. J., Kreestenberg, J. G., and Kruizinga, W. (1979): Hexaclorobenzene-induced stimulation of the humoral immune response in rats. *Ann. N.Y. Acad. Sci.*, 320:535–550.

122. Barnett, J. B., Barfield, L., Walls, R., Joyner, R., Owens, R., and Soderberg, L. S. F. (1987): The effect of in utero exposure to hexachlorobenzene on the developing immune response of Balb/C mice. *Toxicol. Lett.*, 39:263–274.

123. Olufsen, B. (1980): Polynuclear aromatic hydrocarbons in Norwegian drinking water resources. In Polynuclear Aromatic Hydrocarbons: Chemistry and Biological Effects, edited by A. Bjorseth and A. J. Dennis, pp. 333–343. Battelle Press, Columbus, Ohio.

124. National Research Council (1982). Diet, Nutrition and Cancer, 14.25–14.28. National Academy Press, Washington, D.C.

125. Lee, M. L., Novotny, M., and Bartle, K. D. (1976): Gas chromatography/mass spectrometric and nuclear magnetic resonance spectrometric studies of carcinogenic polynuclear aromatic hydrocarbons in tobacco and marijuana smoke condensates. *Anal. Chem.*, 48:405–416.

126. Grimmer, G. (1983): Profile analysis of polycyclic aromatic hydrocarbons in air. In Handbook of PAH, edited by A. Bjorseth, pp. 149–181. Marcel Dekker, New York.

127. Bridbord, K., Finklea, J. F., Wagnoner, J. K., Moran, J. B., and Caplan, P. (1976): Human exposure to polynuclear aromatic hydrocarbons. In Polynuclear Aromatic Hydrocarbons: Chemistry, Metabolism and Carcinogenesis, edited by R. I. Freudenthal and P. Jones, pp. 319–324. Raven Press, New York.

128. Zedeck, M. S. (1980): Polycyclic aromatic hydrocarbons: A review. *J. Environ. Pathol. Toxicol.*, 3:357–537.

129. Dean, J. H., Luster, M. I., Boorman, G. A., and Lauer, L. D. (1982): Procedures available to examine the immunotoxicity of chemicals and drugs. *Pharmacol. Rev.*, 34:137–148.

130. Ball, J. K. (1970): Immunosuppression and carcinogenesis: Contrasting effects with 7,12-dimethylbenz[a]anthracene, benz[a]pyrene, and 3-methylcholanthrene. *J. Natl. Cancer Inst.*, 44:1–10.

131. Wattenberg, L. W. (1973): Inhibition of chemical carcinogen-induced pulmonary neoplasia by butylated hydroxyanisole. *J. Natl. Cancer Inst.*, 50:1541–1544.

132. Hill, W. T., Stanger, D. W., Pizzo, A., Riegeal, B., Shubik, P., and Waitman, W. B. (1951): Inhibition of 9,10-dimethyl-1,2-benzanthracene skin carcinogenesis in mice by polycyclic hydrocarbons. *Cancer Res.*, 11:892–897.

133. Huggins, C., Grand, L., and Fukumishi, R. (1951): Aromatic influences of the yields of mammary cancers following administration of 7,12-dimethylbenz[a]anthracene. PNAS, U.S.A., 51:737–742.

134. DiGiovanni, J., Berry, D. L., Gleason, G. L., Kishore, G. S., and Slaga, T. J. (1980): Time-dependent inhibition by 2,3,7,8-tetrachlorodibenzo-p-dioxin of skin tumorigenesis with polycyclic hydrocarbons. *Cancer Res.*, 40:1580–1587.

135. Wattenberg, L. W., and Leong, J. L. (1970): Inhibition of carcinogenic action of benzo[a]pyrene by flavones. *Cancer Res.*, 30:1922–1925.

136. Zedeck, M. S. (1980): Polycyclic aromatic hydrocarbons: A review. *J. Environ. Pathol. Toxicol.* 3:537–567.

137. Vickers, D. F. H. (1981): Industrial carcinogenesis: *Br. J. Dermatol.*, 105(Suppl. 21):57–61.

138. Stjernsward, J. (1966): Effect of noncarcinogenic and carcinogenic hydrocarbons on antibody-forming cells measured at the cellular level *in vitro*. *J. Natl. Cancer Inst.*, 36:1189–1195.

139. White, K. L. Jr., Lysy, H. H., and Holsapple, M. P. (1985): Immunosuppression by polycyclic aromatic hydrocarbons: A structure activity relationship in B6C3F1 and BBA/2 mice. *Immunopharmacology*, 9:155–164.

140. Ward, E. C., Murray, M. J., Lauer, L. D., House, R. V., Irons, R., and Dean, J. H. (1984): Immunosuppression following 7,12-dimethylbenz[a]anthacene exposure in B6C3F1 mice. I. Effects on humoral immunity and host resistance. *Toxicol. Appl. Pharmacol.*, 75:299–308.

141. Dean, J. H., Luster, M. I., Boorman, G. A., Laurer, L. D., Leubke, R. W., and Lawson, L. (1983): Selective immunosuppression resulting from exposure to the carcinogenic congener of benzopyrene in B6C3F1 mice. *Clin. Exp. Immunol.*, 52:199–206.

142. Ward, E. C., Murray, M. J., and Dean, J. H. (1985): Immunotoxicity of nonhalogenated polycyclic aromatic hydrocarbons. In Immunotoxicology and Immunopharmacology, edited by J. H. Dean, M. I. Luster, A. E. Munson, and H. Amos, pp. 291–303. Raven Press, New York.

143. Sarto, F., Zordan, M., Tomanin, R., Mazzotti, D., Canova, A., Cardin, E. L., Bezze, G., and Levis, A. G. (1989): Chromosomal alterations in peripheral blood lymphocytes, urinary mutagenicity and excretion of polycyclic aromatic hydrocarbon in six psoriatic patients undergoing coal tar therapy. *Carcinogenesis*, 10:329–334.

144. Pallardy, M. J., House, R. V., and Dean, J. H. (1988): Molecular mechanism of 7,12-dimethylbenzene[a]anthracene-induced immunosuppression: Evidence for action via the interleukin-2 pathway. *Mol. Pharmacol.*, 36:128–133.

145. House, R. V., Lauer, L. D., Marray, M. J., and Dean, J. H. (1987): Suppression of T-helper cell function in mice following exposure to the carcinogen 7,12-dimethylbenzene[a]anthracene and its restoration by interleukin-2. *Int. J. Immunopharmacol.*, 9:83–97.

146. Watabe, T., Ishizuka, T., Isobe, M., and Ozawa, N. (1982): A 7-hydroxylmethy sulfate ester as an active metabolite of 7,12-dimethylbenz[a]anthracene. *Science*, 215:403–404.

147. Poland, A., and Glover, E. (1974): Comparison of 2,3,7,8-tetrachlorodibenzo-p-dioxin, a potent inducer of aryl hydrocarbon hydroxylase with 3-methylcholanthrene. *Mol. Pharmacol.*, 10:349–359.

148. Okey, A. B., Bondy, G. R., Masor, M. M., Kahl, G. F., Eisen, H. J., Guenther, T. M., and Nebert, D. W. (1979): Regulatory gene products of the Ah locus. *J. Biol. Chem.*, 254:11636–11648.

149. Merck and Company (1968): The Merck Index, 8th ed., p. 1095. Merck and Company, Rahway, New Jersey.

150. IARC Monographs (1974): Urethan: Evaluation of carcinogenic risk of chemicals to man. 7:111–140, Lyon, France.

151. Lofroth, G., and Gejvall, T. (1971): Diethyl pyrocarbonate: Formation of urethan in treated beverages. *Science*, 174:1248–1250.

152. Fischer, E. (1972): Uber die bildung von carbaminsaureathylester (urethan) in getranken nach behandlung mit pyrokohlensaurediathylester. *Z. Lebensm. Unters. Forsch.* 148:221–222.

153. Mirvish, S. S., (1968): The carcinogenic action and metabolism of urethan and N-hydroxyurethan. *Adv. Cancer Res.*, 11:1–42.

154. Toth, B., Della Porta, G., and Shubik, P. (1961): The occurrence of malignant lymphomas in urethan-treated Swiss mice. *Br. J. Cancer*, 15:322–326.

155. Porta, G. G., Capitano, J., Montipo, W., and Parmi, L. (1963): Studio sull'azimo cancerogena dell'uretano nel topo. *Tumori*, 49:413–428.

156. Tannenbaum, A., and Maltoni, C. (1962): Neoplastic response of various tissues to the administration of urethan. *Cancer Res.*, 22:1105–1112.

157. Klein, M., (1962): Induction of lymphocytic neoplasms, hepatomas and other tumors after oral administration of urethan in infant mice. *J. Natl. Cancer Inst.*, 29:1035–1046.

158. Klein, M. (1966): Influence of age on induction with urethan of hepatomas and other tumors in infant mice. *J. Natl. Cancer Inst.*, 36:1111–1120.

159. Adenis, L., Demaillc, A., and Driesseno, J. (1968): Pouvoir cancerigene de l'urethane chez le rat Sprague. *C. R. Soc. Biol.* (Paris), 162:458–461.

160. Toth, B., Tomatis, L., and Shubik, P. (1961): Multipotential carcinogenesis with urethan in the Syrian golden hamster. *Cancer Res.*, 21:1537–1541.

161. Roe, F. J. C., Millican, D., and Mallett, J. M. (1963): Induction of melanotic lesions of the iris in rats by urethane given during the neonatal period. *Nature* (London), 199:1201–1202.

162. Vesselinovitch, S. D., Mihailovich, N., and Richter, W. R. (1970): The induction of malignant melanomas in Syrian white hamster by neonatal exposure to urethan. *Cancer Res.*, 30:2543–2547.

163. Kawamoto, S., Ida, N., Kirschbaum, A., and Taylor, A. (1958): Urethan and leukemogenesis in mice. *Cancer Res.*, 18:725–729.

164. Kaplan, H. S. (1964): The role of radiation on experimental leukemogenesis. *Natl. Cancer Inst. Monogr.*, 14:207–220.

165. Boyland, E., and Nery, R. (1965): The metabolism of urethane and related compounds. *Biochem. J.*, 94:198–208.

166. Mirvish, S. S. (1966): The metabolism of N-hydroxyurethane in relation to its carcinogenic action: Conversion into urethane and an N-hydroxyurethane glucoronide. *Biochim. Biophys. Acta*, 117:1–12.

167. Luster, M. I., Dean, J. H., Boorman, G. A., Dieter, M. P., and Hayes, H. T. (1982): Immune functions in methyl and ethyl carbamate treated mice. *Clin. Exp. Immunol.*, 50:223–230.

168. Gorelik, E., and Herberman, R. B. (1981): Inhibition of the activity of mouse natural killer cells by urethan. *J. Natl. Cancer Inst.*, 66:543–548.

169. Gorelik, E., and Herberman, R. B. (1981): Susceptibility of various strains of mice to urethan-induced lung tumors and depressed natural killer cell activity. *J. Natl. Cancer Inst.*, 67:1317–1322.

170. Csukas, I., Gungl, E., Fedorcsak, I., Vida, G., Antoni, F., Turloczky, I., and Solymosy, F. (1979): Urethane and hydroxyurethane induce sister-chromatid exchanges in cultured human lymphocytes. *Mutation Res.*, 67:315–319.

171. Boyland, E., and Williams, K. (1969): Reactions of urethane with nucleic acids *in vivo*. *Biochem. J.*, 111:121–127.

172. Dahl, G. A., Miller, J. A., and Miller, E. C. (1978): Vinyl carbamate as a promutagen and a more carcinogenic analog of ethyl carbamate. *Cancer Res.*, 38:3793–3804.

173. Van Duuren, B. L. (1969): Tumor promoting agents in two stage carcinogenesis. *Prog. Exp. Tumor Res.*, 11:31–68.

174. Sivak, A. (1977): Comparison of the biological activity of tumor promotor phorbol myristate acetate and a metabolite, phorbolol myristate acetate in cell culture. *Cancer Lett.*, 2:285.

175. Yuspa, S. H., Lichti, M., Ben, T., Patterson, E., Hennings, H., Slaga, T. J., Colburn, N., and Kelsely, W. (1976): Phorbol esters stimulate DNA synthesis and ornithine decarboxylase activity in mouse epidermal cell culture. *Nature* (London), 262:402–404.

176. Mastro, A. M., and Mueller, G. C. (1974): Synergistic action of phorbol esters in mitogen-activated bovine lymphocytes. *Exp. Cell Res.*, 88:40–46.

177. Suss, R., and Schuster, A. (1974): Tumor-promoting cotton oil factor tetradecanoyl-phorbol-acetate stimulates thymidine incorporation into normal and Con A stimulated lymphocytes, *Experientia*, 30:81.

178. Touraine, J. L., Hadden, J. W., Touraine, F., Hadden, F. M., Estensen, R., and Good, R. A. (1977): Phorbol myristate acetate: A mitogen selective for a T-lymphocyte subpopulation. *J. Exp. Med.*, 145:460–465.

179. Dean, J. H., Luster, M. I., Boorman, G. A., Lauer, L. D., and Ward, K. C. (1983): Immunotoxicity of tumor promoting environmental chemicals and phorbol diesters. In Advances in Immunopharmacology, vol. 2, edited by J. W. Hadden, L. Chedid, P. Dukor, F. Spreafico, and D. Willoughby, pp. 23–31. Pergamon Press, New York.

180. Fuller-Farrar, J., Hilfiker, M. L., Farrar, W. L., and Farrar, J. J. (1981): Phorbol myristate acetate enhances the production of interleukin 2. *Cell. Immunol.*, 58:156–164.

181. Ryffel, B., Henning, C. B., and Huberman, E. (1982): Differentiation of human T-lymphoid leukemia cells into cells that have a suppressor phenotype is induced by phorbol 12-myristate 13-acetate. *PNAS, U.S.A.*, 79:7336–7340.

182. Estensen, R. D., Hill, H. R., Quie, P. G., Hogan, N., and Goldberg, N. D. (1973): Cyclic GMP and cell movement. *Nature* (London), 245:458–460.

183. White, J. G., and Estensen, R. D. (1974): Selective labilization of specific granules in polymorphonuclear leukocytes by phorbol myristate acetate. *Am. J. Pathol.*, 75:45–60.

184. Estensen, R. D., White, J. G., and Holmes, B. (1974): Specific degranulation of human polymorphonuclear leukocytes. *Nature* (London), 248:347–348.

185. Zucker, M. B., Troll, W., and Belman, S. (1974): The tumor promotor phorobol ester (12-0-tetradecanoylphorbol-13-acetate), a potent aggregating agent for blood platelets. *J. Cell Biol.*, 60:325–336.

186. Vassalli, J. D., Hamilton, J., and Reich, E. (1977): Macrophage plasminogen activator: Induction by concanavalin A and phorbol myristate acetate, *Cell*, 11:695–705.

187. Sturm, R. J., Smith, B. M., Lane, R. W., Laskin, D. L., Harris, L. S., and Carchman, R. A. (1983): Antagonist of phorbol ester receptor-mediated chemotaxis in mouse peritoneal macrophages. *Cancer Res.*, 43:4552–4556.

188. Sando, J. J., Hilfiker, M. L., Salomon, D. S., and Farrar, J. J. (1981): Specific receptors for phorbol esters in lymphoid cell populations: Role in enhanced production of T-cell growth factor. *PNAS, U.S.A.*, 78:1189–1193.

189. Lehrer, R. I., Cohen, L. E., and Koeffler, H. P. (1983): Specific binding of [^{3}H]-phorbol dibutyrate to phorbol diester responsive and resistant clones of a human myeloid leukemia (KG-1) line. *Cancer Res.*, 43:3563–3566.

190. Nambu, M., Morita, M., Watanabe, H., Uenoyama, Y., Kim, K., Tanaka, M., Iwai, Y., Kimata, H., Mayumi, M., and Mikawa, H. (1989): Regulation of Fcγ receptor expression and phagocytosis of a human monoblast cell line U937, participation of cAMP and protein kinase C in the effects of IFN-γ and phorbol ester. *J. Immunol.*, 143:4158–4165.

191. Levine, L., and Hassid, A. (1977): Effects of phorbol-12,13-diesters on prostaglandin production and phospholipase activity in canine kidney (MDCK) cells. *Biochem. Biophys. Res. Commun.*, 79:477–484.

192. Bonney, R. J., Wrightman, P. D., Dahlgren, M. E., Davies, P., Kuehl, F. A., and Humes, J. L. (1980): Effect of RNA and protein synthesis inhibitors on the release of inflammatory mediators by macrophages responding to phorbol myristate acetate. *Biochem. Biophys. Acta*, 633:410–421.

193. Grotendorst, G. R., and Schimmel, S. D. (1980): Alteration of cyclic nucleotide levels in phorbol 12-myristate 13-acetate treated myoblasts. *Biochem. Biophys. Res. Commun.*, 93:301–307.

194. Hadden, E. M., Sadlik, J. R., Coffey, R. G., and Hadden, J. W. (1982): Effects of phorbol myristate acetate and a lymphokine on cyclic 3′,5′-guanosine monophosphate levels and proliferation of macrophages. *Cancer Res.*, 42:3064–3069.

195. Kikkawa, M., Takai, Y., Tanaka, Y., Miyake, R., and Nishizuka, Y. (1983): Protein kinase C as a possible receptor protein of tumor-promoting phorbol esters. *J. Biol. Chem.*, 258:11442–11445.

196. Ven der Kerk, G. J. M. (1976): Organotin compounds. New chemistry and applications. Edited by J. J. Zuckerman, p. 186. American Chemical Society, Washington, D.C.

197. Piver. W. T. (1973): Organotin compounds: Industrial applications and biological investigations. *Environ. Health Perspect.*, 4:61–77.

198. Ascher, K. R. S. (1985): Nonconventional biocidal uses of organotins. *Phytoparasitology*, 13:153.

199. Smith, J. (1978): Preservative stains fight fungus, mildew, and rot. *Pop. Sci.*, 212:126.

200. Evans, D. W., and Laughlin, R. B. Jr. (1984): Accumulation of bis(tributyltin) oxide by the mud crab, *Rhithropanopeus harrisii. Chemosphere*, 13:213–219.

201. Alzieu, C. L., Sanjuan, J., Deltreil, J. P., and Borel, M. (1986): Tin contamination in Arachon Bay: Effects on oyster shell anomalies. *Mar. Pollut. Bull.*, 17:494

202. Short, J. W., and Thrower, F. P. (1986): Accumulation of butyltins in muscle tissue of Chinook salmon reared in sea pens treated with tri-n-butyltin. *Mar. Pollut. Bull.*, 17:542.

203. Magee, P. N., Stoner, H. B., and Barnes, J. M. (1957): The experimental production of oedema in the central nervous system of the rat by triethyltin compounds. *J. Pathol. Bacteriol.*, 73:107–124.

204. Barnes, J. M., and Stoner, H. B. (1958): Toxic properties of some dialkyl and trialkyl tin salts. *Br. J. Ind. Med.*, 15:15–22.

205. Gaunt, I. F., Colley, J., Grasso, P., Creasey, M., and Gangolli, S. D. (1968): Acute and short-term toxicity studies on di-n-butyltin dichloride in rats. *Food Cosmet. Toxicol.*, 6:599.

206. Seinen, W., Vos, J. G., Van Spanje, I., Snoek, M., Brands, R., and Hooykaas H. (1977): Toxicity of organotin compounds. II. Comparative *in vivo* and *in vitro* studies with various organotin and organolead compounds in different animal species with special emphasis on lymphocyte cytotoxicity. *Toxicol. Appl. Pharmacol.*, 42:197–212.

207. Krajnc, E. I., Wester, P. W., Loeber, J. G., van Leeuwen, F. X. R., Vos, J. G., Vaessen, H. A. M. G., and van der Heijden, C. A. (1984): Toxicity of bis (tri-n-butyltin) oxide in the rat: I. Short-term effects on general parameters and on the endocrine and lymphoid systems. *Toxicol. Appl. Pharmacol.*, 75:363–386.

208. Pieters, R. H. H., Kampinga, J., Bol-Schoenmakers, M., Lam, B. W., Penninks, A. H., and Seinen, W. (1989): Organotin-induced thymus atrophy concerns the OX-44$^+$ immature thymocytes: Relation to the interaction between early thymocytes and thymic epithelial cells? *Thymus*, 14:79–88.

209. Snoeij, N. J., Penninks, A. H., and Seinen, W. (1989): Thymus atrophy and immunosuppression induced by organotin compounds. *Arch. Toxicol. Suppl.*, 13:171–174.

210. Seinen, W., Vos, J. G., Van Krieken, R., Penninks, A., Brands, R., and Hooykaas, H. (1977): Toxicity of organotin compounds. III. Suppression of thymus-dependent immunity in rats by di-n-butyltindichloride and di-n-octyltindichloride. *Toxicol. Appl. Pharmacol.*, 42:213–224.

211. Seinen, W., Vos, J. G., Brands, R., and Hooykaas, H. (1979): Lymphotoxicity and immunosuppression by organotin compounds. Suppression of graft-versus-host reactivity, blast transformation, and E-rosette formation by di-n-butyltin-dichloride and di-n-octyltindichloride. *Immunopharmacology*, 1:343–355.

212. Vos, J. G., de Klerk, A., Krajnc, E. I., Kruizinga, W., van Ommen, B., and Rozing, J. (1984): Toxicity of bis(tri-n-butyltin) oxide in the rat: II. Suppression of thymus-dependent immune responses and of parameters of nonspecific resistance after short-term exposure. *Toxicol. Appl. Pharmacol.*, 75:387–408.

213. Arakawa, Y., and Wada, O. (1984): Inhibition of neutrophil chemotaxis by organotin compounds. *Biochem. Biophys. Res. Commun.*, 123:543–548.

214. Elferink, J. G. R., Deierkauf, M., and van Steveninck, J. (1986): Toxicity of organotin compounds for polymorphonuclear leukocytes: The effect of phagocytosis and exocytosis. *Biochem. Pharmacol.*, 35:3727–3732.

215. Penninks, A. H., and Seinen, W. (1980): Toxicity of organotin compounds. IV. Impairment of energy metabolism of rat thymocytes by various dialkyltin compounds. *Toxicol. Appl. Pharmacol.*, 56:221–231.

216. Aldridge, W. N., and Cremer, J. E. (1955): The biochemistry of organotin compounds: Diethyltin dichloride and triethyltin sulfate. *Biochem. J.*, 61:406–418.

217. Penninks, A. H., and Seinen, W. (1983): The lymphocyte as target of toxicity: A biochemical approach to dialkyltin induced immunosuppression. In Advances in Immunopharmacology, vol. 2, edited by J. W. Hadden, L. Chedid, P. Dukor, F. Spreafico, and D. Willoughby, pp. 41–60. Pergamon Press, Oxford and London.

218. Penninks, A. H., and Seinen, W. (1984): Mechanisms of dialkyltin induced immunopathology, *Vet. Q.*, 6:209–215.

219. Penninks, A. H., and Seinen, W. (1982): Comparative toxicity of alkyltin and estertin stabilizers. *Food Chem. Toxicol.*, 20:909–916.

220. Cremer, J. E. (1957): The metabolism *in vitro* of tissue slices from rats given triethyltin compounds. *Biochem. J.*, 67:87–96.

221. Cremer, J. E. (1967): Studies on brain-cortex slices: Differences in the oxidation of ^{14}C-labelled glucose and pyruvate revealed by the action of triethyltin and other toxic agents. *Biochem. J.*, 104:212–222.

222. Aldridge, W. N. (1976): The influence of organotin compounds on mitochondrial functions. *Adv. Chem. Ser.*, 157:186–196.

223. Stockdale, M., Dawson, A. P., and Selwyn, M. J. (1970): Effects of trialkyltin and triphenyltin compounds on mitochondrial respiration. *Eur. J. Biochem.*, 15:342–351.

224. Snoeij, N. J., Punt, P. M., Penninks, A. H., and Seinen, W. (1986): Effects of tri-n-butyltin chloride on energy metabolism, macromolecular synthesis, precursor uptake and cyclic AMP production in isolated rat thymocytes. *Biochem. Biophys. Acta.*, 852:234–243.

225. Snoeij, N. J., van Rooijen, J. M., Penninks, A. H., and Seinen, W. (1986): Effects of various inhibitors of oxidative phosphorylation on energy metabolism, macromolecular synthesis, and cyclic AMP production in isolated rat thymocytes. A regulating role for the cellular energy state in macromolecular synthesis and cyclic AMP production. *Biochem. Biophys. Acta*, 852:244–253.

226. Byington, K. H., Yeh, R. Y., and Forte, L. R. (1974): The hemolytic activity of some trialkyltin and triphenyltin compounds. *Toxicol. Appl. Pharmacol.*, 27:230–240.

227. Silberhorn, E. M., Glauert, H. P., and Robertson, L. W. (1990): Carcinogenicity of polyhalogenated biphenyls: PCBs and PBBs. *Crit. Rev. Toxicol.*, 20:439–496.

Clinical Immunotoxicology, edited by
D. S. Newcombe, N. R. Rose, and J. C. Bloom.
Raven Press, Ltd., New York © 1992.

19

Metal-induced Alterations of Immunity

Michael Kowolenko,* Michael J. McCabe, Jr.,†
and David A. Lawrence‡

**Division of Investigative Toxicology, Bristol-Myers Squibb,
Pharmaceutical Research Institute, Syracuse, New York; †Karolinska Institute,
Department of Toxicology, Stockholm, Sweden; ‡Department of
Microbiology and Immunology, The Albany Medical College, Albany, New York*

Heavy metals are known to directly induce pathophysiological changes that affect particular organ systems (40). If the immune system is one of these target systems, these compounds may modulate the host immune system directly or indirectly, resulting in immune activation with subsequent immunopathophysiological changes. Data are presented that demonstrate the capacity of heavy metals to modulate both host resistance and select components of the immune system. Possible biochemical mechanisms of metal-induced alterations of immunoreactivity are discussed.

The ability of the immune system to respond to foreign antigens while not reacting against "self" is the result of dynamic regulatory interactions between its cells. Immunoregulation involves the interaction among lymphocyte subsets (B cells [CD19/20[+]], T-inducer [i] cells [CD4/CD45R[+], Tsi and CD4/CD29[+], Thi] and T-suppressor cells [CD8/CD16[+]]) and accessory cells (antigen-presenting cells, including B cells, macrophages, and dendritic cells). Divergence from a balanced control (as may occur after heavy metal exposure) generally manifests as a pathological disorder. The importance of proper immunoregulation is demonstrated by diseases in which there is a deficiency of one or several components of the immune system. Several pathological conditions are characterized by defects in either T or B cells, the most recognized being the acquired immunodeficiency syndrome (AIDS). Upon infection with human immunodeficiency virus, previously normal individuals acquire a T-helper cell defect that leads to increased morbidity and mortality as a result of an increase in opportunistic infections and/or neoplasms (61,112). Human immunodeficiency virus constituents concomitantly modulate B-cell activities, bypassing T-cell regulation (61). Other conditions of immune deficiency include congenital B-cell defects with resultant recurrent extracellular parasitic infections that can lead to death within the second to third decade of life (102). Patients born without T or B cells generally do not survive their first year of life without immune reconstitution (102). Interestingly, the incidence of neoplasia and autoimmunity increases with age, in contrast to immunoregulated host resistance to infectious diseases, which declines with age (71). Autoimmunity, hyperimmune responsiveness to self-constituents, is the result of altered T-cell activities and/or hyperactive B cells. Autoimmune diseases encompass a variety of immunopathological states and affect most organ systems. Since there is an autoimmune disorder for each of the major organ systems affected by heavy metals, it is reasonable to postulate that heavy metal toxicity may, in part, be due to autoimmunity. This is only a hypothesis, but results with studies with some heavy metals, especially mercury, support this hypothesis. In addition, metals are known inducers of allergic hypersensitivity. All four types of hypersensitivity are caused by sensitized lymphocytes, which are activated by an endogenous or exogenous (environmental) factor and produce antibody responses (types I, II, and III hypersensitivity) or cell-mediated responses (type IV hypersensitivity). As discussed later, the pathological consequences of these processes could be autoimmune disease. Any metal known to produce an allergic response could be a promoter of autoimmunity.

Exposure to heavy metals has the potential of disrupting the body's normal immune homeostasis either by acting directly on the cells of the immune system or by interacting with other cells or organ systems so as to render them immunologically reactive. A direct effect of toxicant exposure on the immune system is quite obvious in that there would likely be changes in lymphocyte subset ratios, altered morphology of immune tissue, decreases in total immune cell numbers, or altered immune functions with or without the above changes (69). The more difficult modulations to assess are the subtle effects of toxicant exposure that cause an imbalance of immune homeostasis, leading to immune activation directed at what the immune system views as "altered self" (6,14,110). Altered self may be the result of newly expressed proteins located on cell surfaces (6,110) or perhaps allosteric changes induced by toxicant-cell surface interactions that result in the immunological appearance of altered self. The formation of structures that are immunogenic (altered self) could result in upregulation of the immune response to unaltered self-molecules as well. Alternatively, the toxicant could cause tissue damage that results in the release of sequestered antigen or higher amounts of tissue antigens, and the immune system would be activated by this new antigen or antigenic dose. These mechanisms for the induction of autoimmunity can lead to further damage to organ systems involving antibody formation against target organ antigens, with subsequent complement activation or immune complex depositions along membranes, leading to autoimmune disease. Further possible mechanisms involve disruption of immunoregulatory circuits. Such alterations could manifest themselves as depressed suppressor cell activity or modification of idiotypic networks. Defective regulatory circuits could allow the overproduction or amplified activity directed against altered self. This could result from activation of T cells producing nonspecific immunoregulatory products that exacerbate responses to modified antigens and initiate responses to bystander antigens (29). Additionally, the toxicant may enhance morbidity, and the higher incidence of infections may aid in establishing autoimmunity. Finally, the metal may directly modulate lymphocyte activation; enhancement of B-cell activity or T-cell activity could lead to autoimmunity.

The interaction of toxicant with cell constituents that leads to immunomodulation is influenced by the genetics of the exposed individual. The ability of animals to respond to peptides and bacterial and viral antigens and the development of tumors or the predisposition to autoimmune disease has been associated with the genes of the major histocompatibility complex (MHC). The MHC molecules associated with these reactivities are the MHC class I and MHC class II cell surface glycoproteins (25). It has been postulated that several autoimmune diseases may be the result of a genetic predisposition to altered self that is triggered by some exogenous environmental factor or pathogen exposure (6,29). It is possible that the toxic effects of heavy metals on organ systems are caused by an induction of autoimmunity in this manner. It therefore would be predicted that the susceptibility of an individual to immunomodulation by a particular heavy metal will vary.

Metals associated with immunomodulation are numerous; this review focuses mainly on cadmium (Cd), mercury (Hg), and lead (Pb). In discussing the immunomodulatory effects of heavy metals, it must be kept in mind that each metal has differential biochemical reactivities and thus is likely to be immunomodulatory via different molecular mechanisms, although some, like thiols, may share some common characteristics, such as an affinity for nucleophils.

Cadmium is often included as a heavy metal; however, it is of period 6, whereas Hg and Pb are period 7 elements; arsenic (11,34), chromium (38), cobalt (36), copper (68), manganese (63), nickel (63), tin (63), and zinc (34) are all immunomodulatory essential trace elements (75,116) and their physiological versus toxic potentials are complex and are not covered in this review. Several heavy metals are used therapeutically. Platinum has found use as an antineoplastic agent that has direct effects on the immune system, among them inhibition of lymphocyte proliferation (2) and humoral immunity (8). Inhibition of macrophage chemotaxis has also been reported (4). Gold treatment for rheumatoid arthritis has been associated with allergic reactions (38,117). Gold-induced immune complex–mediated renal disease has been found in rats (79), guinea pigs (114), and humans (113). Although each therapeutic compound has distinct applications, both platinum and gold react with sulfhydryl groups of cells, as do Hg, Cd, and, to a lesser extent, Pb. Lead, mercury, and cadmium provide good examples of nonessential heavy metals that affect the immune system.

HEAVY METALS AND THE IMMUNE SYSTEM

Many reports of metal-induced immunomodulation display conflicting results. When data are reviewed concerning the immunomodulating potential of a compound, the results obtained often are found to be dependent on the assay employed. Factors implicated in the variances include the dose, duration of exposure, and route of exposure of the compound. In addition, strain, species, and sex differences can be important variables in immunotoxicological testing. Another important variable is the infectious state of the host, that is, whether or not the host has any bacterial, viral, or parasitic infections that could be exacerbated by additional stressors.

Host responsiveness to extracellular or intracellular pathogens tests humoral and cell-mediated immunity, respectively; therefore, the challenge of metal-exposed animals with pathogens provides a reasonable starting place to evaluate the immunotoxic potential of these compounds. However, as noted earlier, it is critical to initiate such studies with "pathogen-free" animals. Exposure of animals to extracellular pathogens leads to T cell-B cell-macrophage activation, culminating in pathogen-specific antibody formation, complement activation, and enhanced phagocytosis and killing. Intracellular pathogen exposure induces T cell-macrophage interactions with concomitant cytokine formation and macrophage activation, followed by enhanced killing of the previously phagocytosed pathogen.

Host resistance to a variety of pathogens is lowered in metal-exposed animals. Although genetic susceptibility has been implicated in metal-induced immunomodulation, there is no apparent strain specificity for lowered host resistance. Lead exposure decreases host resistance in CBA/J, CD-1, SW, NMRI, and S strain mice (35,36,43,51,52,54,65,97). Lowered host resistance to viral challenge has been demonstrated in mice and rabbits exposed to Hg (36,52). The effects of metals on host defenses are often not obvious upon analysis of the components of the immune response. The defect only becomes apparent after pathogenic challenge. For example, CBA/J mice exposed to 0.4 to 10 mM Pb acetate in their drinking water for periods up to 1 year display minimal signs of altered immunity, in that *ex vivo* assessment of humoral (enumeration of antibody [plaque]-forming cells) and cell-mediated immunity (mixed lymphocyte culture response as well as mitogen responses) indicated only slight inhibition (67). However, when mice were treated with 0.4 mM Pb for as little as 2 weeks (resultant blood lead levels being approximately 20 μg/dl) and challenged with *Listeria*, mortality increased significantly (65). It is known that immunity to *Listeria* requires macrophage-T cell interactions (83,115). Macrophages must phagocytose and kill the *Listeria* to keep the infection in check until a cell-mediated immune response is generated. Macrophages from Pb-exposed mice were capable of phagocytosing and killing *Listeria* and secreting interleukin-1 but demonstrated an inhibited ability to present antigen to primed T cells (58). The hematopoietic responses induced by *Listeria* involve the migration of the newly developed macrophages from the bone marrow to the periphery. Mice exposed to Pb have diminished numbers of bone marrow macrophages capable of responding to macrophage colony–stimulating factor while maintaining colony-stimulating activity equal to or above that of control populations (59). Lowered resistance to *Listeria* could result in decreased numbers of macrophages capable of responding to the bacterial insult.

In vitro exposure of mouse bone marrow cells to Pb altered macrophage proliferation and differentiation in response to macrophage colony–stimulating factor (60). Doses as low as 100 nM inhibited colony formation, cell cycle progression, and differentiation as determined by cell adherence. This effect was reversible on removal of cells from the Pb cultures. Growth factor receptors are known to possess large numbers of cysteine residues that may be involved in receptor/ligand interactions (125). Adherent Pb-treated macrophages displayed the greatest degree of morphological changes and decreased growth factor responses on exposure to Pb. Since proliferation and differentiation are associated with morphological changes and adhesion (95), it is possible that Pb interferes with sulfhydryl-rich adhesion proteins (Law 1987), which may influence growth factor responses.

Precursor frequency of stem cells that respond to hematopoietic growth factors may also be affected by metal exposure. Schlick and Friedberg (100) have reported that 1 month of oral administration of Pb caused a significant decrease in the number of pluripotent stem cells. Cadmium exposure also has been reported to decrease the formation of colony-forming cells (42). Although acute exposure of BALB/c mice to Pb or Cd has been associated with increased myeloid/monocytic and blast cells within the bone marrow (12), it is important to note that *in vitro* Pb (1.0 μM) and Cd (0.1 μM) synergistically inhibit macrophage colony-forming units (Table 1). Any modulation of myeloid/monocytic precursor generation, proliferation, or differentiation would be expected to affect host resistance.

Alternatively, host resistance may be lowered because of changes in other parameters required for bactericidal activity. Although acid phosphatase activity has been shown to increase after Pb exposure, it cannot be assumed that all bactericidal factors are increased. Pb has been shown to synergize with endotoxin to alter multiple products and activities of reticuloendothelial cells such as lipid peroxidation, superoxide anion generation, glutathione, and glutathione-associated enzymes (96), and similar modulations could account for alteration of bactericidal activity.

Tests of heavy metal effects on macrophages involve assays of both cell function and capacity. Macrophage populations differ in their location (e.g., alveolar or peritoneal) or activation state. The heavy metals Pb and Cd have been associated with altered oxidative metabolic activity. Cadmium and lead increased oxidative metabolism induced by phorbol myristate acetate, whereas zymosan-induced oxidative activity was deceased after the first hour of *in vitro* exposure of peritoneal macrophages to each metal (44). Castranova and coworkers (15) evaluated the *in vitro* exposure to Cd, Hg, Ni (nickel), and Pb with zymosan-induced rat alveolar macrophages and also demonstrated a decrease in oxidative metabolism. Functional assays of phagocytosis indicate that Pb does not alter *Listeria* phagocytosis but does

TABLE 1. *Synergistic inhibition of macrophage colony-stimulating factor–induced bone marrow[a] colony formation by cadmium and lead*

Cd (μM)	Pb (1 μM)	Number of colonies[b] (% of control)
0	−	68 (100%)
	+	41 (60%)
0.01	−	44 (64%)
	+	25 (36%)
0.1	−	42 (61%)
	+	12 (18%)
1	−	7 (11%)
	+	3 (4%)

[a]Bone marrow cells (10^5) were cultured in macrophage colony-stimulating factor supplemented by soft agar ± Pb and/or Cd.
[b]Colonies (>50 cells) were counted 10 days later.

inhibit phagocytosis of IgG-sensitized sheep red blood cells (51). Because of differences in cell source, stimuli, or activation state, it is difficult to make generalizations about the effects of heavy metals on macrophage capacity or function.

Phagocytosis involves not only macrophages that carry out the process but the generation of complement and immunoglobulins that act as opsonins, enhancing the "attractiveness" of the foreign particle. Altered serum C3 activity has been observed in Pb workers (31,48), but no differences have been reported in Pb-exposed children (43). Both Hg and Pb have been reported to alter complement activities (33). *In vitro*, Au has been shown to inhibit the classic (101) and alternate (13) complement pathways. Cobalt, nickel, and lithium enhanced guinea pig complement activity; mercury, gold, and magnesium enhanced or inhibited it, depending on their concentrations; and gold, manganese, platinum, calcium, barium, strontium, cadmium, lead, zinc, aluminum, copper, chromium, iron, and beryllium were inhibitory (91). A decrease in complement activity could lead to ineffective opsonization of bacteria, with a subsequent lowering of bacterial clearance. Bacterial clearance also is accomplished by the liver. Intravenous administration of Pb has been reported to inhibit clearance of both colloidal carbon and bacterial endotoxin in rats (21,22); however, in NMRI mice, carbon clearance was enhanced or suppressed when 10 to 1,000 μg Pb was given orally for 10 and 30 days, respectively (99).

A decrease in humoral immunity has been suggested to be a factor leading to increased susceptibility to infection. Humoral immunity, the production of antigen-specific cytophilic antibodies, enhances phagocytosis. The data concerning the effect of heavy metals on B cells have indicated both an inhibition (53,55–57) and an enhancement of antibody formation (63,64). Bone marrow cellularity, a possible indication of B-cell development, is reduced by Pb (5), but serum immunoglobulin levels are not altered substantially (31,48). Retrospective studies of preschool children with blood lead levels of 41 to 51 μg/dl demonstrated no difference in IgG, IgA, IgM, or C3 levels when compared with control populations (93). In addition, each child produced high titers to tetanus toxoid after immunization. Lead factory workers (blood lead levels 6.6 to 20.8 μg/dl), in contrast, had below normal levels of IgG, IgA, IgM, and C3 (31,48). Blakely and Archer (10) have reported that *in vivo* Pb exposure inhibits *in vitro* plaque-forming cell responses to the T cell–dependent antigen sheep red blood cells, and that this effect may be the result of impaired macrophage activity. When 2-mercaptoethanol, a sulfhydryl reactive compound, was added to this culture system, plaque-forming cell responses returned to values comparable to those of controls. Decreased B-cell responsiveness has been reported after oral exposure of mice to Pb (56). However, the methods employed in these assays (analysis of C3 receptor-positive cells) did not actually assess B-cell responsiveness or rule out the possibility of the involvement of C3-positive macrophages or a subset of lymphocytes other than B cells. Luster and coworkers (70) have shown that pre- and postnatal exposure of rats to Pb inhibits the plaque-forming cell response, although CBA/J mice exposed for up to 10 weeks (65) or 52 weeks (67) displayed no inhibition of the plaque-forming cell response to sheep red blood cells.

Lipopolysaccharide-induced proliferation of B cells exposed *in vitro* to various metals has provided conflicting data. Lead exposure of CBA/J mouse spleen cells has been reported to moderately enhance lipopolysaccharide responsiveness (65). *In vivo* exposure of CBA/J mice to Pb with subsequent *in vitro* stimulation with lipopolysaccharide produces a slight increase in lipopolysaccharide responsiveness (103). *In vivo* exposure of B6C3F$_1$ mice to Hg has been reported to enhance lipopolysaccharide responsiveness (26). *In vitro* exposure of CBA/J splenocytes to Pb and Ni enhanced whereas zinc inhibited the lipopolysaccharide response (120).

Mitogen response to *Staphylococcus aureus* has been shown to be decreased in Hg-exposed workers (77). In addition, these workers showed a decrease in responsiveness to concanavalin A; however, this appeared to correlate more with the age of the individual than with Hg exposure. There was no difference in the percentage of CD2$^+$, CD4$^+$, or CD8$^+$ cells, but there were fewer CD3$^+$ and sIg$^+$ cells in the Hg-exposed individuals when compared with controls.

Alterations in cell-mediated immunity by metals are often manifested as delayed type hypersensitivity reactions. It is theorized that topical exposure to metals results in an antigenically modified skin protein, which in turn leads to inflammation and macrophage migration. Numerous metals have been reported to induce delayed-type hypersensitivity (30,81). Sinigaglia and coworkers (106) have isolated T-lymphocyte clones from patients with Ni contact dermatitis. These T-cell clones were found to be CD3$^+$, CD4$^+$, and CD8$^-$ and would respond to Ni in the context of MHC class II (HLA) antigens. The cells produced high levels of interferon-gamma and interleukin-2 upon stimulation with Ni and autologous Epstein-Barr virus B cells. Ni and Hg also have been shown to act as mitogens, stimulating DNA synthesis of thymocytes and peripheral blood lymphocytes of children (82). In this study, the mitogenic effect of Hg increased with age, whereas that of Ni decreased. In addition, it appears that Hg may interact with serum constituents in inducing mitogenesis. Correlations between the ability of Ni to induce mitogenesis and the diagnosis of Ni hypersensitivity appears difficult; 63% of Ni-sensitive patients and 30% of the control populations display increased lymphocyte proliferation on *in vitro* stimulation with Ni (9). Although Ni can induce lymphocyte proliferation in apparently all humans, lower doses seem to lead to selective responses that are restricted by MHC class II involvement (104).

When human peripheral blood mononuclear cells were exposed to Pb, Ni, zinc, or Hg, there was increased ^{3}H-thymidine incorporation compared with that of control (no metal) cultures (119). When B and T cells were isolated and exposed to either Pb or zinc, increased proliferation was noted only in T-cell preparations. Cellular thiols, which have been implicated as the target of heavy metals, were increased by 10% to 40% in Pb-, zinc- and Ni-exposed cells, whereas Hg treatment lowered thiol levels by 80% to 90%. The increase in thiol status may reflect an increase in cellular proliferation, in which thiols are known to play a major role, or it may be indicative of metal-induced oxidative stress or metallothionien production.

In vitro analysis of cell-mediated immunity is often evaluated as mixed lymphocyte culture response or concanavalin A responsiveness. *In vitro* Pb, zinc, and Ni have all been shown to enhance the autologous mixed lymphocyte culture response of mouse splenocytes (120,121). Analysis of the cell type responding in the autologous mixed lymphocyte culture response revealed it to be a Thy-1[+], Ly-1[+], Lyt-2[−], L3T4[+] cell that required the presence of an Ia[+] accessory cell. Separation-reconstitution experiments designed to evaluate the effect of Pb on macrophage function demonstrated that either *in vivo* or *in vitro* exposure of the macrophage population to Pb increased the autologous mixed lymphocyte culture response (58). A single intramuscular injection of nickel has been reported to decrease natural killer cell activity in both C57B1/6 and CBA/J mice (107,108). Viral immunity has also been suppressed in both Hg- and Pb-exposed mice (37) and rabbits (51).

In a collaborative study (Table 2), we have analyzed the *in vitro* reactivities of peripheral blood mononuclear cells isolated from venous blood of children (1 to 8 years old) exposed to lead in their urban environment (Bronx, New York). In addition, the peripheral blood mononuclear cells were immunophenotyped by flow cytometric analysis. It is interesting to note that as with the analysis of mice (73), the parameter that approached significantly different was enhancement of MHC class II expression by lead. Although no differences were significant ($p = 0.05$), lead also lowered the number of CD4[+] lymphocytes. To date there have been too few studies evaluating the influence of metals on human immunity. Thus, no conclusive assessment of the potential risk of environmental metal exposures on human health can be made, although it is likely (based on murine studies) that the immune system is another target of the toxic effects of metals, including Pb.

TABLE 2. In vivo *lead effect on various immune parameters of children measured* in vitro[a]

Parameters assayed	Low Pb group[b]	High Pb group	p value[c]
Concanavalin A-induced proliferation	51 ± 5 (n = 19)[d]	57 ± 6 (n = 35)	0.47
PHA-induced proliferation	96 ± 16 (n = 9)	74 ± 8 (n = 27)	0.19
PWM-induced proliferation	29 ± 3 (n = 19)	35 ± 3 (n = 34)	0.21
Autologous MLR	5 ± 1 (n = 19)	7 ± 2 (n = 35)	0.27
PWM-induced IgM synthesis	2.5 ± 0.4 (n = 19)	2.9 ± 0.9 (n = 8)	0.65
Percentage of CD3[+] PBL[e]	62 ± 2 (n = 15)	61 ± 1 (n = 21)	0.23
Percentage of CD4[+] PBL	41 ± 1 (n = 14)	37 ± 1 (n = 8)	0.10
Percentage of CD8[+] PBL	17 ± 1 (n = 13)	20 ± 2 (n = 8)	0.37
Percentage of CD20[+] PBL	11 ± 2 (n = 15)	11 ± 1 (n = 26)	0.76
Percentage of DR[+] PBL	11 ± 1 (n = 10)	15 ± 1 (n = 29)	0.12

[a]Children (nonchelated) between the ages of 1 and 8 years of age were assessed for various immune parameters *in vitro* with use of their venous blood. The blood samples were provided by Dr. J. F. Rosen, Montefiore Medical Center, Albert Einstein College of Medicine, Bronx, N.Y. The proliferative values are ($\times 10^3$) counts per minute, well assessed by incorporation of ^{3}H-thymidine. The IgM values are mg/ml of culture supernatant.

[b]The low Pb group had <25 μg Pb/dl blood (2 to 25 μg/dl); the high Pb group had > 25 μg Pb/dl blood (26 to 49 μg/dl).

[c]The *p* value was calculated by Student's *t*-test.

[d]The values represent the mean ± standard error of the mean.

[e]PBL, peripheral blood lymphocytes, gated by FALS and 90° LS by flow cytometry. PHA, phytohemagglutinin; PWM, pokeweed mitogen; MLR, mixed lymphocyte culture response.

Mercury is the best documented metal to induce autoimmune disease. Mercuric chloride exposure of Brown-Norway rats induces lymphoproliferation, hypergammaglobulinemia, the production of autoantibodies directed against the glomerular basement membrane, and immune complex–induced glomerulonephritis (98). In addition, autoreactive T-cell clones have been isolated from exposed rats that will induce a local graft-versus-host reaction in syngeneic animals (88,89). Adoptive transfer of W3/25[+] T cells obtained from Hg-exposed rats induced autoimmune disease in naive animals (89). Transfer of B cells had no effect. Of particular importance was the observation that the recipients of autoreactive T cells responded with increased proliferation of OX8[+] T (cytotoxic/suppressor) cells. When OX8[+] cells were depleted by *in vivo* treatment with OX8 antibody, the severity of the autoimmunity increased. Animals exposed to Hg did not display increased numbers of OX8[+] cells. The data indicate that autoreactive T-helper cells are induced whereas T-cytotoxic/suppressor cells are inhibited from responding to the increase in autoreactivity. In the mouse, Hg can induce a similar autoimmune process and is known to be restricted to the S haplotype (94). Like Pb and Ni, Hg also is able to augment anaphylaxis, but the mechanism is more apparent for Hg in that Hg has been shown to enhance IgE production (90).

The hypersensitivities induced by heavy metals are proof of their ability to modulate immune reactivity; however, the mechanisms by which they induce autoimmunity have not been fully delineated. Direct interactions of metals with lymphocytes may alter their physiology, resulting in polyclonal activation and/or a hyperactive state (27,45). The direct activation of lymphocytes by heavy metals has been proposed by a number of investigators (16,27). Experimental data have been gathered that support the ability of Pb and Hg to enhance lymphocyte proliferation. Pb, Ni, and zinc have all been shown to induce progression of lymphocytes from G_0 to G_1 of the cell cycle (121). Lead also has been reported to induce proliferation of liver cells (20) and renal tubular cells (18). The mechanisms by which heavy metals influence lymphocyte activation, proliferation, and effector phases of the lymphoid subsets are still unknown. There is evidence that *in vivo* Pb exposure can alter the C3b receptor on some lymphocytes (56), and Pb and Hg are known to modulate numerous cellular enzymes (118). Lead was shown to modulate cyclic adenosine monophosphate and cyclic guanosine monophosphate effects on B cells, both of which are implicated in lymphocyte activation (64).

Although the effects of heavy metals on immune function appear to be quite diverse, it is evident from the data outlined that host resistance is modified. Comparison of data is often complex because of the many variables present in dealing with immunocompetent cells; however, in many cases, MHC class II modulations are posited.

The MHC class II molecules (I-A and I-E, mice; DR, DP, and DQ, humans) play the predominant role in determining immune responsiveness to a particular antigen (25). An obvious question that arises in investigating the effects of heavy metals on immune responsiveness is whether metals alter MHC class II expression. The effects of each metal can vary with the species or strain of animal tested. This, com-

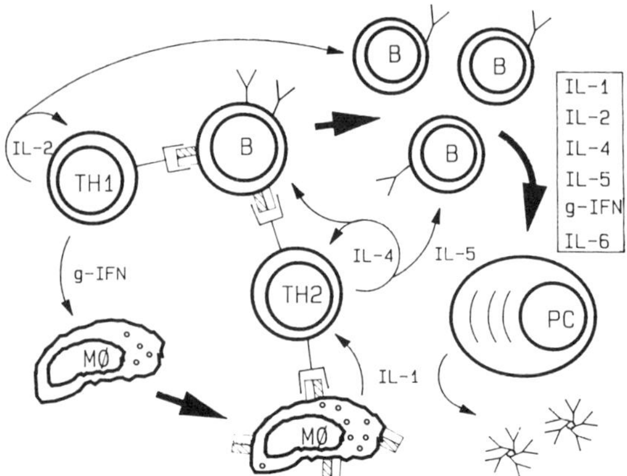

FIG. 1. Immunoregulation by T-helper 1 and T-helper 2 cells. These CD4$^+$ helper T-cell subsets have a preference for particular MHC class II expressing antigen-presenting cells (macrophages, MØ; B cells), have different sensitivities/responsiveness, and produce different regulatory factors.

bined with the knowledge that autoimmune disease is often associated with certain DR phenotypes, leads to the speculation that expression of certain MHC class II molecules renders the animal or patient more susceptible to the immunomodulating effects of heavy metals. An alteration of self MHC class II could result in autoreactivity. Studies of Ia antigens in CBA mice exposed to Pb, zinc, and Ni revealed no difference in the binding of monoclonal antibodies with either I-A or I-E (120). In addition, SDS-PAGE analysis of I-A antigen expressed on activated peritoneal macrophages was not altered in Pb-treated CBA/J mice (58). Furthermore, bone marrow–derived macrophages exposed to Pb in culture demonstrated no significant difference in the binding of a monoclonal antibody directed against I-E (60). However, unlike the effect of Pb on macrophage expression of I-A or I-E, Pb as well as Hg enhances the expression of I-A and I-E on B cells (73). These differential effects of Pb on MHC class II expression are important to note because they probably help to explain the intricate yet subtle way in which Pb as well as other metals may alter immunoregulation. Pb also differentially affects activation of the CD4$^+$ T-cell subsets (74), which are important regulators of all immune responses. Lead appears to inhibit T-helper 1 cell activation but enhances T-helper 2 cell activation. Other toxicants also have been reported to differentially activate these CD4$^+$ T-cell subsets (7,84). Interestingly, T-helper 1 cells and T-helper 2 cells are known to differ in numerous biochemical properties, including sensitivity to cyclic adenosine monophosphate (76) and responsiveness to $[Ca^{2+}]_i$ (123). Lead and cyclic adenosine monophosphate have been reported previously to synergize for the induction of humoral immune responses (64). Although actual modulations of T-helper 1 and 2 cells by Pb at the cellular (biochemical/molecular) level are undelineated, the following correlations should be kept in mind. T-helper 1 and 2 TM$_2$ cells are primarily responsible for upregulation of cell-mediated immunity and HI, respectively (Fig.

1), and Pb preferentially inhibits cell-mediated immunity. Macrophages preferentially present antigen to T-helper 2 cells, whereas B cells seem to preferentially present antigen to T-helper 1 cells. Pb does not appear to alter expression of MHC class II molecules on macrophages, but it does alter their expression on B cells. Although it may usually seem that increased expression of MHC class II molecules should increase antigen presentation, this may not be the case. Lead has been reported to inhibit antigen presentation to a T-helper 1 cell hybridoma (109). The ability of Pb to enhance I-A or I-E was not attributable to increased transcription (74); thus, Pb may alter a translational or posttranslational activity. This does not rule out the possibility that MHC class II molecules are directly affected by heavy metals. Monoclonal antibodies directed against Ia antigen determinants recognize only single epitopes, although many exist. The ability of heavy metals such as Pb to interact with thiol groups could induce changes in MHC class II molecules. Simonis and Cullen have demonstrated that alpha, beta, and invariant chains undergo fatty acid acylation involving thioester or hydroxy ester bonds (105). It is possible that the interaction of MHC class II molecules with fatty acids results in the proper orientation of MHC class II molecules within the cell membrane, allowing for antigen recognition. Heavy metals may interfere with this interaction, resulting in impaired ability to present antigen in the context of self. Alternatively, metals may modify glycosylation of MHC class II molecules; different glycosylation patterns have been suggested to modify MHC class II activities (32).

Major histocompatibility complex gene products are known to regulate Hg-induced renal immunopathologies in mice (94), rats (98), and humans (16). Au induced nephrotic syndrome has been associated with expression of the DR3w phenotype (111,124). Gold-induced thrombocytopenia also was reported to be immunologically mediated and regulated by MHC genes (111). In tests of Pb-poisoned workers (122), it was reported that 21 of 57 individuals with high Pb levels had kidney disease; 15 of these 21 were described as having Pb nephropathy. Eight of these 15 workers with nephropathy were examined for immune involvement and seven tested positive. The study suggests that only 23% of the Pb-burdened workers could get Pb-induced glomerulonephritis. Polak and colleagues (89a) were the first to indicate that sensitization to inorganic metal compounds is under genetic control. Likewise, it has been indicated that many autoimmune diseases are influenced by the genetics of the MHC (25). Altered renal pathology, possibly the result of immune complexes, has been associated with Hg, gold, Cd, and Pb (28,40,72,79) exposure.

The association of metals with protein constituents resulting in altered self is an attractive hypothesis; however, data concerning metal-lymphocyte protein interactions have not materialized. Several metals are associated with proteins in the body. The metallothioniens, a group of cysteine-rich, low molecular weight proteins, have been demonstrated to bind several metals both *in vivo* and *in vitro* (50). Both zinc- and copper-metallothionien complexes are found in humans and may act as a storage depot for these essential trace elements (17). Interestingly, interleukin-1 and interferon-gamma both upregulate the transcription rate of metallothionien (1), indicating that this compound may be influenced by or affect immunoreactivity. Interleukin-1 and interferon-gamma are associated with macrophage activation. The activation of macrophages can lead to the generation of reactive oxygen moieties, which induce cellular damage. Metallothionien may act as a scavenger of free radicals that may work synergistically with glutathione to protect cells against oxidative damage. Heavy metals, with their high affinity for thiol groups, may interact within this system, resulting in an enhanced inflammatory response. Metallothionien recently has been reported to have modulatory effects on lymphocytes, and it is endogenous to lymphocytes (Lynes 1988).

The ability of metals to react with thiols has been well documented (87,118). Lead, mercury, and gold have a high affinity for sulfhydryl (thiol) groups (118), and all are associated with dysregulation of the immune system. The thiol status of lymphocytes appears to be critical for cell activation. Experimental data have shown that modulation of thiols results in a decrease in cell activation by mitogen (80). In addition, the T-suppressor cell subset has a higher level of thiol sensitivity than does the helper cell subset. One could then infer that T-suppressor cells are more prone to the toxic effects of heavy metals. A disruption of helper:suppressor cell ratios could result in polyclonal cell activation, increased immunoglobulin formation to metal-protein antigens, immune complex formation, and basement membrane destruction. Clearly, these are speculative mechanisms of how metals may induce immunopathological changes.

The relationship between the lymphocyte subsets and macrophages is dynamic. Removal of one cell type alters homeostasis and may result in autoimmunity or impaired host resistance. The development of the Brown-Norway rat model of Hg-induced autoimmunity appears to involve an imbalance between T-helper and T-suppressor cells (89). T-cytotoxic/suppressor cells have more cell surface thiols, are more sensitive to permeant thiol blockers, and are more radiosensitive than helper cells (66). A decline in suppressor cell activity and/or an increase in B-cell activity has been suggested to account for the increased incidence of autoimmunity with age (6). Metals, with their high affinity for sulfhydryl groups, may preferentially alter cytotoxic/suppressor cells, inducing a state of autoimmunity or impaired host resistance. Heavy metals, some of which increase in content with age, may accelerate the generation of autoimmune reactions as a result of the combined effects of lowered thiol status and increased body burden of metal.

The mechanisms by which heavy metals induce pathological changes have not been clearly delineated. Immunological parameters could be involved in pathological effects of heavy metals, such as renal, hematopoietic, and central nervous system changes associated with Pb (40). For example, Pb induces renal damage; could this be the result of its effect on the immune system? The possibilities range from a direct effect on basement membranes resulting in antibody deposits and complement activation, or possibly a more nonspecific effect such as Pb-induced alterations of endothelial cells resulting in the generation of mediators of inflammation resulting in macrophage migration, activation, and proliferation. This, in turn, would lead to a chronic inflammatory condition with gradual loss of organ function.

There are many possible scenarios in which the interaction of metals with the immune system and/or target organs could lead to pathological changes. Examples include Hg involvement in Addison's disease (3), Hg- and Pb-induced biochemical changes that may result in autoimmune hemolytic anemia (26), gold-induced thrombocytopenia (19,111), and autoimmune hemolytic anemia (47,111).

The subcellular effects of heavy metals on constituents of the immune system must be investigated. Many experiments describe the phenomenology of metal-induced changes of immune function, but little is known of the mechanisms involved in these alterations. An attractive starting point is the thiol or phospholipid reactivity of the heavy metals. Many biological compounds with immunomodulatory activity are known to react with thiol groups, including cytochalasin B (85), insulin (24), and interferon (49). In addition, many growth factor receptors contain thiol-rich domains that aid in receptor/ligand binding (125). Thiols are involved in cell-cell communications and adherence via the family of proteins known as integrins (62,95). Major histocompatibility complex class II molecules may require thiol groups for proper orientation in the cell membrane (105). Many enzyme systems such as phospholipase A_2 contain thiol domains that are speculated to be involved in orientation on the enzyme in the cell membrane (72a). Thiols are known to be involved in cell transport (41) and DNA synthesis (118). Likewise, all signal transduction is initiated at the cell surface. Thus, plasma membrane modification could be highly regulatory, and metals such as Pb are known to interact with the head groups of phospholipids (46).

Heavy metals also may modify thiols or membranes indirectly by modulating oxidative products. Heavy metals could alter the redox state of the cell, which could affect lipid peroxidation and/or modulate synthesis of immunoregulatory products such as prostaglandins (23) or leukotrienes (86). Of particular interest are the peptidoleukotrienes C_4, D_4, and E_4, which require glutathione for their synthesis (86). These leukotrienes are known to have a wide variety of effects on the immune system; among them, these substances make up slow-reacting substance of anaphylaxis, augment myeloid colony formation, and induce further synthesis of arachidonic acid to its various metabolites (86). Since glutathione is the primary non-protein thiol within the cell, its level may be influenced by heavy metals, which in turn could alter leukotriene synthesis. Other possible targets within the leukotriene system are the metabolizing enzymes (γ-glutamyl transpeptidase and dipeptidase) that convert leukotriene C_4 to leukotriene D_4 to leukotriene E_4. The dipeptidase is a metal-requiring enzyme whose activity can be enhanced by manganese, cobalt, and zinc or inhibited by copper (78,92). Again, an imbalance induced by altered enzyme activity could result in detrimental immunomodulation.

It is obvious that heavy metals alter immunity in certain strains and species. Data reported indicate that all branches of the immune system are affected. The response to any particular metal may enhance some aspects of immunity while suppressing others. The subcellular mechanisms by which metals alter immunity is unknown. Speculation centers on biochemical alterations of cells of the immune system or cells of other organ systems that are under constant immune surveillance, which could trigger immune activation if modified. Genetics plays a pivotal role in immunoregulation and appears to influence metal responses in both animals and humans. Investigations of the subcellular biochemical events involved in lymphocyte activation that could be altered by heavy metals should provide insight into how these metals alter immunity.

ACKNOWLEDGMENT

The research support for the data in the tables was from the United States Environmental Protection Agency, Grant No. R-812977.

REFERENCES

1. Adrian, G. S., Korinek, B. W., Bowman, B. H., and Yang, F. (1986): The human transferrin gene: 5′ region contains conserved sequences which match the control elements regulated by heavy metals, glucocorticoids and acute phase reaction. *Gene*, 49:167–175.
2. Aggarwal, S. K., Broomhead, J. A., Fairlie, D. P., and Whitehouse, M. W. (1980): Platinum drugs: Combined anti-lymphoproliferative and nephrotoxicity assays in rats. *Cancer Chemother. Pharmacol.*, 4:249–258.
3. Alomar, A., Camarasa, J. G., and Barnadas, M. (1983): Addison's disease and contact dermatitis from mercury in a soap. *Contact Dermatitis*, 9:76.
4. Aresta, M., Defazio, F., Fumarulo, R., Giordano, D., Pantaleo, R., and Riccardi, S. (1982): Biological activity of metal complexes. V. Influence of Pd (II), Pt (II), and Rh (I) on the macrophages chemotaxis. *Biochem. Biophys. Res. Commun.*, 104:121–125.
5. Baldwin, J. L., Storb, R., Thomas, E. D., and Mannik, M. (1977): Bone marrow transplantation in patients with gold-induced marrow aplasia. *Arthritis Rheum.*, 20:1043–1048.
6. Battisto, J. R., Claman, H. N., and Scott, D. W. (1982): Immunological tolerances to self and non-self. *Ann. N.Y. Acad. Sci.*, 392:1–435.
7. Baum, C. G., Szabo, P., Siskind, G. W., Becker, C. G., Firpo, A. Clarick, C. J., and Francus, T. (1990): Cellular control of IgE induction by a polyphenol-rich compound. *J. Immunol.*, 145:779–784.
8. Berenbaum, M. C. (1971): Immunosuppression by platinum diamines. *Br. J. Cancer*, 25:208–211.
9. Blomberg-van der Flier, M., van der Burg, C. K. H., Pos, O., van der Plassch-Boers, E. M., Bruynzell, D. P., Garotta, G., and Scheper, R. J. (1987): In vitro studies in nickel allergy: Diagnostic value of dual parameter analysis. *J. Invest. Dermatol.*, 88:362–368.
10. Blakely, B. R., and Archer, D. L. (1981): The effect of lead acetate on the immune response in mice. *Toxicol. Appl. Pharmacol.*, 61:18–26.
11. Blakely, B. R., Sisodia, C. S., and Mukkur, T. K. (1980): The effect of methylmercury, tetraethyl lead and sodium arsenite on the humoral immune response in mice. *Toxicol. Appl. Pharmacol.*, 52:245–254.
12. Burchiel, S. W., Hadley, W. M., Cameron, C. L., Fincher, R. H., Lim, T-W, and Stewart, C. C. (1986): Flow cytometry Coulter volume analysis of lead- and cadmium-induced cellular alterations in bone marrow obtained from young and aged Balb/c mice. *Toxicol. Lett.*, 34:89–94.
13. Burge, J. J., Fearon, D. T., and Austin, K. F. (1978): Inhibition of the alternative pathway of complement by gold sodium thiomalate *in vitro. J. Immunol.*, 120:1626–1630.
14. Burnet, M. (1969): Self and Not-Self. Melbourne University Press, Victoria, Australia.
15. Castranova, V., Bowman, L., Reasor, M. J., and Miles, P. R. (1980): Effects of heavy metal ions on selected oxidative metabolic processes in rat alveolar macrophages. *Toxicol. Appl. Immunol.*, 53:14–23.
16. Charpentier, B., Moullot, P., Faux, N., Manigand, G., and Fries, D. (1981): T lymphocyte functions in mercuric chloride-induced membranous glomerulonephritis in man. Evidence for a defect

of presentation of the histocompatibility class II molecules at the cell surface. *Nephrologie*, 2:153–157.

17. Cherian, M. G., and Goyer, R. A. (1978): Metallothioniens and their role in metabolism and toxicity of metals. *Life Sci.*, 23:1–10.

18. Choie, D. D., and Richter, G. W. (1974): Cell proliferation in mouse kidney induced by lead: I. Synthesis of DNA. *Lab. Invest.*, 30:647–651.

19. Coblyn, J. S., Weinblatt, M., Holdsworth, D., and Glass, D. (1981): Gold-induced thrombocytopenia. A clinical and immunogenetic study of twenty-three patients. *Ann. Intern. Med.*, 95:178–181.

20. Columbano, A., Ledda, G. M., Sirigu, P., Perra, T., and Pani, P. (1983): Liver cell proliferation induced by a single dose of lead nitrate. *Am. J. Pathol.*, 110:83–88.

21. Cook, J. A., Hoffman, E. O., and Di Luzio, N. R. (1975): Influence of lead and cadmium on the susceptibility of rats to bacterial challenge (39117). *Proc. Soc. Exp. Biol. Med.*, 150:741–747.

22. Cook, J. A., and Karns, L. (1978): Effect of RES stimulation and suppression on lead sensitization to endotoxic shock. *J. Reticuloendothel. Soc.*, 24:1A.

23. Cunnane, S. C. (1982): Differential regulation of essential fatty acid metabolism to the prostaglandins: Possible basis for the interaction of zinc and copper in biological systems. *Prog. Lipid. Res.*, 21:73–90.

24. Czech, M. P., Lawrence, J. C., and Lynn, W. S. (1974): Evidence for the involvement of sulfhydryl oxidation in regulation of fat cell hexose transport by insulin. *Proc. Natl. Acad. Sci. U.S.A.*, 71:4173–4177.

25. Dausset, J., and Svejgaard, A. (1977): HLA and Disease. Williams & Wilkins Co., Baltimore.

26. Dieter, M. P., Luster, M. L., Boorman, G. A., Jamieson, C. W., Dean, J. H., and Cox, J. W. (1983): Immunologic and biochemical responses in mice treated with mercuric chloride. *Toxicol. Appl. Pharmacol.*, 68:218.

27. Druet, P., Hirsch, F., Sapin, C., Druet, E., and Bellon, B. (1982): Immune dysregulation and autoimmunity induced by toxic agents. *Transplant. Proc.*, 14:482–484.

28. Druet, P., Teychenne, P., Mandet, C., Bascou., C., and Druet, E. (1981): Immune-type glomerulonephritis induced in the Brown-Norway rat with mercury-containing pharmaceutical products. *Nephron*, 28:145–148.

29. Eastman, A. Y., and Lawrence, D. A. (1982): TNP-modified syngeneic cells enhance immunoregulatory T cell activities similar to allogeneic effects. *J. Immunol.*, 128:926–931.

30. Edwards, F. K., and Edwards, E. K. (1982): Allergic contact dermatitis to lead acetate in a hair dye. *Cutis*, 30:629–630.

31. Ewers, U., Stiller-Winkler, R., and Idel, H. (1982): Serum immunoglobulin, complement C3, and salivary IgA levels in lead workers. *Environ. Res.*, 29:351–357.

32. Ferro, T. J., Monos, D. S., Spear, B. T., Rossman, M. D., Zmijewski, C. M., Kamoun, M., and Daniele, R. P. (1987): Carbohydrate differences in HLA-DR molecules synthesized by alveolar macrophages and blood monocytes. *Am. Rev. Respir. Dis.*, 135:1340–1344.

33. Fonzi, S., and Pengue, L. (1966): Processes of immunization in experimental poisoning with mercury vapors: III. Changes of the complementary power of the serum after active immunization. *Lav. Umano.*, 18:427–429.

34. Gainer, J. H. (1972): Increased mortality in encephalomyocarditis virus-infected mice consuming cobalt sulfate: Tissue concentrations of cobalt. *Am J. Vet. Res.*, 33:2067–2073.

35. Gainer, J. H. (1974): Lead aggravates viral disease and represses the antiviral activity of interferon inducers. *Environ. Health Perspect.*, 7:113–119.

36. Gainer, J. H. (1977): Effects of heavy metals and of deficiency of zinc on mortality rates in mice infected with encephalomyocarditis virus. *Am. J. Vet. Res.*, 38:869–872.

37. Gainer, J. H., and Pry, T. W. (1972): Effects of arsenicals on viral infections in mice. *Am J. Vet. Res.*, 33:2299–2307.

38. Gallagher, K., Matarazzo, W. J., and Gray, I. (1979): Trace metal modification of immunocompetence. II. Effect of Pb^{2+}, Cd^{2+}, and Cr^{3+} on RNA turnover, hexokinase activity, and blastogenesis during B-lymphocyte transformation *in vitro*. *Clin. Immunol. Immunopathol.*, 13:369–377.

39. Geddes, D. M., and Brostoff, J. (1976): Pulmonary fibrosis associated with hypersensitivity to gold salts. *Br. Med. J.*, 1:1444.

40. Goyer, R. A. (1986): Toxic effect of metals. In Toxicology, edited by C. D. Klassen, M. O. Amdur, and J. Doull, pp. 582–635. Macmillan, New York.

41. Hare, J. D. (1975): Distinctive alterations of nucleoside, sugar and amino acid uptake by sulf-hydryl reagents in cultured mouse cells. *Arch. Biochem. Biophys.*, 170:347–352.
42. Hays, E. F., and Margaretten, N. (1985): Long term oral cadmium exposure produces bone marrow hypoplasia in mice. *Exp. Hematol.*, 13:229–234.
43. Hemphill, F. E., Kaeberle, M. L, and Buck, W. B. (1971): Lead suppression of mouse resistance to *Salmonella typhimurium*. *Science*, 172:1031–1032.
44. Hilbertz, U., Kramer, U., De Ruiter, N., and Baginski, B. (1986): Effects of cadmium and lead on oxidative metabolism and phagocytosis by mouse peritoneal macrophages. *Toxicology*, 39:47–57.
45. Hirsch, F., Couderc, J., Sapin, C., Fournie, G., and Druet, P. (1982): Polyclonal effect of $HgCl_2$ in the rat, its possible role in an experimental autoimmune disease. *Eur. J. Immunol.*, 12:620–625.
46. Hoogeveen, J. T. (1970): Thermoconductometric investigation of phosphatidylcholine in aqueous tertiary butanol solutions in the absence and presence of metal ions. In Effects of Metals on Cells, Subcellular Elements, and Macromolecules, edited by J. Maniloff, J. R. Coleman, and M. W. Miller, pp. 207–232. Charles C. Thomas Publisher, Springfield.
47. Hunziker, H. (1978): Gold induced autoimmunohemolytic anemia. *Praxis* 67:702–704.
48. Ito, Y., Kurita, H., Yoshida, T., Shima, S., Niiya, Y., Toriumi, H., Nakayasu, T., Komori, Y., and Sarai, S. (1982): Studies on serum specific protein levels in lead-exposed workers. *Jpn. J. Ind. Health*, 24:390–391.
49. Johnson, H. M. (1980): Similarities in the suppression of the immune response by interferon and by a thiol-oxidizing agent (40882). *Proc. Soc. Exp. Biol. Med.*, 164:380–385.
50. Kagi, J. H. R., Himmehock, S. R., Whanger, P. O., Bethune, J. L., and Vallee, B. L. (1974): Equine hepatic and renal metallothioniens: Purification, molecular weight, amino acid composition and metal content. *J. Biol. Chem.*, 249:3537–3542.
51. Kerkvliet, N. I., and Baecher-Steppan, L. (1982): Immunotoxicology studies on lead: Effects of exposure on tumor growth and cell-mediated tumor immunity after syngeneic or allogeneic stimulation. *Immunopharmacology*, 4:213–224.
52. Koller, L. D. (1973): Immunosuppression produced by lead, cadmium and mercury. *Am. J. Vet. Res.*, 34:1457–1458.
53. Koller, L. D., and Kovacic, S. (1974): Decreased antibody formation in mice exposed to lead. *Nature* (London), 250:148–150.
54. Koller, L. D. (1975): Methylmercury: Effect on oncogenic and nononcogenic viruses in mice. *Am. J. Vet. Res.*, 36:1501–1504.
55. Koller, L. D., Roan, J. G., and Exon, J. H. (1976): Humoral antibody response in mice after single does exposure to lead or cadmium. *Proc. Soc. Exp. Biol. Med.*, 151:339–342.
56. Koller, L. D., and Brauner, J. A. (1977): Decreased B-lymphocyte response after exposure to lead and cadmium. *Toxicol. Appl. Pharmacol.*, 42:621–624.
57. Koller, L. D., Roan, J. G., and Kerkvliet, N. I. (1979): Mitogen stimulation of lymphocytes in CBA mice exposed to lead and cadmium. *Environ. Res.*, 19:177–188.
58. Kowolenko, M., Tracy, L., and Lawrence, D. A. (1988): Effect of lead on macrophage function. *J. Leukocyte Biol.*, 43:357.
59. Kowolenko, M., Tracy, L., and Lawrence, D. A. (1988): Macrophage progenitor cells are altered in lead exposed mice. *FASEB* 33:A665.
60. Kowolenko, M., Tracy, L., and Lawrence, D. A. (1989): *In vitro* effects of lead on macrophage growth and differentiation. *J. Leukocyte Biol.*, 45:198–206.
61. Lane, C. H., and Fauci, A. S. (1985): Immunologic abnormalities in the acquired immunodeficiency syndrome. *Ann. Rev. Immunuol.*, 3:477–500.
62. Law, S. K. A., Gagnon, J., Hildreth, J. E. K., Wells, C. E., Willis, A. C., and Wong, A. J. (1987): The primary structure of the B subunit of the cell surface adhesion glycoproteins LFA-1, CR3 and p150,95 and its relationship to the fibronectin receptor. *EMBO J.*, 6:915–919.
63. Lawrence, D. A. (1981): Heavy metal modulation of lymphocyte activities. I. *In vitro* effects of heavy metals on primary humoral immune responses. *Toxicol. Appl. Pharmacol.*, 57:439–451.
64. Lawrence, D. A. (1981): Heavy metal modulation of lymphocyte activities. II. Lead, an *in vitro* mediator of B-cell activation. *Int. J. Immunopharmacol.*, 3:153–161.
65. Lawrence D. A. (1981): *In vivo* and *in vitro* effects of lead on humoral and cell-mediated immunity. *Infect. Immun.*, 31:136–143.
66. Lawrence, D. A. (1981): Antigen activation of T-cells. In Handbook of Cancer Immunology, edited by H. Waters, pp. 257–320. Garland Press, New York.
67. Lawrence, D. A., Mitchell, D., and Rudofsky, U. (1983): Heavy metal modulation of lymphocyte

and macrophage activity. In Proceedings of the 13th Annual Conference on Environmental Toxicology, AFAMRL-TR-82-101, pp. 63–79.

68. Lipsky, P. E., and Ziff, M. (1980): Inhibition of human helper T-cell function *in vitro* by D-penicillamine and $CuSO_4$. *J. Clin. Invest.*, 65:1069–1076.

69. Luster, M. I., Dean, J. H., and Moore, J. A. (1984): Evaluation of immune functions in toxicology. In Principles and Methods in Toxicology, edited by A. W. Hayes, p. 561. Raven Press, New York.

70. Luster, M. I., Faith, R. E., and Kimmel, C. A. (1978): Depression of humoral immunity in rats following chronic developmental exposure. *J. Envir. Pathol. Toxicol.*, 1:397.

70a. Lynes, M. A., Garvey, J., and Lawrence, D. A. (1988): Metallothionien effects on lymphocyte activities. *FASEB J*, 2:A2741.

71. Makinodan, T., and Kay, M. M. B. (1980): Age influence on the immune system. *Adv. Immunol.*, 29:287–330.

72. Makker, S. P., and Aikawa, M. (1979): Mesangial glomerulonephropathy with deposition of IgG, IgM and C3 induced by mercuric chloride. *Lab. Invest.*, 41:45–50.

72a. Maragnore, J. M. (1987): Structural elements for protein-phospholipid interactions may be shared in protein kinase C and phospholipase A_2. *TIBS*, 12:176–177.

73. McCabe, M. J., and Lawrence, D. A. (1990): The heavy metal lead exhibits B cell stimulatory factor activity by enhancing B cell Ia expression and differentiation. *J. Immunol.*, 145:671–677.

74. McCabe, M. J., and Lawrence, D. A. (1990): Aspects of lead potentiation of B lymphocyte responses and its relationship to immune dysregulation. In Metal Ions in Biology and Medicine, edited by P. Collery, L. A. Poiner, M. Manfait, and J.-C. Etienne, pp. 237–242. John Libbey, London.

75. Mertz, W. (1981): The essential trace elements. *Science*, 213:1332–1338.

76. Munoz, E., Zubiaga, A. M., Merrow, M., Sauter, N. P., and Huber, B. T. (1990): Cholera toxin discriminates between T helper 1 and 2 cells in T cell receptor-mediated activation: Role of cAMP in T cell proliferation. *J. Exp. Med.*, 172:95–103.

77. Mottironi, V. D., Banks, S. M., and Lawrence, D. A. (1986): Analysis of immunologic parameters in mercury workers. *Fed. Proc.*, 46:1318.

78. Nagaoka, I., and Yamashita, T. (1987): Studies on the leukotriene D_4-metabolizing enzyme of rat leukocytes, which catalyzes the conversion of leukotriene D_4 to leukotriene E_4. *Biochem. Biophys. Acta*, 922:8–17.

79. Nagi, A. H., Alexander, F., and Barabas, A. Z. (1971): Gold nephropathy in rats: Light and electron microscopic studies. *Exp. Mol. Pathol.*, 15:354–362.

80. Noelle, R. J., and Lawrence, D. A. (1981): Modulation of T-cell functions. II. Chemical basis for the involvement of cell surface thiol-reactive sites in control of T-cell proliferation. *Cell. Immunol.*, 60:453–469.

81. Norlind, K. (1990): Toxic metals and irritant or allergic skin reactions. In Metal Ions in Biology and Medicine, edited by P. Collery, L. A. Poiner, M. Manfait, and J.-C. Etienne, pp. 252–257. John Libbey, London.

82. Norlind, K., and Henze, A. (1984): Stimulating effect of mercuric chloride and nickel sulfate on DNA synthesis of thymocytes and peripheral blood lymphocytes in children. *Int. Arch. Allergy Appl. Immunol.*, 73:162–165.

83. North, R. J. (1970): The relative importance of blood monocytes and fixed macrophages to the expression of cell mediated immunity to infection. *J. Exp. Med.*, 32:521.

84. Ochel, M., Pfeiffer, C., Vohr, H. W., and Gleichmann, E. (1989): The increased IgE formation inducible by mercuric chloride is inhibited by anti-IL-4. Abstracts. Berlin: 7th International Congress of Immunology, p. 461.

85. Parker, C. W. (1977): Cyclic nucleotides in the immune response. In Cyclic 3′,5′-Nucleotides: Mechanisms of Action, edited by H. Cramer and J. Schultz, pp. 161–187. John Wiley & Sons, New York.

86. Parker, C. W. (1987): Lipid mediators produced through lipoxygenase pathway. *Ann. Rev. Immunol.*, 5:65–84.

87. Passow, H., Rothstein, A., and Clarkson, T. W. (1961): The general pharmacology of the heavy metals. *Pharmacol. Rev.*, 13:185–224.

88. Pelletier, L., Pasquier, R., Hirsch, F., Sapin, C., and Druct, P. (1985): In vivo self reactivity of mononuclear cells to T cells and macrophages exposed to $HgCl_2$. *Eur. J. Immunol.*, 15:460.

89. Pelletier, L., Pasquier, R., Rossert, J., Vial, M.-C., Mandet, C., and Druet, P. (1988): Autoreac-

tive T cells in mercury-induced autoimmunity: Ability to induce autoimmune disease. *J. Immunol.*, 140:750–754.

89a. Polak, L., Barnes, J. M., and Turk, J. L. (1968): The genetic control of contact sensitivity to inorganic metal compounds in guinea pigs. *Immunology*, 14:707–711.

90. Prouvost-Danon, A., Abadie, A., Sapin, C., and Druet, P. (1981): Induction of IgE synthesis and potentiation of anti-ovalbumin IgE antibody response by $HgCl_2$ in the rat. *J. Immunol.*, 126:699–702.

91. Purdy, H. A., and Walbum, L. E. (1922): The action of various metallic salts on hemolysis. *J. Immunol.*, 7:35–45.

92. Raulf, M., Konig, W., Koller, M., and Stunning, M. (1987): Release and functional characterization of the leukotriene D_4 metabolizing enzyme (dipeptidase) from human polymorphonuclear leukocytes. *Scand. J. Immunol.*, 25:305–313.

93. Reigart, J. R., and Graber, C. D. (1976): Evaluation of the humoral immune response of children with low level lead exposure. *Bull. Environ. Contam. Toxicol.*, 16:112–117.

94. Robinson, C. J. G., Balazs, T., and Egorov, I. K. (1986): Mercuric chloride-, gold sodium thiomalate-, and d-penacillamine-induced antinuclear antibodies in mice. *Toxicol. Appl. Pharmacol.*, 86:159–169.

95. Ruoslahti, E., and Pierschbacher, M. D. (1987): New perspectives in cell adhesion: RGD and integrins. *Science*, 238:491–497.

96. Sakaguchi, O., Abe, H., Sakaguchi, S., and Hsu, C. C. (1982): Effect of lead acetate on superoxide anion generation and its scavengers in mice given endotoxin. *Microbiol. Immunol.*, 26:767–778.

97. Salaki, J., Louria, D. B., and Thind, I. S. (1975): Influence of lead intoxication on experimental infections. *Clin. Res.*, 23:417A.

98. Sapin, C., Mandet, C., Druet, E., Gunther, G., and Druet, P. (1981): Immune complex type disease induced by $HgCl_2$; Genetic control of susceptibility. *Transplant. Proc.*, 13:1404–1406.

99. Schlick, E., and Friedberg, K. D. (1981): Influence of low lead doses on the reticuloendothelial system and leukocytes of mice. *Arch. Toxicol.*, 47:197–208.

100. Schlick, E., and Friedberg, K. D. (1982): Bone marrow cells of mice under the influence of low lead doses. *Arch. Toxicol.*, 49:227–236.

101. Schultz, D. R., Volanakis, J. E., and Arnold, P. I. (1974): Inactivation of C1 in rheumatoid synovial fluid, purified C1 and C1 esterase by gold compounds. *Clin. Exp. Immunol.*, 17:395–406.

102. Sell, S. (1987): Immune deficiency disease. In Immunology, Immunopathology and Immunity, edited by S. Sell, pp. 617–654. Elsevier, New York.

103. Shenker, B. J., Matarazzo, W. J., Hirsch, R. L., and Gray, I. (1977): Trace metal modification of immunocompetence. I. Effect of trace metals in the cultures on *in vitro* transformation of lymphocytes. *Cell. Immunol.*, 34:19–24.

104. Silvennoinen-Kassinen, S. (1990): Nickel-induced immune reactions in vitro in cutaneous nickel allergy. In Metal Ions in Biology and Medicine, edited by P. Collery, L. A. Poiner, M. Manfait, and J.-C. Etienne, pp. 258–262. John Libbey, London.

105. Simonis, S., and Cullen, S. E. (1986): Fatty acylation of murine Iaα, β, and invariant chains. *J. Immunol.*, 136:2962–2967.

106. Sinigaglia, F., Scheidegger, D., Garotta, G., Scheper, R., Pletscher, M., and Lanzavecchia, A. (1985): Isolation and characterization of Ni-specific T cell clones from patients with Ni-contact dermatitis. *J. Immunol.*, 135:3929–3932.

107. Smialowicz, R. J., Rogers, R. R., Riddle, M. M., and Stott, G. A. (1984): Immunologic effects of nickel: I. Suppression of cellular and humoral immunity. *Environ. Res.*, 33:413–427.

108. Smialowicz, R. J., Rogers, R. R., Riddle, M. M., Garner, R. J., Rowe, D. G., and Luebke, R. W. (1985): Immunologic Effects of nickel. II. Suppression of natural killer cell activity. *Environ. Res.*, 36:56–66.

109. Smith, K. L., and Lawrence, D. A. (1988): Immunomodulation of in vitro antigen presentation by cations. *Toxicol. Appl. Pharmacol.*, 96:476–484.

110. Smith, H. R., and Steinberg, A. D. (1983): Autoimmunity—A perspective. *Ann. Rev. Immunol.*, 1:175–210.

111. Speerstra, F., Reekers, P., and van de Putte, L. B. A. (1985): HLA associations in aurothioglucose and D-penicillamine induced haematoxic reactions in rheumatoid arthritis. *Tissue Antigens*, 26:35.

112. Talal, N., and Shearer, G. (1983): A clinician and a scientist look at acquired immune deficiency syndrome (AIDS). *Immunol. Today*, 4:180–185.

113. Tornroth, T., and Skrifuars, B. (1974): Gold nephropathy prototype of membranous glomerulone-phritis. *Am. J. Pathol.*, 75:573–584.

114. Ueda, S., Wakashim, Y., Takei, I., Mori, T., Iesato, K., Mori, Y., Wakashim, M., Okuda, K., and Tojos, T. (1980): Autologous immune complex nephritis in gold injected guinea pigs. *Nippon Jinzo Gakkai Shi*, 22:1221–1230.

115. Unanue, E. (1981): The regulatory role of macrophages in antigenic stimulation. Symbiotic relationship between lymphocytes and macrophages. *Adv. Immunol.*, 31:1–136.

116. Underwood, E. J. (1977): Trace Elements in Human and Animal Nutrition. Academic Press, New York.

117. Vaamonde, C. A., and Hunt, F. R. (1970): The nephrotic syndrome as a complication of gold therapy. *Arthritis Rheum.*, 13:826–834.

118. Vallee, B. L., and Ulmer, D. D. (1972): Biochemical effects of mercury, cadmium, and lead. *Ann. Rev. Biochem.*, 41:91–128.

119. Warner, G. L., and Lawrence, D. A. (1986): Effect of heavy metals on human peripheral blood lymphocyte proliferation and cellular thiols. *Fed. Proc.*, 46:1322.

120. Warner, G. L., and Lawrence, D. A. (1986): Stimulation of murine lymphocyte responses by cations. *Cell. Immunol.*, 101:425–439.

121. Warner, G. L., and Lawrence, D. A. (1986): Cell surface and cell cycle analysis of metal-induced murine T cell proliferation. *Eur. J. Immunol.*, 16:1337–1342.

122. Wedeen, R. P., Mallik, D. K., and Betuman, V. (1979): Detection and treatment of occupational lead nephropathy. *Arch. Intern. Med.*, 139:53–57.

123. Williams, M. E., Lichtman, A. H., and Abbas, A. K. (1990): Anti-CD3 antibody induces unresponsiveness to IL-2 in Th1 clones but not in Th2 clones. *J. Immunol.*, 144:1208–1214.

124. Wooley, P. H., Griffin, N., Panayi, G. S., Batchelor, J. R., Welsh, K. I., and Gibson, T. J. (1980): HLA-Dr antigens and the toxic reactions to sodium aurothiomalate and d-penicillamine in patients with rheumatoid arthritis. *N. Engl. J. Med.*, 303:300–303.

125. Yarden, Y., Escobedo, J. A., Kuang, W-J., Yang-Feng, T. L., Daniels, T. O., Tremble, P. M., Chen, E. Y., Ando, M. E., Harkins, R. N., Francke, U., Fried, V. A., Ullrich, A., and Williams, L. T. (1986): Structure of the receptor for platelet derived growth factor helps define a family of closely related growth factor receptors. *Nature*, 323:226.

Clinical Immunotoxicology, edited by
D. S. Newcombe, N. R. Rose, and J. C. Bloom.
Raven Press, Ltd., New York © 1992.

20

The Immunology of Contact Dermatitis

Kristian Thestrup-Pedersen,* Christian Grønhøj Larsen,*
and Jørgen Rønnevig†

*Department of Dermatology, University of Aarhus, Marselisborg Hospital,
Aarhus, Denmark; †Department of Dermatology, University of Oslo,
Rikshospitalet, Oslo, Norway*

Contact dermatitis is the clinical diagnosis of an inflammatory response in the skin caused by external stimuli. It is a frequently occurring disorder in that 5.4% of the Scandinavian adult population have had eczema of the hand at a particular point in time and 2% have continuous problems (18). This chapter does not deal with the external causative factors of contact dermatitis but does concentrate on the inflammatory mechanisms in the skin. Readers are referred to a recent review discussing which allergens or irritants are common causes of contact dermatitis (1).

The clinical signs of contact dermatitis are the appearance of redness and vesicles, followed by scaling and dry skin. There is severe itching in the acute phase and most commonly also in the chronic stage. Histologically, spongiosis and microvesicle formation are present in the epidermis, and there is edema of the upper papillary dermis and a mononuclear cell infiltrate in both the dermis and the epidermis.

Contact dermatitis can be caused by a delayed hypersensitivity reaction involving T lymphocytes sensitized to an allergen. Thus, when contact dermatitis occurs, a search is undertaken for a relevant allergen. The inflammatory response can also be induced by a variety of physical and chemical stimuli, in which an allergen cannot be demonstrated. Allergic and irritant contact dermatitis cannot be differentiated by clinical, histological, or electron microscopic examinations. The demonstration of a type IV immune reaction remains the specific point of difference.

Without exception, allergic contact dermatitis will only develop if molecules are able to penetrate the skin and behave as haptens, i.e., bind to cell surfaces in the epidermis or dermis and induce immunization. A cell-mediated immune reaction to large protein molecules normally is achieved only after injection of the antigen into the skin.

The physiological events in the development of contact dermatitis must involve

1. penetration of the corneal barrier by allergen or irritant;
2. interaction with epidermal or dermal cells;

3. interaction with the immune system; and
4. the inflammatory response.

The initiation of a cell-mediated immune reaction of contact sensitivity includes migration of lymphocytes to sites of antigen challenge, recognition of antigen presented in an immunologically appropriate way, elaboration of mediators to focus on and amplify the inflammatory response, and mechanisms for the control of the intensity of the response.

THE ULTRASTRUCTURE OF THE EPIDERMIS DURING CONTACT DERMATITIS

The cells in the epidermis are keratinocytes (95%), Langerhans' cells (3% to 4%), melanocytes (2% to 3%), and Merkel's cells (< 1%), as estimated by morphological criteria (4–6). Epidermal integrity is maintained through cellular attachments of desmosomes among keratinocytes. Langerhans' cells and melanocytes lack desmosomes but have cytoplasmic filaments protruding into the intercellular spaces. On electron microscopy, Langerhans' cells have distinct Birbeck granules, whereas melanocytes are characterized by melanosomes.

Changes in epidermal cells can be induced by simple, nontraumatic impact on the epidermis. Thus, simple occlusion leads to a temporary intercellular edema, as seen by x-ray microanalysis.

Allergic and irritant reactions have been studied histologically using various allergens or irritants in humans, mice, and guinea pigs (16). The allergic reaction is histologically characterized by pronounced intercellular edema and a pronounced infiltrate of mononuclear cells. Irritant reactions may show epidermal necrosis and less intercellular edema.

The earliest epidermal changes in the allergic reaction seem to start in the stratum basale and the stratum spinosum, where cytoplasmic vacuoles and dilated endoplasmic reticulum are seen. In severe reactions, mitochondria and nuclei become changed, and cytolysis may ensue. Keratinocytes lose contact with each other by breakage of microvilli and retraction or engulfment of desmosomes.

X-ray microanalysis has shown that the ultrastructural changes induced in the epidermis are followed by loss of potassium, phosphorus, and magnesium, concomitant with an increase in total cellular calcium. There is a correlation between the degree of cell injury with dermoepidermal separation and the increase in calcium inside keratinocytes (16). Increase in intracellular calcium is a common mechanism of cell injury and death. The calcium increase can activate phospholipases and will thus increase phospholipid catabolism and cause membrane alterations. Calcium changes also affect cell cohesion. Similar changes may, however, be observed in both irritant and allergic reactions, because enhanced glycerolipid and phospholipid metabolism has been reported following irritant exposure to soap and application of the allergen dinitrochlorobenzene. The impact of these changes on phospholipid

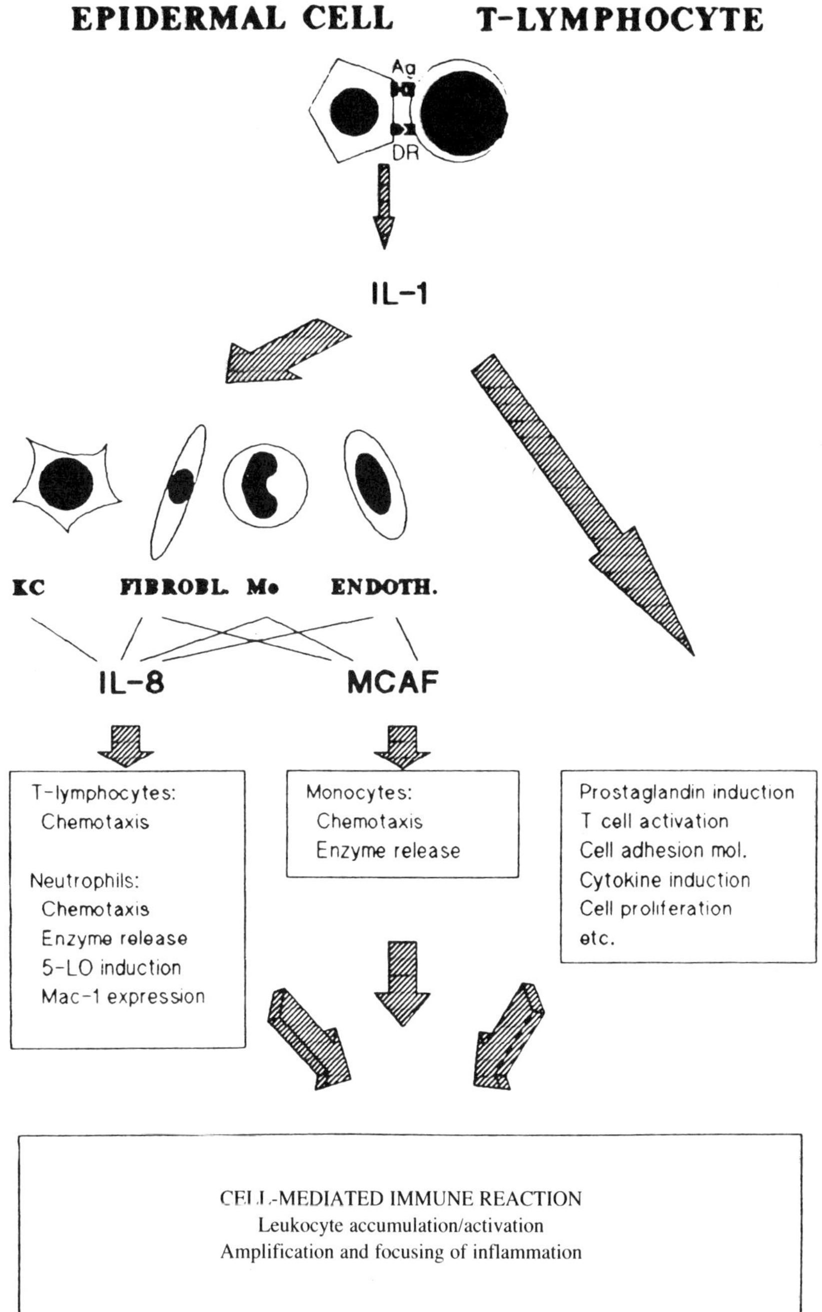

FIG. 1. The principal ways of inducing contact dermatitis reaction, either in an immune specific or in a nonimmune specific way.

metabolism may be important as signals to lymphocytes through leukotriene metabolism.

VASCULAR CHANGES IN CONTACT DERMATITIS

Allergic contact dermatitis shows characteristic vascular changes in the course of an eczematous reaction.

The vascular structure of the skin includes the superficial capillary complex, in the upper papillary part of the dermis, and the superficial venular plexus, consisting of both a superficial and a deeper system of venules lying parallel to the skin surface.

Biopsies in dinitrochlorobenzene-immunized persons at various times after antigen exposure show several distinct changes. Within 8 hours, the superficial capillary complex shows compaction and cell congestion with papillary edema. Extravasation of erythrocytes, a characteristic finding in allergic dermatitis, may also be seen. At 2 to 4 days, interendothelial gaps and plasma products are seen in the surrounding papillary tissue on electron microscopic examination (5).

The superficial venular plexus shows endothelial adherence of lymphocytes and inflammatory cells. The endothelial changes include cell hypertrophy, luminal obstruction, and occasional endothelial cell necrosis. Also, hypertrophy of pericytes and new asymmetrical formation of basal lamina are observed. The endothelial changes include an increased expression of adherence molecules LFA-1, p150.95, and Mac-1, which are most important for the homing of lymphocytes in lymph nodes and Peyer's patches and probably also for the migration of other blood cells (8,15)

MAST CELLS AND BASOPHILS

Mast cells and basophils are clearly involved in contact dermatitis (2). In tuberculin skin reactions and in allergic patch test reactions, mast cells show degranulation, especially the cells in the edematous zone of the papillary dermis and around the superficial venular plexus. After 3 days of antigen challenge, mast cells reappear. Basophils are transiently seen early in contact dermatitis and found immediately below the epidermis rather than in the perivascular region. Basophils and mast cells can release a variety of mediators, such as histamine, serotonin, and leukotrienes. Release can vary differentially, according to the signals given to the cells. Increased histamine levels in the skin of an allergic contact reaction have been reported (24).

Studies in a mouse model have shown that an antihistamine blockade significantly reduces the efferent limb of allergic contact dermatitis. This was also seen following administration of reserpine, which empties the stores of catecholamines and serotonin. Although reserpine has a direct effect on T cells, it also blocks passive cutaneous anaphylaxis, tissue swelling, and leukocyte migration in irritant reactions.

The significance of mast cells for the development of contact dermatitis can only be relative in that mast cell–deficient mice can still express contact sensitivity. Mast cells are a heterogeneous group of cells. The mast cells of the skin behave differently from mucosal mast cells in the gut. Recent findings strongly indicate that there exists a neuroendocrine-immunocyte axis. Thus, mast cells lie in close proximity to nerve fibers, and the neuroendocrine peptides such as substance P, vasoactive-intestinal peptide, and neurotensin seem to influence immunity and hypersensitivity (21). Their eventual role in contact dermatitis remains to be studied.

LEUKOTRIENES

Mast cells and basophils are rich sources of leukotrienes. Leukotrienes may participate in contact dermatitis in several ways. A direct release from basophils and mast cells can lead to attraction of neutrophil granulocytes and lymphocytes (30). Leukotriene B_4 binds to and activates both $CD4^+$ and $CD8^+$ lymphocytes. It can suppress human T-cell functions such as mitogen-induced lymphoproliferation *in vitro*. Its suppressive effect is mediated through direct stimulation of $CD8^+$ cells, which then inhibit mitogen-induced T-cell proliferation by 50%, or through inhibition of $CD4^+$ cells. Blocking of cyclooxygenase with indomethacin and subsequent inhibition of leukotriene formation inhibits the suppressive effect and actually leads to "help." Leukotriene B_4 may also act through monocyte-released prostaglandin or thromboxane.

The importance of leukotrienes for contact dermatitis is, however, controversial. Some of the effects of leukotriene, such as chemotaxis of neutrophils, are not prominent features of contact dermatitis, and leukotriene B_4 has been found in low levels in some but not all positive patch tests (2a). However, leukotriene B_4 may be responsible for the attraction of certain lymphocytes and possibly may influence suppressor mechanisms in contact dermatitis.

CYTOKINES

The term cytokines is used for a heterogeneous group of short-range, cellular-derived peptides, which can be released from a variety of nucleated cells and influence the growth or differentiation of other cells. The induction and release of cytokines are regulated as a cascade reaction, i.e., certain signals induce some cytokines, which then induce other cytokines apart from having certain biological effects.

Cytokine-inducing signals are many: bacterial products such as lipopolysaccharide; serine proteases from *Staphylococcus aureus*; mitogens; or signals that can induce cell damage such as ultraviolet light. Cytokines themselves can induce other cytokines such as interleukin-1, and tumor necrosis factor induces the release of interleukin-8, for example (12a).

Cytokines are present in small amounts and are not specific for any cell type. They are found in many inflammatory disorders and are not specific for any disease.

Therefore, they are probably not of primary importance in the etiology of a disease, but they may significantly influence the inflammatory response. It is possible that quantitative regulation, i.e., transcription of DNA and the release of cytokines, may actually be very important with respect to whether or not an inflammatory response is started, because apart from an immunostimulating activity, they also induce adherence molecules, which enable cells to enter the area (9). Our present knowledge of cytokines in contact dermatitis is presented below; this field is expanding rapidly at present.

INTERFERON

Interferons are polypeptide cytokines released from a variety of cells. All have antiviral activity and increase natural killer cell activity and specific cytotoxic T-cell activity. Perhaps more important in the context of contact dermatitis is that interferon-gamma will induce the expression of class I and class II antigens and intercellular adhesion molecule 1; the latter is responsible for the adhesion between keratinocytes and T lymphocytes (20). The coexpression of adherence molecules and class II antigens creates the immunological background for an immune reaction. These events occur very early in the development of an allergic contact dermatitis reaction.

Leukotrienes may be involved in the release of interferon. Thus, leukotriene B_4 can increase interferon-gamma production from a subpopulation of lymphocytes. In mice, interferon-gamma–releasing cells carry the phenotype Ly 1^-2^+ and need help from T-helper lymphocytes (Ly 1^+2^-) in order to release interferon-gamma upon stimulation. The T-helper signal can be replaced by the addition of leukotriene B_4, leukotriene C_4, or leukotriene D_4 in concentrations as low as 0.2×10^{-9} M. Prostaglandin E_1 and prostaglandin E_2 had no effect in the same experimental study. Prostaglandin E probably suppresses interferon-gamma release as a result of activation of the adenylate cyclase system (cAMP), whereas leukotriene helps through the activation of the guanine cyclase system (cGMP). Interleukin-2, phorbol myristate acetate, and cGMP had a similar interferon-gamma–enhancing effect (9a).

INTERLEUKIN-1

Interleukin is a general term for substances of a peptide nature that augment lymphocyte functions. Interleukin-1 is often identified functionally through its promotion of murine thymocyte proliferation *in vitro*. A comprehensive review has recently been published. A conclusion from this review is that much is still unknown about the exact mechanisms that lead to the release of interleukin-1 from cells and whether interleukin-1 is relevant for *in vivo* immune responses.

Interleukin-1 is released from a large variety of cells, including keratinocytes. Its ability to increase Ia antigen expression on T lymphocytes, its possible chemotactic activity, and its ability to increase the expression of interleukin-2 receptors on T cells may be of utmost importance for the events that occur in contact dermatitis. Interleukin-1 is also able to induce the transcription of interleukin-8 (12).

Addition of as little as 0.04 U/ml of affinity purified human interleukin-1 to human umbilical endothelial cells increases the binding of both human B and T lymphocytes by a factor of approximately 2, and this is because of the enhanced expression of adherence molecules and a first step in lymphocyte migration.

The release of interleukin-1 *in vitro* from lipopolysaccharide-stimulated or non-stimulated human monocytes is increased after the addition of leukotriene B_4 in the range of 10^{-7} to 10^{-8} M. It has also been observed that interleukin-1 release from monocytes *in vitro* is followed by the release of prostaglandins E_2 and I_2, which exert a negative feedback inhibition on interleukin-1 release. This demonstrates that the regulation of interleukin-1 and its eventual participation in immune inflammation may be very delicately balanced.

Recent studies from our laboratory have shown that interleukin-1 is increased threefold in epidermis overlying the area of a positive allergic patch test (13) but not of an irritant skin reaction (14). Time course studies revealed that the increase of interleukin-1 was seen as early as 6 hours after application of allergen, at a time when the clinical reaction was not present (11).

EXPRESSION OF TISSUE ANTIGENS

Tissue antigens (HLA) are important for self-recognition and T-lymphocyte function. All nucleated cells may express HLA antigens. The class II histocompatibility antigens are necessary for lymphocyte-dendritic cell interaction in the induction of immune responses (28). Thus, HLA-D plays a central role in the afferent branch of allergic contact dermatitis.

An increased expression of HLA-D antigen may indicate an ongoing immune response. Its presence may increase the chances for immunization if haptens are present. Several observers have found increased expression of HLA-D antigens in a variety of dermatoses, such as mycosis fungoides, lichen planus, eczematous dermatitis, contact dermatitis, and other disorders of lymphocyte infiltration (6,17).

The wide variety of disorders associated with increased class II antigen expression are all characterized by lymphoid infiltration and proliferation. It is likely that interferon is of importance in such disorders because it is known to be able to increase HLA expression of keratinocytes as well as other epithelial cells. Quantitative variation in Ia antigen expression may be of importance in immunoregulation.

ANTIGEN-PRESENTING CELLS

Dendritic cells are extremely effective in antigen presentation. They release high levels of interleukin-1 and have a high density of Ia antigen molecules, which may be the main reason for their activity. Langerhans' cells are bone marrow–derived, epidermal dendritic cells with receptors for C3b, Fc receptors for IgG, class II antigens, and OKT6 antigen. Silberberg (22) initially showed the central role of the Langerhans' cell in contact dermatitis. Later, many studies confirmed that Langerhans' cells are as capable as monocytes in antigen presentation (haptens, fungal, bacterial, and viral) for T-lymphocyte proliferative responses.

Langerhans' cells are increased in number in immune reactions in the skin. Their presence seems to depend on the age of the reaction. Thus, Langerhans' cells in the epidermis of a tuberculin skin reaction were increased at 41 hours and almost totally gone at 72 hours, with repopulation at 7 days (10). Ultraviolet light can inhibit the number of Langerhans' cells and their HLA-D expression concomitantly with a decrease in immune reactivity of the cells, both *in vitro* and *in vivo*. Thus, it seems likely that Langerhans' cells are of ultimate importance for allergic contact dermatitis (3). However, it has recently been shown that stripping of the skin, with removal of both epidermal keratinocytes and Langerhans' cells, does not prevent an efferent immune response (patch testing), indicating that the interdigitating cells in the dermis can participate in such a response. Also, human dermal fibroblasts have been found to be antigen presenting: interferon can increase their expression of Ia antigen, and they can acquire functional activity in the presence of interleukin-2.

Although Langerhans' cells are important for stimulation of T lymphocytes, keratinocytes can also participate in immune reactions in the skin with the expression of HLA-DR antigens and release of cytokines.

THE CELLULAR INFILTRATE IN CONTACT DERMATITIS

The accumulation of mononuclear cells in the skin and their epidermal infiltration, exocytosis, is an important histological feature of contact dermatitis.

Many studies have tried to determine whether the accumulating cells are antigen-specific. Reinjection of dinitrochlorobenzene-sensitive and labeled T lymphocytes into guinea pigs showed an increased accumulation of hapten-reactive T cells in the positive skin test. Hapten-specific T lymphocytes form a very low percentage of circulating cells, and although they accumulate at an early stage in the skin, most cells seen there are antigen–nonspecific cells. Lymphoblasts migrate more easily to inflammatory skin sites. The release of lymphokines, such as migration inhibition factor, focuses the accumulation of cells. Antibodies raised against migration inhibition factor can inhibit a cutaneous response. However, migration inhibition factor is just one of many factors that are very important for the migration of cells, probably through their effect on the expression of adherence molecules on both endothelial cells and lymphocytes. It has recently been shown that the epidermis overlying a tuberculin skin test contains factors that are chemotactic for T lymphocytes (23) and especially CD4$^+$ T lymphocytes (30). Such factors may be very important because they are able to give discriminating signals to various subpopulations of lymphocytes (5). Readers are referred to two reviews of these important events (4,20). Histological examinations have emphasized the close approximation of lymphocytes to Langerhans' cells in the skin (22). Lymphocytes are also in close contact with macrophages in the dermis. Antigen-specific cells can remain in the area for up to several weeks. This may in part explain flare-up reactions in old test areas of contact sensitivity.

In a positive patch test reaction, OKT4$^+$ lymphocytes are prominent. OKT6$^+$ cells are found in both the epidermis and the dermis. There seems to be no correlation between the size of the reaction, the time of the biopsy, and the ratio between OKT4$^+$ and OKT8$^+$ cells (7).

The histological characteristics of contact dermatitis have been described above. However, some kind of lesion showing cell-mediated immune responses in the skin is associated with epithelioid cell granulomas. This is especially seen in chronic infectious skin diseases, including leprosy, tuberculosis, and syphilis, and is also a feature of sarcoidosis, berylliosis, and sensitivity to zirconium salts. The exact mechanisms by which epithelioid cells develop in these disorders is, however, not known.

SYSTEMIC EFFECTS OF TYPE IV SKIN REACTIONS

The immune system is present throughout the body, except inside the eye. There is ample evidence that an immune reaction in a localized area of the skin can influence other immune functions. This has been documented in many experimental studies, including in humans. In healthy subjects, a tuberculin skin reaction has been found to produce a temporary short-term skin anergy (25), perhaps due to a transient nonspecific suppressor effect of monocytes or a lack of antigen-specific lymphocytes in the blood (25–27).

In contact allergy, opposite effects are present. The excited skin syndrome ("angry back") is well known to dermatologists. The "baboon syndrome" in humans (19) has been observed, as has the red-ear syndrome in guinea pigs undergoing desensitization. Also, patients with cutaneous allergies are more susceptible to new allergies (19a).

SENSITIVITY OR TOLERANCE

The route and dose of antigen administration are important for the development of sensitivity or tolerance. Thus, intravenous, intraperitoneal, or oral administration of antigen, which is used for topical sensitization, can lead to reduced immune reactivity due to suppressor cells. The mechanisms are even more complex in that contra-suppressor cells can arise under certain experimental conditions in mice. These cells release factors that can render proliferating T cells resistant to specific suppressor cell activity (29). The activity of proliferating T cells (T-helper lymphocytes) is dependent on at least two events: (a) very early edema (peak 2 hours), which is related to the presence of antigen-specific T cells and perhaps to serotonin release from mast cells; and (b) later accumulation of other T cells. The T cells responsible for these events belong to different subpopulations. Thus, several consecutive steps are necessary to trigger T lymphocytes to establish a cell-mediated immune response.

ALLERGIC VERSUS IRRITANT CONTACT DERMATITIS

The aforementioned mechanisms are all described in the context of allergic contact dermatitis. What, then, happens in the skin during irritant contact dermatitis, which clinically and histologically is very similar to allergic eczema? Does the immune inflammation in irritant contact dermatitis involve antigen-specific recognition, or could the inflammation be started and sustained through nonspecific mechanisms involving the release of cytokines from damaged and then proliferating epidermal cells?

Theoretically, some of the following possibilities should be considered.

1. Damage to epidermal cells leads to recognition of the cells as foreign. Such mechanisms should explain the similarity to the immune inflammation in allergic contact dermatitis. However, no evidence exists that the epidermis "changes" phenotype.
2. Damage to the epidermis from an immune reaction or from physical or chemical trauma leads to proliferation of keratinocytes. This repair process in eczematous patients may imply an increased release of lymphocyte-activating factors such as interleukin-1 and epidermal lymphocyte chemotactic factor; increased phospholipase activity leading to products that are lymphocyte chemotaxins (e.g., leukotriene B_4); and mast cell release leading to increased blood and lymphocyte flow through the skin.
3. Epidermal proliferation may affect attracted, stimulated T lymphocytes in such a way that the normal suppressor signals do not influence the activated cells.

Thus, a plethora of mediators of inflammation may be responsible for "ignition" of the immune system if the amount of mediator is larger than required or if the normal inhibitor/regulator systems are weakened or disturbed.

REFERENCES

1. Andersen, K. E., Benezra, C., Burrows, D., et al. (1987): Contact dermatitis. A review. *Contact Dermatitis*, 16:55–78.
2. Askenase, P. W. (1977): Role of basophils, mast cells and vasoamines in hypersensitivity reactions with a delayed time course. *Prog. Allergy*, 23:199.
2a. Barr R. M., Brain S. C., Camp R. D., Cilliers J., Greawes M. W., Mallet A. I., Misch K. (1984): Levels of arachidonic acid and its metabolites in the skin in human allergic and irritant contact dermatitis. *Br J Dermatol*, 111:23–29.
3. Cruz, P. D., Tigelaar, R. E., and Bergstresser, P. R. (1990): Langerhans cells that migrate to skin after intravenous infusion regulate the induction of contact hypersensitivity. *J. Immunol.*, 144:2486–2492.
4. Duijvestijn, A., and Hamann, A. (1989): Mechanisms and regulation of lymphocyte migration. *Immunol. Today*, 10:23–28.
4a. Dvorak, A. M., Mihm, M. C., and Dvorak, H. F. (1976): Morphology of delayed-type hypersen-

sitivity reactions in man (II). Ultrastructural alterations affecting the microvasculature and the tissue mast cells. *Lab. Invest.*, 34:179.

5. Dvorak, H. F., Mihm, M. C., Dvorak, A. M., Johnson, R. A., Manseau, E. J., Morgan, E., and Colvin, R. B. (1974): Morphology of delayed-type hypersensitivity reactions in man (I). Quantitative description of the inflammatory response. *Lab. Invest.*, 31:111.

6. Gawkrodger, D. J., Carr, M. M., McVittie, E., Guy, K., and Hunter, J. A. A. (1987): Keratinocyte expression of MHC class II antigens in allergic sensitization and challenge reactions and in irritant contact dermatitis. *J. Invest. Dermatol.*, 88:11.

7. Gawkrodger, D. J., McVittie, E., Carr, M. M., Ross, J. A., and Hunter, J. A. A. (1986): Phenotypic characterization of the early cellular responses in allergic and irritant contact dermatitis. *Clin. Exp. Immunol.*, 66:590.

8. Hamann, A., Jablonski-Westrich, D., Duijvestijn, A., Butcher, E. C., Baisch, H., Harder, R., and Thiele, H.-G. (1988): Evidence for an accessory role of LFA-1 in lymphocyte-high endothelium interaction during homing. *J. Immunol.*, 140:693.

9. Issekutz, T. B. (1990): Effects of six different cytokines on lymphocyte adherence to microvascular endothelium and in vivo lymphocyte migration in the rat. *J. Immunol.*, 144:2140–2146.

10. Kaplan, G., Nusrat, A., Witmer, M. D., Nath, I., and Cohn, Z. A. Distribution and turnover of Langerhans cells during delayed immune responses in human skin. *J. Exp. Med.*, 165:763.

11. Kristensen, M., Larsen, C. G., Zachariae, C. O. C., and Thestrup-Pedersen, K. (1989): ETAF/IL-1 and epidermal lymphocyte chemotactic factor (ELCF) are expressed early in human epidermis during the development of allergic patch test reactions. *J. Invest. Dermatol.*, 93:302 (abstract).

12. Larsen, C. G., Anderson, A. O., Appella, E., Oppenheim, J. J., and Matsushima, K. (1989): The neutrophil-activating protein (NAP-1) is also chemotactic for T lymphocytes. *Science*, 243:1464–1466.

12a. Larsen, C. G., Anderson, A. Q., Oppenheim, J. J., and Matsushima, K. (1989): Production of interleukin-8 by human dermal fibroblasts and keratinocytes in response to interleukin-1 or tumor necrosis factor. *Immunology*, 68:31–36.

13. Larsen, C. G., Ternowitz, T., Larsen, F. G., and Thestrup-Pedersen, K. (1988): Epidermis and lymphocyte interactions during a tuberculin skin reaction (I). Increased ETAF/IL-1 like activity, expression of tissue antigens and mixed skin lymphocyte reactivity. *Arch. Derm. Res.* 280:83.

14. Larsen, C. G., Ternowitz, T., Larsen, F. G., and Thestrup-Pedersen, K. (1988): Epidermis and lymphocyte interactions during an allergic patch test reaction. Increased activity of ETAF/IL-1, epidermal derived lymphocyte chemotactic factor and mixed skin lymphocyte reactivity in persons with type IV allergy. *J. Invest. Dermatol.*, 90:230.

15. Lewis, R. E., Buchsbaum, M., Whitaker, D., and Murphy, G. F. (1989): Intercellular adhesion molecule expression in the evolving human cutaneous delayed hypersensitivity reaction. *J. Invest. Dermatol.*, 93:672–677.

16. Lindberg, M. (1982): Studies on the cellular and subcellular reactions in epidermis at irritant and allergic dermatitis. *Acta Derm. Venereol.*, Suppl. 105.

17. Markey, A. C., Allen, M. H., Pitzalis, C., and MacDonald, D. M. (1990): T-cell inducer populations in cutaneous inflammation: A predominance of T helper-inducer lymphocytes (THi) in the infiltrate of inflammatory dermatoses. *Br. J. Dermatol.*, 122:325–332.

18. Meding, B., and Swanbeck, G. (1987): Prevalence of hand eczema in an industrial city. *Br. J. Dermatol.*, 116:627–634.

19. Mitchell, J. C. (1975): The angry back syndrome: Eczema creates eczema. *Contact Dermatitis*, 1:193.

19a. Moss, C., Friedmann, P. S., Shuster, S., and Simpson, J. M. (1985): Susceptibility and amplification of sensitivity in contact dermatitis. *Clin. Exp. Immunol.*, 61:232.

20. Nickoloff, B. J. (1988): The role of gamma interferon in cutaneous trafficking of lymphocytes with emphasis on molecular and cellular adhesion events. *Arch. Dermatol.*, 124:1835–1843.

21. Payuan, D. G., Levine, J. D., and Goetzl, E. J. (1983): Modulation of immunity and hypersensitivity by sensory neuropeptides. *J. Immunol.*, 132:1601.

22. Silberberg, I. (1973): Apposition of mononuclear cells to Langerhans cells in contact allergic reactions. *Acta Derm. Venereol.*, 53:1–12.

23. Ternowitz, T., and Thestrup-Pedersen, K. (1986): Epidermis and lymphocyte interactions during a tuberculin skin reaction (II). Epidermis contains specific lymphocyte chemotactic factors. *J. Invest. Dermatol.*, 87:613.

24. Theoharides, T. C., Bondy, P. K., Tsakalos, N. D., and Askenase, P. W. (1982): Differential release of serotonin and histamine from mast cells. *Nature*, 297:229.

25. Thestrup-Pedersen, K. (1975): Suppression of tuberculin skin reactivity by prior tuberculin skin testing. *Immunology*, 28:343.
26. Thestrup-Pedersen, K., Dwyer, J. M., and Askenase, P. W. (1977): Studies on the role of the thymus and T cells in the in vivo suppression of delayed hypersensitivity (desensitization): Radio-sensitivity of the mechanism inducing non-specific anergy. *J. Immunol.*, 118:1665.
27. Thestrup-Pedersen, L., Jørgensen, B., Kaltoft, K., and Jensen, J. R. (1985): In vivo and in vitro changes in cell-mediated immunity following tuberculin skin testing in humans. *Br. J. Dermatol.*, 113 Suppl 28:81.
28. Unanue, E. R., Beller, D. I., Lu, C. Y., and Allen, P. M. (1984): Antigen presentation: Comments on its regulation and mechanism. *J. Immunol.*, 132:1.
29. Van Loveren, H., Kato, K., Mead, R., Green, D. R., Horowitz, M., Ptak, W., and Askenase, P. W. (1984): Characterization of two different Ly$^-$ 1$^+$ T cell populations that mediate delayed-type hypersensitivity. *J. Immunol.*, 113:2402.
30. Zachariae, C. O. C., Ternowitz, T., Larsen, C. G., Nielsen, V., and Thestrup-Pedersen, K. (1988): Epidermal lymphocyte chemotactic factor specifically attracts OKT4 positive lymphocytes. *Arch. Dermatol. Res.*, 280:354–357.

Subject Index

National Academy of Sciences-National Research
 Council, Committee on Anesthesia,
 National Halothane Study, 155
Natural antibodies, measurement of, tests for, 18–19
Natural immunity, definition of, 365
Natural killer (NK) cells, 10–13, 212, 288
 activity of
  effect of phorbol myristate acetate on, 386
  effect of polycyclic aromatic hydrocarbons on,
   381–382
  effect of triethylphosphine gold (auranofin) on,
   353–355
 assays of, 21–22
 effects of airborne pollutants on, 237–238
 pulmonary, activity of, effects of ozone on,
  237–238
 suppression of, effects of urethane on, 384
Neoantigens
 57-kDa, identification of, 162
 58-kDa, identification of, 162
 59-kDa, identification of, 161–162
 63-kDa, identification of, 161–162
 80-kDa, identification of, 160–162
 100-kDa, identification of, 160, 162
 chemical determinants of, 211
 halothane-induced
  covalently modified by TFA-CL, antibodies
   against, 159
  identification of, 160–162
  liver microsomal, from halothane-treated rats,
   159
Nephrotic syndrome, Au-induced, 411
Neutropenia, immune, drug-induced, 147–149
Neutrophil chemotactic factor, activity of, in
 asbestosis, 306–307
Neutrophils
 chemotactic activity
  in asthmatics, 291
  in bronchoalveolar lavage, 284–286
  effects of organophosphates on, 352–353
 human, SDS-PAGE autoradiograph of, 358
 tests of, 22
Nickel, 403
 effects of
  on alveolar macrophages, 233
  on immune system, 405–409
 and lung cancer, 231–232
Nickel carbonyl
 and bronchiolitis, 232
 and pneumonitis, 232
Nickel contact dermatitis, 407
Nickel hypersensitivity, 407
Nitrofurantoin
 associated pulmonic syndromes, 191
 and pneumonitis, 192
Nitrogen dioxide
 ambient air quality standards for, 241
 chronic exposures to, effects of, 247
 effects of, 317–318
  on asthmatics, 317
  on humans, 319
  on immune responses of lung, 246–248
  on lung cell populations and functions, 241–243
  on lung defense mechanisms, 244–246
  on susceptibility to infectious agents, 243–244
  on viral infection, 316–317

 exposure to, bronchoalveolar lavage in, 316–319
 immunopathogenesis of, studies of, 319
 and ozone
  comparison of, 241
  mixed exposures of, effects of, 246, 248
Nitrogen oxides, immunosuppressive effects of,
 240–248
Nomifensine, hemolysis associated with, 145
Nonspecific immunity, tests of, 21–22

O

Obesity, and halothane hepatotoxicity, 168
Occupational asthma
 acid anhydride-induced, 199–200
 assessment of, initial approach to, 195–196
 bronchial reactivity in, 208
 bronchoalveolar lavage in, 283–293
 clinical presentations of, 196
 cobalt-induced, 226
 IgE-mediated hypersensitivity in, 203
 initiation and persistence of, 211
 from low molecular weight chemical exposure,
  291–293
 nonimmunological factors that cause, 196–197
 outbreaks of, 195
 pathogenetic mechanisms of, 198–201
  investigations into, 197–198
 platinum-induced, 200
 skin tests for, 206–207, 285–286
 vectors for, 206–207, 285–286, 309
 zinc fume-induced, 310
Occupational dermatitis, 217
OKT3
 antibodies to, 88
 removal of circulating T cells with, 87–88
 toxic effects of, 87–88
OOS-TMP. *See O,O,S*-Trimethyl phosphorothioate
Organophosphates
 and asthma, 197
 effects on neutrophil chemotaxis, 352–353
Organophosphorus binding proteins, in human
 monocytes, 357
Organophosphorus compounds
 commercial applications of, 349
 exposure to, clinical expression of, 349–350
 immunotoxicity of, 349–363
  animal studies, 351–352
  in humans, 349
  mechanisms of, 351
  primary cellular target for, 356
 as inhibitors, 357
 metabolism of, 359
 mutagenic and/or carcinogenic effects of, 358–359
 noncholinergic effects of, 350
Organotins
 immunotoxic effects of, 386–389
  mechanisms for, 388–389
 industrial applications, 386
 toxicity, types of, in animals, 387
Oxacillin, and immune granulocytopenia, 148
Oxidants
 contribution to ozone-induced alterations in immune
  and inflammatory cells, 240